EIGHTH EDITION

LANGE Q&A

SURGICAL TECHNOLOGY EXAMINATION

Carolan Sherman, MSN, CST
Former Director, Surgical Technology Program
Bergen Community College
Paramus, New Jersey

Mary Chmielewski, CST
Clinical Coordinator, Surgical Technology Program
Bergen Community College
Paramus, New Jersey

Mc
Graw
Hill

New York   Chicago   San Francisco   Athens   London   Madrid
Mexico City   Milan   New Delhi   Singapore   Sydney   Toronto

Lange Q&A: Surgical Technology Examination, Eighth Edition

1 2 3 4 5 6 7 8 9   LWI   26 25 24 23 22 21

ISBN 978-1-260-47024-6
MHID 1-260-47024-5

Notice

Medicine is an ever-changing science. As new research and clinical experience broaden our knowledge, changes in treatment and drug therapy are required. The authors and the publisher of this work have checked with sources believed to be reliable in their efforts to provide information that is complete and generally in accord with the standards accepted at the time of publication. However, in view of the possibility of human error or changes in medical sciences, neither the authors nor the publisher nor any other party who has been involved in the preparation or publication of this work warrants that the information contained herein is in every respect accurate or complete, and they disclaim all responsibility for any errors or omissions or for the results obtained from use of the information contained in this work. Readers are encouraged to confirm the information contained herein with other sources. For example and in particular, readers are advised to check the product information sheet included in the package of each drug they plan to administer to be certain that the information contained in this work is accurate and that changes have not been made in the recommended dose or in the contraindications for administration. This recommendation is of particular importance in connection with new or infrequently used drugs.

This book was set in Palatino LT Std by KnowledgeWorks Global Ltd.
The editor was Michael Weitz.
The production supervisor was Catherine Saggese.
Project management was provided by Warishree Pant, KnowledgeWorks Global Ltd.

Library of Congress Cataloging-in-Publication Data

Names: Sherman, Carolan, author. | Chmielewski, Mary, author.
Title: Lange Q & A. Surgical technology examination / Carolan Sherman, Mary
  Chmielewski.
Other titles: Lange Q&A. Surgical technology examination
Description: Eighth edition. | New York : McGraw Hill, [2021] | Includes
  bibliographical references and index. | Summary: "Lange Q&A: Surgical
  Technology Examination, Eighth Edition, has been designed to assist
  surgical technicians planning to take the National Certification
  Examination for Surgical Technologists. The ever-growing body of
  knowledge necessary to prepare the surgical technologist for a
  professional role in the operating room requires that competency be
  measured by an examination that tests both constant and technologically
  up-to-date information. With this in mind, the authors have prepared an
  eighth edition of the review book that has been extensively revised and
  updated to include those advances in technology that have emerged since
  the previous edition" Provided by publisher.
Identifiers: LCCN 2021022830 (print) | LCCN 2021022831 (ebook) | ISBN
  9781260470246 (paperback) | ISBN 9781260470253 (ebook)
Subjects: MESH: Operating Room Technicians | Surgical Procedures, Operative
  | Examination Questions
Classification: LCC RD32.3 (print) | LCC RD32.3 (ebook) | NLM WO 18.2 |
  DDC 617—dc23
LC record available at https://lccn.loc.gov/2021022830
LC ebook record available at https://lccn.loc.gov/2021022831

Contents

Preface

Lange Q&A: Surgical Technology Examination, Eighth Edition, has been designed to assist surgical technicians planning to take the National Certification Examination for Surgical Technologists. Although unable to guarantee a perfect score, a study guide can provide a good deal of assistance in test preparation by enabling the student to review relevant material while becoming familiar with the type of questions that will be encountered on the examination.

The ever-growing body of knowledge necessary to prepare the surgical technologist for a professional role in the operating room requires that competency be measured by an examination that tests both constant and technologically up-to-date information. With this in mind, the authors have prepared an eighth edition of the review book that has been extensively revised and updated to include those advances in technology that have emerged since the previous edition.

The book contains over 1,900 questions that closely correlate in percentage the amount prescribed in the Study Guide for Certification provided by the Liaison Council of the Association of Surgical Technologists. The text is divided into 32 chapters. Following each chapter are questions. Each question has one answer and a full-length explanation; difficulty in a single area indicates a need for individual study emphasis.

Acknowledgments

We would like to give special thanks to Mark Sherman and John Chmielewski for giving us their overwhelming support throughout the process of writing this review book. We also would like to thank all students—past, present, and future—for giving us the inspiration to write this review book, with special thanks to the Smedleys.

Introduction

ORGANIZATION OF THE BOOK

The book is organized into 32 chapters covering the major topic areas found on the Certifying Examination for Surgical Technologists. Each chapter is designed to facilitate your review of the major content areas of surgical technology. Each chapter ends with detailed explanations of each question for reinforcement of knowledge.

HOW TO ANSWER A QUESTION INTELLIGENTLY

Unlike many examinations, which are a composite of several multiple-choice questions, the National Certification Examination for Surgical Technologists uses only one major type of question. Each question will have one correct answer, and the other options are incorrect. However, the remaining three choices may be partially correct, but there can only be one best answer.

When the question reads "EXCEPT," it is to remind you that the correct answer will be the exception to the statement in the question.

Sample Question 1
A left subcostal incision indicates surgery of the:

(A) gallbladder
(B) pancreas
(C) spleen
(D) common bile duct

This question could be answered from rote memory, placing the term "subcostal" with the anatomic structure "spleen." It is more likely that the student will conjure up a picture of the human abdomen and discount gallbladder (choice A) and common bile duct (choice D) immediately because they are located on the right side of the abdominal cavity. Thus, two choices are ruled out as possible answers, improving the odds of selecting the correct answer from 25% to 50%. Although the tail of the pancreas reaches over to the left side of the body and is adjacent to the spleen, spleen is clearly the best choice and the only correct answer.

Sample Question 2
An elderly female, sleeping soundly, arrives in the OR via stretcher with side rails in place and safety strap intact. She is placed alone outside her assigned OR. The woman awakens, climbs off the stretcher, and, falling, receives a deep scalp laceration. The circulating nurse:

(A) can be charged with abandonment
(B) can be charged with simple assault
(C) can be charged with battery
(D) cannot be charged because safety devices were in place

This question is more difficult. Although we clearly see choices B and C as incorrect because the nurse had no physical part in the injury to the patient, the difficulty is now in choosing between the remaining

Table 1. Strategies for Answering Questions[a]

1. Remember that only one choice can be the correct answer.
2. Read the question carefully to be sure that you understand what is being asked.
3. Quickly read each choice for familiarity. (This important step is often not done by test takers.)
4. Go back and consider each choice individually.
5. If a choice is partially correct, tentatively consider it to be incorrect. (This step will help you lessen your choices and increase your odds of choosing the correct choice/answer.)
6. Consider the remaining choices, and select the one you think is the answer. At this point, you may want to quickly scan the stem to be sure you understand the question and your answer.
7. Select the appropriate answer. Even if you do not know the answer, you should at least guess—you are scored on the number of correct answers, so do not leave any blanks.

[a]Note that steps 2 through 7 should take an average of 45–55 seconds total. The actual examination is timed for an average of 45–55 seconds per question.

answers. Choice D may seem correct because the stem of the questions tells us that all safety devices were intact. It is only with knowledge of the legal aspect of OR procedure that we know that the key word *alone* signifies culpability on the part of the nurse. Standard OR procedures claim that one is guilty of abandonment if a patient is left *alone* at any time when in the care of OR personnel and may be charged as such in a court of law.

HOW TO USE THE BOOK

Read the chapter review and then answer the questions at the end of the chapter. Continual notation in this book will provide you with a quick review at the end of the chapter. This will help you determine those areas that require the most emphasis for study and those areas that require additional review. Most of the references are texts that are readily available at your nearest library or that you may already own.

The official source of applications for and information about the surgical technology examination can be obtained from the National Board of Surgical Technology and Surgical Assisting (http://nbstsa.org).

CHAPTER 1

Medical Terminology

- This is the language spoken by health professionals in hospitals, surgicenters, clinics, and physicians' offices.
- You must be able to identify the four basic word parts, construct medical terms by using the word parts, and use the correct pronunciation.
- The four word parts include: root words, prefixes, suffixes, and combining words.
  - Root word—primary meaning
  - Prefix—placed before the root word
  - Suffix—placed after the root word
  - Combining forms—usually an O but can be an I or E
- Example #1: Endocarditis
  - endo—prefix—meaning within
  - card—root word—pertaining to the heart
  - itis—suffix—meaning inflammation of
- Example #2: Osteoarthritis
  - oste—root—pertaining to bone
  - o—combining vowel
  - arthr—root—pertaining to a joint
  - itis—suffix—meaning inflammation of

1. abduction	a.	Supine
2. adduction	b.	Away from the midline of the body
3. dorsal recumbent	c.	Pertaining to the front of the body
4. anterior	d.	Pertaining to the side of the body
5. lateral	e.	Toward the midline of the body

6. proxim/o	a.	Farthest point
7. super/o	b.	Near the point of attachment to the body
8. dist/o	c.	Pertaining to the skull
9. cephalo/o	d.	Pertaining to the head
10. crani/o	e.	Upper, above

11. lumpectomy	a.	Performed in radiology where the mass is identified with a wire
12. radical mastectomy	b.	Excision of a breast lesion with surrounding tissue
13. modified radical mastectomy	c.	First set of nodes closest to the cancerous tumor
14. wire localization	d.	Removal of breast tissue and axillary lymph nodes
15. sentinel lymph node	e.	Removal of breast tissue, muscle, and lymph nodes

16. chrondr/o	a.	Cartilage
17. oste/o	b.	Hand Bones
18. arthr/o	c.	Joint
19. metacarp/o	d.	Tendon
20. tend/o	e.	Bone

21. blephar/o	a.	Retina
22. dacry/o	b.	Iris
23. kerat/o	c.	Cornea
24. retin/o	d.	Tear duct
25. irid/o	e.	Eyelid

26. -cele	a.	Swelling
27. -dyspnea	b.	Difficulty breathing
28. -edema	c.	Inflammation of
29. -itis	d.	Vomiting
30. -emesis	e.	Hernia

31. -megaly	a.	Disease
32. -pathy	b.	Bursting forth
33. -rrhage	c.	Enlargement
34. -oma	d.	Flow, discharge
35. -rrhea	e.	Tumor

36. abruptio placentae
37. ectopic
38. placenta previa
39. atresia
40. rectocele

a. Placenta forms in the lower portion of the uterus and blocks the birth canal
b. Placenta tears away from the uterine wall
c. Lack of a normal body opening
d. Pregnancy outside the uterus
e. Protrusion of the rectum into the vagina

41. cervic/o
42. lapar/o
43. cyst/o
44. gynec/o
45. colp/o

a. Pertaining to the neck, cervix
b. Pertaining to the bladder
c. Pertaining to a female
d. Pertaining to the vagina
e. Pertaining to the abdomen

46. fistula
47. fibroid
48. ovarian cystectomy
49. oophorectomy
50. salpingectomy

a. Benign tumor of the uterus
b. Removal of a cyst on the ovary
c. Removal of the ovary
d. Abnormal passageway that forms between two structures
e. Removal of the fallopian tube

51. mitral valve
52. bradycardia
53. arrhythmia
54. alveoli
55. cyanosis

a. Exchange of oxygen and carbon dioxide occurs here
b. Also called the bicuspid valve
c. Resting heart rate below 60 bpm
d. Condition caused by oxygen deficiency
e. Irregular heart beat

56. atrial septal defect
57. claudication
58. embolism
59. thrombus
60. ischemia

a. Clot composed of blood, air, or fat that moves through the vascular system
b. Stationary clot
c. Abnormally low blood flow to tissues
d. Pain in a limb, usually the leg, caused by poor circulation
e. Congenital condition caused by the septum, between the atria, failing to close, allowing blood to flow back and forth

61. patent ductus arteriosus
62. tetralogy of Fallot
63. hypertension
64. hypotension
65. aneurysm

a. High blood pressure
b. Congenital condition caused by an opening between the pulmonary artery and the aorta that failed to close before birth
c. Bulging of an arterial wall
d. Low blood pressure
e. Congenital defect that consists of four separate cardiac diseases: pulmonary stenosis, ventricular septal defect, incorrect position of the aorta, and ventricular hypertrophy

66. -otomy
67. -pexy
68. -plasty
69. -centesis
70. poly-

a. Surgical repair
b. Puncture to remove fluid
c. Cutting into
d. Many
e. Fixation of

71. pneumothorax
72. pneumoperitoneum
73. apnea
74. thoracocentesis
75. pneumonectomy

a. Surgical removal of the lung or a segment of the lung
b. Temporary loss of breathing
c. Presence of air or gas in the cavity between the lungs and the chest wall, causing collapse of the lung
d. Presence of gas or air in the abdominal cavity
e. Surgical puncture and drainage of the plural cavity

76. encephal/o
77. mening/o
78. -algia
79. -phasia
80. gli/o

a. Pertaining to covering of the brain and spinal cord
b. Pertaining to speech
c. Pertaining to the brain
d. Pertaining to neurological tissue
e. Pertaining to pain

Answers and Explanations

#	Word		Definition
1.	abduction	b	Away from the midline of the body
2.	adduction	e	Toward the midline of the body
3.	dorsal recumbent	a	Supine
4.	anterior	c	Pertaining to the front of the body
5.	lateral	d	Pertaining to the side of the body
6.	proxim/o	b	Near the point of attachment to the body
7.	super/o	e	Upper, above
8.	dist/o	a	Farthest point
9.	cephalo/o	d	Pertaining to the head
10.	crani/o	c	Pertaining to the skull
11.	lumpectomy	b	Excision of a breast lesion with surrounding tissue
12.	radical mastectomy	e	Removal of breast tissue, muscle, and lymph nodes
13.	modified radical mastectomy	d	Removal of breast tissue and axillary lymph nodes
14.	wire localization	a	Performed in radiology where the mass is identified with a wire
15.	sentinel lymph node	c	First set of nodes closest to the cancerous tumor
16.	chrondr/o	a	Cartilage
17.	oste/o	e	Bone
18.	arthr/o	c	Joint
19.	metacarp/o	b	Hand bones
20.	tend/o	d	Tendon
21.	blephar/o	e	Eyelid
22.	dacry/o	d	Tear duct
23.	kerat/o	c	Cornea
24.	retin/o	a	Retina
25.	irid/o	b	Iris
26.	-cele	e	Hernia
27.	-dyspnea	b	Difficulty breathing
28.	-edema	a	Swelling
29.	-itis	c	Inflammation of
30.	-emesis	d	Vomiting
31.	-megaly	c	Enlargement
32.	-pathy	a	Disease
33.	-rrhage	b	Bursting forth
34.	-oma	e	Tumor
35.	-rrhea	d	Flow, discharge

#	Word		Definition
36.	abruptio placentae	b	Placenta tears away from the uterine wall
37.	ectopic	d	Pregnancy outside the uterus
38.	placenta previa	a	Placenta forms in the lower portion of the uterus and blocks the birth canal
39.	atresia	c	Lack of a normal body opening
40.	rectocele	e	Protrusion of the rectum into the vagina
41.	cervic/o	a	Pertaining to the neck, cervix
42.	lapar/o	e	Pertaining to the abdomen
43.	cyst/o	b	Pertaining to the bladder
44.	gynec/o	c	Pertaining to female
45.	colp/o	d	Pertaining to the vagina
46.	fistula	d	Abnormal passageway that forms between two structures
47.	fibroid	a	Benign tumor of the uterus
48.	ovarian cystectomy	b	Removal of a cyst on the ovary
49.	oophorectomy	c	Removal of the ovary
50.	salpingectomy	e	Removal of the fallopian tube
51.	mitral valve	b	Also called the bicuspid valve
52.	bradycardia	c	Resting heart rate below 60 bpm
53.	arrhythmia	e	Irregular heart beat
54.	alveoli	a	Exchange of oxygen and carbon dioxide occurs here
55.	cyanosis	d	Condition caused by oxygen deficiency
56.	atrial septal defect	e	Congenital condition caused by the septum, between the atria, failing to close, allowing blood to flow back and forth
57.	claudication	d	Pain in a limb, usually the leg, caused by poor circulation
58.	embolism	a	Clot composed of blood, air, or fat that moves through the vascular system
59.	thrombus	b	Stationary clot
60.	ischemia	c	Abnormally low blood flow to tissues
61.	patent ductus arteriosus	b	Congenital condition caused by an opening between the pulmonary artery and the aorta that failed to close before birth

#	Word		Definition
62.	tetralogy of Fallot	e	Congenital defect that consists of four separate cardiac diseases: pulmonary stenosis, ventricular septal defect, incorrect position of the aorta, and ventricular hypertrophy
63.	hypertension	a	High blood pressure
64.	hypotension	d	Low blood pressure
65.	aneurysm	c	Bulging of an arterial wall
66.	-otomy	c	Cutting into
67.	-pexy	e	Fixation of
68.	-plasty	a	Surgical repair
69.	-centesis	b	Puncture to remove fluid
70.	poly-	d	Many
71.	pneumothorax	c	Presence of air or gas in the cavity between the lungs and the chest wall, causing collapse of the lung

#	Word		Definition
72.	pneumoperitoneum	d	Presence of gas or air in the abdominal cavity
73.	apnea	b	Temporary loss of breathing
74.	thoracocentesis	e	Surgical puncture and drainage of the pleural cavity
75.	pneumonectomy	a	Surgical removal of the lung or a segment of the lung
76.	encephal/o	c	Pertaining to the brain
77.	mening/o	a	Pertaining to covering of the brain and spinal cord
78.	-algia	e	Pertaining to pain
79.	-phasia	b	Pertaining to speech
80.	gli/o	d	Pertaining to neurological tissue

CHAPTER 2

Microbiology

- ASEPSIS—absence of disease-causing micro-organisms
- STERILE—free of all living microorganisms including spores
- SURGICALLY CLEAN—mechanically disinfected but not sterile
- AERATION—this is the method by which ethylene oxide (a type of sterilization process) is removed from the ETO-sterilized items
- AEROBES—microbes that cannot live and reproduce without oxygen
- FACULTATIVE ANAEROBES—can live in both environments
- ANAEROBES—microbes living in the absence of oxygen
- FOMITE—inanimate object that contains microorganisms
- CELLS—smallest unit of living things
  - MITOCHONDRIA—they are the powerhouse of the cell and provide energy
  - FLAGELLA—provide locomotion to the cell
  - CELL WALL—protects the cell
  - CYTOPLASMIC MEMBRANE—semipermeable membrane within the cell
- BACTERIA—all living cells are classified into two groups:
  - PROKARYOTES—less complex organisms. Single circular chromosome, without a nuclear membrane or membrane-bound organelles
  - EUKARYOTES—complex cellular structure; they include fungi, algae, plant and animal cells. HAS A NUCLEUS
- Bacteria divide by BINARY FISSION—this is the asexual reproduction of a cell by division into two identical daughter cells
- Bacteria are shaped: rod shaped/spherical shaped/spiral shaped
- GRAM-POSITIVE—purple
- GRAM-NEGATIVE—red
- BACTERICIDE—kills gram-positive and gram-negative bacteria
- BACTERIOSTATIC—inhibits (to prevent something from developing) the growth of bacteria
- BIOBURDEN—the amount of microorganisms on an item before sterilization
- BIOLOGICAL INDICATOR—a sterilization monitoring system used to test the effectiveness of the sterilization process used
  - *GEOBACILLUS STEAROTHERMOPHILUS*—is the microbes used in steam sterilization
  - *BACILLUS ATROPHAEUS/GEOBACILLUS SUBTILIS*—are the microbes used for ETO sterilization
- CONTAMINATION—presence of pathogenic microorganisms (disease-causing microorganisms) on animate (living being) and inanimate (nonliving) objects
- DECONTAMINATION—process by which chemical or physical agents are used to clean inanimate objects, NONCRITICAL surfaces
- SSI—SURGICAL SITE INFECTION
- DEEP INCISIONAL SSI—an infection involving deep soft tissue, fascia
- DISINFECTANT—not used on living tissue
- ANTISEPTIC—used on living tissue
- FUNGICIDE—kills fungi
- IMMUNITY—resistant to infection
  - NATURALLY ACQUIRED ACTIVE IMMUNITY—acquired when you get a disease and acquire antibodies

- o ARTIFICIALLY ACQUIRED ACTIVE IMMUNITY—vaccination
- o NATURALLY ACQUIRED PASSIVE IMMUNITY—antibodies from mother to child through the placenta
- o ARTIFICIALLY ACQUIRED PASSIVE IMMUNITY—a short-term immunization by the injection of antibodies, such as gamma globulin, that are not produced by the recipient's cells
- INFECTION—invasion and multiplication of microorganisms in body tissues, causing cellular damage
- SKIN—it is the first line of defense against bacteria
- NOSOCOMIAL INFECTION—an infection that was acquired in the hospital
- PASTEURIZATION—this is not a method of sterilization but a heating process of destroying pathogenic microorganisms such as in milk or wine
- PARASITES—microorganisms that reside on or within living organisms. Some are OBLIGATORY (means they depend on living tissue) and others are FACULTATIVE (meaning they can live on dead tissue)
- PATHOGEN—any disease-producing microorganism
- RESIDENT MICROORGANISMS—these are microorganisms that live deep in the epidermis (outer most layer of skin); they live in the folds and crevices of the skin
- TRANSIENT MICROORGANISMS—these are microorganisms that live on the surface of the epidermis; they have a very short life span and can be removed with a good hand scrub
- VIRUCIDE—kills viruses
- MICROORGANISMS:
  - o *STAPHYLOCOCCUS AUREUS*—commonly found in RESPIRATORY PASSAGES
  - o ENTEROCOCCI—found in the normal flora of the gastrointestinal (GI) tract. These organisms are associated with surgical site infections (SSIs)
  - o STREPTOCOCCI—found in the GI tracts, upper respiratory tracts, and genitourinary tracts
  - o HELMINTHS—parasitic worms (round worms, tape worms). They are acquired by

ingestion of contaminated soil with fecal matter
  - o RICKETTSIAE—they are parasites transmitted by insects
  - o CLOSTRIDIA—produce virulent toxins
    - *CLOSTRIDIUM PERFRINGENS*—GAS GANGRENE (serious infection in body tissue; the severe infection causes a buildup of gas)
    - *C. TETANI*—TETANUS (muscle twitching, cramps that are caused by a problem with the parathyroid glands involving calcium)
    - *C. DIFFICILE*—the normal flora in the intestines is altered, usually caused by the overuse of antibiotics causing severe diarrhea and dehydration
    - *MYCOBACTERIUM TUBERCULOSIS*—it is transmitted directly from the respiratory tract, causing tuberculosis (TB)
    - VIRUSES—some examples of a virus include: HIV, herpes simplex, hepatitis B, C, and D
    - METHICILLIN-RESISTANT *STAPHYLOCOCCUS AUREUS* (MRSA)—this is a particular strain of a virus that is resistant to most all antibiotics; the only antibiotic that works on this virus is VANCOMYCIN
    - CREUTZFELDT–JAKOB DISEASE—this is a fatal neurodegenerative disease of the central nervous system caused by a HUMAN PRION
- PRION/PROTEINACEOUS INFECTIOUS PARTICLE—is the smallest infectious particle; it is neither viral, bacterial, nor fungal. Prions are also responsible for the disease known as mad cow disease. This disease is important for the STSR because there is no sterilization process that kills these prions. When surgery is performed on a patient with this diagnosis, disposable instruments are used
- BIOTERRORIST AGENTS—
  - o Anthrax
  - o Smallpox
  - o Plague (pneumonic, bubonic)
  - o Tularemia (various types of insect bites)
  - o Botulism
- MUTUALISM—is the way two organisms of different species exist in a relationship in which each individual benefits

- COMMENSALISM—when one organism benefits and the other does not benefit but is not harmed
- PARASITISM—a long-term relationship between two species, where one member, the parasite, gains benefits that come at the expense of the host member
- OSMOSIS—when a fluid, usually water, passes through a membrane solution of higher concentration, which equalizes the concentrations of materials on both sides of the membrane
- MITOSIS—division of a single cell into two identical cells. Each cell has an identical number of chromosomes as the parent cell. Each cell contains the same genes
- MEIOSIS—cell division involving sexually reproducing organisms
- CHRONIC INFECTION—there is a continued presence of infection

- ACUTE INFECTION—rapid onset, severe symptoms, and a short course
- EPIDEMIC—it is a quick widespread infectious disease in a certain area, such as the flu
- PANDEMIC—it is a global outbreak of a disease that affects many more people (ie, COVID-19)
- ENDEMIC—a disease connected to a particular group of people in a certain identified area
- MICROSCOPE—an instrument used to view microorganisms that cannot be seen by the naked eye. Invented by Anton Von Leeuwenhoek
- JOSEPH LISTER—father of modern medicine. Discovered antiseptic techniques
- LOUIS PASTEUR—founded the science of microbiology and that diseases are caused by microorganisms

Questions

1. The English surgeon who established the first principles of aseptic technique is:

   (A) Ehrlich
   (B) Madame Curie
   (C) Alexander
   (D) Lister

2. Passage of fluid through a cell membrane is called:

   (A) mitosis
   (B) meiosis
   (C) osmosis
   (D) symbiosis

3. Oxygen-dependent bacteria are said to be:

   (A) anaerobic
   (B) bacillic
   (C) antibiotic
   (D) aerobic

4. The destruction of bacteria by white cells during the inflammatory process is called:

   (A) symbiosis
   (B) mitosis
   (C) lymphocytosis
   (D) phagocytosis

5. Bacteriostatic means:

   (A) inhibit growth of microorganisms
   (B) destroy microorganisms
   (C) control microorganisms
   (D) inactivate microorganisms

6. *Staphylococcus aureus* would most likely be transmitted by:

   (A) urine
   (B) feces
   (C) nose and mouth
   (D) sex organs

7. Microbial death occurs when an organism is:

   (A) reproducing at a slower rate
   (B) reduced in population
   (C) no longer capable of reproduction
   (D) exposed to heat

8. What immune protection is available to the fetus?

   (A) Natural active
   (B) Natural passive
   (C) Active artificial
   (D) Passive artificial

9. The clinical syndrome characterized by microbial invasion of the bloodstream is:

   (A) superinfection
   (B) septicemia
   (C) cross infection
   (D) cellulitis

10. The body's first line of defense against the invasion of pathogens is:

    (A) the immune response
    (B) skin and mucous membrane linings
    (C) cellular and chemical responses
    (D) phagocytosis

11. Rod-like–shaped bacteria are identified microscopically as:

    (A) bacilli
    (B) cocci
    (C) spirilla
    (D) spirochetes

12. Herpes simplex is commonly called:

    (A) cold sore
    (B) shingles
    (C) smallpox
    (D) chickenpox

13. All of the following descriptors refer to the inflammatory process EXCEPT:

    (A) heat
    (B) pain
    (C) vasoconstriction
    (D) edema

14. *Clostridium tetani* causes:

    (A) gangrene
    (B) nosocomial infection
    (C) lockjaw
    (D) malaria

15. A laboratory procedure useful in classifying bacteria using a staining procedure is:

    (A) Gram stain
    (B) iodine stain
    (C) acid-fast stain
    (D) differential stain

16. A fulminating infection arising from necrotic tissue and spreading rapidly is:

    (A) rabies
    (B) gas gangrene
    (C) pasteurellosis
    (D) tetanus

17. A severe allergic reaction possibly resulting in death is called:

    (A) Arthus reaction
    (B) hypersensibility
    (C) anaphylactic shock
    (D) autoimmune disease

18. What organism is responsible for a boil?

    (A) *S. aureus*
    (B) *Clostridium perfringens*
    (C) *Escherichia coli*
    (D) *Neisseria*

19. The organism most frequently found in burns is:

    (A) *C. perfringens*
    (B) *Pseudomonas aeruginosa*
    (C) *C. tetani*
    (D) Hemolytic streptococci

20. Which type of wound would favor the development of gas gangrene?

    (A) Ischemic
    (B) Necrotic
    (C) Dry
    (D) Both A and B

21. Gas gangrene is caused by:

    (A) *Fusobacterium*
    (B) *C. tetani*
    (C) *P. aeruginosa*
    (D) *C. perfringens*

22. The bacteria that are highly resistant to sterilization and disinfection are:

    (A) spores
    (B) fungus
    (C) gram-positive
    (D) *Pseudomonas*

23. The bacteria found in the intestinal tract are:

    (A) *E. coli*
    (B) *Bordetella pertussis*
    (C) *Francisella tularensis*
    (D) *Neisseria gonorrhoeae*

24. The space caused by separation of wound edges is called:

    (A) lag phase
    (B) evisceration
    (C) fibrous scarring
    (D) dead space

25. Which body fluid is least likely to transmit HIV?

    (A) Blood
    (B) Semen
    (C) Saliva
    (D) Spinal fluid

26. Which bacteria are the common cause for postoperative wound infections?

    (A) *S. aureus*
    (B) Rickettsiae
    (C) *Haemophilus influenzae*
    (D) *Candida*

27. Hospital-acquired infections are known as:

    (A) antibiotic resistant
    (B) bacteremia
    (C) nosocomial
    (D) MRSA

28. Methicillin-resistant *S. aureus* (MRSA) is a strain of *S. aureus* that is resistant to most antibiotics. What is the only drug of choice to treat MRSA at this time?

    (A) Vancomycin
    (B) Penicillin
    (C) Gentamicin
    (D) Keflex

29. *E. coli* is part of the normal flora of the _____ of humans.

    (A) skin
    (B) hair
    (C) intestinal track
    (D) None of the above

30. The type of immunity that is acquired by a vaccination is:

    (A) naturally acquired active immunity
    (B) naturally acquired passive immunity
    (C) artificial active acquired immunity
    (D) artificial passive acquired immunity

31. What Gram stain turns red at the end of the staining procedure?

    (A) Gram positive
    (B) Gram negative
    (C) Acid-fast positive
    (D) Acid-fast negative

32. What living cells are more complex, have nuclei, and include protozoa, fungi, and green, red, and brown algae?

    (A) Eukaryotic
    (B) Facultative
    (C) Prokaryotic
    (D) Passive

33. Universal precautions is a previously used term. The term now commonly used is:

    (A) recommended precautions
    (B) evidence-based practice
    (C) occupational precautions
    (D) standard precautions

34. Asepsis means:

    (A) without infection
    (B) destroys bacteria
    (C) clean
    (D) absence of microbes

35. The microbes that reside on the skin and are easily removed are referred to as:

    (A) resident
    (B) transient
    (C) aseptic flora
    (D) None of the above

36. All factors increase the surgical patient's risk for infection EXCEPT:

    (A) location of surgery
    (B) health of the patient
    (C) length of the procedure
    (D) position of the patient

37. What is responsible for bacterial motility?

    (A) Flagella
    (B) Mitochondria
    (C) Cell wall
    (D) RNA

38. Rickettsiae are transmitted by:

    (A) *S. aureus*
    (B) arthropod bites
    (C) tape worms
    (D) fungi

39. When there is a relationship between two organisms that occupy the same space but one organism benefits and the other does not but is unharmed, it is termed:

    (A) mutualism
    (B) commensalism
    (C) parasitism
    (D) None of the above

40. When there is a relationship between two organisms and one benefits at the expense of the other, it is termed:

    (A) mutualism
    (B) commensalism
    (C) parasitism
    (D) fungi

41. The basic structural and functional living unit of the body is known as:

    (A) cell
    (B) tissue
    (C) organ
    (D) mitochondria

42. The biological indicator for ETO is:

    (A) *Bacillus subtilis*
    (B) *Geobacillus stearothermophilus*
    (C) *Bacillus atrophaeus*
    (D) Both A and C

43. Inflammation in which gland may be used to diagnose the disease mumps?

    (A) Sublingual
    (B) Submandibular
    (C) Thyroid
    (D) Parotid

44. What is the term for the division of a reproductive cell into two cells with chromosome cells?

    (A) Binary fission
    (B) Mitosis
    (C) Meiosis
    (D) Osmosis

45. An inanimate object that contains microorganisms is termed:

    (A) fomite
    (B) prion
    (C) obligatory
    (D) flagella

46. Which of the following causes the disease "mad cow"?

    (A) Virus
    (B) Prion
    (C) Spore
    (D) Fungi

47. When there is a continued presence of an infection, it is termed:

    (A) acute
    (B) pandemic
    (C) chronic
    (D) nosocomial

48. The definition of pandemic is:

    (A) disease that has spread throughout a school
    (B) disease that has spread during the winter season
    (C) disease that has spread throughout the world
    (D) disease that has spread quickly and causes serious illness

Answers and Explanations

1. **(D)** In 1867, Lister began the age of chemical control of the atmosphere. He used aqueous phenol to disinfect instruments, soak dressings, and spray the air of surgical rooms.

2. **(C)** Osmosis allows the passage of a solvent, usually water, to pass through the membrane from the region of lower concentration of solute to the region of higher concentration. This tends to equalize the concentration of the two solutions.

3. **(D)** The majority of microbes are aerobes. This means they grow and flourish in the presence of oxygen.

4. **(D)** Leukocytes known as phagocytes rush to a wound to engulf and destroy the bacteria present. Phagocytosis means "cell eating."

5. **(A)** Agents that destroy or inactivate microorganisms are bactericidal. An agent that inhibits the growth of bacteria is known as a bacteriostatic agent.

6. **(C)** *S. aureus* is commonly present on skin and mucous membranes, especially those of the nose and the mouth. It is gram-positive and is the cause of such suppurative conditions as boils, carbuncles, and internal abscesses.

7. **(C)** Microbial death occurs when an organism, or population of organisms, is no longer capable of reproduction.

8. **(B)** In passive natural immunity, maternal antibodies cross the placenta. Infants are immune to the same infectious diseases as their mothers for 6 to 12 months after birth.

Breast-fed babies receive additional protection from the breast milk.

9. **(B)** Microorganisms can multiply in the blood. Infection of bacterial origin carried through the bloodstream is referred to as bacteremia or septicemia. Microorganisms invade from a focus of infection in the tissue.

10. **(B)** The unbroken skin acts as a mechanical barrier to pathogens. Only when it is cut, scratched, or burned can pathogens gain entrance. Mucous membranes entrap invaders.

11. **(A)** Bacteria generally appear in one of several shapes: bacilli are rod shaped, cocci are spherical, and spirilla and spirochetes are corkscrew shaped.

12. **(A)** Herpes simplex, commonly called "cold sores" or fever blisters, is an example of a viral agent capable of latent periods where the virus is not multiplied. It remains intact until stress encourages growth. Its appearance is associated with trauma, sun, hormonal changes, and emotional upset.

13. **(C)** Local irritation causes the small blood vessels to dilate and become more permeable. The tissue spaces become engorged with fluid, and edema results. In inflammation, there is pain, redness, heat, swelling, vasodilation, and disturbance of function.

14. **(A)** *C. tetani* is the causative organism of tetany, or lockjaw. Commonly found in soil contaminated with animal fecal waste. Protection is provided by receiving tetanus toxoid to

stimulate antibodies against tetanus toxins. A booster may be given when a dangerous wound is received.

15. **(A)** The Gram stain is very useful because it classifies bacteria into two large groups: gram-positive and gram-negative. This provides valuable treatment options. Gram-positive bacteria tend to be killed easily by penicillins and cephalosporins. Gram-negative bacteria are generally more resistant.

16. **(B)** When the organisms of gas gangrene are introduced into tissues where conditions permit anaerobic multiplication, they utilize amino acids and carbohydrates freed from dead or dying cells.

17. **(C)** Anaphylactic shock is the state of collapse resulting from injection of a substance to which one has been sensitized. It is a severe allergic reaction. Death may occur if emergency treatment is not given.

18. **(A)** *S. aureus* is associated with skin infections such as boils, carbuncles, furuncles, and impetigo.

19. **(B)** *P. aeruginosa*, most frequently found in burns, presents very difficult problems because the organism is generally resistant to many clinically useful antibiotics.

20. **(D)** An ischemic necrotic wound caused by *C. perfringens* causes gas gangrene.

21. **(D)** Gas gangrene is caused by the microorganism *C. perfringens*.

22. **(A)** The most resistant form of microbial life is the endospore. Spores have a thick wall, making them difficult to destroy. This enables them to withstand unfavorable conditions such as heat. They require a prolonged exposure time to high temperatures to destroy them.

23. **(A)** *E. coli* is by far the best-known enteric bacterium and is found in the intestinal tract of animals and humans.

24. **(D)** Serum or blood clots can form within dead space and prevent healing by keeping the cut edges of the tissue separated. It is the space caused by separation of wound edges that have not been closely approximated.

25. **(C)** Hazardous body fluids include amniotic fluid, blood, pericardial fluid, peritoneal fluid, pleural fluid, semen, spinal fluid, synovial fluid, and vaginal secretions. Saliva has not been implicated in HIV transmission.

26. **(A)** *S. aureus* is the common cause of boils, carbuncles, impetigo, toxic shock syndrome, and postoperative wound infections.

27. **(C)** Hospital-acquired infections are known as nosocomial. They can be acquired due to improper technique.

28. **(A)** Vancomycin destroys bacteria by inhibiting cell wall synthesis and is now the front-line antibiotic therapy used against MRSA.

29. **(C)** *E. coli* is part of the normal flora of the intestinal track of humans; most strains are harmless.

30. **(C)** Artificial active acquired immunity is acquired immunity gained by getting a vaccination.

31. **(B)** Gram-negatives appear red from the safranin stain, and gram-positives remain purple.

32. **(A)** Eukaryotes are more complex and include protozoa; fungi; green, red, and brown algae; and all plant and animal cells including human cells.

33. **(D)** Aseptic technique is among the behaviors and protocols specified in the standard precautions. These evolved from a previous policy called universal precautions established by the Centers for Disease Control and Prevention for control and prevention of disease.

34. **(D)** Asepsis means absence of microbes and infection.

35. **(B)** Transient flora are microbes that reside on the skin and are easily removed.

36. **(D)** Risk factors include location of the surgical site, the health of the patient, condition of tissues and organs, resistance of body tissue, length of the preoperative stay, duration of the procedure, and surgical technique.

37. **(A)** Flagella are responsible for bacterial motility. Mitochondria are known as the "powerhouse of the cell." The cell wall gives shape to the cell and provides a barrier to the outside of the cell. Ribonucleic acid (RNA) is manufactured in the nucleolus and controls cellular protein synthesis.

38. **(B)** Rickettsiae are gram-negative bacteria. They reproduce in the host cell of arthropods (type of invertebrate—insects, spiders, centipedes) and mammals. *S. aureus* is a gram-positive bacterium and is frequently found in the respiratory tract and on the skin. Tape worms are flat worms that live in the intestines of animals. Fungi are part of the group of eukaryotic organisms. They are unicellular and include yeasts and molds.

39. **(B)** Commensalism is the relationship between two organisms that occupy the same space. One organism benefits and the other does not, but neither is harmed. Mutualism is the relationship between two organisms where both benefit. Parasitism is the relationship between two organisms where one benefits at the expense of the other.

40. **(C)** Parasitism is the relationship between two organisms where one benefits at the expense of the other. Mutualism is the relationship between two organisms where both benefit. Commensalism is the relationship between two organisms that occupy the same space; one organism benefits and the other does not, but neither is harmed. Fungi are part of the group of eukaryotic organisms; they are unicellular and include yeasts and molds.

41. **(A)** The smallest structural and functioning unit of an organism is a cell. Tissues are made up of specialized cells that perform a specific function. Organs are made up of tissues and are grouped into systems. Mitochondria are known as the "powerhouse" of the cell.

42. **(D)** The biological indicator for ETO is *Bacillus atrophaeus/subtilis*. *Geobacillus stearothermophilus* is the biological indicator used for steam sterilization.

43. **(D)** The parotid gland is the primary gland that is affected by the mumps. This disease is caused by a virus and is highly contagious. The thyroid gland is an endocrine gland and is found in the neck. Sublingual glands are salivary glands found in the mouth. The submandibular glands are salivary glands located below the lower jaw.

44. **(B)** Mitosis is a type of cell division that results in two daughter cells, each having the same number of chromosomes. Binary fission is when the cell divides into two equal daughter cells. Meiosis is a type of cell division that results in four daughter cells, each with half the number of chromosomes of the parent cell. Osmosis is when liquid passes from a lower concentration through a membrane into an area with a higher concentration to balance them.

45. **(A)** Fomite is an inanimate object that contains microorganisms. A prion is a small proteinaceous, infectious, disease-causing spore. It is not bacterial, fungal, or viral. Prions are responsible for degenerative brain diseases. Obligatory is in regard to bacteria that can grow under aerobic or anaerobic conditions. Flagella are responsible for bacterial motility.

46. **(B)** A prion is responsible for "mad cow" disease. Virus—There are many diseases caused by viruses. Examples include cold, chickenpox, meningitis, and many others. Spores—Two of the major spore-forming diseases include food poisoning caused by *Bacillus cereus* and *C. tetani*, which is found in soil.

47. **(C)** A chronic infection is considered a continued presence of infection. An acute infection is a serious infection with an abrupt onset that progresses rapidly. Pandemic is an outbreak of a disease over a wide geographic area infecting much of the population of that area. Nosocomial is a hospital-acquired infection.

48. **(C)** The definition of a pandemic disease is one that spreads throughout the world. Epidemic is the rapid spread of an infectious disease to a large number of people in a short period of time.

CHAPTER 3

Pharmacology and Anesthesia

- Drug sources include: plants, animals, lab synthesis, and biotechnology
- Pharmacodynamics—what the drug does to the body
- Pharmacokinetics—what the body does to the drug
- Antagonist—a chemical drug that counteracts or blocks the action of another drug
- Synergist agent—one drug works with another drug (boosts the result) to provide the same effect; however, by combining the two drugs, the dose is lower and safer
- Therapeutic effect—the drug is intended to produce a desirable and beneficial effect to the patient
- Side effect—a secondary effect of a therapeutic drug. It is usually undesirable but tolerable
- Adverse effect—an undesirable and potentially harmful effect from a therapeutic drug
- Anaphylaxis—a severe allergic reaction; immediate attention is required or the patient could die
- Toxic effect—undesirable effect that could cause cancer
- Addiction—a dependency on the effect of the drug
- Onset—time required for the drug to work
- Peak effect—period of time when the maximum effect of the drug works
- Duration—how long the medication works

Routes of Administration

• Oral	• By mouth
• Rectal	• Placed in the rectum
• Intradermal	• Placed between the layers of the skin
• Subcutaneous	• Placed in the adipose (fat) tissue under the skin
• Intramuscular	• Placed in the muscle
• Intra-articular	• Placed in a joint
• Intravenous	• Placed into a vein
• Intrathecal	• Placed into the subarachnoid space (spine)
• Intracardiac	• Placed into the heart
• Buccal	• Placed between the cheek and gums (usually dissolved)
• Sublingual	• Placed under the tongue
• Instillation	• Placed in a hollow cavity (bladder)
• Inhalation	• Placed in the lungs through inhalation
• Topical	• Placed on the outer surface (skin)

- FDA—Food and Drug Administration— prescription drugs must go through a review process and an approval process in order to be used in the United States

Drug Forms

• Gas	• Examples: oxygen, nitrous oxide

• Liquid	• Solution
	  ○ Aqueous—water
	  ○ Syrup—sweet water solution
	  ○ Tincture—solution with alcohol
	  ○ Elixir—sweetened alcohol solution
	• Suspension
	  ○ Solid particles are mixed in a liquid and shaken to distribute
	• Emulsion—two liquids that cannot be mixed

• Solid	• Powder within a capsule, tablet, lozenge
• Semisolid	• Creams, foams, gels, lotions

- Controlled substances—drugs that have the potential to cause dependence and abuse
- Medication information
  ○ Trade name/brand name—name assigned by the manufacturer. Example, Advil
  ○ Generic name—shortened name for the chemical name. This is the name on the medication label. Example, ibuprofen

- o Chemical name—chemical composition of the medication. Example, (RS)-2-[4-(2-methylpropyl)phenyl]propanoic acid (this is not on package but on package insert)
- Concentration
  - o How much drug is in a given amount of fluid
  - o The concentration is found on the medication label
  - o For medications that need to be reconstituted (powder mixed with a solution), the instructions will also be on the label
- Dose
  - o The dose of the medication is the amount delivered to the patient
- Application
  - o This applies to the way the medication is being used and how it is delivered to the patient in surgery
  - o Example, lidocaine HCl is commonly used as a local medication to numb a specific area; however, it could also be used to decrease abnormal heartbeats. This medication can be given for two different reasons and administered in two different ways
- Conversions of temperature
  - o Freezing point of water—32°F = 0°C
  - o Boiling point of water—212°F = 100°C
  - o Normal body temperature—98.6°F = 37°C
- The six rights of medication
  - o The *right* patient
  - o The *right* drug
  - o The *right* dose
  - o The *right* route of administration
  - o The *right* time
  - o The *right* labeling/documentation
- Medication identification
  - o Ampule—a little glass container that requires the top to be broken off—contains liquid
  - o Vial—plastic or glass container that has a rubber top—may contain liquid or powder
  - o Preloaded syringe—contains liquid
- Transferring medications onto the sterile field
  - o The circulator and the STSR agree on the medication
  - o The circulator holds the medication so the STSR can see the label; the circulator reads the medication information out loud:
    - ▪ Name of drug

- ▪ Strength of the drug
- ▪ Expiration date
- o As soon as the STSR receives the medication, she must label the container
- o When the STSR fills the syringe, it must be immediately labeled
- o All basins and pitchers containing irrigation fluids, antibiotics, and/or sterile water must be labeled
- o Medications that need to be reconstituted are done by the circulator before transfer to the sterile field
- o Medications can be poured, squeezed, or ejected through a syringe
- All medical cups, glasses, emesis basins and pitchers are placed at the edge of the table by the STSR so the circulator can dispense the fluid without reaching over the sterile field and contaminating the field
  - o The irrigation fluid should be held 12 in above the pitcher when pouring
  - o Irrigation fluids are poured into a pitcher
  - o Transferring medications from a vial onto the sterile field:
    - ▪ Procedure 1—the circulator removes the plastic cap, wipes the top of the vial with an alcohol wipe, draws up the medication in a syringe, and dispenses it onto the sterile field.
    - ▪ Procedure 2—the circulator removes the plastic cap, wipes the top of the vial with an alcohol wipe, and holds the vial upside down. The STSR draws up the medication using a syringe. She then changes the hypodermic needle before passing the syringe to the surgeon just in case there was any contamination.
    - ▪ It is easier to draw up medication with a larger hypodermic needle.
  - o Every time STSRs pass a syringe to the surgeon, they must state:
    - ▪ Name of the drug
    - ▪ Strength and amount
  - o If there is any question about the strength of the drug or name of the drug that has been placed on the sterile field, the drug must be discarded and replaced

Medications Used in Obstetrics and Gynecology

- Oxytocic drugs
  - Oxytocin
  - Pitocin
- Used to induce labor (contractions) and control hemorrhage
- Pitressin
- Injected into the cervix to reduce bleeding
- Rhogam
- An immunoglobulin used when there is a problem with the Rh factor between mother and child; administered to Rh-negative women who are pregnant to prevent sensitization of the maternal immune system when pregnant with an Rh-positive fetus

Medications Used in Orthopedics

- Antibiotic irrigations
  - Polymyxin
  - Bacitracin
  - Cephalosporin
- Irrigation solutions

- Hemostatic agents
  - Gelfoam
  - Avitene
  - Thrombin
  - Bone wax
- Used to control bleeding

- Steroids
  - Decadron
  - Betamethasone/Celestone
- Anti-inflammatory

Cardiovascular Medications

- Heparinized/saline
- Irrigation
- Papaverine HCl
- Lidocaine HCl/Xylocaine
- Oxidized cellulose
  - Oxicell
  - Surgicel
- Intravascular irrigation—thins the blood prevent clotting
- Dilates the blood vessels
- Local anesthetic
- This is used to control bleeding

Neurovascular Medications

- Heparinized saline irrigation
- Papaverine HCl
- Lidocaine HCl
- Gelfoam soaked in thrombin
- Polifeprosan 20 with carmustine (Gliadel wafers)
- Intravascular irrigation—thins the blood to prevent clotting
- Dilates the blood vessels
- Local anesthetic
- Used to control bleeding
- Gliadel wafer is an implant for intracranial use, containing carmustine and polifeprosan. It is an anticancer chemotherapy drug

Ophthalmic Medications

- Mydriatics
  - Neo-Synephrine
- Dilate the pupil but allow the pupil to focus
- Cycloplegics
  - Atropine sulfate
- Dilate the pupil but inhibit focusing
- Miotics
  - Miochol—must be reconstituted immediately before using and must be used within 15 minutes
  - Pilocarpine
  - Miostat
- Constrict the pupil
- Viscoelastics
  - Healon
  - Provisc
  - Viscoat—used to coat the lens before implantation
- Lubricate and maintain a separation between tissues (occupy space)
- Hyperosmotics
  - Mannitol/Osmitrol
- Diuretics—used to reduce intraocular pressure (IOP)
- Anti-inflammatory drugs
  - Dexamethasone
  - Betamethasone/Celestone
  - Prednisolone
- Prevent inflammation
- Antibiotic ointments
  - Gentamycin
  - Tobramycin
  - Erythromycin
  - Ciprofloxacin
- Used to treat ocular infections
- Local anesthetics
  - Tetracaine/Pontocaine
  - Lidocaine HCl—used for retrobulbar blocks
- Irrigation
  - BSS—balance salt solution
- Dyes
  - Fluorescein sodium
- Stain the eye tissue

- Retrobulbar (this block is performed directly into the base of the eyelids or into the back of the globe of the eye)

Medications Commonly Used in the Operating Room

Adrenergics—stimulate the sympathetic nerves

- Epinephrine/adrenalin
- Topical hemostatic drug used to prolong the effects of a local anesthetic
- Neo-Synephrine
- Shrinks mucous membranes before nasal surgery
- Dilates the pupil

Analgesics/Narcotics—Drugs That Relieve Pain, Can Cause Numbness, and Induce a State of Unconsciousness

- Sublimaze
- Provides pain relief
- Used with general anesthesia
- Demerol
- Provides pain relief
- Used with general anesthesia
- Morphine
- Used for severe pain

Analgesics/Antipyretics—Relieve Pain, Nonsteroidal Anti-Inflammatory

- Toradol
  - Short-acting pain reliever
  - Used postoperatively

Benzodiazepines—Antianxiety Drugs That Calm and Relax

- Versed
  - Reduces anxiety
  - Gives an amnesia effect
  - Used in surgery
- Valium/diazepam
  - Reduces anxiety
- Ativan
  - Reduces anxiety

Antiarrhythmics—Used to Suppress Abnormal Rhythms of the Heart

- Lidocaine hydrochloride)/ xylocaine
  - Used for ventricular arrhythmias

Antibiotics—Inhibit or Destroy Bacteria

- Gentamycin/Garamycin
  - Commonly used in genitourinary (GU) and gastrointestinal (GI) surgery
- Penicillins
  - Sepsis
- Cephalosporins
  - Used prophylactically for surgery
  - Ancef/Kefzol
  - Keflex
  - Mefoxin

Antiamebicide—Antifungal

- Flagyl
  - Prevents infection from GI microbes

Miscellaneous Antibiotics

- Bacitracin
  - Orthopedic irrigation
- Neosporin
  - Topical ointment
- Vancomycin
  - Used to treat MRSA—methicillin-resistant *Staphylococcus aureus*

Sulfonamides—Sulfur-Based Antibacterial Drugs

- Silvadene
  - A cream used to treat burns

Anticoagulants—Prevent Blood Clots

- Heparin
  - Commonly used on vascular procedures

Anticoagulant Antagonist—Reverses the Effects of Heparin

- Protamine sulfate
  - Reverses the effects of heparin

Antiemetics—Reduce Anxiety and Reduce Nausea and Vomiting

- Reglan
  - Given perioperatively
- Zofran
  - Given perioperatively

Antihypertensive—Used to Treat Hypertensive Episodes

- Nipride
  - Treats high blood pressure intraoperatively

Cholinergics

- Prostigmin
  - Used to treat myasthenia gravis
  - Reverses the effects of a muscle relaxant used in surgery

Coagulant—Promotes Clot Formation

- Vitamin K
  - Helps form clots

Contrast Media—Used for X-Ray

- Hypaque/diatrizoate sodium
  - Outlines structures for GU and biliary procedures
- Renografin
  - Same as above
- Omnipaque
  - Used for cardiovascular, spinal cord x-rays

Coronary Artery Dilator—Used to Increase Coronary Artery Blood Flow

- Nitroglycerine
  - Prevents angina—chest pain

Diuretics—Used to Treat Pulmonary Edema and Hypertension

- Lasix
  - Maintains urinary output and fluid overload during surgery
- Mannitol/Osmitrol
  - Decreases intraocular pressure and fluid retention

Dyes—Used to Stain an Area of Tissue, for Skin Markings, and to Follow a Tract

- Gentian violet
  - Stains tissue, skin marker, also used to treat fungal infections (thrush)
- Indigo carmine
  - Same as above, commonly used in GU
- Methylene blue
  - Same as above
- Lymphazurin/isosulfan blue
  - Used to identify sentinel lymph nodes

Hemostatic Agents—Promote Clot Formation

- Gelfoam
  - Topical sponge used to stop bleeding, also used with topical thrombin
- Avitene
  - Topical powder, promotes clot formation
- Oxycel/Surgicel
  - Topical material

Histamine Blocker—Inhibits Acid Secretions in the Stomach

- Bicitra
  - Neutralizes gastric acid preoperatively

Immunoglobulin—Treats Rh Sensitization (Rhesus Factor)

- Rhogam
  - Helps to prevent problems with the Rh-negative mother and the Rh-positive fetus during and following birth. It is really harmful for the second child

Malignant Hyperthermia (MH) Antagonist—Interferes with Calcium in Skeletal Muscles, Reducing Contractions

- Dantrolene
  - Only medication used for MH crisis

Narcotic Antagonist—Reverses Narcotic Analgesics

- Narcan
  - Reverses the effects of narcotic drugs. Example, Sublimaze

Oxytocic—Stimulates Uterine Contraction, Helps Control Bleeding

- Pitocin
  - Stimulates labor

Stains—Topical Stains Used on Mucous Membranes (Cervix) to Determine if Cancer Is Present

- Lugol's
  - Shiller's test—used to stain the cervix—the cervix stains brown. Where there is no color change, cancer cells present

Steroids—Decrease Inflammation

- Decadron
  - Anti-inflammatory
- Solu-Medrol
  - Anti-inflammatory
- Celestone/ betamethasone
  - Same as above

Vasoconstrictor—Causes Blood Vessels to Constrict and Decreases Bleeding

- Pitressin
  - Injected into the cervix to control bleeding

Vasodilator—Used to Dilate Vessels During Cardiac and Vascular Procedures

- Papaverine
  - Relaxes the smooth muscles in veins, which helps to reduce blood pressure

Irrigation Solutions—Used to Clean Instruments and to Irrigate Body Cavities

- Sterile water
  - Used to wash instruments and irrigate the bladder
- Normal saline
  - Used to irrigate the body cavity

Hemostasis and blood replacement
- Hemostasis—the technique used to control bleeding during a surgical procedure
- Chemical methods of hemostasis
- Bone wax—a sterile mixture of beeswax used to seal off bleeding on bone
- Absorbable gelatin sponges
  - Made of collagen
  - Gelfoam
  - Gelfilm
- Microfibrillar collagen
  - Avitene—assists in the coagulating process. Must be applied with clean dry gloves or clean forceps
- Oxidized cellulose
  - Surgicel—blood clots and forms a gel. It is applied directly to the bleeding surface
- Silver nitrate
  - It comes in a stick or pencil-like form. Commonly used in the nose or cervix
- Epinephrine
  - It is a vasoconstrictor
  - Mixed with a local anesthetic to prolong the effects and aid in hemostasis
- Thrombin
  - It is a topical hemostatic agent
  - It should never be injected—could cause death
  - Can be used by itself or with a Gelfoam sponge and Cottonoids
- Floseal
  - Used to control bleeding
  - It swells to provide a tamponade (compression) effect
  - It fills the space

- Blood loss in the operating room is monitored through:
  - Suction canisters—irrigation fluid is subtracted and you have an estimated blood loss. Also through sponges
- Blood components
  - Blood components are stored in the blood bank.
  - They must be refrigerated.
  - Before blood products are given, they must be identified by two licensed personnel to identify the correct blood product and the correct patient.
  - All information should match the information on the patient's wrist band, blood bag, and chart.
  - Always check for clots.

Blood is donated by the patient themselves prior to surgery (autologous) or by a donor (homologous).

- Common blood components:

Blood Component	Contents	Use
Whole blood	All components of blood—this is not commonly used	Used to treat trauma—hemorrhage
Packed red blood cells (PRBCs)	Red blood cells after the plasma is removed	To restore oxygen
Fresh-frozen plasma (FFP)	The component of blood containing the clotting factor	Restores the clotting factor, 1 unit of FFP to 4 units of PRBCs
Platelets	Platelets	Replaces the blood's clotting ability

- Autotransfusion
  - Blood products are used to:
    - Increase blood volume
    - Increase the number of red blood cells (RBCs)
    - Increase the number of platelets for clotting
    - Replace the clotting factor that was depleted during surgery
- Autologous blood retrieval system/Cell Saver
  - The Cell Saver is a machine that suctions the blood directly from the wound and filters it to remove debris
  - Mixes with heparinized saline

- Then separates the RBCs from the rest of the fluids
  - The RBCs are pumped into a separate blood bag and infused back into the patient
- Cell Saver blood cannot be used if it contains:
  - Cancer cells
  - Amniotic fluid
  - Hemostatic agents, for example, Avitene
  - Certain antibiotics

GENERAL ANESTHESIA

Methods of anesthetic administration

- The ways anesthetic agents are given:
  - Inhalation agents/gas
  - Injectable agents/intravenous (IV)
  - Instillation agents/the agent is absorbed in a mucous membrane, for example, rectum
- Hypnosis—altered state of consciousness
- Anesthesia—freedom from pain
- Amnesia—lack of recall, memory loss
- Muscle relaxation—neuromuscular blocking agents mixed with inhalation agents provide muscle relaxation
- Anesthesia agents and techniques vary from patient to patient depending on:
  - Physiological status of the patient
  - Current medications
  - Allergies
  - History of substance abuse
  - Emergency conditions
- Phases of general anesthesia

Induction phase	• Loss of consciousness
	• Respiratory depression
	• IV inserted or gas
	• Airway management includes:
	  ◦ Endotracheal tube
	  ◦ Face mask
	  ◦ LMA—laryngeal mask airway
	  ◦ Greatest risk of aspiration
	• Hearing is the last sensation to disappear during induction

Maintenance phase	• Anesthesia is given • Patient is closely monitored throughout surgery
Emergence phase	• Surgery is ending • Reversal agents are given • Patient is waking up
Recovery phase	• Patient is awake • Begins in the operating room to the postanesthesia care unit

Questions

1. A drug that interferes with the blood clotting mechanism is:

   (A) lidocaine
   (B) fentanyl
   (C) heparin
   (D) cefazolin

2. An mg is a measurement of:

   (A) length
   (B) weight
   (C) volume
   (D) temperature

3. The solution used intravenously to replace plasma when plasma is not available is:

   (A) 0.9% NaCl
   (B) dextrose 5% in water
   (C) lactated Ringer's solution
   (D) dextran

4. How many milliliters are in 1 oz?

   (A) 10
   (B) 30
   (C) 75
   (D) 100

5. One gram equals:

   (A) 100 mg
   (B) 1,000 mg
   (C) 100 mL
   (D) 1,000 mL

6. A drug used to increase blood pressure is:

   (A) Avitene
   (B) epinephrine
   (C) heparin
   (D) mannitol

7. The action of an anticholinergic drug is to reduce:

   (A) heart rate
   (B) anxiety
   (C) nausea
   (D) secretions

8. The total volume in a 30-cc syringe is:

   (A) 1 oz
   (B) 2 oz
   (C) 3 oz
   (D) 4 oz

9. Naloxone (Narcan) is an example of a:

   (A) narcotic antagonist
   (B) mydriatic
   (C) histamine
   (D) diuretic

10. Avitene is:

    (A) hemostatic
    (B) adrenergic
    (C) cycloplegic
    (D) mydriatic

11. An absorbable gelatin hemostatic agent that is often soaked in thrombin or epinephrine solution is:

    (A) Avitene
    (B) Oxycel
    (C) Nu-knit
    (D) Gelfoam

12. Each of the following agents must be applied using dry gloves or instruments EXCEPT:

    (A) Gelfoam
    (B) Collastat
    (C) Avitene
    (D) Helistat

13. An anticoagulant given subcutaneously, intravenously, or as a flush is:

    (A) nitroglycerin
    (B) dextran
    (C) heparin
    (D) thrombin

14. A drug that decreases the tendency of blood to clot is:

    (A) warfarin sodium
    (B) diazepam
    (C) lorazepam
    (D) midazolam HCl

15. An antibiotic used intraoperatively is:

    (A) diazepam
    (B) ketorolac
    (C) cyclogyl
    (D) gentamicin

16. A topical antibiotic is:

    (A) bacitracin
    (B) ephedrine
    (C) Ancef
    (D) Keflex

17. Which item is used on cut edges of bone to seal off oozing of blood?

    (A) Electrocautery
    (B) Silver nitrate
    (C) Bone wax
    (D) Epinephrine

18. The most common diuretic is:

    (A) Lasix
    (B) Pronestyl
    (C) Isoptin
    (D) Cefadyl

19. An osmotic diuretic agent used to decrease cerebral edema and intraocular edema is:

    (A) diuril
    (B) furosemide
    (C) papaverine
    (D) mannitol

20. A systemic agent used to control uterine hemorrhage is:

    (A) protamine
    (B) pitocin
    (C) procainamide HCl
    (D) phenylephrine

21. Steroids are used for:

    (A) reduction of fluid in body
    (B) reduction of body's need for oxygen
    (C) reduction of tissue inflammation and swelling
    (D) reduction of uterine constriction and contraction

22. Solu-Medrol is a/an:

    (A) antibiotic
    (B) myotic
    (C) mydriatic
    (D) anti-inflammatory

23. An artificial plasma-volume expander is:

    (A) mannitol
    (B) dextran
    (C) Ringer's solution
    (D) uromatic

24. An anticoagulant used in vascular surgery is:

    (A) protamine sulfate
    (B) heparin
    (C) adrenalin
    (D) papaverine

25. Heparin effects are reversed by:

    (A) pitocin
    (B) phenylephrine
    (C) protamine sulfate
    (D) procainamide HCl

26. Normal saline is used for lap pad moistening and for intraperitoneal irrigation because it is:

    (A) hypotonic
    (B) isotonic
    (C) hypertonic
    (D) hyperkalemic

27. The last sensation to leave the patient during general anesthesia induction is:

    (A) hearing
    (B) sight
    (C) feeling
    (D) smell

28. A short-acting drug useful during intubation to produce paralysis and also to produce muscle relaxation is:

    (A) Sublimaze
    (B) Valium
    (C) Versed
    (D) Anectine

29. Neuroleptanalgesia combines:

    (A) a narcotic and an anticholinergic
    (B) a tranquilizer and narcotic
    (C) an anti-inflammatory and a tranquilizer
    (D) a muscle relaxant and a tranquilizer

30. A sedative/tranquilizer used to reduce anxiety and apprehension of the preoperative patient is:

    (A) Valium
    (B) Marzicon
    (C) Anectine
    (D) Demerol

31. An antimuscarinic:

    (A) controls pain
    (B) prevents nausea
    (C) limits salivation
    (D) reverses muscle relaxation

32. Anesthesia given in a combination of several agents to obtain optimum results is called:

    (A) regional anesthesia
    (B) general anesthesia
    (C) conduction anesthesia
    (D) balanced anesthesia

33. A bolus is:

    (A) a small, intermittent dose intravenously
    (B) a dose injected intramuscularly
    (C) a rapid dose, subcutaneously
    (D) a dose injected all at once, intravenously

34. A drug used to soothe and relieve anxiety is a/an:

    (A) cholinergic
    (B) analgesic
    (C) sedative
    (D) narcotic

35. A Bier block provides:

    (A) anesthesia to a distal portion of an extremity
    (B) anesthesia below the diaphragm
    (C) anesthetic block surrounding a peripheral nerve
    (D) anesthetic block to a nerve group

36. Which inhalation agent is used for short procedures requiring no muscle relaxation?

    (A) Nitrous oxide
    (B) Halothane
    (C) Ethrane
    (D) Forane

37. Halothane is also called:

    (A) Ethrane
    (B) Penthrane
    (C) Forane
    (D) Fluothane

38. A method of anesthesia in which medication is injected into the subarachnoid space, affecting a portion of the spinal cord, is called a:

    (A) Bier block
    (B) field block
    (C) nerve block
    (D) spinal block

39. The indication for an epidural would be:

    (A) anorectal, vaginal, perineal, and obstetric procedures
    (B) Bankart procedure
    (C) upper gastrointestinal procedures
    (D) above the waist procedures

40. Compazine is:

    (A) an antiemetic
    (B) a sedative
    (C) a tranquilizer
    (D) an anticholinergic

41. Which technique can be employed to prevent pain during an operative procedure or to relieve chronic pain?

    (A) Local infiltration
    (B) Bier block
    (C) Nerve block
    (D) Field block

42. The most widely used local anesthetic is:

    (A) Carbocaine
    (B) Marcaine
    (C) prilocaine
    (D) lidocaine

43. Another name for adrenalin is:

    (A) ephedrine
    (B) epinephrine
    (C) lidocaine
    (D) Levophed

44. A vasoconstrictor that, when added to a local anesthetic agent, extends its life is:

    (A) ephedrine
    (B) epinephrine
    (C) aramine
    (D) ethrane

45. The purpose of an LMA is:

    (A) to establish and maintain a patent airway
    (B) to provide patient cooling
    (C) to monitor body temperature
    (D) to evaluate cardiac and venous status

46. Blood oxygenation can be monitored during surgery by means of a/an:

    (A) blood pressure monitor
    (B) arterial catheter
    (C) pulse oximeter
    (D) central venous pressure (CVP) catheter

47. A drug that could be used to reverse the effect of muscle relaxants is:

    (A) Narcan
    (B) protamine sulfate
    (C) Prostigmin
    (D) Valium

48. Arterial blood gases (ABGs) are commonly obtained by accessing the:

    (A) femoral artery
    (B) carotid artery
    (C) radial artery
    (D) renal artery

49. Which piece of equipment is of extreme importance when anesthesia induction begins?

    (A) Oximeter
    (B) Blood pressure apparatus
    (C) Oxygen
    (D) Suction

50. Tablets placed under the tongue for rapid absorption are called:

    (A) oral
    (B) transdermal
    (C) subungual
    (D) sublingual

51. Pharmacokinetics focuses on:

    (A) rejecting drugs
    (B) reacting to drugs
    (C) process by which drugs move through the body
    (D) response to drugs

52. Drug effects that occur predictably and may not cause a problem are:

    (A) adverse reactions
    (B) toxicities
    (C) side effects
    (D) therapeutic effects

53. The patented name of medication is also its:

    (A) chemical name
    (B) proprietary name
    (C) molecular name
    (D) None of the above

54. A capnometer measures:

    (A) O_2 concentration
    (B) CO concentration
    (C) CO_2 concentration
    (D) PO_2 concentration

55. Contrast media for radiographic studies include:

    (A) barium sulfate
    (B) Conray
    (C) Isovue
    (D) All of the above

56. The acronym MAC stands for:

    (A) monitored anesthesia care
    (B) managed airway control
    (C) metabolic analgesia care
    (D) None of the above

57. A drug that constricts the pupil during ophthalmic surgery is:

    (A) Healon
    (B) Miochol
    (C) hyaluronidase
    (D) atropine

58. During general anesthesia, exhaled CO_2 is absorbed by:

    (A) soda lime reservoir
    (B) vaporizer
    (C) ventilator
    (D) breathing bag

59. Cricoid pressure:

    (A) paralyzes the patient
    (B) produces complete anesthesia
    (C) occludes the esophagus
    (D) is done during extubation

60. Extubation occurs during which phase of anesthesia?

    (A) Recovery
    (B) Emergence
    (C) Induction
    (D) Maintenance

61. The drug used to treat malignant hyperthermia is:

    (A) dantrolene
    (B) levophed
    (C) depo-Medrol
    (D) digoxin

62. An example of a depolarizing muscle relaxant is:

    (A) halothane
    (B) fentanyl
    (C) sufentanil
    (D) succinylcholine

63. During ophthalmic surgery, paralysis of the ciliary muscle is achieved by using:

    (A) cycloplegics
    (B) myotics
    (C) mydriatics
    (D) narcotics

64. Zofran is an:

    (A) antiemetic
    (B) sedative
    (C) tranquilizer
    (D) anticholinergic

65. Benzodiazepines produce _____ for up to 6 hours from the onset of the drugs' action.

    (A) pain relief
    (B) hallucinations
    (C) amnesia
    (D) relief from nausea

66. IV lines are preoperatively placed to:

    (A) establish immediate intravenous access for medications
    (B) maintain and manipulate fluid volume
    (C) maintain electrolyte balance
    (D) All of the above

67. There are ____ "rights" to safe medication administration.

    (A) 3
    (B) 4
    (C) 5
    (D) 6

68. The intensity of contractions is increased with the use of:

    (A) oxytocin
    (B) glucagon
    (C) heparin
    (D) Lugol's

69. Drugs used to reduce the reabsorption of water, causing frequent urination, are:

    (A) anticoagulants
    (B) anticholinergics
    (C) diuretics
    (D) colloids

70. A medication that is placed between the lip and the cheek to be absorbed by mucous membranes is:

    (A) parenteral
    (B) buccal
    (C) subungual
    (D) oral

71. The most accurate method used to measure liquid medication is:

    (A) syringe
    (B) measuring cup
    (C) tablespoon
    (D) teaspoon

72. Which name is derived from the molecular formula of a drug?

    (A) Brand
    (B) Proprietary
    (C) Chemical
    (D) Generic

73. An undesirable or intolerable reaction to a drug administered at the normal dosage is a/an:

    (A) toxicity
    (B) allergy
    (C) side effect
    (D) adverse reaction

74. The process whereby the drug enters the bloodstream is known as:

    (A) absorption
    (B) elimination
    (C) distribution
    (D) metabolism

75. One liter is equal to:

    (A) 1,000 mL
    (B) 100 mL
    (C) 10,000 mL
    (D) None of the above

76. One gram is equal to:

    (E) 1,000 mg
    (F) 100 mg
    (G) 10 mg
    (H) 1 mg

77. Medications used to prevent postoperative infections are:

    (A) antiemetics
    (B) antipyretics
    (C) antibiotics
    (D) agonists

78. Drugs with the potential to lead to abuse are:

    (A) narcotics
    (B) prescription
    (C) controlled substances
    (D) All of the above

79. Which organ is primarily responsible for excretion of drugs?

    (A) Kidneys
    (B) Liver
    (C) Gallbladder
    (D) Spleen

80. Anticoagulants such as heparin are used to prevent:

    (A) fevers
    (B) nausea
    (C) allergic reactions
    (D) blood clots

81. The generic name for Marcaine is:

    (A) xylocaine
    (B) bupivacaine
    (C) oxytocin
    (D) lidocaine

82. The phase of anesthesia occurring when surgery is in progress is:

    (A) emergence
    (B) induction
    (C) preinduction
    (D) maintenance

83. Benzodiazepines are categorized as:

    (A) analgesics
    (B) sedatives
    (C) cholinergics
    (D) anticholinergics

84. While under general anesthesia, the anesthesiologist monitors the rate, rhythm, and electrical conduction by:

    (A) electrocardiogram
    (B) oximetry
    (C) ABGs
    (D) blood pressure cuff

85. Drugs classified as antiemetics are used to prevent:

    (A) hypertension
    (B) hypotension
    (C) tachycardia
    (D) nausea

86. A warming blanket that contains warm air and is used on patients during surgery is called:

    (A) Bair Hugger
    (B) SCD
    (C) TED
    (D) hypothermic unit

87. The trade name for xylocaine is:

    (A) Pontocaine
    (B) Marcaine
    (C) Lidocaine
    (D) Sensorcaine

88. The vasoconstrictor used with lidocaine to prolong the effects of the anesthetic is:

    (A) epinephrine
    (B) heparin
    (C) protamine sulfate
    (D) digoxin

89. Which drug is the antagonist to heparin?

    (A) Depo-Medrol
    (B) Papaverine
    (C) Protamine sulfate
    (D) Dantrolene

90. When surgeons perform an intraoperative cholangiogram, they use:

    (A) Renografin
    (B) Conray
    (C) barium sulfate
    (D) gentian violet

91. Another name for Anectine is:

    (E) succinylcholine
    (F) halothane
    (G) fluothane
    (H) fentanyl

92. Malignant hyperthermia can be triggered by:

    (A) succinylcholine
    (B) demerol
    (C) morphine
    (D) Valium

93. A patient is receiving 1 L of 5% dextrose in water as an IV fluid during her 1-hour surgery. The number of grams of dextrose the patient has received during this infusion is:

    (A) 5 g
    (B) 50 g
    (C) 500 g
    (D) 0.5 g

94. The needed medication comes in 100 mg per 1 cc. The surgeon wants 50 mg. Your syringe will draw up _____ of the medication.

    (A) 0.5 cc
    (B) 1 cc
    (C) 2 cc
    (D) 3 cc

95. One ounce is equal to _____ cc.

    (A) 60
    (B) 1
    (C) 30
    (D) 10

96. The vial the circulating nurse is holding is labeled 75 mg per 1 cc. The surgeon wants 150 mg of the medication. You will draw up:

   (A) 0.75 cc
   (B) 1.5 cc
   (C) 2 cc
   (D) None of the above

97. A synergist agent is:

   (A) one drug that works with another drug (boosts the result) to provide the same effect; however, by combining the two drugs, the dose is lower and safer
   (B) a drug that is intended to produce a desirable and beneficial effect to the patient
   (C) a chemical drug that counteracts or blocks the action of another drug
   (D) an undesirable and potentially harmful effect from a therapeutic drug

98. An intrathecal injection is:

   (A) placed between the cheek and gums
   (B) placed in the adipose tissue
   (C) placed into the subarachnoid space
   (D) placed in a hollow cavity

99. Every time STSRs pass a syringe to the surgeon, they must state all of the following except:

   (A) name of the drug
   (B) strength
   (C) amount of the drug
   (D) expiration date

100. A drug used to reverse an overdose of an analgesic is:

   (A) atropine
   (B) demerol
   (C) narcan
   (D) protamine sulfate

101. The drug used to treat ventricular arrhythmias is:

   (A) lidocaine
   (B) marcaine
   (C) sensorcaine
   (D) bupivacaine

102. Which of the following is not a symptom of malignant hyperthermia?

   (A) Muscle contraction
   (B) Bradycardia
   (C) Rigid jaw
   (D) Increased body temperature

103. The biggest risk associated with general anesthesia is:

   (A) aspiration
   (B) inflammation of the esophagus
   (C) breaking of teeth
   (D) overdosing the patient

104. Symptoms of ventricular tachycardia include all of the following EXCEPT:

   (A) changes in the electrocardiogram (ECG)
   (B) heart rate below 100
   (C) heart rate above 120
   (D) arrhythmia

105. Nitrous oxide should never be used during which procedure?

   (A) Shoulder arthroscopy
   (B) Circumcision
   (C) Tympanoplasty
   (D) Closed fracture

106. Which drug has a milky appearance and is sometimes referred to as "milk of amnesia"?

   (A) Narcan
   (B) Pentothal
   (C) Sublimaze
   (D) Propofol

107. A dissociative agent that provides complete unconsciousness and a catatonic state is:

    (A) ketamine
    (B) nitrous oxide
    (C) versed
    (D) anectine

108. Which IV solution is similar to plasma, is water based, and contains sodium, potassium, and calcium?

    (A) Dextrose 5% in water
    (B) Ringer's
    (C) Normal saline
    (D) Lactated Ringer's

109. Induced hypothermia is not used in which of the following surgeries?

    (A) Open heart surgery
    (B) Malignant hyperthermia crisis
    (C) Organ transplant
    (D) Liver biopsy

110. Which instrument aids in positioning the endotracheal, nasotracheal, and nasogastric tubes in the trachea?

    (A) McGill forceps
    (B) Bayonet forceps
    (C) Transfer forceps
    (D) Bozeman forceps

111. During intubation, cricoid pressure is applied in order to occlude the:

    (A) hyoid bone
    (B) trachea
    (C) esophagus
    (D) thyroid gland

112. An A-line is commonly inserted into the:

    (A) jugular artery
    (B) radial artery
    (C) carotid artery
    (D) brachial artery

113. Fast breathing for short periods of time, followed by apnea, is termed:

    (A) dyspnea
    (B) tachypnea
    (C) Cheyne-Stokes
    (D) eupnea

114. Which of the following refers to Korotkoff sounds?

    (A) The first tapping sound heard when taking a blood pressure
    (B) Soft whistling sound as cuff is deflated
    (C) Rhythmic tapping sound as the cuff is deflated
    (D) All of the above

Answers and Explanations

1. **(C)** Heparin and warfarin are anticoagulant drugs that interfere with blood clotting mechanism.

2. **(B)** Kilograms, grams, milligrams, and micrograms are the metric weight designations.

3. **(D)** Dextran, artificial plasma, is used when plasma is not available.

4. **(B)** An ounce (fluid, apothecaries) is a measure for liquids. It is equal to 29.6 mL; thus, 30 mL.

5. **(B)** One gram (g) is equal to 1,000 mg.

6. **(B)** Epinephrine is an adrenergic that increases blood pressure.

7. **(D)** Anticholinergics block secretions; an example is atropine or scopolamine.

8. **(A)** One fluid ounce equals 29.573 mL. One milliliter equals 1 cc. Thus, 30 cc equals 1 oz.

9. **(A)** A narcotic antagonist is given to reverse the effects of a narcotic.

10. **(A)** Avitene is a microfibrillar collagen hemostatic agent. It is an adjunct to hemostasis when conventional methods are ineffective. It is an absorbable topical agent of purified bovine collagen, and it must be applied in its dry state.

11. **(D)** Gelfoam is an absorbable hemostatic agent that aids in clot formation and absorbs 45 times its own weight in blood. It is frequently soaked in thrombin or epinephrine solution before being handed to the surgeon.

12. **(A)** Gelfoam can be used wet or dry. Each of the others must be applied dry.

13. **(C)** Heparin prolongs clotting time and may be given simultaneously, intravenously, and as a flush to keep IV lines open or to flush the lumen of a blood vessel (1 mL heparin in 100 mL normal injectable saline).

14. **(A)** Warfarin sodium is a Coumadin derivative that depresses blood prothrombin and decreases the tendency of blood platelets to cling together, thus decreasing blood clotting. The others are either sedatives or help provide a calm, hypnotic state preoperatively.

15. **(D)** An antibiotic used intraoperatively is gentamicin.

16. **(A)** Bacitracin is a topical antibiotic ointment.

17. **(C)** Bone wax, made from refined and sterilized bee's wax, is used on cut edges of bone to seal off oozing blood. Soften by kneading before use.

18. **(A)** Lasix (furosemide) increases the amount of urine secreted and is a common diuretic.

19. **(D)** Mannitol, an osmotic diuretic, is given prophylactically to prevent renal failure. It is also used to decrease intracranial and intraocular pressure.

20. **(B)** Pitocin is a trademark for an oxytocic (oxytocin), a hormone produced by the pituitary gland, which is prepared synthetically for therapeutic injection. In labor and delivery, it is given to contract the uterus after placenta delivery or systemically to control

uterine hemorrhage. It is also given to induce contractions.

21. **(C)** Steroids reduce tissue inflammation and postoperative swelling. Examples are Decadron and Cortisporin ophthalmic ointment. In eye surgery, they are applied topically to reduce postoperative swelling. In plastic surgery, they are applied in and around the site in patients who tend to form keloids.

22. **(D)** Methylprednisolone (Medrol) is an adrenal corticosteroid drug. Corticosteroids prevent the normal inflammatory response; thus, they are anti-inflammatory. In eye surgery, they reduce the resistance of the eye to invasion by bacterial viruses and fungi.

23. **(B)** Dextran is an artificial volume expander that acts by drawing the fluid from the tissues. It remains in the circulation for several hours. It is used in emergency situations to treat shock by increasing blood volume.

24. **(B)** Heparin is the most common drug used in vascular surgery to anticoagulate the patient. Protamine reverses heparin.

25. **(C)** Heparin is reversed by protamine. It should be given.

26. **(B)** Normal saline is used because it is isotonic (contains an amount of salt equal to that of intracellular and extracellular fluid) and thus will not alter sodium, chloride, or fluid balance.

27. **(A)** During the induction phase, the patient retains an exaggerated sense of hearing until the last moment. Thus, it is essential that all personnel in the room remain as quiet as possible.

28. **(D)** Succinylcholine (Anectine) is an ultra-short-acting agent with rapid onset and is useful to produce paralysis during intubation as well as continuing muscle relaxation when used in a dilute solution.

29. **(B)** The combination of a narcotic (potent analgesic) and a tranquilizer (neuroleptic) produces neuroleptanalgesia. When these are reinforced with an inhalation anesthetic, it is call neuroleptanesthesia.

30. **(A)** Valium and Versed are examples of benzodiazepines (sedative tranquilizers) and are used in two ways: to reduce the anxiety and apprehension of the patient and as an adjunct to general anesthesia to reduce the amount and concentration of other more potent agents.

31. **(C)** Antimuscarinics (formerly known as anticholinergics) act as blockers of cholinergic effects and thus limit salivation and bradycardia; examples are atropine sulfate and glycopyrrolate.

32. **(D)** Balanced anesthesia is a technique whereby the properties of anesthesia (hypnosis, analgesia, and muscle relaxation) are produced in varying degrees by a combination of agents.

33. **(D)** A bolus is a rapid medication dose injected all at once intravenously.

34. **(C)** Sedatives are drugs that soothe and relieve anxiety. The only difference between a hypnotic and a sedative is one of degree. A hypnotic produces sleep, whereas a sedative provides mild relaxation. It is quieting and tranquilizing.

35. **(A)** A Bier block provides anesthesia to the distal portion of the upper extremity by injecting an anesthetic agent into a vein at a level below a tourniquet (double cuffed). The limb is exsanguinated with Esmarch, and the cuff is inflated.

36. **(A)** Nitrous oxide has a rapid induction and recovery. It is used on short procedures, when muscle relaxation is unimportant.

37. **(D)** A widely used halogenated hydrocarbon is Fluothane, also known as halothane. It is nonflammable and provides smooth induction.

38. **(D)** Spinal anesthesia is an extensive nerve block, sometimes called a subarachnoid block. It affects the lower spinal cord and nerve roots. It is used for lower abdominal or pelvic procedures.

39. **(A)** An epidural is used for anorectal, vaginal, perineal, and obstetrical procedures. Injection is made into the space surrounding the dura mater within the spinal canal (the epidural space).

40. **(A)** Compazine is an antiemetic that minimizes nausea and vomiting.

41. **(C)** Nerve blocks may be used preoperatively, intraoperatively, and postoperatively to prevent pain or therapeutically to relieve chronic pain. In a field block, the surgical site is blocked off with a wall of anesthetic drug.

42. **(D)** Lidocaine hydrochloride (Xylocaine) is the most widely used local anesthetic. It is potent, has rapid onset, and lacks local irritation effects. Allergic reactions are rare.

43. **(B)** Adrenalin is another name for epinephrine.

44. **(B)** Epinephrine is added to a local anesthetic when a highly vascular area is to be injected. It causes vasoconstriction at the operative site. This holds the anesthetic in the tissue, prolongs its effect, and minimizes local bleeding.

45. **(A)** LMA (laryngeal mask airway) is a device placed into the laryngopharynx through the mouth to form a low-pressure seal (with an inflated balloon) around the laryngeal inlet. It is a simple, effective way of establishing a patent airway.

46. **(C)** The pulse oximeter measures blood oxygenation. The fingertip is commonly used. It is a continuous, rapid, and easy means of assessment.

47. **(C)** Neostigmine, also known as Prostigmin, reverses the effect of muscle relaxants.

48. **(C)** ABGs involve invasive monitoring of pH, oxygen saturation, and CO_2 levels. A common site is the radial artery (arterial line or A-line). Direct blood pressure monitoring may also be performed this way.

49. **(D)** Suction must always be available and ready, along with assistance to the anesthesiologist, as induction begins for the safety of the patient.

50. **(D)** When a tablet is placed under the tongue, this is sublingual.

51. **(C)** Pharmacokinetics is the movement of a drug through the tissues and cells of the body, including the processes of absorption, distribution, and localization in tissues.

52. **(C)** Anticipated effects of a drug other than those intended are side effects.

53. **(B)** The patented name given to a drug by its manufacturer is its proprietary name.

54. **(C)** Expired CO_2, which is a product of ventilation, is measured. The exhaled gas is analyzed and the results displayed in wave form on a monitor. This is capnography.

55. **(D)** These are all examples of radiopaque solutions introduced into body cavities to outline their inner surfaces.

56. **(A)** MAC is monitoring of vital functions during regional anesthesia to ensure patients' safety and comfort.

57. **(B)** Miochol is a cholinergic that rapidly constricts the pupil and is used in the intraocular space during anterior segment surgery and is reconstituted immediately before surgery.

58. **(A)** Exhaled CO_2 captured from the system is measured and absorbed by a soda lime reservoir.

59. **(C)** Cricoid pressure is digital occlusion of the esophagus by applying external pressure over the cricoid cartilage during intubation.

60. **(B)** The emergence phase is the cessation of the anesthetic. Reversal drugs may be administered, and the patient regains consciousness.

61. **(A)** Dantrolene relieves symptoms of malignant hypothermia by acting on the sarcoplasmic reticulum to block calcium release, which relieves muscle spasticity.

62. **(D)** Succinylcholine is a neuromuscular blocking agent.

63. **(A)** Cycloplegics are drugs that cause paralysis of the ciliary muscle.

64. **(A)** Zofran is an agent that blocks serotonin receptors, including on afferent vagal neurons in the upper GI tract.

65. **(C)** Benzodiazepines cause amnesia, which is loss of recall of events, for up to 6 hours from the onset of the drugs' action.

66. **(D)** All of these are achieved by inserting an intravenous line.

67. **(D)** In addition to the right drug, the right dose, the right route, the right patient, and the right time, there is a sixth right that applies to medications used on the surgical field. It is the right surgical label.

68. **(A)** Drugs that enhance uterine contractions are called uterotropics. The most common is oxytocin.

69. **(C)** A diuretic is an agent that promotes urine secretion. These drugs are prescribed to rid the body of excess fluid.

70. **(B)** Buccal is defined as pertaining to or directed toward the cheek.

71. **(A)** A syringe is the most accurate instrument used when measuring and dispensing a liquid.

72. **(C)** Chemical names are derived from the molecular formula of a drug following the International Convention.

73. **(D)** An adverse reaction is an undesirable or intolerable reaction to a drug administered at the normal dosage.

74. **(A)** Absorption is the process by which a drug enters the bloodstream following administration. Absorption usually involves chemical and physical breakdown of the drug.

75. **(A)** One liter is equal to 1,000 mL.

76. **(A)** One gram is equal to 1,000 mg.

77. **(C)** An antibiotic is a chemical compound produced by and obtained from certain living cells, especially bacteria, yeast, and mold, or an equivalent synthetic compound that is an antagonist to some other form of life, especially pathogenic or noxious organisms. Antibiotics are used to reduce the chance of infection after an operation.

78. **(D)** All of these have the potential for abuse. These are rated according to their risk potential.

79. **(A)** Drugs are mainly eliminated or cleared from the body through the kidneys.

80. **(D)** Anticoagulants are used to prevent the coagulation/clotting of blood.

81. **(B)** Bupivacaine is the generic name for Marcaine.

82. **(D)** Maintenance is the phase involving continuation of the anesthetic agent; unconsciousness is maintained with the inhalation agent and adjunct agents.

83. **(B)** Benzodiazepines (sedatives) are a group of drugs that prevent and relieve anxiety.

84. **(A)** Electrocardiography is the graphic recording from the body surface of the potential of electric currents gathered and generated by the heart.

85. **(D)** An antiemetic is an agent used to cease or prevent vomiting.

86. **(A)** A Bair Hugger is a blanket that connects to a hose that blows hot air in order to maintain the patient's body temperature.

87. **(C)** Lidocaine is the trade name for xylocaine.

88. **(A)** The vasoconstrictor used with lidocaine to prolong the duration of lidocaine is epinephrine.

89. **(C)** Protamine is given to reverse the effects of heparin.

90. **(A)** Renografin is a contrast medium used to outline hollow organs or vessels before radiographs are obtained.

91. **(A)** Anectine or succinylcholine produces a state known as depolarizing neuromuscular blockage.

92. **(A)** Malignant hyperthermia is a rare, potentially fatal condition that can be triggered by succinylcholine and other inhalation anesthetics as well.

93. **(B)** Medications described by percentages describe grams per 100 cc. 5% = 5 g per 100 cc of fluid. This is 1 L of 1,000 cc total, so this is equal to 10×5.

94. **(A)** If 1 cc contains 100 mg, 50 mg equals one-half that amount, or 0.5 cc.

95. **(C)** One ounce is equal to 30 cc.

96. **(C)** If 1 cc contains 75 mg, then 2 cc equals 150 mg.

97. **(A)** A synergist is a drug that works with another drug to boost the result to provide the same effect; however, by combining the two drugs, the dose is lower and safer.

   A therapeutic affect is intended to produce a desirable and beneficial effect on the patient.

   A drug that counteracts or blocks the action of another drug is an antagonist. An adverse effect is an undesirable and potentially harmful effect from a therapeutic drug.

98. **(C)** An intrathecal injection is placed into the subarachnoid space. Buccal is placed between the cheek and gums. Subcutaneous is placed in the adipose under the skin. Instillation is placed in a hollow cavity.

99. **(D)** The expiration date is confirmed by the STSR and circulator. It is not necessary to repeat this to the physician.

100. **(C)** Narcan is the drug of choice used to reverse an overdose of an analgesic. Atropine is an anticholinergic. Demerol is an analgesic. Protamine sulfate reverses heparin.

101. **(A)** Lidocaine is used to treat ventricular arrhythmias. Marcaine, Sensorcaine, and bupivacaine are not used because they cannot be given intravenously.

102. **(B)** Bradycardia is a heart rate below 60 bpm. Malignant hyperthermia causes muscle contraction, rigid jaw, increased body temperature, and tachycardia.

103. **(A)** Although all are possible risks associated with general anesthesia, aspiration is the most severe.

104. **(B)** A heart rate below 100 bpm is not a symptom of ventricular tachycardia (VT). VT is an arrhythmia; there are definitive changes in the electrocardiogram, and the heart rate is above 120 bpm.

105. **(C)** Nitrous oxide cannot be used on a tympanoplasty because it causes pressure in enclosed spaces. Nitrous oxide can be used during any of the other procedures.

106. **(D)** Propofol has a white and milky appearance. Narcan, Pentothal, and Sublimaze are clear liquids.

107. **(A)** Ketamine causes a catatonic state while the patient remains awake. Nitrous oxide is a sedative agent mixed with O_2 during anesthesia. Versed is a sedative used to relieve anxiety and provide an amnesic affect. Anectine is a muscle relaxant.

108. **(B)** Ringer's solution is a water-based solution similar to plasma containing sodium, potassium, and calcium. Dextrose 5% in water is used to treat hypoglycemia. Normal saline is a salt solution commonly used when blood products are given. Lactated Ringer's is also a salt solution that contains electrolytes.

109. **(D)** Induced hypothermia is not necessary for a liver biopsy. It is commonly used during open heart surgery, malignant hyperthermia crisis, and organ transplant to lower the body temperature.

110. **(A)** McGill forceps is the instrument used to position the endotracheal, nasotracheal, and nasogastric tubes. Bayonet forceps are commonly used in neurosurgery. Transfer forceps are used to remove a sterile item from the steam autoclave by a nonsterile person to place the item on the sterile back table. Bozeman forceps are packing forceps used in gynecology.

111. **(C)** Cricoid pressure is applied to the tracheal cartilage to occlude the esophagus to avoid aspiration.

112. **(B)** An A-line is commonly inserted into the radial artery. The femoral artery is the second most common site for cannulation.

113. **(C)** Cheyne-Stokes breathing consists of fast breathing for short periods of time followed by apnea. Dyspnea is difficulty breathing. Tachypnea is rapid breathing, and eupnea is normal breathing.

114. **(D)** Korotkoff sounds are the first tapping sound heard when taking a blood pressure. Korotkoff sounds occur in five phases; a soft whistling sound as the cuff is deflated is one of the phases. As the cuff is deflated, you can hear a rhythmic tapping sound.

CHAPTER 4

Blood Values

- COMPLETE BLOOD COUNT—used as a general screening for your health and to diagnose diseases. It includes:
  - WHITE BLOOD CELL COUNT—the total number of white blood cells in your blood. These cells protect your body against infection
    - 5,000–10,000 adult male/female
  - WHITE BLOOD COUNT DIFFERENTIAL— each of these white blood cells helps protect your body against disease and provide information about diseases by determining the correct numbers of these cells. They include:
    - Neutrophils
    - Lymphocytes
    - Monocytes
    - Eosinophils
    - Basophils
  - RED BLOOD CELL (RBC) COUNT—RBCs carry oxygen from the lungs to the rest of the body and CO_2 back to the lungs to be exhaled
    - 4.7–6.1 adult male
    - 4.2–5.4 adult female
  - HEMOGLOBIN (HGB)—gives blood its red color and carries oxygen
    - 14–18 adult male
    - 12–16 adult female
  - HEMATOCRIT (PACK CELLS)—this test measures the amount of volume RBCs take up in the blood
    - 0.42–0.52 adult male
    - 0.37–0.47 adult female
  - PLATELETS (THROMBOCYTES)—are important in blood clotting
    - 150–400 adult male/female

- BLOOD TYPES
  - O negative—UNIVERSAL DONOR
  - A—can donate to type A and AB
  - B—can donate to type B and AB
  - AB—UNIVERSAL PLASMA DONOR—can only donate to AB, but can receive from all others
  - RH factor/RHESUS FACTOR—these are antigens found on the surface of RBCs. If you have the antigen, you are Rh positive; if you do not have the antigen, you are Rh negative. This becomes very important when involving blood transfusions and pregnancy.
- BLOOD TRANSFUSION—a blood transfusion is performed to replace blood loss. It can be the patient's own blood, donor blood, and/or blood products.
  - AUTOLOGOUS—patient's own blood
  - HOMOLOGOUS—someone else's blood

Table 4–1.

		Blood Donor							
		O–	O+	B–	B+	A–	A+	AB–	AB+
R E C I P I E N T	AB+	♥	♥	♥	♥	♥	♥	♥	♥
	AB–	♥		♥		♥		♥	
	A+	♥	♥			♥	♥		
	A–	♥				♥			
	B+	♥	♥	♥	♥				
	B–	♥		♥					
	O+	♥	♥						
	O–	♥							

- ARTERIAL BLOOD GASES
  - Arterial blood gases (ABGs) are diagnostic tests performed on blood taken from an artery that contains oxygen and carbon dioxide.
  - ABGs measure how well the lungs can provide adequate oxygen to the body and subsequently remove carbon dioxide.

Normal ABG Figures	
PH	7.35–7.45
PO$_2$	80–100
PCO$_2$	35–45
HCO$_3$	22–28

pH LEVELS

- A pH level below 7.35 indicates that acidosis is present, indicating a buildup of carbonic acid in the blood.
- A pH level above 7.45 indicates alkalosis is present, which indicates the buildup of bicarbonate (bases) in the blood.

PCO$_2$ LEVEL

- Is the level of carbon dioxide in your blood
  - The condition of respiratory alkalosis is present if the PCO$_2$ is below 35 mm Hg. This indicates that there is too little carbon dioxide in the blood. A person with this condition may be breathing very fast (hyperventilating).
  - The condition of respiratory acidosis is present if the PCO$_2$ is above 45 mm Hg. This is an indication that there is too much carbon dioxide in the blood. A person with this condition can be confused or restless and have a low heart rate.

HCO$_3$ LEVEL

- This is the renal component in the acid-base balance.
  - An HCO$_3$ level below 24 mEq/L indicates metabolic acidosis. When in a state of metabolic acidosis, the body cannot produce enough bicarbonates to keep up with the carbonic acid in the blood. This can be caused by many conditions including dehydration and kidney disease.
  - An HCO$_3$ level above 26 mEq/L indicates metabolic alkalosis. There are too many bicarbonates in the blood. Hyperventilation is the common cause, but it is also seen in many other conditions including Cushing's disease and long-term steroid therapy.

PROTHROMBIN TIME

- Prothrombin time (PT) is a blood test that measures the time it takes for the liquid portion (plasma) of your blood to clot.
- If you are taking warfarin/Coumadin or Plavix, your health care provider will check your PT regularly.
  - The normal range is 11.0–13.5 seconds.

CELL SAVER

- Blood is suctioned directly from the surgical field into the machine; it washes the blood and prepares it to be given back to the patient.
- You should not use the Cell Saver in the presence of bacterial contamination, malignancy, or anticoagulants.

Questions

1. Who is the universal blood donor?

   (A) AB

   (B) A

   (C) B

   (D) O negative

2. Who is the universal plasma donor?

   (A) AB

   (B) A

   (C) B

   (D) O

3. Type A positive blood can donate to:

   (A) A positive

   (B) B positive

   (C) AB positive

   (D) Both A and C

4. Homologous refers to:

   (A) one's own blood

   (B) donated blood

   (C) blood products

   (D) synthetic blood products

5. If you are Rh positive:

   (A) you do NOT have the antigen on the surface of RBCs

   (B) you can donate blood to all patients

   (C) you do have the antigen found on RBCs

   (D) you CANNOT receive O negative blood

6. The test used to determine the total number of white blood cells in your blood is:

   (A) platelet count

   (B) white blood cell count

   (C) white count differential

   (D) complete blood count

7. Autologous refers to:

   (A) your own blood

   (B) recipient blood

   (C) blood products

   (D) a specific blood product

8. What gives red blood its color?

   (A) Platelets

   (B) Neutrophils

   (C) Hemoglobin

   (D) Hematocrit

9. All of the following are types of white blood cells EXCEPT:

   (A) neutrophils

   (B) lymphocytes

   (C) astrocytes

   (D) monocytes

10. What is the normal white blood cell count in an adult male?

    (A) 5.0–6.0

    (B) 5,000–10,000

    (C) 14–18

    (D) 150–400

11. When is the Cell Saver contraindicated?

    (A) When there is a malignancy
    (B) When anticoagulants are used
    (C) When bacteria are present
    (D) All of the above

12. Blood gas analysis is called:

    (A) BGA
    (B) SAT rate
    (C) ABG
    (D) ABO

13. Cross-matching of blood:

    (A) determines patient's blood type
    (B) determines Rh factor of both patient and donor
    (C) determines suitability of donor by mixing donor RBCs with recipient serum
    (D) determines blood group of donor

14. The highly specialized blood cell whose function is oxygen transportation is:

    (A) RBC
    (B) white blood cell
    (C) blood plasma
    (D) fibrinogen

15. A differential count provides an estimate of:

    (A) the amount of hemoglobin
    (B) the volume percentage of red cells
    (C) the percentage of each type of white cell
    (D) electrolyte percentages

16. Mixing of incompatible bloods may result in:

    (A) agglutination
    (B) infectious hepatitis
    (C) leukocytosis
    (D) hyperglycemia

17. Platelets are essential for:

    (A) coagulation of blood
    (B) controlling infection
    (C) carrying oxygen
    (D) combating histamine effects

18. In a normal adult, the average number of leukocytes per cubic millimeter of circulating blood is:

    (A) 1,000–4,000
    (B) 3,000–8,000
    (C) 5,000–10,000
    (D) 10,000–15,000

19. Blood or fluid can be quickly delivered to a patient via:

    (A) rapid infusion pump
    (B) SARA
    (C) Bair Hugger
    (D) Doppler

20. Blood oxygenation can be monitored during surgery by means of a:

    (A) blood pressure monitor
    (B) arterial catheter
    (C) pulse oximeter
    (D) central venous pressure (CVP) catheter

21. The universal donor blood that may be given in extreme emergencies until the patient can be typed and cross-matched is:

    (A) A
    (B) B
    (C) O
    (D) AB

Answers and Explanations

1. **(D)** O negative is the universal blood donor. See Table 4–1.

2. **(A)** AB is the universal plasma donor.

3. **(D)** A positive can donate to both A positive and AB positive recipients. See Table 4–1.

4. **(B)** Homologous blood refers to blood donated from another person. One's own blood is autologous.

5. **(C)** An antigen is found on RBCs. Most people are Rh positive. If you are Rh positive, you do have the antigen on your RBCs. If you are Rh negative, you do not have the antigen on your RBCs.

6. **(B)** White blood cell (WBC) count is the test used to determine the total number of WBCs in the blood. Platelets are needed for clotting. The differential white count determines correct numbers of a specific WBC, which can help to determine certain diseases. Complete blood count (CBC) is a general screening of blood components.

7. **(A)** Autologous refers to one's own blood.

8. **(C)** Hemoglobin carries the oxygen that gives blood its red color. Platelets are needed for clotting. Hematocrit is the amount of volume RBCs take up in your blood. Neutrophils are a component of WBCs.

9. **(C)** An astrocyte is not a WBC. It is a glial cell of the nervous system. Neutrophils, lymphocytes, and monocytes are three types of WBCs.

10. **(B)** 5,000–10,000 is the normal WBC count for both adult males and females.

11. **(D)** The Cell Saver should not be used when there is a malignancy present, anticoagulants such as Avitene are used, or bacteria are present.

12. **(C)** Arterial blood gas assesses the oxygen and carbon dioxide in arterial blood, measured by various methods to assess the adequacy of ventilation and oxygenation and the acid-base status.

13. **(C)** In a cross-match of blood, the donor RBCs are mixed with the recipient's serum. If agglutination does not occur, the recipient does not have antibodies that will attack the donor RBCs. If no agglutination (clumping) occurs, the donor's blood may be safely transfused to the recipient, provided all the other criteria have been met.

14. **(A)** RBCs contain the oxygen-carrying protein hemoglobin. They are also called erythrocytes.

15. **(C)** The differential white count (an estimate of the percentage of each type of WBC) is done using a stained blood slide. Some blood diseases and inflammatory conditions can be identified this way.

16. **(A)** Incompatibility of blood transfusions may be attributable to either the plasma or red cells of the donor's blood. The red cells of the donor's blood may become clumped or held together in bunches. This process is called agglutination.

17. **(A)** Platelets are formed by the red bone marrow and are essential for the coagulation of blood and in maintenance of hemostasis.

18. **(C)** A normal adult has an average of 5,000 to 10,000 leukocytes per cubic millimeter of circulating blood, or about 1 leukocyte to 700 erythrocytes. A high WBC count is indicative of infection.

19. **(A)** A rapid infusion pump aids in rapidly delivering blood or other fluids by means of a pressurized cuff around the administration bag to exert external force. It may also have a fluid warmer component.

20. **(C)** The pulse oximeter measures blood oxygenation. The fingertip is commonly used.

21. **(C)** Type O blood is the universal donor blood. The four main types are A, B, O, and AB.

CHAPTER 5

Aseptic Technique

- Asepsis—without infection
- Sterility—completely free of all viable microorganisms including spores
- Sterility is maintained by aseptic technique.
- Preoperative—all duties that are required prior to the incision
- Intraoperative—this phase is from the incision to closure.
- Postoperative—all duties from the time the surgery is finished and the dressings are applied
- Masks should be changed between each case.
- Masks cannot hang; they are either on or off.
- Sterile people must always wear protective eyewear—either a mask with a face shield or goggles that protect the eyes from contamination.
- The gown is sterile from the midchest to the waist level; the sleeves circumferentially to 2 in above the elbow.
- The white cuffs of the gown are considered unsterile because they are permeable.
- Due to evidence-based practice, all operating room personnel must double glove on all cases. It also makes it easier if you contaminate yourself and must change gloves. When double gloving, it is recommended to wear a half size larger for the first pair and normal size for the second.
- Closed gloving is performed after the surgical scrub and after the gown has been donned.
- If the STSR gets contaminated during the procedure, the first choice is that another sterile team member reglove the STSR.
- Sterile gloves are also worn for other procedures, not just for surgery (eg, urinary catheterization).
- When the STSR is standing at the operating room (OR) table, the top of the OR table and the top of the back table are considered sterile.

If anything falls below these areas, it is considered contaminated.
- You should not gown and glove off the back table. A separate surface should be used.
- The STSR should never sit unless the procedure is performed sitting down.
- When entering the OR, wipe down all horizontal surfaces and the overhead OR lights with a disinfectant.
- Before opening sterile supplies, check integrity of the item for holes and water spots.
- If the item falls to the floor, check for air implosion and make sure the area that touched the floor is clean and dry. If the item is good, you may open it now for that case only. If you do not use it on that case, the item must be discarded and not put back on the shelf.
- If the item is double wrapped or or in a container, check the chemical indicators (tape/plastic indicator) to determine whether there has been a color change.
  - Steam tape—cream-colored lines turn brown when sterilized.
  - ETO tape is green—the lines turn brown when sterilized.
- If there is a color change, it still does not mean the item is sterile. It only means the sterilant has met the parameters of the item. Once sterile, you must check the internal indicators before placing the item on your sterile field.
- It is recommended that the gown and gloves be opened on the Mayo stand or small gown and glove table.
- Check integrity of all sterile packages for holes and moisture.
- The inner edge of a peel pack is the line between sterile and unsterile.

- When opening an envelope-type sterile wrapper, open the first flap away from you.
- The inside of paper wrappers containing sterile items is considered sterile except for 1 in around the outside edge of the wrapper.
- Never reach over a sterile field.
- Two methods of the surgical scrub
  - Timed method (5–10 minutes depending on the institution)
  - Counted brushstroke method
- Two types of microbes we are trying to control:
  - Transient—live only on the surface of the skin—we can remove these
  - Resident—live deeper in the skin—we cannot remove these but can only reduce the microbial count
- When rinsing hands, use a unidirectional motion.
- The circulator will assist in turning the gown. Hand her the tie, and she will proceed around you. You do not want to turn your back to the sterile field.
- The sterile field should be set up as close as possible to the procedure time.
- The sterile solutions should be poured into the sterile container that has been placed toward the edge of the table for easier access for the circulator. When pouring the solution, it must be held 12 in above the sterile field. You may never recap a solution.
- When opening sharps, the correct method is to directly pass the object to the STSR. They may be flipped onto another area; however, it must be stated to the STSR where the item is to avoid injury or loss of item.
- The sterile field must be broken down if the case has been canceled. You cannot cover the sterile field with a sterile drape and move to another OR.
- When draping a nonsterile surface, always place hands inside a cuff.
- When an STSR is draping a nonsterile surface, the drape should be opened toward you first and the second away from you.
- The top of a back table, when draped, is the only part of the table that is sterile.
- Sterile drapes can never be repositioned.
- Strike through—moisture soaking through a sterile barrier
- When clamping a tubing with a metal clamp that perforates the drape, you must consider the tips of the clamp contaminated as well as the drape it is attached to. They should not be removed until the end of the surgical procedure.
- A nonsterile person should remain 12 in from the sterile field.
- Drapes are considered a physical barrier. Antiseptic prep solutions are considered chemical barriers.
- Sterile team members should pass front to front and back to back.
- When removing your gown and gloves, remove your gown first, followed by gloves, and lastly, your mask, touching the ties only.
- Sterile gloves should be removed glove to glove and skin to skin.

Questions

1. The minimum distance a nonsterile person should remain from a sterile field is:

   (A) 6 in
   (B) 1 ft
   (C) 2 ft
   (D) 3 ft

2. Which of the following is NOT a safe practice?

   (A) Discard opened sterile bottles.
   (B) Sterile persons drape first toward themselves and then away.
   (C) Sterile persons face sterile areas.
   (D) Sterile tables may be covered for later use.

3. Tables are considered sterile:

   (A) on the top and 2 in below the table level
   (B) up to 2 ft off the ground
   (C) on the top and in the area that has been pulled close to the sterile field
   (D) only on the top

4. At the end of the case, drapes should be:

   (A) pulled off and placed in a hamper
   (B) rolled off and placed on the floor so they can be checked for instruments
   (C) rolled off and placed in a hamper
   (D) checked for instruments, rolled off, and placed in a hamper

5. If a solution soaks through a sterile drape:

   (A) discard drape and replace it
   (B) cover wet area with impervious sterile drape or towel
   (C) cover wet area with at least two layers of fabric
   (D) fill out an incident report at the end of the case

6. Which of the following is not an acceptable wrapper for gas sterilization?

   (A) Nylon
   (B) Muslin
   (C) Paper
   (D) Plastic

7. Which of the following is the only acceptable plastic that can be used for a steam sterilization wrapper?

   (A) Polyethylene
   (B) Polypropylene
   (C) Polyamide
   (D) Polyvinyl chloride

8. All of the following statements regarding muslin wrappers are true EXCEPT:

   (A) Muslin must be laundered, even if unused, in order to rehydrate it.
   (B) A 140-thread count of unbleached muslin is used for wrappers.
   (C) Muslin is flexible and easy to handle.
   (D) Small holes can be repaired by stitching on a patch.

9. Packages wrapped in muslin must have:

    (A) one thickness
    (B) two thicknesses
    (C) three thicknesses
    (D) four thicknesses

10. The maximum storage life for a muslin-wrapped item in a closed cabinet is:

    (A) 7 days
    (B) 14 days
    (C) 21 days
    (D) 30 days

11. An item dropped on the floor is considered safe only if:

    (A) it is wrapped in woven material
    (B) it is enclosed in an impervious material
    (C) it is used right away
    (D) it is inspected carefully

12. When using a pour solution:

    (A) a portion may be poured and the cap replaced
    (B) the contents must be used or discarded after the bottle is opened
    (C) the cap may be replaced if it has not been placed on a nonsterile surface
    (D) the solution may be used on the same case if the cap is not replaced

13. What is the standard safety margin on package wrappers?

    (A) Up to the edge
    (B) Less than 1 in
    (C) 1 in
    (D) None of the above

14. When opening a wrapper, the circulator should open the top flap:

    (A) toward self
    (B) away from self
    (C) after the sides
    (D) over the sterile field

15. When the scrub nurse drapes a basin stand:

    (A) the side nearest the body is opened first
    (B) the side nearest the body is opened last
    (C) the lateral areas are done first
    (D) Both A and B

16. When flipping a sterile item onto the field, the circulator may:

    (A) lean over the sterile field to shake item out of package
    (B) project item without reaching over the sterile field
    (C) shake item into sterile basin stand
    (D) lean over sterile linen pack and drop item onto it

17. Gowns are considered sterile only from:

    (A) waist to neck level in front and back and the sleeves
    (B) waist to shoulder, front and back, and the sleeves
    (C) neck to thighs in front and the sleeves
    (D) only in front from chest to sterile field level and sleeves from elbow to cuffs

18. An acceptable action when drying the hands and arms after the surgical scrub is to:

    (A) dry from elbow to fingertip
    (B) dry thoroughly, cleanest area first
    (C) keep the hands and arms close to the body, at waist level
    (D) dry one hand and arm thoroughly before proceeding to the next

19. All of the following statements regarding gowning another person are true EXCEPT:

    (A) Open the hand towel and lay it on the person's hand.
    (B) Hand the folded gown to the person at the neckband.
    (C) Keep hands on the outside of the gown under a protective cuff.
    (D) Release the gown once the person touches it.

20. Which statement regarding the scrub procedure is NOT true?

    (A) It reduces the microbial count.
    (B) It leaves an antimicrobial residue.
    (C) It renders the skin sterile.
    (D) It removes skin oil.

21. If the scrub nurse needs to change a glove during an operation:

    (A) the scrub must also regown
    (B) the circulator pulls the glove off
    (C) the scrub pulls the glove off
    (D) the scrub uses the closed gloved technique to reapply gloves

22. Which statement regarding the removal of gown and gloves does NOT meet safe criteria?

    (A) The gloves are removed before the gown.
    (B) The gown is pulled off inside out.
    (C) The gown is untied by the circulator.
    (D) The gloves are removed inside out.

23. An effective surgical scrub procedure is the:

    (A) time method
    (B) brushstroke method
    (C) 3-minute anatomic method
    (D) Both A and B

24. Regarding the surgical scrub, which statement would violate acceptable practice?

    (A) Fingernails should only reach the tip of the finger.
    (B) Nail polish may be worn if freshly applied.
    (C) It is okay to scrub with a cut or abrasion.
    (D) A non–oil-based hand lotion may be used to protect the skin.

25. Eyewear, goggles, and/or face shields should be worn:

    (A) on every case
    (B) on orthopedic cases
    (C) on vascular cases
    (D) on HIV-positive cases

26. The surgical scrub is:

    (A) sterilization of the skin
    (B) mechanical cleansing of the skin
    (C) chemical cleansing of the skin
    (D) mechanical washing and chemical antisepsis of the skin

27. Scrub technique ends

    (A) 2 in below the elbow
    (B) just below the elbow
    (C) at the elbow
    (D) 2 in above the elbow

28. Which statement regarding the surgical scrub indicates INAPPROPRIATE preparation by the scrub?

    (A) Wearing artificial nails is acceptable.
    (B) Nail polish may be worn, if not chipped.
    (C) Finger nails should not reach beyond fingertips.
    (D) Skin should be protected with a non–oil-based product.

29. Which statement best describes an effective surgical hand scrub?

    (A) Time, no anatomical sequence
    (B) Number of strokes, no anatomical sequence
    (C) Time or number of strokes, hand to elbow sequence
    (D) Number of strokes, elbow to hand sequence

30. The brushstroke method of scrubbing prescribes the number of strokes required. Indicate the number for each: nails, fingers, hands (back and palm), and arms.

    (A) 40, 30, 30, 30
    (B) 40, 40, 20, 20
    (C) 30, 20, 20, 20
    (D) 30, 20, 10, 10

31. Evidence-based practice (EBP) relies on:

    (A) opinion and tradition
    (B) past evident practices
    (C) current practices
    (D) science and evidence

32. Standard precautions evolved from a practice called:

    (A) universal precautions
    (B) aseptic technique
    (C) EBP
    (D) the method of thinking and doing

33. When water comes in contact with a sterile drape or gown, it can cause:

    (A) strike-through contamination
    (B) a slippery surface
    (C) resident flora
    (D) a potential fire hazard

34. Standards during surgery include all of the following EXCEPT:

    (A) nonsterile team members do not pass between two sterile fields
    (B) sterile gowns are only considered sterile from the waist to the axillary lines, from hands to shoulders
    (C) movement should be kept to a minimum
    (D) if there is any doubt about the sterility of the item, consider it contaminated

35. When removing sterile attire, arrange the following in proper order: (1) remove your gloves, (2) remove your gown, (3) remove your mask

    (A) 1, 2, 3
    (B) 1, 3, 2
    (C) 2, 1, 3
    (D) 3, 2, 1

36. When opening sterile supplies, all of the following are proper techniques EXCEPT:

    (A) do not readjust the table drape after it has been opened
    (B) open the first flap away from you on an unwrapped item
    (C) remember not to lean over the sterile field
    (D) when opening items in a peel pouch, slowly allow the item to slide out of the package onto the sterile field

37. When opening supplies for a case, what should be passed directly to the scrub or flipped in an area where they are clearly visible?

    (A) Medications
    (B) 10-cc syringes
    (C) Peanuts
    (D) Blades

38. How should sterile personnel pass each other?

    (A) Right to left
    (B) They should never pass each other
    (C) Back to back, front to front
    (D) It does not really matter because gowns that wrap around are used

39. What is known as the center of your sterile field?

    (A) Back table
    (B) Mayo
    (C) Surgeon
    (D) Draped patient

40. If there is a break in sterile technique during the procedure, the STSR should tell:

    (A) the surgeon
    (B) the person who broke technique
    (C) the circulator
    (D) everyone in the lounge

41. Which condition regarding sterile technique is NOT recommended?

    (A) Sterile tables are set up just before the operation.
    (B) Sterile tables may be set up and safely covered until the time of surgery.
    (C) Once sterile packs are open, someone must remain in the room to maintain vigilance.
    (D) Sterile persons pass each other back to back.

42. Which of the following conditions is NOT an acceptable aseptic technique?

    (A) Scrub nurse stands on a platform or standing stool.
    (B) Scrub nurse keeps hands below shoulder level.
    (C) Scrub nurse folds arms with hands at axillae.
    (D) Scrub nurse's hands are at or above waist level.

43. When a sterile item is hanging or extending over the sterile table edge, the scrub nurse:

    (A) must watch closely so that no one comes near it
    (B) does not touch the part hanging below table level
    (C) should pull it back onto the table so it does not become contaminated
    (D) may use the item

44. Which of the following is considered a break in technique?

    (A) A sterile person turns his or her back to a nonsterile person or area when passing.
    (B) Sterile persons face sterile areas.
    (C) A sterile person sits or leans against a nonsterile surface.
    (D) Nonsterile persons avoid sterile areas.

45. In which situation should sterility be questioned?

    (A) If a sterilized pack is found in an unsterile workroom
    (B) If the surgeon turns away from the sterile field for a brow wipe
    (C) If the scrub drapes a nonsterile table, covering the edge nearest the body first
    (D) If the lip of a pour bottle is held over the basin as close to the edge as possible

46. When handing skin towels to the surgeon, where should the scrub person stand in relation to the surgeon?

    (A) On the opposite side of the table
    (B) On the same side of the table
    (C) At the foot of the table
    (D) Any position is acceptable

47. According to Centers for Disease Control and Prevention (CDC) guidelines, each of the following actions by a scrub person prevents wounds and punctures EXCEPT:

    (A) use an instrument to remove blades
    (B) recap injection needles
    (C) account for each needle as surgeon finishes with it
    (D) protect sharp blades, edges, and tips

48. Which of the following is NOT an acceptable technique when draping a patient?

    (A) Hold the drapes high until directly over the proper area.
    (B) Protect the gloved hands by cuffing the end of the drape over them.
    (C) Unfold the drapes before bringing them to the OR table.
    (D) Place the drapes on a dry area.

49. The procedure to follow if a hair is found on the operative field is to:

    (A) notify circulator
    (B) complete an incident report
    (C) remove it with a clamp and cover over area
    (D) no action is necessary

50. If the floor or wall becomes contaminated with organic debris during a case, the circulator:

    (A) calls housekeeping stat
    (B) decontaminates promptly
    (C) decontaminates after case is complete
    (D) defers for terminal cleaning

Answers and Explanations

1. **(B)** All nonsterile persons should remain at least 1 ft from any sterile field.

2. **(D)** Sterile tables should be set up just before the surgical procedure. Covering of tables is not recommended.

3. **(D)** A sterile draped table is considered sterile only on the top. The edges and sides extending below table level are considered nonsterile.

4. **(D)** Check drapes for instruments. Roll drapes off the patient to prevent sparking and airborne contamination. Wet areas should be placed in the center to prevent soaking through the laundry bag.

5. **(B)** If a solution soaks through a sterile drape to a nonsterile area, the wet area is covered with impervious sterile drapes or towels.

6. **(A)** Nylon is not used for ethylene oxide (EO) sterilization because of inadequate permeability; however, muslin, nonwoven fabric, paper, and plastic are safely used. Items wrapped for gas sterilization should be tagged to avoid inadvertent steam sterilization.

7. **(B)** Polypropylene film of 1- to 3-mm thickness is the only plastic acceptable for steam sterilization. It is used in the form of pouches presealed on two or three sides. The open sides are then heat sealed.

8. **(D)** Small holes can be heat sealed with double-vulcanized patches; they can never be stitched because this will leave needle holes in the muslin.

9. **(D)** Muslin wrappers must have two layers of double thickness (four thicknesses) to serve as a sufficient dust filter and microbial barrier. A 140-thread count muslin is used for wrappers.

10. **(D)** The storage life for muslin is 30 days maximum in closed cabinets. Muslin wets easily and dries quickly, so water stains may not be obvious. On open shelving, the storage life is 21 days.

11. **(B)** If a sterile package is dropped, the item may be considered safe for immediate use only if it is enclosed in an impervious material and the integrity of the package is maintained. Dropped items wrapped in woven materials should not be used.

12. **(B)** After a sterile bottle is opened, the contents must be used or discarded. The cap cannot be replaced without contamination of the pouring edges. The edges of anything that encloses sterile contents are considered nonsterile.

13. **(C)** A 1-in safety margin is usually considered standard on package wrappers. After a package is open, the edges are nonsterile.

14. **(B)** The top flap is opened away from self, and the sides are turned under and secured. The last flap is pulled toward the person opening the package.

15. **(A)** When a scrub nurse is draping a ring stand, the side nearest the body is opened first. The portion of the drape then protects

the gown, enabling the nurse to move closer to the table to open the opposite side.

16. **(B)** When flipping a sterile item onto a sterile field, the circulator may never reach over the sterile field and shake the item from the package.

17. **(D)** Gowns are considered sterile only in front from chest to level of sterile field, and the sleeves from elbow to cuffs.

18. **(B)** The STSR should bend forward slightly at the waist, holding hands and elbows away from the body. Dry both hands and arms independently starting at the fingertips, which are the cleanest area, and moving to 2 in above the elbow.

19. **(B)** Before handing a gown to another person, unfold it carefully, holding it at the neckband.

20. **(C)** The surgical scrub removes skin oil, reduces the microbial count, and leaves an antimicrobial residue on the skin. The skin can never be rendered sterile (aseptic). It is considered surgically clean.

21. **(B)** To change a glove during an operation, the scrub nurse must turn away from the sterile field. The circulator pulls the glove off inside out, and the open-glove technique is used to don a new pair of gloves.

22. **(A)** The gown is always removed before the gloves. It is pulled downward from the shoulders, turning the sleeves inside out as it is pulled off the arms. Gloves are turned inside out, using the glove-to-glove then skin-to-skin technique as they are removed. The circulating nurse unfastens the gown at the neck and waist.

23. **(D)** Either the time method or brushstroke method is effective if properly executed. Studies have shown that a vigorous 5-minute scrub with a reliable agent is as effective as the 10-minute scrub with less mechanical action.

24. **(C)** Persons with an open wound/abrasion should not scrub.

25. **(A)** Eye protection or masks with face shields should be worn on all surgical cases to avoid direct contact with blood and body fluids.

26. **(D)** The surgical scrub is the process of removing as many microorganisms from the hands and arms as possible by mechanical washing and chemical antisepsis.

27. **(D)** The arm is scrubbed, including the elbow and the antecubital space to 2 in above the elbow.

28. **(A)** Artificial nails are never acceptable in the operating room.

29. **(C)** Time varies with the frequency of the scrub, the agent used, and the method used. The procedure may be time method or counted brushstroke, each of which follows an anatomical pattern of scrub ending 2 in above the elbow. All steps begin with hands and end with elbow, with the hands having most direct contact.

30. **(C)** The nails are scrubbed for 30 strokes; all sides of each finger, 20 strokes; the back of the hand and palm, 20 strokes; and the arms, 20 strokes to 2 in above the elbow.

31. **(D)** Scientific investigation and discovery supersede old practices; EBP considers only the best of current study and evidence. An example is double gloving: in the past, double gloving was only done on orthopedic cases. The current practice is for all surgical personnel to double glove for all cases. This is due to EBP.

32. **(A)** Standard precautions evolved from a policy called universal precautions. They were originally established to prevent the spread of HIV and AIDS.

33. **(A)** This occurs when moisture from either side of the drape serves as a vehicle for

bacteria to infiltrate the drape from a nonsterile surface.

34. **(B)** Sterile gowns are considered sterile only in the front from the axillary lines to the waist, from the hands to the elbows.

35. **(C)** Gown first, then gloves, and mask last.

36. **(D)** Items wrapped in peel pouches are delivered directly to the scrub.

37. **(D)** Scalpel blades and other sharps should be passed directly to the scrub or flipped onto an open area where they are visibly seen.

38. **(C)** Sterile personnel pass each other back to back or front to front.

39. **(D)** The draped patient is the center of your sterile field during surgery.

40. **(B)** If there is a break in technique during a procedure, the person who broke technique should be told and correct actions should be taken.

41. **(B)** Covering sterile tables for later use is not recommended because it is difficult to uncover a table without contamination.

42. **(C)** Hands are kept at or above waist level, away from the face and arms, and never folded, because there may be perspiration in the axillary region.

43. **(B)** Anything falling or extending over a table edge is unsterile. The scrub person does not touch the part hanging below table level.

44. **(C)** Sitting or leaning against a nonsterile surface is a break in technique because a sterile person should keep contact with nonsterile areas to a minimum.

45. **(A)** If the sterility of anything is in doubt, consider it not sterile. Do not use a pack, even if it appears to be sterile, if it is found in a nonsterile workroom.

46. **(B)** The scrub who hands the drapes to the surgeon should stand on the same side of the table in order to avoid reaching over the unsterile OR table.

47. **(B)** Do not recap used injection needles.

48. **(C)** Drapes should be carried to the OR table folded to prevent them from coming in contact with unclean items in transport.

49. **(C)** A hair found on a drape must be removed with a hemostat; hand instrument off of field and cover the area with a suitable drape.

50. **(B)** Decontaminate the floor and walls promptly during operation if contaminated by organic debris. Use a broad-spectrum detergent disinfectant and wear gloves. This action helps prevent microorganisms from drying and becoming airborne.

CHAPTER 6

Sterilization and Disinfection

- Asepsis—absence of disease-causing micro-organisms
- Sterile—free of all living microorganisms including spores
- Surgically clean—mechanically disinfected but not sterile
- Strike-through contamination—contamination of the sterile field with fluid through a puncture or absorbing through the drapes
- Aeration—this is the way ethylene oxide is removed from the sterilized items
- Aerobes—microorganisms that cannot live without oxygen
- Anaerobes—microorganisms that are able to survive without oxygen
- Bacteria—all living cells are classified into two groups:
  - Prokaryotes—divide by the process of binary fission. No nucleus
  - Eukaryotes—include fungi, algae, and plant and animal cells. Have a nucleus
  - Bacteria divide by binary fission
- Binary fission—asexual reproduction of a cell by division into two identical cells
- Bactericide—kills bacteria
- Bacteriostatic—prevents the growth of bacteria
- Bioburden—amount of microorganisms on an item before sterilization
- Biological indicator—sterilization monitoring system used to test the effectiveness of the sterilization process used
- Contamination—presence of microorganisms on animate living and nonliving objects
- Decontamination—process by which chemical or physical agents are used to clean inanimate objects, noncritical surfaces

- SSI—surgical site infection. Factors that increase SSI infections include:
  - Age
  - Obesity
  - General health
- Shaving a patient should be performed the day before surgery to avoid SSI.
- Using an electrical razor is preferred over using a razor to prevent cuts that can become infected.
- Deep incisional SSI—an infection involving deep tissue
- Disinfection—not used on tissue. Chemical or physical process of destroying most forms of pathogenic microorganisms, used for inanimate objects
- High-level disinfection—the process that destroys all microorganisms if the contact time with the item is sufficient
- Intermediate-level disinfection—the process that destroys inactive vegetative bacteria and most fungi and viruses but not bacterial endospores
- Low-level disinfection—the process that destroys most bacteria, some viruses, and some fungi but not bacterial endospores
  - Always use sterile distilled water to rinse items.
- Flash sterilization—a sterilization process that is used for immediate patient use using the steam sterilization method. It is usually done in the substerile room autoclave
- Fungicide—kills fungi
- Immunity—resistant to infection
  - Naturally acquired active immunity—when you are exposed to and get the disease and, as a result, you become immune

- Artificially acquired active immunity—when you receive a vaccine and become immune
- Artificially acquired passive immunity—when you receive an immunization such as a gamma globulin. It is a short-term immunization
- Naturally acquired passive immunity—this occurs during pregnancy when a pregnant woman passes the antibodies to her fetus through the bloodstream
- Infection—invasion of microorganisms in body tissues causing damage
- Nosocomial infection—an infection that was acquired in the hospital; they include:
  - Urinary tract infection (UTI)
  - SSI
  - Lung infection
  - Infection in the blood
- Pasteurization—heating process that destroys pathogenic microorganisms such as in milk or wine
- Parasites—microorganisms that live on or within living organisms. Some are:
  - Obligatory—means they depend on living tissue
  - Facultative—means they can live on dead tissue
- Pathogen—any disease-producing microorganisms
  - Resident microorganisms—microorganisms that live deep in the epidermis
  - Transient microorganisms—microorganisms that live on the surface of the epidermis
- Mutualism—when different organisms exist and benefit from each other
- Commensalism—when one organism benefits from the other and neither is harmed
- Parasitism—when one organism benefits from the other and harms the host
- Virucide—kills viruses
- Viruses—some examples include HIV, herpes simplex, hepatitis B, C, D
- MRSA—methicillin-resistant *Staphylococcus aureus*—this is a virus that is resistant to most antibiotics; the only antibiotic that works on this virus is vancomycin. MRSA is highly contagious
- Creutzfeldt-Jakob disease—a fatal neurodegenerative disease of the central nervous system (brain) caused by a human prion

- Prion—the smallest infectious particle; it is not viral, bacterial, or fungal
  - Prions are also responsible for the disease known as mad cow disease. There is no known form of transmission.
  - This prion causes holes in the brain.
  - There is no sterilization process that kills these prions. When surgery is performed on these patients, we use disposable instruments so they can be thrown away.
  - They have no DNA/RNA.
- *Staphylococcus aureus*—these microorganisms are found in the respiratory tract, in nasal passages, and in skin. These are gram-positive microbes.
- Gram-positive—purple
- Gram-negative—red
- Enterococci—found in the normal flora of the gastrointestinal (GI) tract and female genital tracts
- Streptococci—found in the GI tracts, upper respiratory tracts, and genitourinary tracts
- Clostridia
  - *Clostridium perfringens*—responsible for gas gangrene
  - *C. tetani*—tetanus
  - *C. difficile*—the normal flora in the intestines is altered usually as a result of the overuse of antibiotics, causing severe diarrhea, dehydration, and in some cases, death. Very contagious
- *Mycobacterium tuberculosis*—transmitted directly from the respiratory tract, causing tuberculosis (TB)
- The most common bioterrorist agents include:
  - Anthrax
  - Smallpox
  - Plague (pneumonic, bubonic)
  - Tularemia (types of insect bites)
  - Botulism
- New infectious diseases emerging in the United States include:
  - SARS—severe acute respiratory syndrome
  - West Nile virus
  - Avian influenza
  - H1N1 virus—flu
- Central processing department—made up of a decontamination area, instrument room, sterile processing area, and sterile storage area

- Personnel in this department wear PPE (personal protective equipment), which includes:
  - Waterproof aprons
  - Caps
  - Face shields
  - Gloves that are used for chemical disinfection; these are not surgical gloves or patient care gloves
- Spaulding's classification of patient care items—Spaulding was a microbiologist who developed a method of classifying the levels of processing equipment to be used on patient care items
  - Critical items—they must be sterile because they enter sterile body tissue and the vascular system; examples include:
    - Surgical instruments
    - Endoscopic equipment that cuts tissue
    - Catheters
    - Implants
    - Needles
  - Semicritical items—require high-level disinfection because they come in contact with skin and mucous membranes and go into the mouth and urinary tract. Examples include:
    - Respiratory equipment
    - Anesthesia equipment
    - Bronchoscopes
    - Colonoscopes
    - Gastroscopes
    - Cystoscopes
- Noncritical items—require low-level disinfection because they only come in contact with skin. Examples include:
  - Blood pressure cuffs
  - Furniture
  - Linens
- Chemical disinfectants
  - Alcohol—used in housekeeping to damp dust lights, furniture, etc.
    - Intermediate-level disinfection
    - Used on semicritical items
  - Chlorine compounds—they are limited to housekeeping disinfection for spot cleaning of blood and body fluids
    - Household bleach—sodium hypochlorite
  - Low-level disinfectant—can be high level depending on concentration and pH
    - Used on noncritical items
  - Formaldehyde—high-level disinfectant used for surgical instruments
    - Kills TB and viruses when items soak for 10 minutes
    - Sporicidal when soaking for 12 minutes
    - Fumes irritate the eyes and mucous membranes. All items that come in contact with formaldehyde must be rinsed with sterile distilled water
    - High-level disinfectant
    - Used on critical items
  - Glutaraldehyde—Cidex
    - Used on surgical instruments; can also be used on rubber and plastic
    - A 2% solution is considered a high-level disinfectant
    - Kills bacteria, fungi, virus, HIV
    - Kills hepatitis B virus (HBV) when soaked for 10 minutes
    - Kills TB when soaked for 45–90 minutes
    - Kills spores in minimum of 10 hours
    - Odor and fumes are irritating to mucous membranes, eyes, respiratory tract
    - The solution can be reused; it is kept in a basin with a cover
    - Has a shelf life of 14–30 days (manufacturer instructions)
    - Instruments must be washed first, rinsed with sterile water, dried, and totally submerged in the solution. All lumens must also be filled with the solution. After the appropriate time for disinfection, the instruments must be rinsed again with sterile water
    - High-level disinfectant
    - Used on critical/semicritical items
  - Iodophors—iodine compound, used for housekeeping
    - Low-level disinfectant
    - Used on noncritical items
  - Quaternary ammonium compounds—known as quats—kill bacteria, fungi
    - Low-level disinfectant
    - Used on noncritical items
  - Hydrogen peroxide—kills bacteria, fungi, virus, TB
    - Low-level disinfectant
    - Noncritical items
- Instrument cleaning—combines manual, mechanical, chemical, and physical decontamination process

- Washer-sterilizer/decontaminator:
  - All bioburden must be washed and rinsed from the instruments by hand
  - Instruments are then reassembled—all box locks on instruments are open, and instruments disassembled such as the Balfour retractor, blade, and wing nuts
  - Instrument sets are placed in the washer-sterilizer and the cycle begins
- Ultrasonic cleaner:
  - The ultrasonic cleaner works by cavitation (high-frequency sound waves). This removes small organic particles that the washer-sterilizer cannot reach
- Power equipment—should never be submerged in water or a cleaning solution or placed in any of the mechanical decontaminating machines. Proper cleaning includes:
  - Keep cords attached to drill while cleaning to prevent any solutions from entering into the cord or drill
  - Wash cord and drill with neutral detergent. Never use alcohol on these items as it will harden and crack the cord
  - Rinse all components with distilled water and dry
- Instruments with lumens—trocars, nondisposable tonsil suction tips
  - Flush the lumen with hydrogen peroxide until it runs clear and rinse with distilled water
  - Hand clean the outside with neutral detergent
  - The inside with a brush
- Decontamination of endoscopes
  - Rigid
    - Clean all lumens as noted above and soak rigid scope in an enzymatic solution
    - Using a water pressure gun, rinse and dry the instrument
    - Do not hit the lens, and do not tightly wind or kink the light cord or you will break the fibers in the cord
  - Flexible endoscope
    - Ports are cleaned with a small brush
    - Soak in enzymatic solution with the ports open
    - Wash the outside manually with neutral detergent
    - Be careful with lens and cords and scope itself
    - Dry all scopes before storing
    - Basins

- Must be separated by a cloth towel when sterilized together
- Never place sponges in the basin when sterilizing
- Place basins on their sides when sterilizing
- They should not weigh more than 7 lb
- Drape packs
  - Must not exceed a maximum of 12 × 12 × 20
  - Must not weigh more than 20 lb
  - Are placed on their side close to the edge when sterilizing
- Rubber and plastics
  - Tubing, catheters, and drains require a residual of distilled water in their lumens when sterilizing
  - Tubing should not be kinked
- Wood products—should be packaged and sterilized separately; an example would be:
  - An orthopedic instrument with a wooden handle
  - Repeated sterilization cracks the wood
- Oils/petroleum products/talcs—sterilized by dry heat sterilizers. Examples include:
  - Convection oven
  - Gravity convection oven
- Rubber goods—tubing, catheters, and drains must have a residual of sterile distilled water in their lumen
  - All tubing that is coiled must not have kinks
  - Most of this equipment is disposable and is the preferred method
- Peel packs
  - Choose the correct size wrapper
  - The pack should be heat sealed unless it has an adhesive tape. If it does, it may be used
  - Never use staples/rubber bands
  - Write only on the plastic
  - Instruments/equipment with sharp edges should have protective paper and foam sleeves to prevent the sharp tip from coming through the pack
  - Peel packs are placed on their side in the autoclave
- Julian date indicates the date of sterilization
  - It is attached to the item with a labeling gun
  - Example—February 27, 2012, is the date of sterilization; the Julian date is 58 (count from January 1 to February 27 = 58)
- Woven fabrics
  - Reusable, also called muslin or linen

- Made of 100% cotton, muslin
- After each use and wash, they must be inspected for holes
- You cannot stitch the material if there is a hole; it will make more holes; a patch is used
- 140-thread count is used
- Not moisture resistant and requires double wrapping
- When using muslin wraps, the recommended maximum size of a linen pack is 12 × 12 × 20 (12 in high × 12 in wide × 20 in long)
- Nonwoven fabrics
  - Disposable wrappers for single use only
  - Come in a variety of sizes to accommodate different items to be sterilized
  - Paper is a type of nonwoven material difficult to work with because it has extreme memory
- Chemical indicators
  - Autoclave tape on the outside of wrapped items (tape changes colors when exposed to the sterilant and temperature)
    - Steam-sensitive tape is tan and reveals dark stripes when exposed to steam sterilization
    - Gas-sensitive tape is light green and reveals dark stripes when exposed to gas sterilization
  - Internal steam indicators are placed on the inside of the instrument sets
  - Rigid containers have a plastic indicator that is attached to the outside locking devices; a black dot appears when exposed to the sterilant and temperature
- Biological indicator—this is the only true indication that all sterilization conditions have been met
  - The biological microorganism used in steam sterilizers is *Geobacillus stearothermophilus*
  - The biological microorganism used for ethylene oxide (ETO) is *Bacillus atrophaeus/Geobacillus subtilis*
  - The biological indicator is placed in the most difficult area in the autoclave for the sterilant to reach
  - Incubation period is 48 hours
- Chemical sterilization
  - ETO—ethylene oxide gas sterilization
    - Used to sterilize items that are sensitive to heat and moisture
    - The process interferes with the microorganisms' metabolism and results in cell death

- ETO must be carefully regulated because it is highly toxic, explosive, and flammable
- Aeration is required after every cycle
- Radiation sterilization—gamma ray and beta particle sterilization
  - Cobalt-60 is a type of isotope that produces gamma rays used for sterilization
  - Back table covers and all manufactured packs are sterilized by cobalt-60
- Bowie-Dick test—chemical indicator used with a prevacuum sterilizer to test if the air has been removed from the cycle
- Flash sterilization—fast sterilizing process for unwrapped instruments that are to be used immediately
  - Minimum exposure time to the sterilization process is 270–275°F for 3 minutes for instruments and 4 minutes for porous items
- Gravity displacement sterilizer—steam sterilizer that uses a downward motion to remove air from the sterilizing chamber. Air is pushed down near the front lower chamber
  - Air is heavier than steam and pushes the air out
  - Minimum exposure time to the sterilization process is:
    - 15 minutes at 250–254°F
    - 15–17 psi (pounds per square inch)
    - Time/temperature/pressure
  - The total cycle is about 30 minutes
  - No living thing can withstand steam at 270°F for 15 minutes
- Indicators
  - Biological indicators—the best and most effective indicators to prove sterility; they are living spores
    - The bacterial spore used in the biological indicator for steam sterilization is *G. stearothermophilus*
    - This test is performed daily and when implants are used
    - Indicator is placed in the most difficult area for the sterilant to reach. This is known as the coldest point/front bottom of the chamber. The color is red. If after sterilization the liquid remains red, it is a negative (the sterilization process was successful and the spores were destroyed). If the liquid turns yellow, it is positive (the spores were not destroyed)

- Prevacuum sterilizer—fast steam sterilizer that removes air by a vacuum before filling the chamber with steam
  - Time, temperature, and pressure are the three components needed for sterilization
  - The complete cycle time is shorter in the prevacuum sterilizer than in the gravity displacement sterilizer
    - Gravity displacement: 30 minutes
    - Prevacuum: 15–20 minutes
  - Exposure time:
    - 270–276°F for a minimum of 4 minutes
    - 27 psi
- ETO gas sterilization—used on items that cannot be sterilized with heat and moisture (eg, plastics, some scopes, cameras)
  - Highly flammable, explosive, and toxic
  - ETO is mixed with carbon dioxide to reduce its flammability
  - For ETO to be highly effective, it depends on four parameters:
    - Concentration of the gas
    - Temperature
    - Humidity
    - Time
  - Sterilization takes 3–5 hours depending on the size of the chamber and load
  - Aeration is essential because ETO can be toxic to humans
  - The items must be aerated for 8 hours at 140°F
  - The biological indicator must be incubated for 48 hours before it is read
- Dry heat sterilization—not used in the operating room
  - Used for oils (mineral oil is used for dressings), petroleum products, and talc
  - Biological indicator used for dry heat ovens is *B. atrophaeus*
  - Examples include:
    - Mechanical convection ovens
    - Gravity convection ovens
- Hydrogen peroxide plasma sterilization—a cloud or glow of pink plasma covers the items to be sterilized; kills all microorganisms including spores

---

Gravity displacement steam sterilizer
- Bowie-Dick test—used to make sure air is out of chamber
- sterility indicators
  - mechanical—on the machine
  - chemical—yellow tape/lines turn dark brown-black, indicators in the sets
  - orange plastic clips on the outside of sets
  - biological—only true indicator that the items are sterile. *Geobacillus stearothermophilus* are the microbes used in steam sterilizers
- instrument with lumens—sterile distilled water inside lumen
- steam enters top back
- air exits front bottom
  wrapped instruments:
  - 250°F, 15 psi 30 minutes
  - 270°F, 27 psi 15 minutes
  unwrapped instruments:
  - 270°F, 27 psi 3 minutes
  unwrapped instruments with lumens:
  - 270°F, 27 psi 10 minutes

Prevacuum steam sterilizer/dynamic air removal steam sterilizer
- air is heavier than steam
- Bowie-Dick test—used to make sure air is out of chamber
- sterility indicators
  - mechanical—on the machine
  - chemical—yellow tape/lines turn dark brown-black, indicators in the sets
  - orange plastic clips on the outside of sets
  - biological—only true indicator the items are sterile. *G. stearothermophilus* are the microbes used in steam sterilizers
- instrument with lumens—sterile distilled water inside lumen
- steam enters top back
- air exits front bottom
  wrapped instruments:
  - 270°F, 27 psi 4 minutes
  unwrapped instruments:
  - 270°F, 27 psi 3 minutes
  unwrapped instruments with lumens:
  - 270°F, 27 psi 4 minutes

ETO chemical (gas) sterilizer
- used on items that cannot be sterilized with steam
- kill microbes by permeating the cell wall and causing cell death
- aeration is required
- instruments with lumens must be dry (air blown) because when the ETO comes in contact with water, it will bind and create a toxin—ethylene glycol
- chemical indicator tape is green; lines turn brown when exposed to the chemical
- biological indicator—only true effective way to prove sterility. The microbe used is *Bacillus atrophaeus/Geobacillus subtilis*
- incubation 48 hours; can be read after 24 hours
  temperature:
  - 85–145°F
  humidity:
  - 30–80%

Questions

1. The amount of pressure necessary in a steam sterilizer set at 250°F is:

   (A) 15–17 lb
   (B) 20–22 lb
   (C) 22–25 lb
   (D) 25–27 lb

2. Positive assurance that sterilization conditions have been achieved can only be obtained through:

   (A) biological control test
   (B) heat-sensitive tape
   (C) color change monitor
   (D) mechanical indicator

3. A wrapped tray of instruments is sterilized in a gravity displacement sterilizer at 250°F for:

   (A) 10 minutes
   (B) 15 minutes
   (C) 30 minutes
   (D) 40 minutes

4. The minimum exposure time for unwrapped instruments in a flash sterilizer that is set at 270°F (132°C) is:

   (A) 2 minutes
   (B) 3 minutes
   (C) 5 minutes
   (D) 7 minutes

5. When steam is used to sterilize rubber tubing or a catheter:

   (A) the lumen must be dried thoroughly before the process begins
   (B) a rubber band may be placed around it so it does not unwind
   (C) it should be fanfolded before wrapping
   (D) a residual of distilled water should be left inside the lumen

6. To be sterilized effectively, a linen pack must not weigh more than:

   (A) 12 lb
   (B) 14 lb
   (C) 16 lb
   (D) 18 lb

7. Gravity displacement utilizes _____ to destroy microorganisms.

   (A) gas
   (B) radiation
   (C) gamma rays
   (D) steam

8. The process called cavitation occurs in the:

   (A) moist heat sterilizer
   (B) ultrasonic cleaner
   (C) high-speed pressure sterilizer
   (D) washer-sterilizer

9. All of the following statements regarding instrument sets are true EXCEPT:

    (A) instruments must be placed in perforated trays
    (B) heavy instruments are placed on the bottom
    (C) all instruments must be closed
    (D) all detachable parts must be disassembled

10. All of the following statements regarding steam sterilization are true EXCEPT:

    (A) flat packages are placed on the shelf on edge
    (B) small packages, placed one on top of the other, are crisscrossed
    (C) basins are placed on their sides
    (D) solutions may be autoclaved along with other items as long as they are on a shelf alone

11. Wrapped basin sets may be sterilized by steam under pressure at 250°F for a minimum of:

    (A) 5 minutes
    (B) 10 minutes
    (C) 15 minutes
    (D) 20 minutes

12. Which of the following statements regarding the sterilization of basin sets is TRUE?

    (A) Basins must be separated by a porous material if they are nested.
    (B) Sponges and linen may be packaged inside the basin to be sterilized.
    (C) Basins are placed flat in the autoclave.
    (D) Basins must always be placed on the top shelf of the autoclave in a combined load.

13. Why would gas sterilization be chosen over steam sterilization?

    (A) It is less expensive.
    (B) It is less damaging to items.
    (C) It is faster.
    (D) It is more effective.

14. The chemical agent used in gas sterilization is:

    (A) ethylene glycol
    (B) ethacrynate sodium
    (C) ethyl chloride
    (D) ethylene oxide

15. What chemical system uses peracetic acid as the sterilant?

    (A) Ozone gas sterilization
    (B) STERIS
    (C) Sterrad
    (D) Vapor phase sterilizer

16. The lumen of a tubing undergoing ethylene oxide (ETO) sterilization is:

    (A) well lubricated
    (B) dried thoroughly
    (C) prepared with a residual of distilled water
    (D) prepared with a NaCl flush

17. The commercial name for glutaraldehyde is:

    (A) peracetic acid
    (B) phenol
    (C) Quats
    (D) Cidex

18. Who is responsible for transporting instrumentation postoperatively to the decontamination room following the surgical procedure:

    (A) STSR
    (B) circulator
    (C) first assistant
    (D) All of the above

19. Which organization regulates the production of biological sterilization test packs in house?

    (A) Centers for Disease Control and Prevention (CDC)
    (B) Food and Drug Administration (FDA)
    (C) American Medical Association (AMA)
    (D) Association for the Advancement of Medical Instrumentation (AAMI)

20. What is the shelf life of Cidex?

    (A) 14 days
    (B) 7 days
    (C) 1 month
    (D) Indefinite

21. In which procedure would the use of a high-level disinfectant be acceptable instrument preparation?

    (A) Suction lipectomy
    (B) Tracheotomy
    (C) Cystoscopy
    (D) Mediastinoscopy

22. In a high-speed flash sterilizer, unwrapped instruments are exposed for a minimum of:

    (A) 1 minute
    (B) 3 minutes
    (C) 5 minutes
    (D) 10 minutes

23. To kill spores, an item must be immersed in a 2% aqueous solution of glutaraldehyde for:

    (A) 20 minutes
    (B) 2 hours
    (C) 10 hours
    (D) 24 hours

24. When placing tubing in an activated glutaraldehyde solution, one should:

    (A) use a shallow container
    (B) be certain that the interior of the tubing is completely filled
    (C) moisten it thoroughly before submersion
    (D) Both B and C

25. What is the role of moisture in ETO sterilization?

    (A) The items will dry out during the process if no humidity is added.
    (B) The sterilizer will deteriorate from gas over a period of time if no moisture is added.
    (C) Dried spores are resistant to the gas, so they must be hydrated.
    (D) Moisture is not an essential element in gas sterilization.

26. "Slow exhaust" in a gravity displacement steam sterilizer is used for:

    (A) plastics
    (B) solutions
    (C) rubber
    (D) drape packs

27. What is the function of an aerator in ETO sterilization?

    (A) After the sterilization process, aeration is necessary to remove the toxic gas.
    (B) Recommendations are for the sterilizer and aerator to be part of the same machine.
    (C) It is used to aerate items before sterilization.
    (D) Both A and B

28. ETO destroys cells by:

    (A) interfering with the normal metabolism of the protein and reproductive processes
    (B) coagulating cell protein
    (C) converting ions to thermal and chemical energy, causing cell death
    (D) shrinking the cell

29. Activated glutaraldehyde is used to disinfect endoscopes for:

    (A) 5 minutes
    (B) 10 minutes
    (C) 20 minutes
    (D) 60 minutes

30. Toxic anterior segment syndrome (TASS) can be attributed to:

    (A) contaminated ultrasonic machines
    (B) enzymatic residue left on eye instrumentation
    (C) incomplete instrument cleaning
    (D) All of the above

31. The chemical sterilant used in the STERIS method of sterilizing is:

    (A) formaldehyde
    (B) Cidex
    (C) ETO
    (D) peracetic acid

32. How should basins be positioned in the autoclave for sterilization?

    (A) Stacked on top of each other
    (B) On their sides
    (C) Upside down
    (D) Does not matter

33. Gravity displacement steam sterilizers operate on the principle that:

    (A) air is heavier than steam
    (B) air and steam have equal weight
    (C) steam is heavier than air
    (D) water is heavier than air

34. The process of terminal decontamination follows every surgical case. Decontamination of the walls consists of:

    (A) cleaning all walls up to 3 ft
    (B) cleaning all walls up to 1 ft
    (C) spot cleaning where soiled
    (D) always cleaning with alcohol

35. Which of the following kills bacterial spores?

    (A) Sterilant
    (B) Germicide
    (C) Antiseptic
    (D) Fungicide

36. Instrumentation and equipment are processed according to their level of risk. This system is known as:

    (A) evidence-based practice
    (B) the Spaulding method
    (C) reprocessing
    (D) central monitoring

37. According to the Spaulding system, what risk is assigned to sterile body tissue, including the vascular system?

    (A) Critical
    (B) Semicritical
    (C) Noncritical
    (D) Intermediately critical

38. What method of sterilization is used on objects that cannot tolerate heat, moisture, and the presence of steam sterilization?

    (A) Gravity displacement
    (B) ETO
    (C) Hydrogen peroxide
    (D) Cidex

39. Glutaraldehyde is a high-level disinfectant, that is, a sporicidal, a bactericidal, and a viricidal. At a 2% concentration for _____, it is also a tuberculocidal.

    (A) 10 minutes
    (B) 15 minutes
    (C) 20 minutes
    (D) 40 minutes

40. Chemical monitors are placed inside and outside of all packs to be sterilized. These monitors show that:

    (A) the item is sterile
    (B) proper packaging is achieved
    (C) parameters, such as heat and pressure, have been reached
    (D) the proper time has been met

41. To achieve 270°F, the required pressure is:

    (A) 15 psi
    (B) 20 psi
    (C) 27 psi
    (D) 40 psi

42. Why is ETO diluted with an inert gas?

    (A) It increases its effective sterilization.
    (B) It adds convenience and speed.
    (C) It adds humidity.
    (D) It helps with aeration.

43. Bioburden refers to:

    (A) the degree of microbial contamination
    (B) a hospital-acquired infection
    (C) a chemical agent
    (D) high-level disinfectant

44. Sterility was previously measured by time, but this is now considered invalid. The principle now used is:

    (A) carefully checking sterile indicators
    (B) event-related sterility
    (C) terminal sterilization
    (D) Both B and C

45. All of the following statements regarding wrapping materials are true EXCEPT:

    (A) Disposable nonwoven wrappers are intended for one use only.
    (B) You can use two 140-thread count per square inch.
    (C) You can use one 280-thread count per square inch.
    (D) Peel pouches can be used on all instruments including large heavy instruments and micro instruments.

46. Gastrointestinal endoscopes are characterized as _____ under the Spaulding sterilization system.

    (A) critical
    (B) noncritical
    (C) semicritical
    (D) Scopes are not considered in the Spaulding system

47. All of the following are environmental disinfectants used for low-level disinfection and terminal decontamination EXCEPT:

    (A) glutaraldehyde
    (B) hypochlorite
    (C) quaternary ammonium compound
    (D) alcohol

48. Personal protective equipment (PPE) includes all of the following EXCEPT:

    (A) protective eyewear
    (B) facemask
    (C) surgical and/or patient care gloves
    (D) full protective body suit or gown

49. Most packaged sterilized equipment from a manufacturer such as sutures, sponges, and disposable drapes is sterilized by means of:

    (A) ETO
    (B) cobalt-60 (ionizing radiation)
    (C) gravity displacement sterilizer
    (D) quaternary ammonium compounds

50. Which of the following is not a method of sterilization but is a heating process that destroys microorganisms at a temperature and exposure time and does not alter their chemical makeup?

    (A) Decontamination
    (B) Pasteurization
    (C) Hydrogen peroxide plasma sterilization
    (D) ETO gas sterilization

51. Which type of immunity occurs when you are exposed to the disease and as a result you become immune?

(A) Naturally acquired active immunity

(B) Artificially acquired active immunity

(C) Artificially acquired passive immunity

(D) Naturally acquired passive immunity

52. An obligatory parasite is:

(A) a type of prion

(B) a type of microorganism that depends on living tissue to survive

(C) a type of microorganism that depends on dead tissue to survive facultative parasite

(D) All of the above

53. The only antibiotic that treats MRSA is:

(A) gentamycin

(B) amoxicillin

(C) tobramycin

(D) vancomycin

54. All of the following are true regarding prions EXCEPT:

(A) They cause Creutzfeldt-Jakob disease.

(B) They contain DNA/RNA.

(C) They are not viral, bacterial, or fungal.

(D) When performing surgery on a patient that is infected with a prion, disposable instruments should be used.

55. _____ is when different organisms exist and benefit from each other. _____ is when one organism benefits from the other and neither is harmed. _____ is when one organism benefits from the other and harms the host.

1. Parasitism, 2. Mutualism, 3. Commensalism

(A) 1, 2, 3

(B) 3, 2, 1

(C) 2, 3, 1

(D) 1, 3, 2

56. Bioterrorist agents include all of the following EXCEPT:

(A) anthrax

(B) botulism

(C) smallpox

(D) bubonic plague

57. New infectious diseases emerging in the United States include:

(A) SARS

(B) West Nile virus

(C) avian influenza

(D) All of the above

58. The chemical name for common household bleach is:

(A) sodium hypochlorite

(B) quaternary ammonium compounds

(C) petroleum products

(D) hydrogen peroxide

59. All of the following apply to immediate-use steam sterilization (IUSS) EXCEPT:

(A) items used for IUSS must always be wrapped

(B) implants should never be sterilized immediately before use except in a documented emergency situation when there is no other option

(C) immediate use sterilizers must be located where sterile items can be transported directly from the autoclave to the sterile field (ie, substerile room)

(D) items used for IUSS are never wrapped unless specified by the manufacturer

60. Instruments and equipment are processed according to their level of risk. This system is known as:

(A) ETO sterilization

(B) event-related sterility

(C) the Spaulding method

(D) instrument cleaning and disinfection

61. What is the test that is used to check for air trapped in the prevacuum sterilizer?

    (A) Biological indicator
    (B) Bowie-Dick test
    (C) Chemical indicator
    (D) Prevacuum test

62. The bacterial spore used in the biological indicator for steam sterilization is *Geobacillus stearothermophilus*. This is placed in the bottom front of the sterilizer, also known as the coldest point of the sterilizer. Following the sterilization process, the biological indicator is removed, crushed, and incubated. What should the color of the growth medium be if the spores were killed and the sterilization process was successful?

    (A) Fluorescent yellow
    (B) Red
    (C) Blue
    (D) It remains red for 60 minutes and then turns fluorescent yellow

63. All of the following are true of dry heat sterilization EXCEPT:

    (A) the indicator used for dry heat ovens is *B. atrophaeus*
    (B) it is used only in an emergency in the operating room
    (C) sterilization occurs in mechanical convection ovens
    (D) sterilization occurs in gravity convection ovens

64. Hydrogen peroxide plasma sterilization utilizes:

    (A) a cloud or glow of pink plasma sterilization
    (B) a chamber much like a microwave
    (C) a hydrogen peroxide solution
    (D) All of the above

65. In a gravity displacement sterilizer, steam enters the chamber at the _____.

    (A) bottom
    (B) bottom back
    (C) top rear
    (D) top front

66. ETO is mixed with carbon dioxide to:

    (A) increase antimicrobial effect
    (B) reduce flammability of ETO
    (C) reduce temperature requirement
    (D) increase microbial killing rate

67. How long should the ETO biological indicator be incubated before the reading is recorded?

    (A) 24 hours
    (B) 48 hours
    (C) 12 hours
    (D) 3 hours

68. For ETO sterilization, how long must instruments remain in the aerator being operated at 140°F?

    (A) 8 hours
    (B) 6 hours
    (C) 4 hours
    (D) 2 hours

69. What spore is used to test steam under pressure (steam sterilizer)?

    (A) *Clostridium perfringens*
    (B) *G. stearothermophilus*
    (C) *Treponema pallidum*
    (D) *Staphylococcus aureus*

70. All of the following apply to the daily air removal test (DART) test EXCEPT:

    (A) it is a preassembled type of Bowie-Dick test monitor
    (B) it is used in a prevacuum sterilizer
    (C) this test is done to determine that sterilization has occurred
    (D) this test is done daily to check for air removal and air entrapment

71. The bacteria used for the biological monitor in ETO is:

    (A) *G. stearothermophilus*
    (B) *Bacillus atrophaeus*
    (C) *Bacillus subtilis*
    (D) Both B and C

72. All of the following apply to the prevacuum autoclave EXCEPT:

    (A) it is also called a dynamic air removal autoclave
    (B) the vacuum pump located in the bottom front removes the air from the chamber
    (C) the Bowie-Dick test must be used to confirm air removal
    (D) the most common temperature used with the prevacuum sterilizer is 250°F 27 psi

73. Following a surgical procedure, the first step in the intraoperative decontamination process is for the STSR to rinse off the instruments with water and use a lap pad or towel to remove blood and debris. Once taken to the decontamination room, how soon should the instruments be cleaned?

    (A) Within 20 minutes
    (B) Within 1 hour
    (C) There is no set time constraint
    (D) According to manufacturer's instructions

Answers and Explanations

1. **(A)** Fifteen to seventeen pounds of pressure are necessary in the steam sterilizer set at 250°F. It is 27 psi if set at 270°F.

2. **(A)** Positive assurance that sterile conditions have been achieved by steam, ETO, or dry heat sterilization can be obtained only through a biological control test. These should be done at least weekly. The most dependable is a preparation of living spores resistant to the sterilizing agent.

3. **(C)** Instruments wrapped as a set in double-thickness wrappers are autoclaved at a setting of 250°F for 30 minutes.

4. **(B)** In a flash (high-speed pressure) sterilizer set at 270°F, the minimum exposure time is 3 minutes for unwrapped items. With this cycle, the entire time for starting, sterilizing, etc., is 6–7 minutes.

5. **(D)** Rubber tubing should not be folded or kinked because steam can neither penetrate it nor displace air from folds. A residual of distilled water should be left in the lumen. Rubber bands must not be used around solid items because steam cannot penetrate through or under rubber.

6. **(A)** Linen packs must not weigh more than 12 lb. Linen must be freshly laundered. Items must be fanfolded or loosely rolled.

7. **(D)** Gravity displacement utilizes steam under pressure to effect moist heat sterilization.

8. **(B)** The ultrasonic cleaner (which is not a sterilizer) utilizes ultrasonic energy and high-frequency sound waves. Instruments are cleaned by cavitation. In this process, tiny bubbles are generated by high-frequency sound waves. These bubbles generate minute vacuum areas that dislodge, dissolve, or disperse soil.

9. **(C)** Hinged instruments must be open with box locks unlocked to permit steam contact on all surfaces. All detachable parts should be disassembled.

10. **(D)** Solutions are sterilized alone on a slow exhaust cycle to prevent them from boiling over. The pressure gauge must read 0°F before opening the door. This is so the caps will not pop off.

11. **(D)** Wrapped basin sets are sterilized at 250°F for a minimum of 20 minutes. They are placed on their sides to allow air to flow out of them. This also helps water flow out.

12. **(A)** Basins and solid utensils must be separated by a porous material if they are nested to permit permeation of steam around all surfaces and condensation of steam from the inside during sterilization. Sponges and linen are not packaged in basins.

13. **(B)** ETO gas is an effective substitute for most items that cannot be sterilized by heat or that would be damaged by repeated exposure to heat. It is noncorrosive and does not damage items. It completely penetrates porous materials.

14. **(D)** ETO gas is used to sterilize items that are either heat or moisture sensitive. It kills microorganisms, including spores, by interfering with the normal metabolism of protein and reproductive processes.

15. **(B)** A proprietary (STERIS) chemical formulation of peracetic acid, hydrogen peroxide, and water causes cell death by inactivating the cell systems.

16. **(B)** Any tubing or other item with a lumen should be blown out with air to force dry before packaging because water combines with ETO gas to form a harmful acid, ethylene glycol.

17. **(D)** Glutaraldehyde, a high-level disinfectant, is known commercially as Cidex.

18. **(A)** The surgical technologist in the scrub role is responsible for transporting dirty instrumentation, equipment, and supplies to the decontamination room.

19. **(D)** The AAMI develops standards for the safety, use, and management of medical devices and health technologies. In regard to sterilization, it provides guidance to health care personnel who use steam for sterilization (the test packs containing the vial with the bacterial spore). The CDC provides health information on disease control and prevention. The FDA is responsible for protecting the public by providing information and regulating drugs, biological products, medical devices, food, cosmetics, and many other products. The AMA provides medical education.

20. **(A)** Glutaraldehyde must be renewed after 14 days because it becomes ineffective after that time.

21. **(C)** In cystoscopy, sterilization of instruments with steam or ETO provides the greatest elimination of the risk of infection; however, it is not essential. High-level disinfection is recommended and provides reasonable assurance that items are safe to use.

22. **(B)** The minimum exposure time at 270°F with 27 psi is 3 minutes for unwrapped nonporous items.

23. **(C)** Immersion in a 2% aqueous solution of activated, buffered alkaline glutaraldehyde is

sporicidal (kills spores) within 10 hours. It is chosen for heat-sensitive items that cannot be steamed or if ETO gas is unavailable or impractical.

24. **(B)** Lumens of instruments or tubing must be completely filled with solution. All items should be placed in a container deep enough to completely immerse them. All items should be dry before immersion so that the solution is not diluted.

25. **(C)** Moisture is essential in gas sterilization. Desiccated or highly dried bacterial spores are resistant to ETO gas; therefore, they must be hydrated in order for the gas to be effective.

26. **(B)** Solutions are sterilized alone on slow exhaust so solutions will not boil over and so caps will not blow off.

27. **(D)** An aeration process is essential for the ETO machine to remove the toxic gas. The most favorable situation is for them to be located in the same machine.

28. **(A)** ETO is a chemical agent that kills microorganisms, including spores. It interferes with the normal metabolism of protein and reproductive processes, resulting in cell death.

29. **(C)** A minimum of 20 minutes is used to kill vegetative bacteria, fungi, hepatitis B, and HIV. A minimum of 45 minutes is required for tuberculocidal activity.

30. **(D)** TASS is an acute inflammatory condition affecting the anterior segment of the eye containing the cornea, iris, ciliary body, and lens. It is seen postoperatively after cataract surgery. The condition is attributed to improper instrument reprocessing, including contaminated ultrasonic machines, enzymatic residue left on eye instrumentation, and incomplete instrument cleaning.

31. **(D)** Peracetic acid or acetic acid mixed with a solution of salts (Bionox) kills microorganisms. It is used only in the STERIS system for heat-sensitive and immersible instruments.

Processing is 20–30 minutes, and temperature is controlled at 131°F; it is cost effective and environmentally friendly.

32. **(B)** Basins, jars, cups, or other containers should be placed on their sides with the lid ajar so that air can flow out and steam can enter.

33. **(A)** Gravity displacement steam sterilizers operate on the principle that air is heavier than steam. Steam is forced into the inner chamber. Any air in the inner chamber blocks the passage of pressurized steam and prevents sterilization.

34. **(C)** Walls, doors, surgical lights, and ceilings are spot cleaned if they are soiled with blood tissue or body fluids.

35. **(A)** Spores are not killed unless an item is sterilized.

36. **(B)** The Spaulding system assigns a risk category that is specific to the regions of the body in which a device is to be used.

37. **(A)** Critical risk is assigned to sterile body tissues including the vascular system.

38. **(B)** ETO is used to sterilize objects that cannot tolerate heat, moisture, and the pressure of steam sterilization.

39. **(C)** Two percent glutaraldehyde is a tuberculocidal when an item is sterilized for 20 minutes.

40. **(C)** Subjecting items to the process of sterilization does not ensure that the item is sterile, but only that the parameters such as heat and pressure have been met.

41. **(C)** The laws of physics tell us that to raise the temperature of steam, we must also raise the pressure in the closed sterilization chamber; to achieve 270°F, the required pressure is 27 psi.

42. **(A)** When blended with inert gas, ETO produces effective sterilization by destroying DNA and the protein structure of microorganisms.

43. **(A)** Bioburden is the number and type of live bacterial colonies on the surface before it is sterilized.

44. **(D)** Event-related sterility or terminal sterilization is based on the principle that sterilized items are assumed sterile between uses unless environmental conditions or events interfere with the integrity of the package.

45. **(D)** Peel pouches are intended for lightweight instruments and devices.

46. **(C)** Gastrointestinal scopes come in contact with mucous membranes or nonintact skin. They are semicritical items.

47. **(A)** Environmental disinfectants that are used for routine low-level disinfection and terminal decontamination include phenolics, quats, hypochlorites, and alcohol. Glutaraldehyde is a high-level disinfectant known as Cidex commonly used on instruments.

48. **(C)** All staff members who work in the decontamination area must wear PPE in compliance with government regulations. Only gloves approved for contact with chemical disinfectants are used. Surgical gloves and patient care gloves are not permitted.

49. **(B)** Most equipment available that is packaged from the manufacturer has been sterilized by cobalt-60 or ionizing radiation. This process is restricted to commercial use because of its expense.

50. **(B)** Pasteurization is a heating process that destroys microorganisms at a certain temperature and exposure time but does not alter their chemical makeup.

51. **(A)** Naturally acquired active immunity is when you are exposed to the disease and as a result become immune. Artificially acquired active immunity is when you receive a vaccine and become immune. Artificially acquired passive immunity is when you receive immunization such as gamma globulin. It is a

short-term immunization. Naturally acquired passive immunity occurs during pregnancy when a pregnant woman passes the antibodies to her fetus through the bloodstream.

52. **(B)** An obligatory parasite is a type of microorganism that depends on living tissue to survive.

53. **(D)** Vancomycin is the antibiotic used to treat MRSA.

54. **(B)** Prions do not contain DNA/RNA.

55. **(C)** Mutualism, commensalism, and parasitism.

56. **(D)** Anthrax, botulism, and smallpox are bioterrorist agents.

57. **(D)** SARS, West Nile virus, and avian flu are all infectious diseases emerging in the United States.

58. **(A)** Sodium hypochlorite is the chemical name for household bleach.

59. **(A)** Items sterilized by IUSS should never be wrapped unless specified by the manufacturer. There are very strict guidelines for this.

60. **(C)** The Spaulding method is used to rate the level of risk when processing equipment.

61. **(B)** The Bowie-Dick test is used to check for air trapped in the prevacuum sterilizer. The biological indictor is the most effective indicator to prove sterility. A chemical indicator is tape used in the autoclave.

62. **(B)** The bacterial spore should remain red following the sterilization process. If it turns yellow, the results are positive, meaning the sterilization conditions were not met and the items are considered NOT sterile. The items in the load must immediately be recalled and reprocessed, and the autoclave must be checked for a malfunction.

63. **(B)** Heat sterilization is not just used during emergencies.

64. **(A)** Hydrogen peroxide plasma sterilization utilizes a cloud or glow of pink plasma covering the items to be sterilized.

65. **(C)** In the gravity displacement autoclave, steam enters at the top rear and displaces the air and exits through a drain at the front bottom of the chamber.

66. **(B)** ETO is mixed with carbon dioxide to reduce the flammability of the ETO.

67. **(B)** ETO biological indicators should be incubated for 48 hours before reading.

68. **(A)** Instruments must remain in the aerator cycle of the ETO at 140°F for 8 hours.

69. **(B)** *G. stearothermophilus* is the spore used to test steam under pressure sterilizers.

70. **(C)** The DART test is performed daily in a prevacuum sterilizer to make sure air is properly removed for the sterilization process to be performed properly.

71. **(D)** *B. atrophaeus* and *B. subtilis* can both be used for ETO; *G. stearothermophilus* is used in steam sterilization

72. **(D)** Prevacuum autoclaves are also called dynamic air removal autoclaves. A vacuum pump is used to evacuate the air, which is why a Bowie-Dick/DART test is required to make sure the air is removed. Prevacuum autoclaves work at higher temperatures of 270°F and 27 psi, and gravity sterilizers work at lower temperatures 250°F and 15–17 psi.

73. **(A)** Instruments should be washed within 20 minutes of arriving to the decontamination room to prevent blood and tissue from totally drying on the instruments, which makes the sterilization process more time consuming.

CHAPTER 7

Operating Room Environment

OPERATING ROOM ENVIRONMENT/SPECIALTY EQUIPMENT/FURNITURE

- Electrical outlets—operating rooms use 110- and 220-volt outlets. They must be mounted off the floor. They must be grounded and explosion proof
  - An example of a grounding system includes cords with a three-prong plug:
    - Current comes from the two upper prongs, and the third prong on the bottom is for grounding
- Suction—used during surgery and by anesthesia during intubation and extubation to remove blood, body fluids, and irrigation during surgery. It consists of:
  - Vacuum device—this can come from the ceiling, wall, or a portable unit
    - Neptune mobile suction unit—to remove waste, the unit can be relocated to a waste disposal area through a docking station
  - Each operating room should have at least two suction outlets, one for surgery and one for anesthesia
  - Collection canisters come as single or double canisters that are positioned in a carousel. They are used to collect and monitor the amount of body fluids and irrigation during the surgical procedures
  - Tubing from the surgical field and anesthesia is connected to the canister, and an additional tubing is connected to the suction device
  - The suction power can be adjusted according to what it is being used for
  - There are several types of suction tips and specialty equipment. They come as nondisposable and disposable

- Poole suction tip—commonly used for suctioning large amounts of fluid and irrigation in the abdomen
- Yankauer/tonsil suction tip—commonly used by anesthesia and also in other parts of the body
- Frazier suction tip—this is an angled tip with a small hole on the handpiece used to control the amount of suction needed. Fraziers also have a flexible stylet that is inserted into the lumen to clean the inside of the suction tip if it gets clogged. They come in various sizes
- Smith and Nephew Coblator—this instrument cauterizes, irrigates, and has a suction device attached to the instrument. Used on tonsils
- Special long suction tips are used on endoscopic procedures
- Gas outlets—these lines are piped into the operating rooms and must have manual shut-off valves outside the operating room
  - They can be wall-mounted, ceiling-mounted, and on a boom
  - Each line is specifically color coded, as follows:
    - Vacuum for suction
    - Oxygen—green
    - Nitrogen—black
    - Nitrous oxide—blue
    - Compressed air—yellow
- Overhead operating room lights—designed to be nonglaring with a blue-white beam to prevent eye fatigue
  - The lights have an intensity control on the light itself covered with a sterile light handle

so the light may be manipulated at the surgical field
- They are adjustable to many positions
- They should be damp dusted every morning prior to the first surgical procedure
- Ventilation systems—these systems remove:
  - Airborne contamination
  - Toxic fumes
  - Anesthesia gas
- Laminar air flow
  - This is a positive air pressure, unidirectional air flow
  - The air pressure in the operating room is kept at a higher pressure than the hallways; when the operating room door is opened, air is pushed out of the operating room instead of the air coming in and spreading airborne contaminates
- HEPA filters—High-efficiency particulate air
  - They remove dust particles and filter air
  - Air enters through the ceiling and exits from the grills near the floor
  - They remove bacteria particles in the air that are larger than 0.3 mm. It can remove bacteria as large as 0.5–5 mm
  - Air exchange should be:
    - Between 20 and 25 air exchanges per hour
    - No less than 15 air exchanges per hour
    - 20% should be fresh air from the outside that is filtered in
- X-ray viewing box—used to view patients' films prior to and during surgery
- OR table—operating room beds—should be positioned under the center of the operating room lights and away from the doors to prevent contamination from the outside corridors
  - They can be controlled manually or electrically
  - They have break points at the head, waist, knee, and foot
  - Weight limits vary
  - Special tables are used for bariatric patients
  - Parts of the operating room bed include:
    - Head piece/body/foot piece
    - Neuro/ortho attachments:
      - Mayfield headrest
      - Gardner-Wells tongs
      - Horseshoe headrests
  - Special operating room tables
    - Orthopedic fracture table

- Andrews—used for laminectomy procedures in the knee-chest position
- Jackson—used for cervical, thoracic, and lumbar procedures
- Wilson—used to support the patient's upper body for laminectomies, discectomies, and bladder stimulators
- Cystoscopy table—covered in Genitourinary (GU) chapter
- Hand table
- Pneumatic tourniquet—the tourniquet is used to create a bloodless surgical field by restricting blood flow to the operative site.
  - The tourniquet cuff is inflated with nitrogen or air
  - The widest cuff should be used and is determined by:
    - The size and weight of the patient
    - Size of the limb
    - Preexisting conditions of the patient
    - Type of surgery
  - The tourniquet should not be used on patients with:
    - Traumatic injury
    - Peripheral vascular disease
    - An infected limb
    - Deep vein thromboses (DVTs) in the operative limb
    - Poor skin conditions on the operative limb
    - On a limb that has an arteriovenous (AV) fistula/AV shunt
  - Protect the patient's skin by wrapping a lint-free padding around the limb and making sure the padding is free of wrinkles
  - Place the tourniquet cuff on the patient and connect the tubing to the inflation machine
  - The limb is exsanguinated first by elevating the limb for approximately 2 minutes and wrapping an Esmarch bandage—distal to proximal
  - The extremity is prepped and draped
  - The tourniquet is inflated at the pressure the surgeon decides. Surgeon should be notified when the cuff is inflated and notified after the first 60 minutes
    - The cuff on an upper limb can be inflated for 60 minutes
    - The cuff on a lower limb can be inflated for 90 minutes
  - Once the time limit has been reached, it is recommended practice that the tourniquet be

deflated for approximately 15 minutes before the limb is re-exsanguinated and the tourniquet reinflated
  - The recommended guidelines for tourniquet pressure are:
    - 50 mm Hg above the patient's systolic blood pressure for upper extremity
    - 100 mm Hg above the patient's systolic blood pressure for lower extremity
- Wall-mounted clock should have a start–stop timer and second hand if they need to track time on arterial occlusion, tourniquet, or cardiac arrest
- Intercom system—allows communication with the outside; examples include the front desk and pathology
  - It should have a floor-mounted intercom switch for the sterile members of the surgical team in the room
- Computers—computers, printers, and fax machines are at the front desk, and each operating room has its own computer. They are used to access patient records, films, and lab work. The circulator and surgeon use computers for patient charting, to communicate with other departments, to access surgeons' preference cards, and to access the operating room schedule, and so the patient's family can track the patient's progress in the operating room
  - Switch on the computer; startup process is termed "booting"
  - Screen background is termed "wallpaper"
  - Surfing the internet—allows you to look at different webpages and switch them
  - Scrolling—term used for moving up and down on a document
  - Word processing is the term for creating a document
  - Hard drive—the internal part of the computer that stores information
  - CD-ROM/DVD
  - Modem—helps send information
  - Task bar—shows documents; allows you to switch documents
  - Mouse—allows scrolling through documents; moves the cursor to different areas on the screen
  - Monitor—screen
  - Keyboard—enters characters and commands into the computer
  - WWW—World Wide Web—allows browsing the internet

  - E-mail—allows you to send a message and receive a message or forward a message
  - Computers allow you to:
    - Create, save, and print a document
    - Check spelling
    - Cut, copy, paste—move words and documents to another place on the document or to another document
    - Fonts—different styles of letters—you can change their color, make them bold, and change their size. The standard type size is 11/12
    - Bullets—can be designs or letters; allow you to list words and sentences
- TV systems—(closed-circuit) TVs can be mounted at the front desk and used to view what is going on in each operating room
  - They are also used to view endoscopic procedures and communicate with other departments so that procedures can be seen from other locations
- Microscopes—used to magnify the surgical field
  - Microscopes can be floor-mounted, ceiling-mounted, wall-mounted, and/or mounted to the operating room bed
  - They should be damp dusted prior to surgery
  - The microscope is draped by the STSR and the circulator. A clear drape is placed over the top part of the microscope and secured to the oculars with sterile lens covers and rubber bands
  - The microscope has two types of lenses. They include:
    - Objective lens
    - Ocular lens
  - The objective lens—closest to the object
  - The ocular lens—the eyepiece the surgeon looks through
  - Zoom lens—allows the surgeon to change the magnification at the surgical field; it is foot controlled
  - Illumination/lighting system
    - Coaxial illuminator—uses fiberoptics to transmit light. This light is cool to touch to protect patient tissues
    - Paraxial illuminator—uses light tubes, halogen bulbs, and focusing lenses
  - Beam splitter—allows the microscope to transmit the same image to the assistant's field of vision

- Magnifying power—ability of the microscope to magnify the image
- Resolving power—allows the microscope to differentiate and clarify details at the surgical field
- The surgeon uses a special chair when working with the microscope. The chair is on wheels, has hydraulic foot pedals to raise and lower as needed, and attached armrests to support surgeon's forearms for stability
- The STSR must carefully place instruments in the surgeon's hands and guide toward the surgical field because surgeon's field of vision is restricted. The surgeon does not want to take eyes off the surgical site
- C-arm—a mobile image intensifier used to take pictures
  - The fluoroscopy allows films to be taken while still and with movement in real time. It is controlled by a foot pedal
  - It is called a C-arm because of its obvious shape
  - X-rays can be taken in lateral or anterior positions
  - Both the patient and staff must wear a lead apron to protect the testicles and ovaries. A thyroid collar is worn to protect the thyroid. Do not turn your unprotected back to the C-arm
  - Do not bend or twist lead aprons as that could damage the lead
  - The C-arm delivers high doses of radiation. The surgeon and staff should limit the time their hands are exposed or wear lead gloves
  - All personnel working with fluoroscopy should be monitored for exposure time. An x-ray badge is worn at the neck and routinely checked
  - While the fluoroscopy is in use, it is recommended to stand at least 1 ft from the machine, or further if possible
  - A special drape is used to protect the surgical field from contamination
- Mini C-arm—smaller version of the original C-arm commonly used on hands and feet
- Head light—adjustable head piece worn by the surgeon to provide a concentrated beam of light to the surgical field. The head piece is connected to the light source by a fiberoptic cord. It is important for those who handle this piece

of equipment not to overbend the cord because the fiberoptics can be damaged
- ESU—electrosurgical unit. Bipolar electrocautery/bipolar cautery—the current is delivered to the surgical site and returned to the generator by forceps. The current passes between the tips of the forceps. One tip is active; the other is inactive
- Monopolar electrosurgery—current flows from the generator to the active electrode (Bovie handpiece), to the patient, to the inactive dispersive electrode, and back to the generator
- Coagulating current—current that passes through the active electrode (Bovie handpiece) with intense heat to burn and control bleeding vessels
- Cutting current—current used to cut tissue
- Blended current—current that can be used to provide hemostasis to tissue and cut tissue
- Generator—power source; the machine that produces the current by using high-frequency radio
- Inactive dispersive electrode—pad used to return the current back to the generator. Also referred to as the grounding pad, inactive electrode, or return electrode
- Active electrode—handpiece or active electrode directs the current to the target tissue
- Smoke evacuator—used to suction large amounts of smoke from ESU or laser
  - It has a filtration system that can trap particles and toxic plumes. The filters should be changed between patients because they are considered biohazard materials
  - The suction tip should be held as close to the target area as possible (2 in) for effectiveness
- Doppler—used to access blood flow through a vessel by sound. It can be used pre-, intra-, or postoperatively. A sterile drape is used to cover the probe when used during a surgical procedure
- Booms—ceiling-mounted arms that contain surgical equipment
- Cabinets—contain operating room supplies. They should always remain closed. Patient care gloves should be removed before entering the cabinet for additional supplies
- Doors—should always be kept closed except when the patient is entering or exiting the operating room to prevent traffic and outside contamination

OPERATING ROOM FURNITURE

- Back table—it is used to create the sterile field for the surgical procedure. The sterile pack is opened on the back table, and operating room sterile supplies and instruments are set up on the back table. They come in various sizes and heights, with some being double-tiered
- Mayo stand—used for instruments and supplies that are being used immediately for the surgical procedure. It is moved to the operative field and placed over the patient. It has an adjustable height and can be raised simply by pulling it up
- Utility table, prep table, gown and glove table—used for all of the above-mentioned purposes
- Kick bucket—used for sponges that have been used during the surgical procedure—not garbage. They are low on the floor and maneuvered with your foot
- Ring stands—come single or double and hold basins that contain solutions used during the surgical procedures
- Standing stool/sitting stool—should be positioned before opening the sterile field to avoid contamination
- Trash containers and linen hampers—have foot control pedals so the STSR can open them
- IV poles
- Lead door—used to protect staff from x-rays
- Cautery machine—explained in the chapter on electricity

Questions

1. The room temperature in an operating room (OR) should be:

   (A) below 50°F
   (B) below 60°F
   (C) between 68°F and 76°F
   (D) between 80°F and 86°F

2. The most effective protection from the radiation of x-rays is a:

   (A) lead apron
   (B) double-thick muslin apron
   (C) 3-ft distance from machine
   (D) 3-ft distance from patient

3. It is considered good technique to:

   (A) change your mask only if it becomes moistened
   (B) hang the mask around the neck
   (C) crisscross the strings over the head
   (D) handle the mask only by the strings

4. Electrical cords should be:

   (A) removed from outlets by the cord
   (B) wrapped tightly around equipment
   (C) removed from pathways so equipment is not rolled over them
   (D) disconnected from the unit before disconnection from the wall

5. Scatter radiation effects are directly related to:

   (A) when the beam interacts with the patient's body and spreads out in different directions
   (B) accumulation of radioactive substances in the OR
   (C) a break in the lead apron
   (D) orthopedic surgical procedures

6. Room temperature for infants and children should be maintained as warm as:

   (A) 70°F
   (B) 80°F
   (C) 85°F
   (D) 95°F

7. Areas needing cleaning attention on a weekly basis include:

   (A) OR furniture
   (B) air vents and heating ducts
   (C) mounted lighting tracks, ceilings, walls
   (D) both B and C

8. A glass suction bottle should ideally be:

   (A) rinsed with tap water between each case
   (B) cleaned with a disinfectant solution and autoclaved before reuse
   (C) rinsed with sterile distilled water between each case
   (D) autoclaved daily

9. Storage shelves must be cleaned with a germicide:

   (A) each case
   (B) each day
   (C) each week
   (D) each month

10. While a surgical case is in progress:

    (A) doors remain open so that staff can easily move in or out
    (B) doors should remain closed
    (C) doors remain open to circulate air
    (D) doors may be opened or closed

11. When cleaning the floor between cases for routine decontamination, the procedure is:

    (A) to use a disinfectant and wet vacuum
    (B) to use a two-bucket system: one detergent and one clear water
    (C) that buckets should be emptied and cleaned between cases
    (D) to use a clean mop head

12. If a sterile item falls to the floor:

    (A) it may be used immediately only if the wrapper has no implosion holes and the floor is clean and dry
    (B) it may be used or returned to the shelf if there are no implosion holes and the floor is clean and dry
    (C) it may be used or returned to the shelf if it is double wrapped in muslin
    (D) it can never be used

13. The following comply with the protocol for protective eyewear EXCEPT:

    (A) impervious face shields can be worn
    (B) goggles can be worn
    (C) prescribe eyeglasses
    (D) all eye covers must extend from the front to the side

14. Which statement regarding OR attire is true?

    (A) Head caps and hoods must be worn to reduce contamination from hair and dander onto the field.
    (B) Long sleeve, nonsterile cover jackets are worn by nonsterile personnel to prevent contamination by bacterial shedding of their arms.
    (C) The scrub suit is worn by both sterile and nonsterile personnel.
    (D) All of the above

15. All of the following statements are true in preparing nonsterile equipment EXCEPT:

    (A) make sure the OR table is positioned directly under surgical lights
    (B) arrange the room according to how the surgical tech likes it
    (C) place furniture so that draped sterile tables are no closer than 12–18 in to a nonsterile surface
    (D) pretest suction lines for adequate pressure

16. All are recommendations for opening a case EXCEPT:

    (A) when opening packages sealed with tape, break the tape rather than tearing it
    (B) open the scrub gown on to the back table
    (C) never unwrap a heavy item while holding it in mid air
    (D) when opening instruments in closed sterilization trays, break the seal and lift top straight up and away from the tray

17. Excessive exposure to radiation can affect the:

    (A) integumentary system
    (B) brain
    (C) reproductive organs
    (D) stomach

18. Radiation exposure of the staff is monitored with:

    (A) a homing device
    (B) a Holter monitor
    (C) film badges
    (D) a notation on each operative record

19. During a craniotomy procedure, a specialty instrument falls to the floor. The physician wants the instrument sterilized immediately (immediate-use steam sterilization [IUSS]). Why is this not considered an acceptable practice?

    (A) The autoclave is located in a room adjacent to the OR, and transferring the instrument may not be safe.
    (B) Items used for IUSS may be required to be wrapped, and there are no wrappers available.
    (C) Only specific instruments may be sterilized.
    (D) The manufacturer guidelines are not the same for all instruments.

20. An OR hazard that has been linked to increased risk of spontaneous abortion in female OR employees is exposure to:

    (A) x-ray control
    (B) radium
    (C) sterilization agents
    (D) waste anesthetic gas

21. While using this mixture, a scavenging system is used to collect and exhaust or absorb its vapors. The mixture is called:

    (A) glutaraldehyde
    (B) polypropylene
    (C) methyl methacrylate
    (D) halon

22. How is inhalation of the laser plume best prevented?

    (A) Double mask worn by scrub team
    (B) Filter on suction
    (C) Laser on standby whenever possible
    (D) Mechanical smoke evacuator on field

23. A Cavitron unit is used for:

    (A) ultrasonic ablation and aspiration in tumor surgery
    (B) ultrasonic energy for the destruction of cataracts
    (C) freezing and removing abnormal tissue
    (D) treating glaucoma

24. The power source for Hall's power equipment is:

    (A) carbon dioxide
    (B) nitrous oxide
    (C) nitrogen
    (D) electricity

25. The power source for air-powered dermatomes is:

    (A) compressed nitrogen
    (B) nitrous oxide
    (C) air
    (D) either A or C

26. Suction tubing should be processed in the following way:

    (A) residual of distilled water in lumen, steam sterilize, tubing coiled
    (B) residual of saline in lumen, ethylene oxide sterilization (ETO), tubing coiled
    (C) lumen dried thoroughly, ETO, tubing banded
    (D) either A or B

27. The suction tip that is right angled and is used for small amounts of fluid such as in brain surgery is:

    (A) Poole
    (B) Ferguson-Frazier
    (C) Yankauer
    (D) Tungsten

28. Which suction tip has an angle and is used in the mouth or throat?

(A) Ferguson
(B) Ferguson-Frazier
(C) Poole
(D) Yankauer

29. A tourniquet is used in the OR to:

(A) prevent nerve damage
(B) minimize blood loss during the surgical procedure
(C) provide a bloodless field and better visualization of the surgical site
(D) both B and C

30. Exsanguination of a limb before tourniquet inflation is accomplished with wrapping the elevated extremity with:

(A) Kling
(B) Esmarch
(C) Stockinette
(D) Webril

31. The amount of pressure used to inflate a tourniquet depends on all of the following EXCEPT:

(A) patient's age
(B) size of extremity
(C) depth of surgical incision
(D) systolic blood pressure

32. A regional block that uses the tourniquet is a/an:

(A) Bier block
(B) intrathecal block
(C) peridural block
(D) field block

33. The tourniquet is contraindicated if:

(A) patient's circulation to distal part of extremity is poor
(B) patient is elderly
(C) patient is obese
(D) patient has epidural anesthesia

34. At what point should the surgeon be informed of the time of tourniquet application?

(A) After 15 minutes, then every 5 minutes
(B) After 1 hour, then every 15 minutes
(C) After 2 hours, then every hour
(D) After 3 hours, then every 15 minutes

35. When would the use of Esmarch be contraindicated?

(A) Patient has had previous anesthesia.
(B) Patient has had recent injury.
(C) Patient has had recent cast.
(D) Both B and C

36. Which agent or power source is NOT used with the pulse lavage irrigator?

(A) Nitrogen
(B) Battery powered
(C) Electrical
(D) Oxygen

37. A precaution necessary when using a pneumatic tourniquet is:

(A) limb must be continually elevated
(B) tourniquet time must not exceed 20 minutes
(C) solutions must be prevented from pooling under tourniquet
(D) inflation is done before prep and draping

38. In which procedure would a tourniquet be contraindicated?

(A) Tendon repair, child
(B) Arthroscopy, adult
(C) Bunionectomy
(D) Gangrenous toe amputation

39. All of the following statements regarding a grounding plate for electrosurgery are true EXCEPT:

(A) the plate must have good contact with the patient's skin

(B) the plate must be lubricated with electrosurgical gel

(C) the plate must be placed directly over a bony prominence

(D) the grounded pathway returns the electrical current to the unit after the surgeon delivers it to the operative site

40. A grounding pad is not required for the electrocautery in:

(A) a cutting current setting

(B) a coagulation current setting

(C) a monopolar unit

(D) a bipolar unit

41. The inactive electrode of the cautery is the:

(A) grounding pad

(B) electrocautery pencil

(C) cable connecting pad to pencil

(D) blade tip pencil

42. The electrical circuit of the electrocautery is complete when:

(A) current flows from generator to inactive electrode, through tissue, and back to generator

(B) current flows from active electrode to generator, to tissue, and returns

(C) current flows to and from the generator to patient via the active electrode

(D) current flows from the generator to active electrode, through tissue, and back to generator via the inactive electrode

43. Why must the electrocautery tip be kept clean?

(A) To ensure electrical contract effectiveness

(B) To avoid fire via accidental drape ignition

(C) To prevent burn injuries to staff

(D) To prevent circuit overload

44. In electrosurgery, "buzzing" refers to:

(A) coagulation of vessel via a metal instrument touching the active electrode

(B) coagulation of tissue via a metal instrument touching the inactive electrode

(C) cutting current

(D) blended current (cutting and coagulating simultaneously)

45. Which electrosurgical unit provides precise control of the coagulated area?

(A) Monopolar

(B) Blended

(C) Bipolar

(D) Bovie

46. Which condition is MOST acceptable when using electrocautery?

(A) Ground pad placed on scar or hairy area

(B) Ground pad placed on patient's forearm

(C) Ground pad placed on skin over metal implant

(D) Ground pad placed close to operative site

47. When using the phacoemulsifier:

(A) ultrasonic energy is used to fragment, irrigate, and aspirate the cornea in the eye

(B) the machine uses cavitation

(C) aspirated fluids are replaced with irrigation of balanced salt solution to maintain the anterior chamber

(D) both B and C

48. A cautery would not be used:

(A) when Betadine skin prep is used

(B) in cases requiring irrigation

(C) in neck or nasopharynx surgery if nitrous oxide is used

(D) in hernia repair if an epidural is used

49. Why are only moist sponges utilized during electrocautery use?

   (A) To prevent snagging of sponges on a cautery tip
   (B) To prevent fire
   (C) To reflect beam
   (D) None of the above

50. HEPA filters exchange the air in the OR how many times per hour?

   (A) Between 10 and 15
   (B) Between 15 and 25
   (C) 10
   (D) Less than 10

51. Fulguration via the resectoscope is accomplished by the use of a/an _____ tip.

   (A) electrode
   (B) ball
   (C) blade
   (D) needle

52. Fiberoptic lighting is:

   (A) a cool light
   (B) made of plastic fibers
   (C) of low intensity
   (D) powered by battery

53. All are precautions when handling fiberoptic cables EXCEPT:

   (A) light cables should be dropped or swing free when carried
   (B) cables are coiled loosely, with no kinking
   (C) heavy items are not laid on cables
   (D) cables are only gas sterilized

54. Fiberoptic cable integrity is questionable when:

   (A) illumination is bright
   (B) dark spots are evident
   (C) tubing has been coiled
   (D) tubing is scratched

55. When using a fiberoptic cable, how are burns and fires prevented?

   (A) The cable is kept away from drapes when disconnected from the endoscope.
   (B) Personnel should not lean on a cable end that is disconnected but is still on.
   (C) The cable end is kept on a moist towel when disconnected from endoscope.
   (D) All of the above

56. Loupes are used for:

   (A) tissue retraction
   (B) magnification
   (C) hemostasis
   (D) patient transfer

57. Resolving power of an operating microscope means:

   (A) the ability to discern detail
   (B) the ability to enlarge the image
   (C) the adaptation of operative procedure to individual patient requirements
   (D) the ratio of image size on viewer's retina with and without magnification

58. Which item in the optical lens system is responsible for magnification?

   (A) Oculars
   (B) Paraxial illuminators
   (C) Objective lens
   (D) Both A and C

59. The range of focal lengths of the objective lenses in the operating microscope is:

   (A) 0–100 mm
   (B) 100–200 mm
   (C) 100–400 mm
   (D) 5–25 mm

60. A continuously variable magnification system is afforded to the eye surgeon by the:

    (A) broadview viewing lens
    (B) microadapter
    (C) zoom lens with foot control
    (D) couplings

61. The purpose of the "slit" lamp in eye surgery is:

    (A) defining depth perception
    (B) focusing ability
    (C) magnifying power
    (D) discerning detail

62. The operating microscope that visually employs fiberoptics for its light source is:

    (A) halogen
    (B) tungsten
    (C) coaxial illuminators
    (D) paraxial illuminators

63. Care of the microscope would include all of the following EXCEPT:

    (A) damp dust external surfaces with detergent-disinfectant before use
    (B) damp dust lenses with detergent-disinfectant before use
    (C) enclose in an antistatic plastic cover when not in use
    (D) clean casters before each use

64. The purpose of the beam splitter in an operating microscope is to:

    (A) coincide the assistant's field of view with the surgeon's
    (B) increase light intensity
    (C) decrease vibration
    (D) narrow the beam of light

65. The colpomicroscope affords a view of the:

    (A) fallopian tube
    (B) intraperitoneal structures
    (C) cervix
    (D) uterine endometrium

66. The procedure that uses a self-retaining laryngoscope and microscope is called a/an:

    (A) indirect laryngoscopy
    (B) direct laryngoscopy
    (C) suspension microlaryngoscopy
    (D) laser microlaryngoscopy

67. The binocular microscope provides stereoscopic vision. This refers to:

    (A) the view afforded by double eyepieces
    (B) the color projected on the field
    (C) the magnification capability
    (D) the illumination process

68. Which magnifying powers are available for the microscope eyepieces?

    (A) 1×, 2×, 3×, and 4×
    (B) 10×, 20×, 30×, and 40×
    (C) 10×, 12.5×, 16×, and 20×
    (D) 300 mm, 400 mm, 500 mm, and 600 mm

69. Which procedure is inappropriate when caring for optic lenses?

    (A) Blood, water, and irrigating solutions are removed with cotton-tipped applicators and distilled water.
    (B) Lens is always cleaned in a circular motion, beginning at the center.
    (C) Oil or fingerprints are removed by soaking in solvent for 10 minutes and drying with a cotton ball.
    (D) Lint or dust is removed with a lens brush or rubber bulb syringe.

70. The OR bed may have a metal crossbar between the two upper sections, which may be raised to elevate the:

    (A) kidney
    (B) breast
    (C) gallbladder
    (D) both A and C

71. The smallest diameter on a French scale is a:

    (A) 3
    (B) 5
    (C) 7
    (D) 9

72. Which of the following is a motorized device whose action prevents venous stasis and reduces risk of deep vein clotting in high-risk patients?

    (A) Pneumatic antishock garment
    (B) Military antishock trousers (MAST)
    (C) Thromboembolic-deterrent stockings
    (D) Sequential pneumatic compression boots

73. A blood flow detector is a:

    (A) Doppler
    (B) Gruentzig
    (C) Moretz
    (D) Warren

74. All apply to cryotherapy EXCEPT:

    (A) it uses liquid nitrogen, Freon, or CO_2
    (B) the insulated probe uses extreme heat to destroy diseased tissue
    (C) the insulated probe uses extreme cold to destroy diseased tissue
    (D) both A and C

75. The mobile suction unit is called:

    (A) Neptune
    (B) Smith and Nephew
    (C) Andrews
    (D) Saturn

76. What is the all-in-one instrument used to cauterize, irrigate, and suction simultaneously?

    (A) Yankauer
    (B) Coblator
    (C) Neptune
    (D) Poole

77. What color is the gas outlet used for oxygen?

    (A) Blue
    (B) Yellow
    (C) Black
    (D) Green

78. All pertain to laminar air flow EXCEPT:

    (A) maintains positive pressure
    (B) maintains negative pressure
    (C) has unidirectional airflow
    (D) maintains a higher pressure in the OR

79. HEPA filters remove bacterial particles that are:

    (A) larger than 0.3 mm
    (B) smaller than 0.3 mm
    (C) 0.3–0.5 mm
    (D) both A and C

80. HEPA filters exchange the air in the OR how many times per hour?

    (A) Between 20 and 25
    (B) Between 10 and 15
    (C) 10
    (D) Less than 10

81. All are facts regarding OR tables EXCEPT:

    (A) they have break points at head, waist, knee, and foot
    (B) they can be controlled manually or electrically
    (C) there is no weight limit
    (D) they are positioned under the OR lights and away from main door

82. Neurosurgery attachments include all EXCEPT:

    (A) Mayfield
    (B) Gardner-Wells
    (C) Horseshoe
    (D) Alvarado

83. Special OR tables used for spine surgery include all EXCEPT:

    (A) Andrews
    (B) fracture table
    (C) Jackson
    (D) Wilson

84. When is the standing stool positioned?

    (A) Before the opening of the sterile field to avoid contamination
    (B) After the surgical prep and prior to draping
    (C) Prior to incision
    (D) There is no specific time to position the stool.

85. Chest rolls are used to:

    (A) help secure the patient
    (B) assist with respirations
    (C) prevent pressure wounds
    (D) assist patients with back injuries

86. Which of the following apply to electrical accidents and/or their prevention?

    (A) The most common injury to the STSR is the ESU.
    (B) All electrical equipment must be grounded.
    (C) Always turn the electrical equipment on/off before unplugging from the power plug.
    (D) All of the above

87. Staff who must remain in the OR when using ionizing radiation should maintain a distance of how many feet from the radiation beam?

    (A) 3 ft
    (B) 4 ft
    (C) 5 ft
    (D) At least 6 ft

88. The device used to measure cumulative radiation exposure is called a:

    (A) radiograph monitor
    (B) dosimeter
    (C) film badge
    (D) both B and C

89. A fire requires three main components. Which is NOT considered a component?

    (A) Oxygen
    (B) Fuel
    (C) Temperature
    (D) Source of ignition

90. Proper body ergonomics include all EXCEPT:

    (A) do not bend at the knees when lifting a heavy object
    (B) when you need to reach upward, never twist your body or balance on one foot
    (C) pushing an object is the preferred method of moving objects rather than pulling
    (D) musculoskeletal injury can result from stress, lack of balance, repetitive motion, and overexertion

Answers and Explanations

1. **(C)** Room temperature is maintained within a range of 68–76°F.

2. **(A)** Lead-lined aprons should be worn to protect the staff from radiation, especially during the use of an image intensifier. Thyroid collars are also particularly useful for protection.

3. **(D)** Masks should be handled only by the strings, thereby keeping the facial area of the mask clean. The mask should never be worn around the neck. Upper strings are tied at the top of the head; lower strings are tied behind the neck because crisscrossing distorts mask contours and makes the mask less efficient.

4. **(C)** Electrical cords should not be kinked, curled, or tightly wrapped. They should be handled by the plug, not the cord, when disconnecting. Always remove cords from pathways before rolling in equipment because this can break the cord.

5. **(A)** Scatter radiation occurs in the OR when the beam interacts with the patient's target tissue and spreads out in different directions.

6. **(C)** Infants and children are kept warm to minimize heat loss and prevent hypothermia; 85°F should be maintained.

7. **(D)** Weekly cleaning in the operating room includes ceilings, walls, and floors inside outside of the OR room, mounted lighting tracks and fixtures, air vents and grill ducts, supply cabinets and shelving, and supply rooms and linen rooms.

8. **(B)** Glass suction bottles should be thoroughly cleaned with a disinfectant solution and autoclaved before reuse.

9. **(C)** Storage areas should be cleaned at least weekly to control dust.

10. **(B)** Doors should be closed during and in between cases to reduce the microbial count.

11. **(A)** A wet vacuum system is the best. However, if mopping is to be utilized, a clean mop is used. Each time the mop is used, a two-bucket system is recommended (detergent germicide and clear water), and the buckets must be emptied and cleaned between uses.

12. **(A)** It may be used immediately only if the item was not compromised with an implosion hole and the floor was clean and dry. It should never be put back into the cabinet. It MUST be used immediately.

13. **(C)** Protocol for the eyes say eyes must be covered from the brow to the top of the surgical mask and must extend over the temples. Prescription eyeglasses are not protocol.

14. **(D)** All of the above statements are true.

15. **(B)** OR furniture should be arranged in a manner that prevents contamination of sterile surfaces by traffic and by nonsterile equipment and also to prevent clutter.

16. **(B)** The scrub person's gown and gloves should be opened on a small table or Mayo stand, not a back table.

17. **(C)** Exposure to radiation can cause genetic changes, cancer, cataracts, injury to bone marrow, burns, tissue necrosis, and spontaneous abortion and congenital anomalies.

18. **(C)** Film badges are the most widely used monitors measuring total REMs of accumulated exposure. Data are reviewed.

19. **(D)** The manufacturer's guidelines are not the same for all instruments. Exposure time and temperature may vary. Unless you have the manufacturer's guidelines for that particular instrument, you should not do it.

20. **(D)** Waste anesthetic gas is gas and vapor that escape from the anesthesia machine and equipment, as well as gas released through the patient's expiration. The hazards to personnel include an increased risk of spontaneous abortion in females working in the OR, congenital abnormalities in their children as well as in the offspring of unexposed partners of exposed male personnel, cancer in females administering anesthesia, and hepatic and renal disease in both males and females. This problem can be reduced by a scavenging system that removes waste gases.

21. **(C)** Methyl methacrylate, bone cement, is mixed at the sterile field. Vapors are irritating to eyes and respiratory tract. It may be a mutagen, a carcinogen, or toxic to the liver. It can cause allergic dermatitis. A scavenging system is used to collect vapor during mixing and exhaust it to the outside or absorb it through activated charcoal.

22. **(D)** A mechanical smoke evacuator or suction with a high-efficiency filter removes toxic substances including carcinogens and viruses from the air. Personnel should not inhale the fumes.

23. **(A)** Cavitron ultrasonic surgical aspirator (CUSA) is used for ablation and aspiration in tumor surgery. Phacoemulsification uses ultrasonic energy for the destruction of cataracts. Cryosurgery uses extreme cold to destroy abnormal tissues such as tumors.

Cyclodialysis is a surgical treatment option for glaucoma.

24. **(C)** The power source is inert, nonflammable, and explosion-free gas. Compressed nitrogen is the power source for all air-powered equipment.

25. **(D)** Dermatomes may be electric or air powered with compressed nitrogen or air.

26. **(A)** A residual of distilled water should be left in the lumen of any tubing to be sterilized by steam. Tubing should be coiled without kinks and disassembled from suction tips. Rubber bands prevent steam penetration.

27. **(B)** A right-angled tube with a small diameter used for small amounts of fluid such as in brain, spinal, plastic, or orthopedic surgery is Ferguson-Frazier.

28. **(D)** The Yankauer tonsil tip is a hollow tube, with an angle, used in the mouth and throat.

29. **(D)** The two main purposes of the tourniquet for surgery are to minimize the amount of blood loss during the surgical procedure and to create a bloodless field. Nerve damage can be caused by improper placement of the cuff or excessive tourniquet pressure.

30. **(B)** While elevated, the extremity is wrapped distally to proximally with an Esmarch rubber bandage to exsanguinate the limb. The tourniquet is then inflated.

31. **(C)** The patient's age, the size of extremity, and the patient's systolic pressure are all factors to be considered when applying a tourniquet. The depth of the incision is of no consequence.

32. **(A)** A Bier is a regional intravenous injection of a local anesthetic to an extremity below the level of the tourniquet. The extremity remains painless as long as the tourniquet is in place.

33. **(A)** A tourniquet should never be used when direct circulation in the distal part of an

extremity is impaired. It could cause tissue injury, shutting off blood supply to the part below and causing gangrene and loss of the extremity.

34. **(B)** Tourniquet application and removal times are recorded. The surgeon is informed when the tourniquet has been on for 1 hour and then every 15 minutes.

35. **(D)** If the patient has had a traumatic injury or casting, danger exists that thrombi might be in vessels because of injury or stasis of blood. These could become dislodged and result in emboli.

36. **(D)** The pulse lavage irrigator is powered by nitrogen, is battery powered, and uses electrical energy to irrigate a traumatic or surgical wound.

37. **(C)** Caution must be taken to prevent solution from pooling under a tourniquet. Apply tourniquet and drape position before tourniquet is inflated.

38. **(D)** Tourniquets are not used if circulation is compromised. Arthroscopy, bunionectomy, and tendon repair on a child would be indications for use.

39. **(C)** The ground plate or inactive electrode is lubricated with an electrosurgical gel and is placed in good contact with a fleshy, nonhairy body surface. It should not be placed over a bony prominence. The grounded pathway returns the electrical current to the unit after the surgeon delivers it to the operative site.

40. **(D)** Bipolar units provide a completely isolated output with negligible leakage of current between the tips of the forceps. The need for a dispersive pad is eliminated.

41. **(A)** The dispersive pad is the inactive electrode. It is placed as close to the operative site as possible, on the same side of the body as the operative site and over a large muscle if possible. Bony prominences and scar tissue should be avoided. Good contact is essential.

42. **(D)** To complete the electric circuit to coagulate or cut tissue, current must flow from a generator (power unit) to an active electrode, through tissue, and back to the generator via the inactive electrode.

43. **(A)** The tip is kept clean, dry, and visible. Charred or coagulated tissue is removed by wiping with a tip cleaner or scraping with the back of a knife blade. Charred tissue on the electrode absorbs heat and decreases effectiveness of current.

44. **(A)** Vessels are coagulated when any part of the metal instrument is touched with the active electrode. It is known as buzzing.

45. **(C)** The bipolar cautery provides extremely precise control of the coagulated area.

46. **(D)** The ground plate should be as close as possible to the site where the active electrode will be used to minimize current through the body.

47. **(D)** The opacified lens in cataract surgery is fragmented, irrigated, and aspirated by cavitation (ultrasonic energy). Aspirated fluids are replaced with irrigation of balanced salt solution to maintain the anterior chamber.

48. **(C)** Electrosurgery is not used in the mouth, around the head, or in the pleural cavity when high concentrations or oxygen or nitrous oxide are used because of fire and explosion hazards.

49. **(B)** Only moist sponges should be permitted on a sterile field while the electrosurgical unit is in use to prevent fire.

50. **(B)** The air exchange per hour with HEPA filters is between 15 and 25.

51. **(A)** Fulguration of a tumor is accomplished by use of a cutting electrode to destroy tissue. It both cuts and coagulates.

52. **(A)** Fiberoptic lighting is an intense cool light that illuminates body cavities via a bundle

of thousands of coated glass fibers. It is nonglaring.

53. **(A)** Light cables should never be dropped or swung while carrying.

54. **(B)** A simple test for the integrity of the cable is to hold one end of the cable to a bright light and inspect the opposite end. Dark spots are an indication that some of the fibers are broken.

55. **(D)** Light is cold, meaning that the heat is not transmitted throughout the scope and tissue is not damaged. The ends, however, can get hot and should be kept out of contact with patient and personnel skin. Keep cable away from drapes, or place on moist towel to prevent burns and fires.

56. **(B)** Loupes are glasses with telescopic lenses used for magnification in microvascular surgery and nerve repair.

57. **(A)** The ability to discern detail is known as resolving power or resolution.

58. **(D)** The optical combination of the objective lens and the oculars determines the magnification of the microscope.

59. **(C)** Objective lenses are available in various focal lengths ranging from 100 to 400 mm with intervening increases by 25-mm increments. The 400-mm lens provides the greatest magnification.

60. **(C)** A continuously variable system of magnification for increasing or decreasing images is possible with zoom lens, usually operated with a foot control to free the surgeon's hands from the task.

61. **(A)** The slit aperture permits a narrow beam of light to be brought into focus on the field. This slit image assists the surgeon in defining depth perception (relative distance of objects within the field).

62. **(C)** Usually fiberoptic, coaxial illumination provides intense, cool light. Paraxial illuminators contain tungsten or halogen bulbs.

63. **(B)** Microscopes should be damp dusted before use. All external surfaces, except the lenses, are wiped with detergent-disinfectant solution. Casters are also cleaned. It is kept dust free with an antistatic cover.

64. **(A)** A beam splitter takes the image from one of the surgeon's oculars and transmits it through an observer tube, thereby providing the assistant with an identical image of the surgeon's view.

65. **(C)** The culpomicroscope illuminates and permits identification of abnormal cervical (ectocervical, lower cervical canal, and vaginal wall) epithelium to target for biopsies.

66. **(C)** The laryngoscope becomes self-retaining by suspension in a special appliance placed over the patient's chest, thus enabling the surgeon freedom of his or her hands to use a microscope and perform procedures.

67. **(A)** A microscope is monocular or binocular. The binocular has two telescopes mounted side by side that give stereoscopic vision.

68. **(C)** Eyepieces are interchangeable and are available in four magnifying powers: 10×, 12.5×, 16×, and 20×.

69. **(C)** A, B, and D are appropriate techniques. Oil or fingerprints are removed with a solvent or lens-cleaning solution or 50% denatured alcohol; however, solvents should be used sparingly so that cemented surfaces are not destroyed.

70. **(D)** Some tables have a metal crossbar or body elevator between the two upper sections that can be raised to elevate a gallbladder or kidney.

71. **(A)** Instruments and catheters are measured on a French scale; the diameter (in millimeters) is multiplied by 3. The smallest is 1 mm in diameter times 3, or 3 French.

72. **(D)** Inflatable, double-walled vinyl boots use alternating compression and relaxation to reduce risk of deep vein clotting in legs of high-risk patients undergoing general anesthesia.

73. **(A)** The Doppler is a blood flow detector. Ultrasonic imaging records flowing blood.

74. **(D)** Cryotherapy is performed using an insulated probe to deliver extreme cold to target diseased tissue without damaging surrounding tissue.

75. **(A)** The mobile suction unit is called the Neptune. It removes waste and can be relocated to a waste disposal area through a docking station.

76. **(B)** Smith and Nephew coblator cauterizes, irrigates, and suctions simultaneously. It is commonly used in tonsil surgery.

77. **(D)** The tubing for oxygen is green. Nitrous oxide is blue. The tubing for compressed air is yellow, and the tubing for nitrogen is black.

78. **(B)** Laminar maintains positive pressure not negative. It has a unidirectional flow and maintains a higher pressure in the OR.

79. **(D)** HEPA filters remove dust particles and bacteria as small as 0.3–5 mm in the OR.

80. **(A)** The air exchange per hour with HEPA filters is 20–25 exchanges.

81. **(C)** There is a weight limit for OR tables. All tables in the OR have weight limits.

82. **(D)** The Alvarado is not a neuro attachment but used as a foot holder in total joints.

83. **(B)** The fracture table is used for hip and leg fractures.

84. **(A)** The standing stool should be positioned before opening the sterile field to avoid contamination.

85. **(B)** Chest rolls are used to allow the patient to expand their lungs or chest.

86. **(D)** All of the above information applies to prevention of electrical accidents.

87. **(D)** Staff who must remain in the room during exposure to ionizing radiation should maintain a distance of at least 6 ft from patient (beam).

88. **(B)** The dosimeter is the correct name for the radiation-measuring device.

89. **(C)** The three components needed to start a fire are oxygen, fuel, and a source of ignition.

90. **(A)** Always bend at the knees when lifting or lowering a heavy object as it eases pressure off the lower back. B and C are examples of proper body mechanics as musculoskeletal injury is caused by poor body mechanics, stress, lack of balance, repetitive motion and over exertion.

Transportation and Positioning

Patient transport, transfer to the operating room (OR) table, operating table attachments, and positioning prior to surgery: vital signs/blood pressure/urethral catheterization/sequential compression devices (SCDs)

- Patient transport to the OR
  - The patient should be transported through the hallways feet first and enter the elevator head first
  - Side rails should be up and patient advised to keep hands and feet in
- Transfer and positioning
  - Four people are required to move an immobile patient
  - Two people for an ambulatory/mobile patient
  - The stretcher should always be locked before moving the patient
  - Anesthesia determines when it is time to move the patient. They are also responsible for moving the head/neck
  - Once the patient is centered on the OR bed, a safety strap is placed 2 in above the knee
  - Arms are placed on arm boards not to exceed 90 degrees. This prevents nerve damage to the brachial plexus
  - The patient's feet should not extend beyond the end of the OR bed to avoid foot drop
  - The patient should always be covered when possible to protect the patient's privacy and keep the patient warm
- Once the patient is properly positioned on the OR bed, provide normothermia to keep the patient comfortable; this includes:
  - Warming of the OR suite until the prep is performed and dries
  - Blankets from the warmer

  - Bair Hugger—air-forced warming blankets
    - They should never be placed directly next to the patient's skin because it can cause burns
  - Warming lamps
  - Blanketrol warmers that contain water or alcohol
    - Used to circulate warm or cool water through the coils to control the patient's body temperature
  - Fluid warmers are used to warm intravenous (IV) solutions
  - Irrigation fluid warmer is used to warm irrigation fluids
- Heat loss in the OR occurs four ways; they include:
  - Radiation—patient loses heat through the surrounding environment. The patient is brought from a warm environment to a cold OR
  - Convection—patient loses heat through air currents
  - Conduction—patient loses heat by direct contact with the patient's skin
  - Evaporation—liquid on skin evaporates and causes heat loss; loss through perspiration
- Hypothermia—a drop in normal body temperature where your body loses heat faster than it can produce heat. When your body temperature drops, your heart, nervous system, and other organs cannot function properly, which can cause failure of the heart and respiratory system. Symptoms include:
  - Increased oxygen—shivering
  - Compromise of the cardiovascular and nervous systems

- Increased blood pressure
- Bradycardia
- When a patient is undergoing cardiac surgery, hypothermia is a desired effect
- Antiembolic device/SCD (sequential compression device)
  - These are stockings placed on the patient prior to surgery in order to pump blood back up to the heart while the patient is immobile. This avoids blood clots. Venous stasis occurs due to long periods of immobility. The superficial and deep veins in the legs do not get a normal blood flow and can develop pooling of the blood and clots
  - The SCD massages the legs and moves the blood in an upward direction to prevent venous stasis
  - SCDs come in various sizes
  - SCDs are placed on the patient, after the patient is transferred to the OR table
  - The device should never be turned off or removed without permission from the anesthesiologist or surgeon
- Vital signs include:
  - Temperature
  - Pulse
  - Respiration
  - Blood pressure
- Temperature
  - Noninvasive temperature monitors include:
    - Temperature monitoring disc—this is placed on the patient's forehead to monitor temperature during surgery
  - Invasive temperature monitors include:
    - Oral, rectal
    - Esophageal—used during radiofrequency ablation of atrial fibrillation
    - Bladder—commonly used in the intensive care unit. It is a heat-sensitive indwelling urinary catheter
  - Normal body temperature
    - Oral—98.6°F (37°C)
    - Rectal—99.6°F (37.6°C)
    - Axillary—97.6°F (36.4°C)
  - Pulse
    - Pulse is taken at the radial artery 1 in proximal to the thumb
    - Apical pulse—a pulse taken at the apex of the heart with a stethoscope

- Measure the pulse rate for 15 seconds and multiply by four to get the heart rate
  - Normal heart rates
    - Birth—130–160 bpm
    - Infants—110–130 bpm
    - Children—80–120 bpm
    - Adults—60–80 bpm
  - Tachycardia—heart rate over 100 bpm can be caused by:
    - Stress
    - Drugs
    - Exercise
    - Congestive heart failure (CHF)
  - Bradycardia—less than 60 bpm; this includes:
    - Athletes
    - Cerebral hemorrhage
    - Heart block
    - Drugs
    - Hypoxia (decrease in oxygen reaching body tissues)
  - Respirations—breathing is the exchange of oxygen and carbon dioxide in the cells
    - Pulse oximeter (oxygen saturation device)—measures the amount of oxygen in the hemoglobin portion of blood. The device clips onto the patient's finger or toe
    - Apnea—cessation of breathing
      - Brought on by anesthesia
      - Foreign body stuck in the airway
    - Bradypnea—decreased rate of breathing
    - Cheyne-Stokes—the patient's breath is deeper and faster followed by decrease in breathing. They can sometimes stop breathing for a short time. This pattern repeats itself. It is commonly found in patients with heart failure or brain damage
    - Dyspnea—shortness of breath and/or difficulty breathing. This can occur during exercise or if the patient has a history of heart/lung disease
    - Tachypnea—rapid breathing. Occurs in patients with a high fever
    - Kussmaul—fast, deep, labored breathing
- Blood pressure—when your heart beats, it contracts and pushes blood through the arteries to the rest of the body. This force is called systolic blood pressure and is the top number. Diastolic blood pressure is the bottom number. It is the pressure in the arteries when the heart is at rest

- Blood pressure can be taken manually or with an electric recording sphygmomanometer
- Blood pressure is measured in millimeters of mercury (mm Hg)
- The cuff is placed around the upper portion of the arm and inflated, and arterial blood flow is stopped
- A stethoscope is placed on the brachial artery, and the air in the cuff is slowly released
- Korotkoff's sounds—these are the first tapping sounds you hear. These sounds take place in five phases:
  - □ Systolic pressure—the first tapping sounds you hear
  - □ Soft whistling sound as the cuff is deflated
  - □ Rhythmic tapping sound as the cuff is deflated
  - □ Fading tapping sound as the cuff is deflated
  - □ Diastolic pressure—the point where the sounds disappear altogether
- Normal blood pressure—less than 120/less than 80 mm Hg
- Hypertension—140–159/90–99 mm Hg
  - ○ An arterial line/art-line/A-line—thin catheter inserted into an artery. It is most commonly used in intensive care and during surgery where the anesthesiologist can monitor the patient's status with a blood sample. The blood pressure is also monitored
    - This can also be used to obtain blood gases
    - An arterial line can be inserted in:
      - □ Wrist: radial artery
      - □ Elbow: brachial artery
      - □ Groin: femoral artery
      - □ Foot: dorsalis pedis artery
- *Bispectral index monitor—used to monitor of the depth of anesthesia in the surgical patient*
  - ○ Urethral catheterization—performed by non-sterile team members; however, it is a sterile procedure requiring aseptic technique to prevent a urinary tract infection. Always check for patient allergies to latex
  - ○ Performed to drain the bladder and for irrigation; the bladder is drained:
    - To prevent injury
    - For better visualization

- To monitor urine output
- To obtain a sterile specimen
- To relieve urinary retention
- They are made of latex, silicone, and Teflon
  - ○ Foley catheter is commonly used and comes in various sizes (8–30 Fr)
  - ○ 16-French 5-cc Foley balloon catheter is commonly used on adults
    - The catheter balloon is tested with 10 mL of sterile water. Saline breaks down the catheter, and air can leak. Not commonly done anymore because the catheter can lose its integrity (always follow manufacturer's instructions)
  - ○ Coude catheter (this catheter has a bend at the tip)—can be used as an indwelling catheter or a straight catheter. This is used on male patients with an enlarged prostate
  - ○ A Robinson catheter is a straight catheter used in a dilation and curettage procedure
  - ○ Urinary catheter drains by gravity. The catheter bag must be kept below bladder level
  - ○ When performing a urethral catheterization on a female patient:
    - Female patient—frog leg position
    - Open the catheter pack by using sterile technique (four-quadrant)
    - Put on sterile gloves
    - Test the catheter—follow manufacturer's instructions
    - Use the nondominant hand to hold the labial fold open
    - Prep the area—urethra down
    - Place the tip of the catheter in lubricant and insert catheter
    - Connect the catheter to the drainage bag. When urine begins to flow, you know the catheter is in the bladder
  - ○ When performing this procedure on a male patient:
    - The patient is positioned supine
    - Procedure same as above except the catheter is inserted into the male urethra
- Patient positioning—patient positioning takes place following anesthesia induction. Everyone involved in patient positioning should have the knowledge of positioning to prevent damage to skin, nerves, joints, cardiovascular system, respiratory system, and other body parts

- Patient positioning provides visualization of the surgical site and the best access to the surgical site
  - You must slowly and carefully position when the patient is asleep; they cannot tell you what is hurting them or react to pain
  - You must keep the range of motion within the body's limits to avoid damage to a limb
  - You must be aware of the position of the IV, Foley catheter, and other patient care devices so as not to accidently pull them out
  - Protect pressure points and boney prominences by using padding
  - The patient's skin should not come in contact with metal parts of the table as it can cause burns from the electrosurgical unit (ESU)
  - Confirm that patient's legs are not crossed
- Positioning aids include:
  - OR beds—they should be positioned under the center of the OR lights and away from the doors to prevent contamination from the outside corridors
    - Weight limits vary
    - Special tables are used for bariatric patients
    - Parts of the OR bed include head piece/ body/foot piece
    - Neuro/ortho attachments:
      - Mayfield headrest
      - Gardner-Wells tongs
      - Horseshoe headrests
  - Special OR tables
    - Orthopedic fracture table
    - Andrews—used for laminectomy procedures, knee-chest
    - Jackson—used for cervical, thoracic, and lumbar procedures
    - Wilson—used to support the patient's upper body for laminectomies or disc removal
    - Hand table
  - Arm boards
  - Shoulder braces
  - Foot boards
  - Stirrups
    - Candy cane
    - Allen
  - Patient transfer devices
    - Roller
    - Toboggan
    - Flexible air mattress for bariatric patients

- Ergonomics—using proper body mechanics when moving or positioning the surgical patient. This is important to prevent injury to the health care worker
- Supine position—dorsal recumbent
  - The patient is always in supine position when anesthesia is induced
  - Patient is flat on their back with their legs straight
  - Arms on arm boards, palms facing up and not extending 90 degrees. Overextension can cause injury to the brachial plexus
  - Elbows must be carefully positioned to avoid damage to the ulnar nerve
  - Arms can be positioned at the patient's sides if needed; arms and hands must be positioned carefully to avoid injury. When tucking the patients' arms at their side with a draw sheet, you must not tuck the draw sheet under the mattress but under the patients themselves
  - Padding is placed under the head. There are several varieties of headrests
  - Safety strap is placed 2 in above the knee
  - Supine position is used in surgery of:
    - Chest/breast
    - Abdomen
    - Pelvis
    - Anterior extremities
- Trendelenburg position—a modification of the supine position where head and upper body are tilted downward
  - Used to displace the pelvic organs for better exposure
  - This position is used in treatment for shock
  - Shoulder braces can be used to prevent the patient from sliding off the table
- Reverse Trendelenburg—a modification of the supine position where the head and upper body are positioned upward
  - Displaces the abdominal organs
  - Foot board can be used to prevent the patient from sliding off the table
- Fowler's/sitting position—the upper body is at a 90-degree angle
- Semi-Fowler's—same as above except the upper body is at about an 85-degree angle
  - This position reduces blood flow from the upper body and facilitates respiration. A major concern is an air embolism

- o Used for surgery on the breast, head/neck, and shoulder
- o Arms may be positioned on arm boards or across the abdomen
- o Padded foot board is used to prevent the patient from sliding off the table
- Lithotomy position
  - o Various positioning devices can be used
    - Candy cane stirrups
    - Yellofins/Allen stirrups
  - o Stirrups must be equal height and length
  - o Arms are on arm boards or at patient's side tucked under the patient using a draw sheet that is tucked under the patient
  - o Raise and lower legs slowly and simultaneously. Two people are required to avoid blood pressure changes
  - o Buttocks must be positioned on the edge of the bed. Do not have legs hanging off the bed as this can cause a back injury
  - o Return the patient to supine position as soon as possible to avoid cardiovascular and respiratory problems
  - o Surgery includes—vagina, perineum, anus, rectum, and urethra
- Prone position
  - o The anesthesiologist induces the patient while they are in supine position before positioning in prone
  - o You need padding to prevent compression on the vena cava and abdominal aorta
  - o Use padding: axillary rolls, chest rolls to provide expansion of chest so lungs can expand
  - o Position the breasts and male genitalia carefully
  - o Be careful in positioning the arms to prevent injury to the shoulder
  - o Lower and rotate arms for placement on an arm board with palms facing downward, or tuck along the side of the body with palms facing inward
  - o Surgeries performed—posterior cranium, dorsal body, spine, and/or posterior extremities

- Sims' position
  - o This is a modification of left lateral position
  - o Used for endoscopies (colonoscopy)
  - o The left leg is straight, and the right leg is bent
  - o Usually, the patient can position themselves
- Kraske/jackknife
  - o This is a modification of prone position
  - o Used for surgery on the anus and rectum
  - o Patient's hips (iliac crest) are positioned at the table break
  - o Safety strap is placed proximal to the knees
  - o Same applies to positioning the arms as with prone position
- Lateral position/lateral recumbent/lateral decubitus
  - o Right lateral position—the right side of the body is down, exposing the left side of the body. Same for the left lateral position
  - o Same precautions as prone position
  - o Use padding: axillary rolls or chest rolls to provide expansion of chest to ease respirations
  - o Lower leg is bent and upper leg is straight with a pillow between them
  - o Blood pressure should be measured from the lower arm
  - o A Mayo stand is used to support the upper arm
  - o The lower arm is on the arm board with the palm facing up, and the upper arm is positioned on the mayo stand with the palm facing downward
  - o A bean bag can be used to stabilize the upper body
- Kidney position
  - o Modification of lateral position
  - o The kidneys must be properly placed on the kidney bar/rest so they are able to be elevated
- Knee-chest position
  - o Similar to the jackknife position, but the legs are bent at the knee at a 90-degree angle
  - o Used for spine surgery

Questions

Transportation

1. When using a patient roller, how many people are necessary to move the patient safely and efficiently?

    (A) Two
    (B) Three
    (C) Four
    (D) Five

2. When moving the patient from the operating room (OR) table, who is responsible for guarding the head and neck from injury?

    (A) Circulating nurse
    (B) Scrub nurse
    (C) Anesthesiologist
    (D) Surgical technician

3. To move the patient from the transport stretcher to the OR table:

    (A) one person stands at the head, one at the foot, while the patient moves over
    (B) one person stands next to the stretcher, one adjacent to the OR table, while the patient moves over
    (C) one person stands next to the stretcher, stabilizing it against the OR table, while the patient moves over
    (D) one person may stand next to the OR table and guide the patient toward him or her if stretcher wheels are locked

4. When moving a patient with a fracture in the OR, all of the following are true EXCEPT:

    (A) extra personnel are necessary
    (B) the extremity should be supported from above and below the fracture site
    (C) the surgeon should be the one supporting the fracture during the transfer and positioning
    (D) personnel on the affected side support the fracture

5. Which statement is false regarding the position on the OR table?

    (A) Elbow should not rest against the metal table
    (B) Feet should be uncrossed
    (C) Pillows provide support and comfort to prevent strain
    (D) Safety strap is 4 in below the knee

6. To avoid compromising the venous circulation, the restraint or safety strap should be placed:

    (A) at knee level
    (B) at the mid-thigh area
    (C) 2 in above the knee
    (D) 2 in below the knee

7. When transporting a patient with an underwater seal drainage system, the drainage system:

   (A) should be placed at the patient's side and disconnected
   (B) should be above the patient's body level attached to suction
   (C) should be clamped off and placed below the patient's chest level
   (D) can be placed by using any of the above methods

Positioning

8. Crossing the patient's arms across his or her chest may cause:

   (A) pressure on the ulnar nerve
   (B) interference with circulation
   (C) postoperative discomfort
   (D) interference with respiration

9. A precaution always taken when the patient is in the supine position is to:

   (A) place the pillows under the knees for support
   (B) place the safety strap 3–4 in below the knee
   (C) place the head in a headrest
   (D) protect the heels from pressure on the OR table

10. During lateral positioning:

    (A) a pillow is placed between the legs
    (B) a sandbag is placed between the knees
    (C) a rolled towel is placed under the bottom leg
    (D) a sheet is folded flat between the legs

11. To prevent strain to the lumbosacral muscles and ligaments when the patient is in the lithotomy position:

    (A) the buttocks must not extend beyond the table edge
    (B) the legs must be placed symmetrically
    (C) the legs must be at equal height
    (D) a pillow should be placed under the sacral area

12. The lithotomy position requires all of the following EXCEPT:

    (A) patient's buttocks rests along the break between the body and leg sections of the table
    (B) stirrups are at equal height on both sides of the table
    (C) stirrups are at the appropriate height for the length of the patient's legs to maintain symmetry
    (D) each leg is raised slowly and gently as it is grasped by the toes

13. All of the following are requirements of the Kraske position EXCEPT:

    (A) patient is prone with hips over the break of the table
    (B) a pillow is placed under lower legs and ankles
    (C) a padded knee strap is applied 2 in above knees
    (D) arms are tucked in at sides

14. When using an arm board, the most important measure to take is to:

    (A) support the arm at the intravenous site
    (B) strap the patient's hand to the board securely
    (C) avoid hyperextension of the arm
    (D) avoid hypoextension of the arm

15. Anesthetized patients should be moved slowly in order to:

    (A) prevent fractures
    (B) prevent circulatory overload
    (C) allow the respiratory system to adjust
    (D) allow the circulatory system to adjust

16. If the patient is in a supine position, the circulator must always:

    (A) place a pillow between the knees
    (B) place a pillow under the knees
    (C) confirm that ankles and legs are not crossed
    (D) pad the thoracic area adequately

17. Extreme positions of the head and arm can cause injury to the:

    (A) cervical plexus
    (B) radial nerve
    (C) ulnar nerve
    (D) brachial plexus

18. Ulnar nerve damage could result from:

    (A) poor placement of legs in stirrups
    (B) hyperextension of the arm
    (C) using mattress pads of varying thickness
    (D) placing an arm on an unpadded table edge

19. In the prone position, the thorax must be elevated from the OR table to prevent:

    (A) compromised respiration
    (B) pressure areas
    (C) circulatory impairment
    (D) brachial nerve damage

20. The anesthesiologist closes the eyelids of a general anesthetic patient for all of the following reasons EXCEPT:

    (A) to prevent drying of the eye
    (B) to prevent the patient from seeing the procedure
    (C) to prevent eye trauma
    (D) to protect the eye from anesthetic agents

21. Which position would be the most desirable for a pilonidal cystectomy or a hemorrhoidectomy?

    (A) Lithotomy
    (B) Kraske
    (C) Knee-chest
    (D) Modified prone

22. A position often used in cranial procedures is called:

    (A) Fowler's
    (B) Kraske
    (C) Trendelenburg
    (D) lithotomy

23. In positioning for laminectomy, rolls or bolsters are placed:

    (A) horizontally, one under the chest and one under the thighs
    (B) longitudinally to support the chest from axilla to hip
    (C) longitudinally to support the chest from sternum to hip
    (D) below the knees

24. The position used for a patient in hypovolemic shock is:

    (A) modified Trendelenburg
    (B) reverse Trendelenburg
    (C) supine
    (D) dorsal recumbent

25. A Mayfield headrest would be used for which type of surgery?

    (A) Ophthalmic
    (B) Gynecological
    (C) Neurological
    (D) Urological

26. Good exposure for thyroid surgery is ensured by all of the following EXCEPT:

    (A) modified dorsal recumbent with shoulder roll
    (B) hyperextension of the neck
    (C) utilization of skin-stay sutures
    (D) firm retraction of the laryngeal nerve and surrounding structures

27. A procedure requiring the patient to be positioned supine in modified lithotomy is:

    (A) colonoscopy
    (B) abdominoperineal resection (APR)
    (C) marsupialization of pilonidal cyst
    (D) ileostomy

28. In which procedure may the patient be placed in a supine position with the right side slightly elevated by a wedge to tilt the patient to the left?

    (A) Cerclage
    (B) Marsupialization of Bartholin's cyst
    (C) Shirodkar
    (D) Cesarean section

29. The position for most open-bladder surgery would be:

    (A) lithotomy
    (B) supine position
    (C) reverse Trendelenburg
    (D) Fowler's, modified

30. In which position could the patient sustain injury to the pudendal nerves?

    (A) Positioned on the fracture table
    (B) Positioned in lateral chest
    (C) Positioned in lithotomy
    (D) Positioned on the urological table

31. Which factor is important to consider when positioning the aging patient?

    (A) Skeletal changes
    (B) Limited range of motion of joints
    (C) Tissue fragility
    (D) All of the above

32. When positioning the patient for a procedure, which of the following provides maximum patient safety and maximum surgical site exposure?

    (A) Patient's body does not touch metal on table
    (B) Equipment, Mayo stand, or personnel are not resting on the patient
    (C) Bony prominences are padded
    (D) All of the above

33. What position would be used for an abdominoperineal resection?

    (A) Supine, slight reverse Trendelenburg
    (B) Low lithotomy
    (C) Sims
    (D) Kraske

34. All are ways to identify a patient EXCEPT:

    (A) address patient by their full name and state the surgery they are having
    (B) examine the patient's identification band and compare with the name and number on the chart
    (C) ask the patient to state their full name, do not call the patient by their name before asking
    (D) ask the patient to tell you what procedure they are having

35. To assist a falling patient, you should:

    (A) support the patient's weight with your body
    (B) ease the patient to the floor while protecting their head
    (C) run and get assistance once the patient is down
    (D) none of the above

36. Intravenous (IV) lines and fluids should be:

    (A) lower than the patient's body
    (B) level with the patient's arm
    (C) higher than the patient's body
    (D) it really does not matter

37. What is the position called when the OR bed is tilted with feet down?

    (A) Trendelenburg
    (B) Low lithotomy
    (C) Hyperflexion
    (D) Reverse Trendelenburg

38. Antiembolism devices or SCDs are placed on the patient's legs prior to surgery to:

    (A) prevent thromboembolus
    (B) prevent cramping
    (C) provide protection from metal parts of the OR table
    (D) assist in the range of motion

39. The dorsal recumbent position is a slight modification of what position?

    (A) supine
    (B) prone
    (C) right lateral
    (D) Kraske

40. When the patient is positioned in supine, the arm board must not be:

    (A) flexed more than 90 degrees
    (B) adducted more than 90 degrees
    (C) abducted more than 90 degrees
    (D) There are no specific criteria

41. The position that allows greater access to the lower abdominal cavity and pelvic structures due to gravity is:

    (A) reverse Trendelenburg
    (B) lithotomy
    (C) Trendelenburg
    (D) supine

42. The orthopedic fracture table provides:

    (A) circumferential access
    (B) horizontal traction
    (C) exposure to the ankle
    (D) both A and B

43. What position is occasionally used for facial, cranial, or reconstructive breast surgery?

    (A) Sims'
    (B) Fowler's
    (C) Reverse Trendelenburg
    (D) Anterolateral

44. What position would be used for a surgical procedure requiring a transurethral approach?

    (A) Supine, Trendelenburg
    (B) Supine, reverse Trendelenburg
    (C) Lithotomy
    (D) Lateral kidney

45. Thoracic outlet syndrome can occur when there is pressure on:

    (A) the thoracic artery
    (B) the brachial plexus
    (C) subclavian artery
    (D) both B and C

46. Ulnar neuropathy results from:

    (A) improper padding
    (B) continuous pressure from the edge of the OR table
    (C) when the elbow is tightly flexed
    (D) all of the above

47. The following is a risk when positioning the patient on the OR table:

    (A) hyperextension of limbs
    (B) pressure on bony prominences
    (C) improper padding
    (D) all of the above

48. When transferring an unconscious or immobile patient from the stretcher to the OR table, ideally how many people are required?

    (A) Two or three
    (B) Four to six
    (C) One or two
    (D) None of the above

49. When removing a patient from lithotomy position:

    (A) lower the legs separately
    (B) lower the legs quickly
    (C) lower the legs together
    (D) lower stirrups, then remove legs

50. All of the following help to maintain normothermia during surgery EXCEPT:

    (A) warm the OR until the prep is performed and dries
    (B) blankets from the warmer are used
    (C) SCD is applied
    (D) fluid warmers are used to warm IV solution

51. Heat loss caused by convection occurs when:

    (A) patient loses heat through the surrounding environment—from warm environment to a cold OR
    (B) the liquid (due to perspiration) on their skin evaporates and causes heat loss
    (C) patient loses heat by direct contact with an object or another body (cold)
    (D) patient loses heat through air currents

52. Symptoms of hypothermia include all EXCEPT:

    (A) tachycardia
    (B) increased shivering
    (C) compromised cardiovascular and nervous systems
    (D) increased blood pressure

53. The device used by the anesthesiologist to measure the amount of oxygen in the hemoglobin component of the blood is:

    (A) pulse oximeter
    (B) oxygen saturation device
    (C) sphygmomanometer
    (D) both A and B

54. Cheyne-Stokes breathing is defined as:

    (A) shortness of breath and breathing difficulty
    (B) breaths are deeper and faster followed by a decrease in breathing. The breathing can sometimes stop for a short time.
    (C) rapid breathing as in patients with a high fever
    (D) fast deep labored breathing

55. Korotkoff's sounds are:

    (A) observed during Cheyne-Stokes breathing
    (B) the first tapping sounds heard when taking a blood pressure
    (C) observed when using the bispectral index monitor
    (D) the sounds noted when using a Doppler

56. An arterial line can be inserted into the:

    (A) radial artery
    (B) brachial artery
    (C) femoral artery
    (D) all of the above

57. A bispectral index monitor is used to:

    (A) monitor the depth of anesthesia in the surgical patient
    (B) monitor blood pressure
    (C) measure the amount of oxygen in blood
    (D) monitor the body temperature

58. The neuro/ortho headrest attachments include all EXCEPT:

    (A) Mayfield headrest
    (B) Gardner-Wells tongs
    (C) horseshoe headrest
    (D) Andrews headrest

59. OR tables commonly used in spinal surgery include:

    (A) Andrews
    (B) Wilson
    (C) Jackson
    (D) All of the above

60. Which statement is incorrect when the patient is in Fowler's position?

    (A) The upper body is at a 90-degree angle.
    (B) Blood flow from the upper body is reduced and facilitates respirations.
    (C) A padded shoulder board is used to prevent the patient from sliding off the table.
    (D) It is used for surgery on the breast, head, neck, or shoulder.

61. Positioning aids used for lithotomy position include:

    (A) candy cane stirrups
    (B) Yellofins stirrups
    (C) Allen stirrups
    (D) all of the above

62. All of the following statements are true regarding the Sims' position EXCEPT:

    (A) used for spine procedures
    (B) left leg is straight, and right leg is bent
    (C) this is a modification of left lateral position
    (D) used for endoscopic procedures

63. All apply to a lateral position EXCEPT:

    (A) padding, axillary rolls, and chest rolls are used to improve respirations
    (B) a Mayo stand should not be used to support the upper arm
    (C) lower leg is bent and upper leg is straight with a pillow in between
    (D) blood pressure should be measured from the lower arm

64. The desirable position for better visualization in the lower abdomen or pelvis is:

    (A) Fowler's
    (B) reverse Trendelenburg
    (C) Trendelenburg
    (D) Kraske

65. In which of the following positions is a patient placed for a right nephrectomy:

    (A) left lateral
    (B) right lateral
    (C) left lateral kidney
    (D) right lateral kidney

66. Which of the following positions is used for a total hip arthroplasty?

    (A) Fowler's
    (B) Lithotomy
    (C) Kraske
    (D) Lateral

67. In what position is the patient placed for an anterior total hip arthroplasty?

    (A) Supine
    (B) Lithotomy
    (C) Lateral
    (D) Fowler

68. If a patient is having a procedure performed on the Allen table, when would they be intubated and what position would be used?

    (A) After the patient has been positioned prone
    (B) When the patient is on the stretcher in supine position
    (C) When the patient is positioned on the OR bed in supine
    (D) The decision on how the patient is to be intubated for this procedure is determined by the anesthesiologist

69. What position is the patient put in following extubation after a tonsillectomy?

    (A) Supine
    (B) Fowler's
    (C) Sims'
    (D) Lateral

70. All pertain to a shearing injury EXCEPT:

 (A) intense friction placed on the patient's skin

 (B) it is more common in a debilitated patient or the elderly who have compromised skin

 (C) it is caused when the patient is transported from the stretcher to OR bed or OR bed to stretcher

 (D) it is caused by hyperflexion of the muscle and facia when moving the patient from one surface to another

71. What position most commonly results in an eye injury in patients?

 (A) Lateral

 (B) Prone

 (C) Supine

 (D) Dorsal recumbent

Answers and Explanations

Transportation

1. **(C)** Four people are needed to move the patient safely when using a roller. One lifts the head, one lifts the feet, one is beside the stretcher, and one is beside the OR table.

2. **(C)** It is the responsibility of the anesthesiologist to guard the neck and head. It also puts him or her in a better position to observe the patient. Four people are needed, and the action must be synchronized.

3. **(B)** There should be an adequate number of personnel to safely transfer the patient to the OR table. One person should stand next to the stretcher to stabilize it against the adjacent OR table. Another receives the patient from the opposite side of the table.

4. **(D)** Fractures should be handled gently. Additional personnel are necessary to aid in the transfer and positioning for the patient's safety. The fracture should be supported by the surgeon and others, if necessary, from above and below the fracture.

5. **(D)** The safety strap is 2 in above the knee and not too tight but secure.

6. **(C)** The safety strap should be applied securely but loosely about 2 in above the knee. This is to avoid compromise of venous circulation or pressure on bony prominences or nerves.

7. **(C)** The drainage system should be placed below the patient's chest level, clamped off, and disconnected from suction. This prevents a pneumothorax and reentry of drainage into the thoracic cavity.

Positioning

8. **(D)** Patient's arms should not be crossed on the chest in order to prevent hindrance of diaphragmatic movement and airway. This is essential to maintain respiratory function, to prevent hypoxia, and to facilitate inhalation anesthesia induction.

9. **(D)** In the supine position, heels must be protected from pressure on the table by a pillow, ankle roll, or doughnut. The feet must not be in prolonged flexion; the soles are supported to prevent foot drop.

10. **(A)** When a patient is positioned on his or her side, a pillow is placed lengthwise between the legs to prevent pressure on blood vessels and nerves.

11. **(A)** The buttocks should be even with the table edge but should not extend over the edge; otherwise, it could cause strain to the lumbosacral muscles and ligaments because the body weight rests on the sacrum.

12. **(D)** Legs are raised simultaneously by two people who grasp the sole of a foot in one hand and support the knee area with the other. Stirrups must be of equal height and appropriate for the size of the patient's leg.

13. **(D)** The requirements of the Kraske position are as follows: patient is prone with hips over break of table, wide arm board is under head of mattress to support arms, pillow is under

lower legs and ankles, padded knee strap is 2 in above knees, table is flexed to acute angle, and small rolled towel is under each shoulder.

14. **(C)** When using an arm board, caution should be taken so that the arm is not hyperextended or the infusion needle dislodged. Hyperextension can cause nerve damage.

15. **(D)** The anesthetized patient and the elderly patient must be moved slowly and gently. This allows the circulatory system to adjust. This is for patient safety.

16. **(C)** The patient must not have ankles or legs crossed as this could create pressure on blood vessels and nerves. A normal reaction for a supine patient is to cross his or her legs before going to sleep.

17. **(D)** Injury to the brachial plexus can result from extreme positions of the head and arm. This can be avoided with proper care and careful observation.

18. **(D)** Ulnar nerve damage can occur from pressure from the OR table edge. The arm resting on an unpadded surface places pressure on the ulnar nerve as it transverses the elbow. This can be prevented by the use of padding, by fastening the arm securely with a lift sheet, or by placing the arms on arm boards.

19. **(A)** The thorax is elevated when the patient is in the prone position in order to facilitate respiration. This is accomplished with supports, rolls, elevating pads, body rests, or braces.

20. **(B)** The patient's eyes may remain open even when the patient is under anesthesia. This exposes them to drying or trauma from drapes or instruments. They can be protected with ophthalmic ointment or taped closed.

21. **(B)** The Kraske (jackknife) position is used for procedures in the rectal area such as pilonidal sinus or hemorrhoidectomy. Feet and toes are protected by a pillow. The head is to the side, and the arms are on arm boards.

22. **(A)** In the Fowler's position, the patient lies on his or her back with knees over the lower break in the table. A footboard is raised and padded. The foot of the table is lowered slightly, flexing the knees. The body section is raised. Arms rest on a pillow on the lap. This position is used in some cranial procedures with the head supported by a headrest.

23. **(B)** The patient is in prone position with lumbar spine over the center break of the table; two laminectomy rolls (or other firm padding) are placed longitudinally to support the chest from axilla to hip. Additional padding protects bony prominences.

24. **(A)** A modified Trendelenburg position is used for patients in hypovolemic shock. This may aid in venous return and cardiac output.

25. **(C)** A Mayfield is a special neurosurgical overhead instrument table.

26. **(D)** The patient is in modified dorsal recumbent position with a rolled sheet to extend the neck and raise the shoulders. Skin flaps may be held away with stay sutures. The laryngeal nerve is identified and carefully preserved.

27. **(B)** For an abdominoperineal resection, the patient is initially positioned supine in modified lithotomy providing simultaneous exposure of both abdominal and perineal fields.

28. **(D)** In a cesarean section procedure, a bolster is inserted under the right flank to prevent uterine compression on the right flank and the vena cava. Compression on the vena cava can cause hypotension and compromise fetal circulation. The use of a bolster will maintain fetal well-being.

29. **(B)** For most open-bladder surgeries, the patient is placed in the supine position. Trendelenburg may be desired to allow viscera to fall toward the head, allowing excellent pelvic organ exposure.

30. **(A)** On the orthopedic fracture table, the patient is positioned supine with the pelvis stabilized against a well-padded vertical post. Pressure on the genitalia from the perineal post can injure the pudendal nerves.

31. **(D)** The aging patient's skin integrity is very important. Aging decreases range of motion of joints. Elderly people cannot fully extend the spine, neck, or upper and lower extremities. Pillows, padding, and support devices compensate for the skeletal changes to ensure patient comfort and ensure against postoperative pain or injury.

32. **(D)** Maximum patient safety is accomplished by padding all bony prominences, protecting the brachial plexus in the axillary region from strain or pressure, ensuring that the legs are not crossed to prevent pressure on nerves and blood vessels, supporting and securing extremities to prevent them from falling off the bed, ensuring that no part of the patient's body touches metal on the OR bed, and making certain no equipment, Mayo, or personnel rest on the patient.

33. **(B)** Low lithotomy provides access to the perineal area.

34. **(A)** All are ways to identify a patient except addressing the patient by their full name and stating the surgery they are having.

35. **(B)** If a patient is walking unsteadily, you should use a wheelchair. If he or she is falling down, ease the patient to the floor while protecting their head, and immediately call for assistance while remaining with the patient. Do not abandon the patient under any circumstances.

36. **(C)** IV lines and fluids should always be higher than the patient's body.

37. **(D)** Reverse Trendelenburg or foot down position is used when the surgeon requires unobstructed access to the upper peritoneal cavity and the lower esophagus.

38. **(A)** SCDs reduce the risk of blood pooling or stasis and thrombus formation.

39. **(A)** The dorsal recumbent position is a slight modification of the supine position, although it is commonly referred to as the supine position. The patient is lying on their back with their legs moderately flexed. Pillows are placed to lift the feet and heels off of the mattress/table.

40. **(D)** To protect the brachial plexus, arm boards must not be abducted more than 90 degrees.

41. **(C)** Trendelenburg provides greater access to lower abdominal cavity and pelvic structures by allowing gravity to retract the organs.

42. **(D)** The fracture allows circumferential access and horizontal traction during the surgical procedure.

43. **(B)** The position used for facial, cranial, or reconstructive breast surgery is the Fowler's position.

44. **(C)** The lithotomy position or low lithotomy position would be used for a procedure such as a transurethral resection of the prostate, which requires a transurethral approach.

45. **(D)** Thoracic outlet syndrome is a rare condition in which the brachial plexus and the subclavian artery are compressed.

46. **(D)** The ulnar nerve passes through the condylar groove of the elbow. It is only covered by skin and subcutaneous tissue. The nerve is subject to compression injury when the elbow is tightly flexed or there is direct pressure from the edge of the OR table.

47. **(D)** All of the above. The patient can be seriously and permanently injured as a result of improper positioning. Only personnel specifically trained and competent to position the patient should assist in this task.

48. **(B)** Transferring the patient who is unable to control movement to the OR table requires four to six people.

49. **(C)** Sudden shifts in blood pressure and spinal injury can occur during positioning and removal from stirrups. To prevent this injury, both legs must be lowered together slowly.

50. **(C)** SCDs do not provide warmth to the patient. They are used to prevent deep vein thrombosis.

51. **(C)** Convection is when the patient loses heat through air currents. Radiation is when the patient loses heat through the surrounding environment. The patient is brought from a warm environment to a cold OR. Conduction is when the patient loses heat by direct contact with an object or another body, and evaporation is when the liquid on the patient's skin from perspiration evaporates and causes heat loss.

52. **(A)** Bradycardia is a symptom of hypothermia.

53. **(D)** The pulse oximeter and oxygen saturation device both measure the amount of oxygen in hemoglobin.

54. **(B)** Cheyne-Stokes is when the patient's breathing is deeper and faster followed by a decrease in breathing. They can stop breathing for a short time. This pattern repeats itself. Dyspnea is shortness of breath or difficulty breathing. Tachypnea is rapid breathing, and Kussmaul is fast deep labored breathing.

55. **(B)** Korotkoff's sounds are the first tapping sounds that are heard during blood pressure reading and take place in five phases.

56. **(D)** An arterial line can be inserted into the radial artery, brachial artery, femoral artery, or dorsalis pedis artery.

57. **(A)** A bispectral index monitor is used to monitor the depth of anesthesia in the surgical patient. A pulse oximeter measures the amount of oxygen in the hemoglobin.

58. **(D)** The Andrews table is used for spinal surgery.

59. **(D)** All mentioned tables can be used for spinal surgery.

60. **(C)** A padded foot board is used to prevent the patient from sliding off the table.

61. **(D)** Yellofins and Allen stirrups are used when the patient is in lithotomy position.

62. **(A)** Sims' position is not used for spinal surgery; it is commonly used for patients undergoing a colonoscopy.

63. **(B)** A Mayo stand is used to support the upper arm with proper padding. The lower hand that is placed on the arm board is supinated (palm facing upward), and the upper hand placed on the mayo stand is pronated (palm facing downward).

64. **(C)** The Trendelenburg position is used for procedures in the lower abdomen or pelvis in which it is desirable to tilt the abdominal viscera away from the pelvic area for better exposure. The entire table is tilted downward (about 45 degrees at table head) while the foot is also lowered the desired amount.

65. **(A)** When referring to the lateral position, the side down is the *nonoperative* side. Left lateral position would be used for the surgical procedure being performed on the right kidney.

66. **(D)** The patient is placed in lateral position. The body is supported using a bean bag or padded table attachments positioned anteriorly and posteriorly. The affected leg/hip is draped freely, and padding is placed between the legs.

67. **(A)** The patient is positioned in the supine position with slight variations to their legs.

68. **(B)** If a patient is positioned on an Allen table, they are most likely having surgery on their spine. The patient would remain on the stretcher in supine position while being intubated and flipped into prone position.

69. (D) The patient would be placed in lateral position with their head slightly elevated to prevent aspiration and continue to monitor their respiratory function.

70. (D) All of the above pertain to a shearing injury except hyperflexion. This is a greater than normal flexion causing a stretching injury. This can cause loss of mobility and nerve damage.

71. (B) Accidental eye injuries most commonly occur when the patient is in prone position. This can happen when the patient is being positioned and comes in contact with a part of the OR bed or a person aiding in the positioning. To protect the eye, patients are lubricated and taped when being intubated in the supine position.

CHAPTER 9

Counts

- The scrub tech and circulating nurse are responsible for counting items before, during, and after the surgical procedure because the surgeon relies on their accuracy for patient safety and legal reasons
- Counts are performed:
  - Before the skin incision is made
  - Before closing a hollow organ; example: uterus
  - Any time there is a change of shift in the room
  - When additional supplies are added to the sterile field, they must be counted
  - When closing the peritoneum
  - When closing skin
- When counting, the scrub tech will touch each item and count out loud with the circulating nurse watching
- When performing a closing count, the order is as follows:
  - Surgical field
  - Mayo stand
  - Back table
- The only time a count may be omitted is in an extreme emergency situation
  - The omitted count must be documented
  - The surgical technologist and circulator individually do the best they can to keep track of everything
  - At the end of the case, there will be a final count, and if requested by the surgeon, an x-ray can be taken

SPONGES

- All sponges on the sterile field should be radiopaque
- Bar coding—radiofrequency sponges that are counted with a scanner have a small black encoded tag attached
- 4 × 4's—come in packs of 10—they should be individually separated and counted
- Laparotomy pads/lap pads
  - They come square and oblong in packs of five with a radiopaque blue twill tape sewn on one corner
  - They may also come with five plastic or radiopaque rings. When using the lap pad with rings in the abdominal or thoracic cavities, the rings must remain outside of the body
- Peanut sponges—small, radiopaque, rolled gauze sponges
  - Commonly used for blunt dissection and absorption of fluid
  - Come in packs of five
  - Attached to the tip of a clamp using a Kelly or an Adson
- Kittner dissector—similar to a peanut, made from heavy cotton dental tape
  - Commonly used for blunt dissection
- Tonsil sponges—soft, cotton-filled gauze in the shape of a ball with a cotton string attached
  - They come in groups of five
  - Commonly used on T&A surgery
- Cottonoid patties—small, square- or rectangle-shaped strips of compressed cotton or rayon used for hemostasis
  - Commonly used on neurological procedures of the spine and brain
  - Are moistened with various solutions including topical thrombin
  - The surgeon uses bayonet forceps to pick up the patty
- Cloth towels—not commonly counted but, when used to pack the abdomen, it is the responsibility of the surgical technologist and

circulator to keep count of them going in and out of the abdomen

- All of the above types of sponges should be handled and counted one by one by the surgical technologist and circulator

SPECIAL CONSIDERATION WHEN USING SPONGES

- Secure sponges in a safe area away from other supplies so as not to accidently grab one and drag it into the wound
- Never cut sponges on the surgical field
- Never remove the radiopaque marker
- Never pass off a specimen on a surgical sponge; use a piece of Telfa
- Pass off the dirty sponges into the kick bucket; do not keep on your field
- Once the abdomen is opened, all small sponges should be removed from the Mayo stand
- Use Raytec sponges on sponge forceps if used on an open abdomen
- Lap pads should be counted going into the abdomen and when coming out of abdomen
- They should be handed to the surgeon on an exchange basis

COUNTING SHARPS

Needles
- Needles are counted while in the package. As they are opened for use, the count is verified
- Needles should be left in their package until the surgeon requests the suture
- No needle should be on the Mayo stand without a needle holder attached
- Needles are handed on an exchange basis with the neutral zone/no-hand technique
- When the surgeon returns the needle to the surgical technologist, it should be placed on the needle board immediately
- All hypodermic needles should be counted
- The electrosurgical unit (ESU) tip should be counted

Blades
- Blades should be handed directly to the STSR, or STSR should be told immediately where the blade has been flipped to

- Blades should be loaded onto the handle with a heavy needle holder
- If a blade breaks, all parts must be counted
- The skin blade should only be used for skin. Once handed back, it should be isolated
- The scalpel should be passed to the surgeon by the neutral zone technique or the no-hand technique

INSTRUMENT CONTAINERS

- Instruments are first counted and documented on a count sheet in sterile processing
- When counting the instruments in the operating room (OR), the STSR hands the count sheet off the sterile field to the circulator
- Instruments should be counted on the back table before they are placed on the Mayo stand
- Instruments should be counted one at a time
- All instruments should be visually and verbally counted by the surgical technologist and the circulator
- The surgical technologist should touch each instrument when counting
- Instruments that have multiple parts are counted individually

POTENTIAL PROBLEMS WITH COUNTS

- If the count sheet does not match the actual number of instruments, change the numbers on the count sheet
- Always count twice if there is a discrepancy
- If the patient is not yet in the OR and you have an incorrect sponge count, remove the sponges from the sterile field, bag them, and remove them from the room
- If the patient is in the OR and you have an incorrect sponge count, you must remove the sponges from the sterile field, bag them, and isolate them in the room
- The Mayo stand and back table should remain sterile until the patient has left the room
- The correct steps when experiencing an incorrect closing count are as follows:
  - Notify the surgeon immediately
  - Count again
  - Check drapes and incision

- The circulator looks through all garbage, linen hampers, under the OR furniture, and on the floor
- After all search efforts are complete and the item is still missing, call for x-ray
- The incident must be documented and an incident report completed

DOCTRINE OF RES IPSA LOQUITUR

- This means "The thing speaks for itself"
- This doctrine applies to a negligent act in the OR. An example is a retained foreign object in the patient

Questions

1. When are counts done in the OR?

   (A) At beginning and end of case
   (B) Before beginning of case, at beginning of wound closure, and at skin closure
   (C) As case begins and when case is in progress
   (D) Before beginning of case and after end of case

2. Soiled sponges are:

   (A) never touched with bare hands
   (B) left in the kick bucket until the count begins
   (C) removed from the room once the peritoneum is closed
   (D) counted and stacked on a towel or sheet on the OR floor

3. The initial count requires:

   (A) a count of both plain and radiopaque sponges
   (B) that counts be done in the right-hand corner on the back table
   (C) that the count be done aloud by circulator and scrub
   (D) the scrub to count each item and report to the circulator for recording

4. If a sponge pack contains an incorrect number of sponges once the patient is in the room, the circulating nurse:

   (A) should isolate the pack, put it in bag, and not remove it from the room
   (B) does not need to perform any documentation
   (C) should use it after adding or subtracting the correct number
   (D) should remove it from the room

5. In an instrument count:

   (A) all instruments and parts must be counted
   (B) precounted sets eliminate the need for precase count
   (C) large bulky instruments need not be counted
   (D) count only instruments that will be used

6. All of the following statements concerning sponges are true EXCEPT:

   (A) only radiopaque sponges should be used on the sterile field
   (B) sponges should be counted from the folded edge
   (C) a pack containing an incorrect number of sponges is discarded
   (D) a count is unnecessary in a vaginal procedure

7. The following statements regarding counts are true EXCEPT:

   (A) the relief scrub or circulator does not need to repeat count if only one of them is relieved
   (B) all counts are verified before person being relieved leaves room
   (C) persons taking final count are held accountable
   (D) persons taking final count must sign the count record

8. During the closure count, a discrepancy:

   (A) is noted on patient's chart
   (B) is reported to surgeon
   (C) is reported to supervisor
   (D) is reported to anesthesiologist

9. The following statements regarding counting sponges are true EXCEPT:

   (A) sponges are counted at folded edge
   (B) fan pack to separate sponges
   (C) separate each sponge and number aloud while placing it in a pile on table
   (D) an incorrect number of sponges in a pack should be compensated for on count sheet with a notation

10. Instruments added to the sterile field after the case is in progress:

    (A) are counted by STSR and circulator
    (B) are counted by STSR and first assist
    (C) do not need to be counted
    (D) are included in final count

11. Counted items include:

    (A) sponges
    (B) umbilical tapes
    (C) suture reels
    (D) all of the above

12. The closing counts are done in what order?

    (1) Mayo stand
    (2) Back table
    (3) Sterile field
    (4) Items discarded from the sterile field
    (A) 1, 2, 3, 4
    (B) 3, 2, 1, 4
    (C) 3, 1, 2, 4
    (D) 2, 3, 1, 4

13. If the count is incorrect, which is the proper order of the following procedural steps?

    (1) Radiograph is taken
    (2) Search is initiated
    (3) Notify surgeon and repeat count
    (A) 3, 2, 1
    (B) 1, 2, 3
    (C) 2, 3, 1
    (D) 1, 3, 2

14. When performing a C-section, the first count is initiated:

    (A) before closing the body cavity
    (B) before closing the uterus
    (C) before the closing suture is given
    (D) when the shift change occurs

15. The first closing count is performed on which abdominal layer?

    (A) Skin
    (B) Subcutaneous
    (C) When the surgeon requests
    (D) Peritoneum

16. When can dressing sponges be flipped onto the sterile field?

    (A) Prior to the first count
    (B) Following the first count
    (C) After the final closing count
    (D) Never

17. What is the correct way to count radiopaque 4 × 4 sponges?

    (A) Keep the tab on the 4 × 4's, give a slight shake, and count while holding
    (B) Remove the tab and count by 2's
    (C) Remove the tab and count each sponge individually
    (D) Lay them out and let the circulator count them and proceed with your setup

18. Prior to the beginning of the surgical procedure, the ideal situation to count instruments is:

    (A) from the back table when all instruments and their parts are all in one area
    (B) once you have set up your back table and Mayo stand
    (C) after you have assembled all instrument parts to assure all are working properly
    (D) at any time prior to the incision

19. When would a count be omitted?

    (A) Never
    (B) In an emergency situation
    (C) On a small procedure
    (D) On procedures where the peritoneum is not entered

20. What is included in a sharps count?

    (A) Needles, suture, and hypodermics
    (B) Blades
    (C) ESU tip
    (D) All of the above

Answers and Explanations

1. **(B)** The first count is performed before the surgical procedure begins. The second count is performed before closure of the peritoneum, and the third count is performed before skin closure. In the case of a C-section and exchange of personnel during any case, four counts are required. Additional counts must be performed when supplies and instrumentation are added to the sterile field.

2. **(A)** Soiled sponges should never be touched with bare hands. Sponges should be counted in units and bagged in a waterproof plastic bag or transferred to a moisture-proof surface until the final count is completed. This is done to avoid hepatitis or pathogenic organism transmission.

3. **(C)** The scrub nurse and the circulator count each item aloud and together. The nurse then records the number. Count additional items away from already counted items. Counting should be uninterrupted.

4. **(A)** If a pack contains an incorrect number of sponges, it is the responsibility of the circulator to isolate it, and it is not used. The danger of error is great if attempts are made to correct or compensate for discrepancies.

5. **(A)** Each item used must be considered a foreign object that can cause unnecessary harm should it be left inside the patient. Detachable parts of instruments must be counted. This ensures that part of an instrument does not remain in the wound.

6. **(D)** Sponge and instrument counts are very important in vaginal procedures. Sponges should be secured on sticks in deep areas. This prevents loss in hard-to-see areas.

7. **(A)** The relief of either the scrub or the circulator by another person necessitates the verification of all counts before the person being relieved leaves room. Persons taking final counts are held accountable and must sign the record.

8. **(B)** During the closure count, the scrub person reports counts as correct or incorrect to the surgeon.

9. **(D)** If a pack contains an incorrect number of sponges, scrub hands pack to circulator. Attempts should not be made to correct errors or compensate for discrepancies. Pack is isolated and not used.

10. **(A)** Recommended procedure for counts includes sponges, sharps, instruments, and special equipment, which requires at least a licensed registered nurse and an STSR.

11. **(D)** Counted items include sponges, sharps, instruments, retraction devices (umbilical tapes, vessel loops, bolsters, sutures, reels), and any other small item that is used on the sterile field.

12. **(C)** The closing count begins with the sterile field and then moves to the Mayo stand, back table, and, finally, items that were discarded from the field.

13. **(A)** When the count is incorrect, the surgeon is notified and the count is repeated. A search is initiated, and finally, an x-ray is taken.

14. **(B)** The first count performed during a C-section is done before closing the uterus, which is a hollow organ.

15. **(D)** The first closing count is performed when the peritoneum is being closed.

16. **(C)** Dressing sponges should not be flipped onto the sterile field until the wound is closed and the final closing count is performed. Dressing sponges do come in some of the back-table packs. When this occurs, they should immediately be isolated somewhere safe. An example would be under the basin.

17. **(C)** The tab holding the Raytec 4 × 4 sponges should be removed and each sponge counted individually.

18. **(A)** The ideal time to count your instruments is when all instruments and supplies are still on the back table.

19. **(B)** Counts may be omitted in an emergency situation. It must be documented, and the STSR and circulator should do their best to keep track of everything entering the body. At the end of the case, a final count may be performed and an x-ray taken. Examples of emergency situations include a ruptured abdominal aneurysm and an emergency C-section.

20. **(D)** All needles, including suture and hypodermics, scalpel blades, and the ESU tip should be considered sharps and must be counted.

CHAPTER 10

Specimens

- Biopsy—excision of tissue or aspirated fluid
- Histology—study of tissue
- Cytology—study of cells
- All tissue and objects removed from the patient are considered specimens and must be sent to pathology
- Permanent specimens are sent in formalin or saline. The fluid is drained and replaced with paraffin. This is a type of wax that helps to keep the tissue hard or together so it can be cut and viewed under a microscope at a later date
- Frozen sections are sent immediately to the lab and placed in a dry container
- Urine specimens
- Clean catch—urethral meatus is cleaned, and the patient urinates in a sterile specimen cup midstream upon voiding
- Urine specimens are obtained under sterile conditions and sent in a sterile specimen container
- The STSR must confirm the specimen with the surgeon before handing it off the field
- The circulator must confirm with the STSR and surgeon to confirm proper labeling before sending it out of the room. "Write down and read back"
- The surgeon may mark specimens with suture/clips/margin markers to identify the correct orientation of the specimen when taken from the body
- Bullets—must be handled with gloved hands, not instrumentation, because instruments can leave a scratch or indentation in the bullet, and forensics will not be able to make an accurate match. All guns have markings in the barrel, and the bullet should have identical markings; an instrument could alter these markings
- Removed prosthesis—kept clean and dry before sending to pathology
- Amputated limbs are sent dry to pathology
- Breast specimens that are sent for frozen section are sent dry (no formalin)
- Gallstones and kidney stones should go dry to pathology as the preservative can alter the specimens
- Smear and/or brush biopsy specimens are commonly used for endoscopic procedures (bronchoscopy)
- Fluid and cells are obtained with a small brush and placed on a slide for the cells to be examined
- Specimens are placed on Telfa or in a basin; never place on a surgical sponge that is counted
- Incisional biopsy—removal of a portion of the lesion for frozen section
- Gram stain—used to identify bacteria. Stains used include:
  ○ Blue/purple—gram positive
  ○ Red/pink—gram negative
- Cerebrospinal fluid (CSF)—obtained by performing a spinal tap. CSF is withdrawn from the lumbar region of the spinal column for analysis
- Thoracentesis—a needle is placed into the pleural space and fluid is withdrawn for diagnosis
- Lukens tube—collection tube used to obtain specimens from the lungs and stomach during procedures

Questions

1. Who is directly responsible for receiving and handling the specimen on the sterile field?

    (A) STSR
    (B) Circulator
    (C) Anesthesiologist
    (D) Surgeon

2. Damage to or loss of specimens results in:

    (A) an incorrect diagnosis
    (B) repeat or needless surgery
    (C) delayed treatment
    (D) all of the above

3. What type of biopsy is performed during a flexible endoscopic procedure?

    (A) Incisional biopsy
    (B) Needle biopsy
    (C) Brush biopsy
    (D) Fine-needle aspiration

4. Stones are sent to pathology in:

    (A) formalin
    (B) dry container
    (C) sterile saline
    (D) not sent to pathology

5. Which of the following is considered a foreign body?

    (A) A nontissue item
    (B) Wood
    (C) An implant
    (D) All of the above

6. An amputated limb is sent:

    (A) to the morgue
    (B) to pathology
    (C) in formalin
    (D) to be discarded

7. What type of specimen requires immediate analysis?

    (A) Stones
    (B) Foreign body
    (C) Frozen section
    (D) All of the above

8. Bacteria cultures obtained during surgery are:

    (A) arterial blood gases (ABGs)
    (B) aerobic
    (C) anaerobic
    (D) both B and C

9. The term describing the removal of a specimen in one piece is:

    (A) in situ
    (B) en bloc
    (C) colon resection
    (D) none of the above

10. Foreign bodies removed from a patient must go to pathology.

    (A) True
    (B) False

11. Urine specimens do NOT need to be obtained under sterile conditions.

    (A) True
    (B) False

12. Prior to labeling the specimen, the circulator must:

    (A) ask the STSR what the specimen is
    (B) ask the anesthesiologist what the specimen is
    (C) ask the surgeon what the specimen is
    (D) none of the above

13. Specimens should never be placed on:

    (A) Raytec 4 × 4
    (B) Telfa
    (C) emesis basin
    (D) none of the above

14. Histologic examination is also known as:

    (A) study of tissue
    (B) study of cells
    (C) both A and B
    (D) none of the above

15. What is considered improper procedure for handling a bullet specimen?

    (A) Handle as little as possible.
    (B) Use tissue forceps to gently grasp the bullet.
    (C) Do not drop bullet into metal basin or bowl.
    (D) Do not use an instrument to grasp the bullet.

16. When sending a frozen specimen to the lab:

    (A) send immediately for analysis
    (B) send in a dry container
    (C) verify with the surgeon before handing it off the sterile field
    (D) all of the above

17. Permanent specimens are sent to pathology:

    (A) immediately for a diagnosis
    (B) in a dry container
    (C) in a container with formalin or saline
    (D) they do not need to go to pathology and can be discarded

18. A femoral implant removed from the patient's body is sent:

    (A) clean in formalin
    (B) clean in a dry container
    (C) to be discarded
    (D) clean wrapped in a lap and placed in a dry container

19. Which describes an incisional biopsy?

    (A) The entire mass with surrounding tissue
    (B) A small portion of tissue is incised and sent for examination
    (C) Sent as a permanent specimen
    (D) Sent in formalin

20. Which describes thoracentesis?

    (A) A needle is placed into the pleural space and fluid is withdrawn for diagnosis.
    (B) A Lukens is used to obtain a thoracentesis specimen.
    (C) A brush instrument is used to obtain the specimen.
    (D) It is a video-assisted thoracoscopic surgery (VATS) procedure.

21. A specimen obtained in one piece is termed:

    (A) in situ
    (B) en bloc
    (C) frozen
    (D) none of the above

22. The color of a gram-positive bacteria stain is:

    (A) red/pink
    (B) green
    (C) blue/purple
    (D) yellow

23. When obtaining CSF for a specimen:

    (A) it is termed a spinal tap
    (B) it is retrieved from the lumbar region
    (C) it is sent as a frozen specimen
    (D) both A and B

24. Cultures obtained during surgery:

    (A) are handled as any other specimen
    (B) are passed off the sterile field into a bag or container held by the circulator
    (C) should be kept warm or sent to the laboratory immediately
    (D) should be handled only by the scrub nurse

25. How is a frozen section sent to the laboratory?

    (A) In formalin
    (B) In saline
    (C) In water
    (D) Dry

26. Which of the following specimens is NOT placed in preservative solution?

    (A) Stones
    (B) Curettings
    (C) Tonsils
    (D) Uterus

Answers and Explanations

1. **(A)** The STSR is directly responsible for receiving the specimen on the sterile field.

2. **(D)** If a specimen is lost or damaged, the result can be an incorrect diagnosis, repeat or needless surgery, and delayed treatment.

3. **(C)** A brush biopsy is performed during a flexible endoscopic procedure. A fine brush is used to collect cells on the surface of mucous membranes.

4. **(B)** Stones removed from the urinary tract, salivary ducts, and the gallbladder are sent in a dry container to pathology.

5. **(D)** A nontissue item, wood, and an implant are all considered foreign bodies.

6. **(B)** Initially, the limb must be sent for analysis to pathology like any specimen and then sent to the morgue.

7. **(C)** Frozen section requires immediate analysis. This is accomplished by freezing the tissue and making fine sectional slices that can be examined microscopically.

8. **(D)** The two types of bacteria cultures taken intraoperatively are aerobic and anaerobic.

9. **(B)** En bloc is when the specimen is removed all in one piece.

10. **(A)** All specimens, including foreign bodies, must be sent to pathology.

11. **(B)** All urine being sent for specimen must be collected under sterile conditions.

12. **(C)** The circulator must ask the surgeon how to label the specimen.

13. **(A)** Specimens can never be placed on a Raytec sponge because it is a counted item and cannot leave the room.

14. **(A)** Histologic examination is the study of tissue. Cytologic examination is the study of cells.

15. **(B)** Instruments can damage the bullet. Marks on the bullet need to be examined to match the gun. Any alteration to the bullet can distort that test.

16. **(D)** All of the above facts are true regarding frozen sections.

17. **(C)** Permanent specimens go to pathology in formalin or saline.

18. **(B)** After removal of a prosthesis, the item must go in a clean dry container.

19. **(B)** An incisional biopsy is a small portion of tissue that is removed. Excisional biopsy is removal of the entire mass. This biopsy is never sent as permanent or in formalin.

20. **(A)** A needle is inserted into the pleural space to remove fluid. A Lukens is used for peritoneal washings. Brush instruments are used in cytology. This procedure is done without video assistance.

21. **(B)** En bloc refers to all pieces of specimen to remain attached when it is removed. In situ is a specimen that is in its original position.

Frozen specimen is tissue that is sent immediately to pathology.

22. **(C)** The color of the stain in gram-positive specimens is blue/purple. Gram-negative specimens turn red/pink.

23. **(D)** Obtaining CSF is done through a spinal tap and is taken from the lumbar region.

24. **(B)** Cultures are obtained under sterile conditions. The tips must not be contaminated by any other source. The circulating nurse can hold open a small bag for the scrub nurse to drop the tube into if it is handled on the sterile field. This protects personnel and prevents the spread of microorganisms.

25. **(D)** Frozen section specimens are not placed in solution because they can react with tissue and affect the pathologist's diagnosis. A frozen section is the cutting of a thin piece of tissue from a frozen specimen. This permits examination under a microscope.

26. **(A)** Stones are placed in a dry container to prevent dissolving. Stones are sent for additional study to determine their composition.

CHAPTER 11

Medical, Ethical, and Legal Responsibilities

MEDICAL/ETHICAL/LEGAL FOR THE REVIEW BOOK

- We are all responsible for our own actions
- Scope of practice—this is a term given that identifies the knowledge and skills required for the professional (STSR) to provide effective and reliable care. This is based on:
  - Education
  - Experience
  - National credentialing
- The STSR performs tasks in the operating room (OR) under the authority of the surgeon
  - We can only do what we are legally trained to do. If someone asks us to do something we were not trained to do—do not do it!!!!! Often in the OR, you will see people performing tasks that they shouldn't do, and you will be asked to do tasks you shouldn't do either. Politely say, "I'm sorry I can't do that."
- When faced with a task that you feel is not in your scope of practice, ask yourself these questions:
  - "Was the task taught in our surgical technology program?" If the answer is yes, then you may do it. If the answer is no, then do not do it.
  - "Am I willing to take full responsibility for what I am about to do?"
- Licensure
  - Most restrictive
  - Registered nurses are licensed
- Certification—surgical technology students are credentialed by certification
  - NBSTSA—National Board of Surgical Technology and Surgical Assisting—administers the national certification examination

  - Surgical technologists must pass the examination in order to work in New Jersey, Texas, Illinois, Indiana, South Carolina, and Tennessee
  - Accreditation—in order to sit for the national certification examination, you must come from an accredited program
  - CAAHEP—Commission on Accreditation of Allied Health Education Programs—sets the standards for the surgical technology program
  - Core Curriculum—the guide that outlines the mandatory curriculum for the surgical technology program
  - ARC/STSA—Accreditation Review Council on Education in Surgical Technology and Surgical Assisting—directly oversees the educational part of the program. They assist accredited programs prepare for site visits
- Legal terms
  - Accountability—to be held responsible for your actions
  - Affidavit—sworn written statement of facts (confession)
  - Allegation—a claim that someone has done something illegal or wrong, usually made without any proof
  - Bona fide—sincere without intention to deceive
  - Guardian—court-appointed guardian to care for someone who cannot take care of themselves
    - Minor children
    - Incapacitated adults
  - Iatrogenic injury—an injury caused by a health care worker

- o Liability—obligation to do something or not to do something. Being responsible for doing something or not doing something
- o Malpractice—when a medical professional does something or doesn't do something that causes injury to the patient.
  - ▪ Abandonment—leaving the patient at any given time without proper protection for the patient
- o Negligence—carelessness but no intention to do harm. Failure to use reasonable care; another professional would not do the same thing in the circumstance. Examples include:
  - ▪ Something left in the body during surgery
  - ▪ Poor positioning that injured a patient
  - ▪ Patient burns from prep solution or the cautery
  - ▪ Performing surgery on the wrong side or site
- o Standard of care—the conduct that is expected of a health care professional in given circumstances
  - ▪ Health professionals must recognize responsibility to patients first and to other health professionals
  - ▪ Provide competent medical care
  - ▪ Respect human dignity and human rights
- Tort—a wrongful act that results in injury to another's person, property, or reputation, and the injured party is entitled to compensation. Torts can be intentional or unintentional
  - o Intentional torts
    - ▪ Assault—threat of bodily harm with the intent to actually cause bodily harm
    - ▪ Battery—intentional unlawful touching of someone without their consent. You actually want to cause harm
    - ▪ Defamation—oral or written statement about someone that is untrue and can damage to their reputation
    - ▪ Invasion of privacy—discussing private information about a patient without their consent
  - o Unintentional torts
    - ▪ Patient misidentification
    - ▪ A patient's wrist band should never be removed until they leave the hospital
    - ▪ Transport should check the ID bracelet before bringing the patient into the OR
    - ▪ The preoperative nurse in the holding area should check the name on the bracelet with the name on the chart

- ▪ The patient is requested to state their name, and it should match the ID bracelet
- ▪ Circulator, anesthesiologist should do the same
- ▪ The last is the surgeon in the OR
- o Aeger primo—the patient first
- o Primum non nocere—above all, do no harm
- o Res ipsa loquitor—the thing speaks for itself
- o Respondeat superior—let the master answer
- Time out
  - o Anyone can initiate the time out; however, it is usually the circulator
  - o Everyone in the room must stop and pay close attention to the time out
  - o Everyone in the room should be in agreement with the information and verbally agree to it
- Time out includes:
  - o Confirming the patient's name, procedure, and where the incision will be made (specific right, left side)
  - o Allergies
  - o Anesthesia has addressed any patient concerns
  - o Have antibiotics been given prophylactically?
  - o Estimated blood loss
  - o All films, supplies, equipment ready
  - o Are there any patient specific concerns?
  - o All agree?
- Foreign bodies left in the patient—counts must be completed between the STSR and the circulator verbally and visually:
  - o Before the case begins
  - o When closing a hollow cavity (eg, uterus, C-section)
  - o Peritoneum
  - o Skin
- Patient burns—burns in the OR include:
  - o Hot instruments—cool off instruments from the autoclave with cool sterile water
  - o Placing the return electrode improperly
  - o The electrosurgical unit (ESU) should be placed in its holder when not in use. Do not clamp the ESU cord with a metal instrument because if the electrical cord has a cut or tear in it, the current will travel and cause a burn
  - o Electrical equipment should be tested prior to use
  - o Improper use of lasers and neglect of laser safety
  - o Pooled prep solutions under the patient

- Hot irrigation solutions
- Anesthesia flammable gases
- Light cords that are placed on the patients drapes
- Falls or improper patient positioning
  - Side rails should be up when transferring the patient, and all extremities should be kept inside the bed rails
  - The stretcher and OR table should be locked when transferring the patient
  - Proper amount of people when moving the patient include:
    - Two—mobile patient
    - Four—immobile patient
    - Anesthesia controls the head and time of transfer
  - Immediately place safety strap 2 in above the knee as soon as the patient is on the OR table
  - Ensure proper padding
  - Understand positioning techniques and work together
- Incorrect administration of drugs
  - The STSR and the circulator should verify verbally and visually the correct drug, expiration date, and amount
    - The STSR MUST label the med cup/pitcher/syringe as soon as the drug is received and the syringe is filled
    - When passing the syringe to the surgeon, the STSR should state the medication and the percentage
- Always check equipment before use and follow manufacturer's directions
- Loss or damage of patient property—the RN in the holding area should remove patient's personal property, place it in a labeled bag, and keep it with the patient's chart. If it gets past her, the circulator in the OR should follow protocol
- Be responsible for any breaks in sterile technique you make. Surgical site infections (SSIs) are caused by breaks in technique. They can be traced back to someone who does not follow sterile technique
- The STSR is under the direct authority of the surgeon; however, we should not do anything that is out of our scope of practice. It is illegal

Questions

1. A patient was burned on the lip with a hot mouth gag. Which of the following actions would have prevented this incident?

   (A) The circulator cooled the item in the sterilizer.
   (B) The scrub nurse warned the surgeon that the item was hot.
   (C) The scrub nurse cooled the item in a basin with sterile water.
   (D) The surgeon had checked the item before using it.

2. A patient signs a permission form for surgery, but because of a language barrier, he or she does not fully understand what he or she has signed. This could constitute a liability case for:

   (A) assault and battery
   (B) lack of accountability
   (C) improper documentation
   (D) invasion of privacy

3. If a patient falls because he or she was left unattended, the OR team member could be cited in a lawsuit for:

   (A) misconduct
   (B) assault
   (C) doctrine of respondeat superior
   (D) abandonment

4. The legal doctrine that mandates every professional nurse and technician to carry out their duties according to national standards of care practiced throughout the country is the:

   (A) doctrine of res ipsa loquitor
   (B) doctrine of respondeat superior
   (C) Nurse Practice Act
   (D) doctrine of reasonable man

5. The doctrine of respondeat superior refers to:

   (A) the legal terms for assault and battery
   (B) invasion of privacy
   (C) employer liability for employee's negligent conduct
   (D) professional misconduct

6. Liability is a legal rule that:

   (A) applies only in criminal actions
   (B) holds the hospital responsible for its personnel
   (C) holds each individual responsible for his or her own acts
   (D) has no significance in malpractice suits

7. Criteria that identify, measure, monitor, and evaluate patient care are:

   (A) audits
   (B) automated information systems
   (C) quality control circles
   (D) quality assurance programs

8. Failing to observe or act in a situation that the individual should have known about and acted on is called:

(A) negligence

(B) abandonment

(C) guilt

(D) defamation

9. A document in which a person gives instructions about his or her medical care in the event that the individual cannot speak is a/an:

(A) hospital policy

(B) administrative law

(C) ethical deposition

(D) advanced directive

10. The legal document signed by the patient before surgery is a/an:

(A) operative report

(B) safe medical act

(C) ethical policy

(D) informed consent

11. The operative paperwork completed by the RN contains:

(A) sponges, sharps, and instrument counts

(B) specimens

(C) medications given

(D) all of the above

12. The Latin phrase aeger primo refers to:

(A) patient first

(B) do no harm

(C) breathe

(D) it speaks for itself

13. Events requiring an incident report include:

(A) bullying

(B) equipment failure

(C) incorrect count

(D) all of the above

14. Accreditation for surgical technology programs is done by:

(A) ARC/STSA

(B) CAAHEP

(C) AORN

(D) JACHO

15. The code of ethics of the Association of Surgical Technologists includes:

(A) to follow the principles of asepsis

(B) to report any unethical conduct or practice to proper authorities

(C) to respect and practice the patient's legal and moral rights for quality patient care

(D) all of the above

16. The American Hospital Association's (AHA) Patient's Bill of Rights was adopted in what year?

(A) 1972

(B) 1985

(C) 1990

(D) 1960

17. Ethics is defined as:

(A) a legal obligation that one person owes another person

(B) a moral obligation that one person owes another person

(C) laws

(D) what the patient requests

18. When you pass the CST exam, the certification is described as:

(A) a formal process by which qualified individuals are listed in a registry

(B) a legal right granted by a government agency that complies with a statute that authorizes the activities of the profession

(C) a recognition by an appropriate body that an individual has met a predetermined standard

(D) able to perform according to the facility guidelines

19. The Health Insurance Portability and Account-ability Act (HIPAA):

    (A) gives patients the right to have elective surgery
    (B) are privacy standards to protect the patient's medical records
    (C) gives patients the right to sue their doctor
    (D) allows patients to see any physician they chose

20. Risk management objectives for a hospital include:

    (A) minimize risks to patients and employees
    (B) control financial loss
    (C) collect data to decrease harm to patients and staff
    (D) all of the above

21. When a negligence suit is filed against the hospital, who is named?

    (A) The surgeon
    (B) The RN
    (C) The STSR
    (D) Every person that has played a part in that surgery

Answers and Explanations

1. **(C)** It is the responsibility of the scrub nurse to cool an instrument in cool sterile water before handing it to the surgeon. Burns are one of the most frequent causes of lawsuits.

2. **(A)** Lack of consent is an aspect of assault and battery. Consent must be given voluntarily with full understanding of the implications. The procedure must be explained fully, in understandable language, so that the patient fully comprehends what will be done.

3. **(D)** Abandonment may be a cause for a lawsuit if an unattended patient falls from a stretcher or an OR table. It is the responsibility of a staff member to stay with the patient at all times.

4. **(D)** The doctrine of reasonable man means that a patient has the right to expect all professional and technical nursing personnel to utilize knowledge, skill, and judgment in performing duties that meet the standards exercised by other reasonable, prudent persons involved in a similar circumstance.

5. **(C)** An employer may be liable for an employee's negligent conduct under the respondeat superior master–servant employment relationship. This implies that the master will answer for the acts of the servant.

6. **(C)** An unconditional general rule of law is that every person is liable for the wrongs he or she commits that cause injury, loss, or damage to any person's property. Liability means to be legally bound, answerable, and responsible. A patient or family member may institute a civil action against the person who caused the injury, loss, or damage.

7. **(D)** Quality assurance (QA) establishes the criteria for measuring, monitoring, and evaluating patient care as well as setting standards for improvement.

8. **(A)** Negligence is legally defined as the omission to do something that a reasonable person, guided by those ordinary considerations that regulate human affairs, would do.

9. **(D)** An advanced directive is a document giving someone instructions pertaining to medical care in the event the person cannot make decisions on their own.

10. **(D)** Informed consent is a legal document that states the patient procedure, risks, consequences, and benefits of the surgery.

11. **(D)** This paperwork includes patient assessment, care plan, equipment, and devices used during the procedure. It counts specimens, medications, and the names of all perioperative personnel who participated in the procedure.

12. **(A)** The Latin term aeger primo means patient first.

13. **(D)** Many events require an incident report, including medication errors, bullying, equipment failure, and incorrect counts.

14. **(B)** CAAHEP accredits programs upon recommendation of the ARC/STSA. The ARC/STSA provides educational standards and recommendations required for the accredited program of surgical technology and surgical first assisting.

15. **(D)** All of the above are part of the code of ethics and many more.

16. **(A)** The AHA adopted the Bill of Rights in 1972.

17. **(B)** Ethics is defined as the moral obligation one person owes to another.

18. **(C)** Certification is described as being recognized by an appropriate body stating that the person has met the required standards.

19. **(B)** HIPAA assures privacy standards in regard to a patient's medical condition and medical records.

20. **(D)** The risk management department is responsible for minimizing risks to patients and employees, avoiding or minimizing the financial loss to the institution, and collecting data to avoid future injuries.

21. **(D)** When a negligence suit is filed, everyone in contact with that patient will be named in the suit.

CHAPTER 12

Diagnostic Procedures

DIAGNOSTIC IMAGING

- Radiography/roentgenography—term used to describe producing images of internal structures of the body; they include:
- Portable x-ray machine—can be used in the operating room. It uses:
  - Cassette—this can placed under the patient or on a wheel-mounted machine that can be placed alongside the patient covered with a sterile drape sheet
  - Once the film is taken, it is processed to be viewed
- Contrast media—chemical substances used in x-ray. When the contrast media is injected, it makes the images on the film look dense, and the target structure stands out. They include:
  - Renografin
  - Hypaque/sodium diatrizoate
  - Cystografin
  - These chemical substances can be introduced into the body:
    - Intravenously
    - Intra-arterially
    - Intrathecally—injected into the spine
    - Intra-abdominally
- C-arm—a mobile image intensifier used to take pictures
  - Contrast media can be used
  - The fluoroscopy allows films to be taken still and with continuous movement in real time. It is controlled by a foot pedal
  - It is called a C-arm because of its obvious shape
  - X-rays can be taken in lateral or anterior positions
  - Both the patient and staff must wear a lead apron to protect the testicles and ovaries and

a thyroid collar to protect the thyroid. Do not turn your unprotected back to the C-arm
  - Lead apron thickness: 0.5 mm of lead
  - Do not bend and twist lead aprons; it could damage the lead
  - The C-arm delivers high doses of radiation. The surgeon and staff should limit the time their hands are exposed or wear lead gloves
  - All working with fluoroscopy should be monitored regarding the amount of exposure; an x-ray badge called a dosimeter is worn at the neck and routinely checked
  - While the fluoroscopy is being used, it is recommended to stand at least 1 ft from the machine or even further if possible
  - A special drape is used to protect the surgical field from contamination
- Mini C-arm—a smaller version of the original C-arm; commonly used on hands and feet
- Mammography—an x-ray taken of the soft tissue of the breast to diagnose breast tumors. The x-ray can take many different angles to view the breast tissue
- Myelography—an x-ray of the spine. Contrast media is used
- Angiography—an imaging technique used to view the inside of vessels. Contrast media is injected and the vessels outlined
- Cardiac catheterization—the process of injecting the contrast media whereby the coronary arteries are outlined. The invasive cardiologist can now diagnose which of the coronary arteries is obstructed. A stent may be placed in the coronary artery that is obstructed. This stent keeps the artery open
  - A cut-down procedure is performed, a catheter is introduced into the vessel, and contrast

media is injected; depending on which part of the heart they are focusing on, they can use the:

- Femoral vessel
- Brachial vessel

- Electrocardiogram (ECG)—performed to test the electrical activity of the heart. Electrodes are placed on the skin—trunk, arms, and legs
- Pulmonary angiography is primarily performed to detect pulmonary embolism or pulmonary artery aneurysms
- Cholangiography—can be performed preoperatively or intraoperatively; the contrast media is injected preoperatively through an IV and intraoperatively directly into the common bile duct to visualize stones or an obstruction
- Ventriculography—an x-ray of the ventricles in the brain
- Arthrography—an x-ray of the inside of a joint using contrast media or gas (air or carbon dioxide)
- Gastrointestinal (GI) x-ray
  - Upper GI tract—a barium drink is used as the contrast media while fluoroscopy is used to visualize the esophagus, stomach, and small intestines
  - Lower GI tract—a barium is given while fluoroscopy is used to visualize the large intestines
- X-rays of the genitourinary (GU) tract
  - Cystography—x-ray of the bladder
  - Cystourethrography—x-ray of the urethra and bladder
  - KUB—x-ray of the kidneys, ureters, and bladder to obtain information regarding the size, shape, and position of the structures
  - Intravenous pyelogram (IVP)/intravenous urogram (IVU)—contrast media is injected through an IV and x-rays are taken of the entire GU system
- Computed axial tomography scan (CAT/CT)—a specialized x-ray machine that takes pictures in cross-sections or slices. The CT scan uses radiation, and contrast media can be used via an IV
- Magnetic resonance imaging (MRI)—this type of x-ray does not use radiation. It uses radiofrequency waves and a magnetic field. The patient is slid into a tubular magnetic type of machine. MRI also takes pictures of the body in slices, but

they can be taken from any direction and provides a detailed picture. Contrast media can also be used by introducing media through an IV
- Positron emission tomography (PET)—this type of x-ray uses a radioactive substance called a "tracer," which is introduced into the body through a vein. The organs in your body absorb the tracer, and the physician can interpret how your organs and tissues are working
- Ultrasound—uses high-frequency sound waves to create an image of organs inside of the body. A water-soluble gel is placed on the skin to provide an airtight connection, and a transducer probe transmits images to the screen. This is commonly used for images of:
  - Stomach
  - Liver
  - Heart/echocardiogram—this type of ultrasound provides a two-dimensional image of the structures and function of the heart
  - Tendons
  - Muscles
  - Joints
  - Blood vessels
  - Fetus
  - Cannot be used on the lungs because it cannot pass through organs with air
- Radionuclide scan—in this type of scan, a radioactive chemical is administered by oral ingestion or through an IV. The radioactive chemical (eg, iodine) is used to produce an image of the structure and function of body organs. This is performed in nuclear medicine
- Biopsy—performed to diagnose a disease by excising tissue and/or fluids for examination with a microscope. Types of biopsies include:
  - Incisional biopsy—a portion of the target tissue is excised and sent to pathology for a diagnosis. They can be sent:
    - Frozen—immediate diagnosis
    - Permanent—this study will be performed at a later time
    - Specimens are covered more in depth in the Specimens chapter
  - Aspiration biopsy—fluid is removed from target tissue through a syringe and sent to pathology for diagnosis
  - Smear or brush biopsy—cells are placed on a microscope slide and sent for examination

- Gram stains—performed to identify bacteria for examination. A dye is applied, and the bacteria are cultured
  - Gram positive—retains a violet/blue dye
  - Gram negative—retains a pink/red dye
- Spinal tap—performed to remove cerebrospinal fluid (CSF) through a lumbar puncture for diagnosis
- Electromyography (EMG)—performed to study the electrical activity of muscles. A probe is inserted through the skin, and an electrical impulse is introduced to see how the muscles contract and relax
- Doppler—used to access blood flow through a vessel by sound. It can be used pre-/intra-/postoperatively. A sterile drape is used to cover the probe when used during a surgical procedure

- Plethysmography—performed to measure changes in vessels. A pressure-sensitive instrument or a pressure cuff is placed around a limb and records the changes. It does not measure blood flow in a particular vessel but blood flow of the entire area that the cuff is placed on
- Thoracentesis—performed to remove fluid from the pleural cavity for diagnosis and/or therapeutic treatment
- Electroencephalography (EEG)—performed to measure the electrical activity of the brain. Leeds are placed on the scalp and measure brain waves and determine how the brain functions
- Blood work—discussed in Blood Values chapter
- Urinalysis—discussed in GU chapter

Questions

1. Contrast media includes all EXCEPT:

   (A) Renografin
   (B) sodium hypochlorite
   (C) Hypaque
   (D) Cystografin

2. Contrast media can be introduced into the body by which route?

   (A) Intravenously
   (B) Injected into the spine
   (C) Intrathecally
   (D) All of the above

3. All pertain to C-arm procedures EXCEPT:

   (A) a dosimeter is used to monitor the amount of x-ray exposure from the fluoroscopy machine
   (B) the x-ray badge is worn at the bottom hem area of the lead apron
   (C) it is recommended to stand at least 6 ft from the fluoroscopy x-ray beam
   (D) lead apron thickness is 0.5 mm of lead

4. An x-ray of the spine is termed:

   (A) mammography
   (B) ECG
   (C) myelography
   (D) IVU

5. During a cardiac catheterization, the vessels used to introduce the catheter and inject the contrast media are:

   (A) femoral
   (B) popliteal
   (C) carotid
   (D) cephalic

6. When performing a cholangiogram, the contrast media is introduced into the:

   (A) cystic artery
   (B) cystic vein
   (C) CBD
   (D) cystic duct

7. A ventriculography is an x-ray of the:

   (A) ventricles in the brain
   (B) vessels of the body
   (C) cross-sections of the body
   (D) varicosities

8. What type of x-ray uses high-frequency sound waves to create an image of organs inside of the body?

   (A) CT scan
   (B) PET scan
   (C) Ultrasound
   (D) All of the above

9. A biopsy is performed to diagnose a disease by excising tissue and fluids for examination; the type of biopsy that requires an immediate diagnosis is termed:

   (A) permanent
   (B) frozen
   (C) brush
   (D) none of the above

10. Gram stains are performed to identify bacteria for examination; a stain that is gram positive is:

   (A) violet/blue
   (B) red
   (C) pink/blue
   (D) pink

11. When performing a spinal tap to retrieve CSF, the puncture is performed in which space?

   (A) Cervical
   (B) Thoracic
   (C) Lumbar
   (D) Sacral

12. The first step in determining the origin of a patient's illness is:

   (A) x-rays
   (B) history and physical
   (C) ultrasound
   (D) PET scan

13. The test used to view and evaluate pain in the spine, neck, back, or leg is:

   (A) electrocardiogram
   (B) cystogram
   (C) myelogram
   (D) spinal tap

14. The procedure performed to measure changes in blood vessels is termed:

   (A) plethysmography
   (B) ventriculography
   (C) radionuclide scan
   (D) ECG

15. Thoracentesis:

   (A) is performed to remove fluid from the pleural cavity
   (B) is a test to visualize whether the tumor is hard or fluid filled
   (C) uses ultrasonic sound waves to produce an image containing fluid
   (D) is performed to remove fluid from the abdominal cavity

16. An x-ray performed of the entire mouth in one film is termed:

   (A) EEG
   (B) panoramic
   (C) audiometry
   (D) basic x-ray

17. ECG is:

   (A) a stress test of the heart
   (B) used to assess blood flow through a vessel
   (C) used to measure electrical activity of the brain
   (D) used to measure electrical activity of the heart

Answers and Explanations

1. **(B)** Sodium hypochlorite is household bleach.

2. **(D)** Contrast media can be introduced into the body by all routes.

3. **(B)** The x-ray badge is called a dosimeter. It is recommended to be worn at the neck level.

4. **(C)** Myelography is an x-ray of the spine.

5. **(A)** During a cardiac catheterization, the vessels used to introduce the catheter to inject contrast are the femoral vessels.

6. **(D)** The cystic duct is the area where the contrast is introduced.

7. **(A)** Ventriculography is an x-ray of the brain. Angiography is x-ray of vessels. A CT scan produces cross-sections of the body. Varicosities are thrombosed veins.

8. **(C)** An ultrasound uses high-frequency sound waves to create an image. PET scan uses a radioactive substance called a tracer. CT scan uses radiation and contrast media.

9. **(B)** A specimen that is sent to pathology for an immediate diagnosis is a frozen section.

10. **(A)** Gram stains that are gram positive turn violet/blue.

11. **(C)** A spinal tap retrieves CSF from the lumbar space.

12. **(B)** Performing a history and physical is the first thing a physician does prior to ordering any diagnostic tests.

13. **(C)** A myelogram is done to view and evaluate pain in the spine, neck, back, or leg.

14. **(A)** Plethysmography is used to measure changes in blood flow.

15. **(A)** Thoracentesis is performed to remove fluid in the pleural cavity.

16. **(B)** Panoramic views include the entire mouth.

17. **(D)** ECG is done to measure the electrical activity of the heart.

CHAPTER 13

Consents

- Informed consent—an oral and written consent that is signed before a patient has a surgical procedure
  - The informed consent is obtained by the surgeon. The information regarding the consent includes:
    - Patient's name
    - Surgeon's name
    - Procedure
    - Signature of the patient and witness
    - Date of the signatures
- The surgeon is responsible for obtaining the consent; he should clearly explain:
  - The procedure
  - Risks involved
  - Benefits
  - Alternatives
  - Complications
- The patient must receive this information in terms that they understand. If the patient does not fully understand what the physician informed them about the procedure because they have a language barrier and something goes wrong, then this could constitute assault and battery
- Information prior to the patient signing the consent includes:
  - Exactly who will perform the procedure and who will assist
  - The consent must be signed before the patient has received any preoperative medication
  - The circulating nurse should ensure that this process has taken place before the patient is admitted to the operating room
- Patients should sign the consent themselves unless they are:
  - Minors
  - Unconscious
  - Mentally incompetent
  - In a life-threatening situation; if this is the case, the next closest relative is authorized to sign
  - If the patient is a minor, the parent or guardian must sign
  - Illiterate person—may sign with an X
  - Unconscious person—a responsible relative or guardian
  - Mentally incompetent—the legal guardian
  - If the patient is incompetent because they are under the influence of alcohol or drugs, the closest relative may sign if it is an emergency; if it is not an emergency, wait for the patient to detox
- General consent form is signed upon admission to the health care facility
  - This is signed to perform generalized day-to-day treatment
  - An additional informed consent is required for surgery
- Consent in an emergency
  - Phone consent—two nurses must monitor the call and sign a legal form
  - Two surgeons (not part of the patient's care team) may be called in to witness that the patient is in a life-threatening situation and needs the surgery; they sign a legal form
- Witnessing the consent—may be a nurse or other facility employees. The witness must verify:
  - Patient's signature
  - That the signature was made voluntarily
  - That the patient had a sound mental state
- Every patient has the right to refuse a surgical procedure at any time. The surgeon and nurse document the patient's refusal for surgery, and all sign. This will relieve the hospital and health care team from any liability

- Advanced directives—a document that allows the patient to give instructions about their medical care in the event they become incapacitated and cannot speak for themselves. Additional information can include information on organ donation
- Living will—a document that specifies the type of medical intervention that the patient does not want; examples include:
  - Feeding tubes
  - Ventilator
- Power of attorney—a document that authorizes a designated person to make decisions for a patient if they are incapacitated and cannot make decisions for themselves

- DNR—do not resuscitate. No cardiopulmonary resuscitation (CPR)
- Incident report—a written statement regarding an accident involving a patient or employee. The details should be written as statement of facts without your opinion
  - This should be reported to the nurse manager. Examples include:
    - Needle sticks
    - Falls
    - Loss of instruments

Questions

1. In the event that a child needs emergency surgery and the parents cannot be located to sign the permission:

    (A) no permission is necessary

    (B) permission is signed by a court of law

    (C) permission is signed by the physician

    (D) a written consultation by two physicians other than the surgeon will suffice

2. The patient is scheduled for an appendectomy. After completing this procedure, the surgeon decides to remove a mole from the shoulder while the patient is still under anesthesia. No permission was obtained for this. The circulating nurse should:

    (A) report it to the anesthesiologist

    (B) report it to the chief of surgery

    (C) report it to the supervisor or proper administrative authority

    (D) let the surgeon proceed because it is his or her responsibility to obtain the consent

3. The surgical consent form can be witnessed by each of the following EXCEPT:

    (A) the surgeon

    (B) a nurse

    (C) an authorized hospital employee

    (D) the patient's spouse

4. The patient is premedicated and brought to the operating room (OR) for a cystoscopy and an open reduction of the wrist. Upon arrival in the OR, it is observed that the patient has only signed for the cystoscopy. The correct procedure would be to:

    (A) cancel surgery until a valid permission can be obtained

    (B) have the patient sign for the additional procedure in the OR

    (C) ask the patient verbally for consent and have witnesses attest to it

    (D) let the surgeon make the decision as to whether surgery could be done

5. A general consent form is:

    (A) a form authorizing all treatments or procedures

    (B) a form for all patients having general anesthesia

    (C) a form for all patients having hazardous therapy

    (D) another name for an operative permit

6. The ultimate responsibility for obtaining consent lies with the:

    (A) OR supervisor

    (B) circulating nurse

    (C) surgeon

    (D) unit charge nurse

7. The surgical consent is signed:

   (A) before induction
   (B) in the holding area
   (C) the morning of surgery
   (D) before administration of preoperative medications

8. An informed consent:

   (A) authorizes routine duties carried out at the hospital
   (B) protects patient from unratified or unwanted procedures
   (C) protects the surgeon and the hospital from claims of an unauthorized operation
   (D) both B and C

9. Implied consent:

   (A) is the preferred option for consents
   (B) is allowed by law in emergencies when no other authorized person may be contacted
   (C) is never legally valid
   (D) is the permission for surgical action

10. Which statement regarding the withdrawal of a consent by a patient is NOT true?

    (A) The surgeon informs the patient of the dangers if the procedure is not carried out.
    (B) The surgeon informs the hospital administration of the patient's refusal.
    (C) The surgeon obtains a written refusal from the patient.
    (D) The surgeon may do the procedure if he or she documents that it is necessary as a lifesaving measure.

11. Conditions of signing a consent form include:

    (A) signed voluntarily
    (B) patient must be competent
    (C) patient must sign before preoperative medications are given
    (D) all of the above

12. Consents are required for:

    (A) anesthesia
    (B) blood and blood products
    (C) experimental treatments
    (D) all of the above

13. The patient must receive information regarding consent, and the patient must understand the procedure. If the patient does not fully understand what the physician informed them about due to a language barrier and something goes wrong during the procedure, this could constitute:

    (A) assault and battery
    (B) atonement
    (C) neglect
    (D) defamation of character

14. Which document allows the patient to give instructions regarding their medical care in the event they become incapacitated and cannot speak for themselves:

    (A) living will
    (B) power of attorney
    (C) advanced directive
    (D) DNR

15. What is the protocol for consent forms for illiterate persons who cannot write?

    (A) The closest relative can sign for them.
    (B) Explain the situation and omit a signature.
    (C) Two physicians unrelated to the case must be in agreement that surgery is required.
    (D) They can sign with an X.

16. Living wills include statements on which of the following?

    (A) Feeding tubes
    (B) Ventilators
    (C) IVs
    (D) All of the above

Answers and Explanations

1. **(D)** In a dire emergency, the patient's condition takes precedence over the permit. Permits may be accepted from a legal guardian or responsible relative. Two nurses should monitor a telephone consent and sign the form; it is then signed by the parent, guardian, or spouse upon arrival. A written consultation by two physicians, not including the surgeon, will suffice until the proper signature can be obtained.

2. **(C)** If the surgeon intends or wants to perform a procedure not specified on the permission or consent form, the OR nurse assumes the responsibility of informing the surgeon and/or the proper administrative authority of the discrepancy.

3. **(D)** The patient's (or suitable substitute's) signature must be witnessed by one or more authorized persons. They may be physicians, nurses, or other hospital employees authorized to do so. The witness is attesting to the proper identification of the patient and the fact that the signing was voluntary.

4. **(A)** The patient giving his or her consent must be of legal age, mentally alert, and competent. The patient must sign before premedication is given and before going to the OR. This protects the patient from unratified procedures and also protects the surgeon and the hospital.

5. **(A)** The general consent form authorizes the physician in charge and hospital staff to render such treatments or perform such procedures as the physician deems advisable. It applies only to routine hospital procedures. The consent document for any procedure possibly injurious to the patient should be signed before the procedure is performed.

6. **(C)** The ultimate responsibility for obtaining permission is the surgeon's. The circulating nurse (RN or charge nurse) and the anesthesiologist are responsible for checking that the consent is on the chart and is properly signed and that the information on the form is correct.

7. **(D)** All consent forms must be signed before the administration of preoperative medications. This is to ensure that the patient fully understands what the procedure is. If the permission is signed incorrectly, it may not be revised until the preoperative medication has worn off.

8. **(D)** An informed consent (operative permit) protects the patient from unratified procedures and protects the surgeon and the hospital from claims of an unauthorized operation. A general consent authorizes the physician and staff to render treatment and perform procedures that are routine duties normally carried out at the hospital.

9. **(B)** Implied consent is never the preferred action. Law allows it in emergency situations when no other authorized person can be contacted or when conditions are discovered during a surgical procedure.

10. **(D)** The patient has a right to withdraw written consent if it is voluntary and if he or she is in a rationale state. The surgeon explains consequences, obtains a written refusal, and informs hospital and administration. The surgery is postponed.

11. **(D)** All of the above are conditions for signing a consent.

12. **(D)** All of the above require written consents, in additions to placing central venous catheters and other vascular devices and performing an elective sterilization process.

13. **(A)** The physician can be charged with assault and battery.

14. **(C)** Advanced directives give instructions on how to proceed should the patient become incapacitated.

15. **(D)** The patient may sign with an X if they cannot write due to illiteracy.

16. **(D)** Living wills include statements regarding the feeding tube, ventilator, or whether the patient wants an IV started

CHAPTER 14

Skin Preparation and Draping

Prepping and draping the patient for the Review Book

- Skin prep is performed to remove transient flora and reduce the amount of resident flora and hinder the growth of microbes during the surgical procedure to prevent infection
- Prep solutions include:
  - Povidone-iodine/Betadine—must be allowed to dry at least for 2 minutes prior to draping
    - Less irritating to skin than other prep solutions
    - Should not be used on the patient with allergies to iodine and shellfish
    - Betadine can be used on the face and around the eyes and ears
    - When used as a hand scrub, the iodine compounds are mixed with a detergent and should be rinsed off the skin, unlike the prep solution, which is left to dry on the skin
  - Chlorhexidine gluconate/Hibiclens—can be used for a surgical had scrub and a skin prep
    - When applying as a skin prep, it should be applied properly for approximately 2 minutes and towel dried, with this step repeated
    - Has a residual effect for 5–6 hours following application
    - Is an eye irritant and ototoxic
  - Alcohol—these solutions should contain 70% isopropyl alcohol as an effective prep solution
    - Works fast
    - Should not be used on mucous membranes, the eyes, and open wounds
    - Should be dry prior to placing the drape sheets
    - Is extremely flammable

- Dura-Prep—solution contains 70% isopropyl alcohol and iodophor solution
  - Fast acting and lasts for 12 hours on the skin
  - Should be dry prior to draping
  - Comes in self-contained applicators
- You must follow manufacturer's instructions before warming a prep solution. It is not recommended because warming can change the chemical properties of solutions and reduce their effectiveness regarding destroying microbes

Prior to performing the surgical prep

- Hair removal—If a shave prep is ordered, it should be performed as close to the time of surgery as possible in order to reduce the risk for microbial growth in the case of a break in the skin, which can cause an infection
  - The shave prep should be performed in the patient holding area not the operating room
  - It is recommended that an electric clipper be used not a razor to prevent cutting the patient's skin
  - Eyebrows should never be shaved
  - Long eyelashes should be carefully trimmed using small scissors and a water-soluble jelly
  - When hair is removed for a craniotomy procedure, the patient's hair should go into a secure bag that is labeled with the patient's name and identification number. This is property of the patient and should be kept with the chart
- Surgical prep
  - The night before or the morning prior to surgery, the patient should shower/bathe; the surgeon may order a special antiseptic wash be used
  - The skin prep is performed using sterile technique

- This should always be performed from clean to dirty
- The skin prep begins at the planned incision site and is carried to the periphery, using a circular motion; never return over the clean area with a sponge
- The boundaries of the skin prep should be much wider than the planned incision to allow the incision to be extended if needed
- Sterile towels should be placed to prevent pooling of the prep solution and prevent a chemical burn or a burn from the electrosurgical unit (ESU)
- Each sponge must be discarded once used
- You must avoid contamination when performing the prep
- When holding a limb during a prep, always don sterile gloves to prevent contamination
- Preps that require two separate preps
  - Abdominal perineal prep—the perineal area should be prepped first and covered with a sterile towel to avoid contamination of the abdominal area, and the abdominal area is prepped last
  - Preps for donor and recipient sites—the donor site is prepped first usually using a colorless solution so the surgeon can see the skin clearly; the recipient site is prepped next
- Special considerations when performing the skin prep for contaminated areas include:
  - Umbilicus—even though the umbilicus is considered contaminated, it should be cleaned first with a cotton-tipped applicator and antimicrobial solution, which should then be discarded
  - Cancer prep—the prep should be applied gently to avoid spreading the cancer cells
  - Stomas
    - If the stoma is included in the surgical procedure, it should be covered with an adhesive drape; the incision site is prepped and the drape is removed and the stoma is prepped last
    - If the stoma is not part of the surgical procedure, an adhesive drape should be placed and left on until the procedure is complete
  - Vagina/perineal area/anus—these areas should be prepped last, with each sponge used only once and discarded
  - Traumatic wounds/open wounds

- Sometimes an incision and drainage is performed first
- The wound is then packed with sterile saline–soaked gauze sponges, and the area around the wound is prepped
  - Axilla/hairline—these areas have a high microbial count and need to be prepped last

Anatomical boundaries, preps

- Abdominal
  - Nipple line to symphysis pubis
  - Lateral to sides of the bed
- Thoracoabdominal—patient is in lateral position
  - Chest/axilla down to the iliac crest
  - Beyond the midline anterior and posterior
- Breast
  - From the incision site to anterior neck to operating room (OR) table on affected side, arm and shoulder are elevated, and upper arm to the elbow is prepped circumferentially
  - Prep continues down to the to the symphysis pubis and lateral to the OR table on the affected side
  - Axilla prepped last
- Face
  - Place cotton balls in the ears
  - Hairline to behind the ears
  - Neck to both sides of the OR table
- Eyes
  - Be careful not to allow the prep solution to enter the patient's eyes
  - Center of the lid to the eyebrow to the cheek
- Neck
  - Neck laterally to both sides of the OR table
  - Up to the chin and
  - Down to the chest and shoulders laterally to both sides of the OR table
- Shoulder
  - Patient's head is turned to the opposite direction of affected shoulder
  - The arm is held and the shoulder is elevated off the OR table, and the prep begins at the shoulder to the base of the neck
  - Over the shoulder, scapula, and chest to the midline
  - Upper arm to below the elbow circumferentially
  - Axilla last
- Elbow and forearm
  - The arm is held by the hand

○ Prep extends from the hand to the shoulder circumferentially

○ Axilla is prepped last

- Hand
  ○ The arm is held above the elbow; also can be placed on a bolster and supported
  ○ The hand to above the elbow is prepped circumferentially
- Ankle/foot
  ○ The leg is held at the knee
  ○ Prep extends from the foot to the knee circumferentially
- Leg—lower leg and knee
  ○ The leg is held by the foot
  ○ Prep includes the foot to the upper thigh, circumferentially
- Thigh
  ○ The leg is held at the foot
  ○ The entire leg is prepped circumferentially from the foot to above the hip and buttocks laterally to the OR table on the affected side
  ○ Groin area last
- Hip
  ○ The leg is elevated at the knee
  ○ Prep begins at the hip up to the abdomen on the affected side
  ○ Over the buttock laterally to the OR table on the affected side
  ○ Down to the knee
  ○ Groin area last
- Vaginal and perineal prep
  ○ The prep begins at the pubic symphysis down over the genitalia area
  ○ Anus is last
- Always remember the following when the surgery involves the abdominoperineal areas:
  ○ The perineal area is prepped first and covered
  ○ The abdominal area is prepped last to prevent contamination from below
  ○ They are considered two separate preps

Drapes

- Drapes are used to preserve the sterile field and create a sterile barrier
- Draping sequence varies from hospital to hospital and surgeon to surgeon
- Drapes must be:
  ○ Fluid and blood resistant
  ○ Antistatic and flame resistant
  ○ Lint free

○ Tear and puncture proof

○ Porous so that the patient's body temperature is not affected

○ Nonreflective to OR lights

○ Toxic free

Drape materials

- Nonwoven disposable
  ○ Synthetic made of nylon, rayon, and polyester
- Woven fabric—reusable drapes
  ○ These drapes must be hospital laundered
  ○ Inspected routinely for wear and tear and holes
  ○ 270–280 thread count
- Fenestrated drapes—drapes with an opening (hole) placed over the incision site; they include:
  ○ Laparotomy drape sheet—has a large opening, commonly used on the abdomen
  ○ Laparoscopy drape sheet—a combination of a laparotomy sheet and a lithotomy, perineal drape sheet; commonly used in gynecological (GYN) procedures
  ○ Transverse drape sheet—rectangular sheet commonly used for pelvic GYN and kidney procedures
  ○ Pediatric drape sheet—sheet with a smaller fenestration
  ○ Lithotomy/perineal drape sheet—used for the patient in lithotomy position
    ▪ Leg drapes accompany this drape sheet; there is a folded cuff to protect your hands from contamination
- Aperture drape—a fenestrated drape sheet with adhesive that surrounds the opening to help secure the drape
- Incise drape—the entire drape is a clear plastic sticky drape that is applied to the skin. The incision is made directly through the drape
  ○ These drapes can also be impregnated with an iodophor-containing adhesive
- Split sheet/U-drape—(these drape sheets are very similar and used the same way) this drape is split up the middle, with adhesive tape along each side of the slit; used to wrap around a limb or body part
- Drape sheets—sheets without a fenestration that come in various sizes:
  ○ Used as additional drapes for multiple parts of the body

- o Provide an extra thickness to the fenestrated drape sheet
- o Can be used to drape OR furniture or be used as reinforcement to the furniture drapes
- Towel drape/utility drape—small drape with a straight adhesive band

Rules of draping

- Always check the surgeon's preference card for draping instruction
- Organize drapes on your back table in order of use prior to the surgical procedure to be more efficient
- Never hand a drape across the sterile field
- Always keep a distance when maneuvering around the sterile field to avoid contamination
- Don't let the drape fall below table level
- Never adjust a drape sheet that has been improperly placed
  - o The circulator will remove the drape by peeling it from the sterile field without contaminating any other drapes
  - o If contamination occurs, the patient should be prepped and draped again
- Utility drapes (disposable)—the order to be handed to the surgeon is:
  - o First drape is handed on the same side as the surgeon
  - o Second drape is handed and placed superior
  - o Third drape is handed and placed inferior
  - o Fourth drape is placed opposite the first drape
- Cloth towels—same principles as above apply
  - o Towel clips are to be carried with the towels
  - o Folded edge goes down
  - o Nonperforating towel clips should be used to secure the drapes
  - o If sutures are used to secure a drape, the needle holder, suture, and scissor should be discarded
  - o Once a towel clip or clamp has been fastened to a drape and goes through the drape, it cannot be removed until the end of the case to avoid contamination
  - o If the clip must be removed, it should be immediately handed off the field and covered with another drape sheet
- If a hole is discovered, it should immediately be covered with another drape sheet
- If a hair is found on the sterile drape, it should be removed with a clamp and handed off the sterile field; immediately cover the area with another drape sheet

Questions

1. The main purpose of the skin prep is to:

   (A) remove resident and transient flora
   (B) remove dirt, oil, and microbes, and reduce the microbial count
   (C) remove all bacteria from the skin
   (D) sterilize the patient's skin

2. Which is the antiseptic solution of choice for a skin prep?

   (A) Cipex
   (B) Staphene
   (C) Povidone-iodine
   (D) Zephiran

3. When preparing a patient for a breast biopsy, a breast scrub is either eliminated or done very gently because of:

   (A) patient anxiety
   (B) dispersal of cancer cells
   (C) contamination
   (D) infection

4. The ideal place for the patient's shave prep to be done prior to surgery is:

   (A) patient's room
   (B) operating room (OR) suite
   (C) holding area of the OR
   (D) OR where the surgery will be performed

5. Any area that is considered contaminated:

   (A) should be scrubbed last or separately
   (B) should not be scrubbed at all
   (C) should be scrubbed first
   (D) needs no special consideration

6. In preparation for the surgical procedure, the surgeon prepped the patient with Betadine prep solution. Skin should be washed and painted:

   (A) from the incision site to the periphery in a circular motion
   (B) from the periphery to the incision site in a circular motion
   (C) in a side-to-side motion
   (D) in an up-and-down motion

7. Preliminary preparation of the patient's skin begins:

   (A) with a preoperative shower
   (B) with the shave preparation
   (C) in the OR
   (D) in the holding area

8. Suction tubing is attached to the drapes with a/an:

   (A) nonperforating towel clip
   (B) nonmetal, nonperforating clamp
   (C) Kocher clamp
   (D) Kelly clamp

9. All of the following statements regarding sterility are true EXCEPT:

   (A) wrapper edges are unsterile
   (B) instruments or sutures hanging over the table edge are discarded
   (C) sterile persons pass each other back to back
   (D) a sterile person faces a nonsterile person when passing

10. When draping a table, the scrub nurse should drape:

(A) back to front
(B) front to back
(C) side to side
(D) either A or B

11. A seamless, stretchable material often used to cover extremities during draping is:

(A) Esmarch
(B) ace bandage
(C) Kling
(D) stockinette

12. Drapes are:

(A) adjusted after placement for correct position
(B) unfolded before being carried to OR table
(C) passed across the table to surgeon along with towel clips
(D) placed on a dry area

13. Which statement demonstrates a break in technique during the draping process?

(A) Gloved hands may touch the skin of the patient.
(B) Discard a drape that becomes contaminated.
(C) Discard a sheet that falls below table level.
(D) Cover or discard a drape that has a hole.

14. A head drape consists of:

(A) medium sheet, towel, towel clip
(B) two medium sheets, towel clip
(C) one small sheet, one medium sheet, towel clip
(D) towel, fenestrated sheet

15. When the scrub person is draping a nonsterile table, he or she must:

(A) cover the back edge of the table first
(B) use a single-thickness drape
(C) be sure the drape touches the floor
(D) cuff the drape over his or her gloved hands

16. When covering a Mayo stand, the scrub person should:

(A) use a wide cuff
(B) use no cuff
(C) open the cover fully before placement
(D) ask the circulator to pull on the cover

17. If a sterile field becomes moistened during a case:

(A) nothing can be done
(B) extra drapes are added to area
(C) the wet sections are removed and replaced with dry sections
(D) the wet sections are covered with a plastic adherent drape

18. Which of the following actions by the scrub person is NOT an acceptable sterile technique principle?

(A) Discarding tubing that falls below sterile field edges without touching the contaminated part
(B) Reaching behind sterile team members to retrieve instruments so they do not collect on the patient
(C) Facing sterile areas when passing them
(D) Stepping away from the sterile field if contaminated

19. Which antiseptic agent is safe for ophthalmic use and in a face prep?

(A) Alcohol
(B) Betadine
(C) Chlorhexidine
(D) Triclosan

20. When prepping a contaminated area, such as a colostomy, the procedure includes:

(A) contaminated area is prepped first and covered with sterile gauze, and clean prep sponges are used to clean surrounding area

(B) contaminated area is prepped first, and clean sponges are used to prep the surrounding area

(C) prep the clean surrounding area first, and then with clean sponges, prep the contaminated area

(D) all of the above can be done

21. Why should prep solutions dry before applying drapes?

(A) To prevent strike-through contamination

(B) Because they stick better

(C) To enhance the antiseptic effect

(D) To avoid staining the drapes

22. Risks associated with prep solutions pooling under a patient include:

(A) causes no harm to patient

(B) chemical burn

(C) blistering and skin loss

(D) both B and C

23. Betadine is categorized as a/an:

(A) alcohol

(B) chlorhexidine gluconate

(C) iodophor

(D) sterilant

24. A prep that includes from the chin to the nipple line or the waist and around the side of the body to the OR table on each side is indicated for what type of surgery?

(A) Breast

(B) Neck (radical)

(C) Shoulder

(D) All of the above

25. How is rectal surgery prep done?

(A) Patient is prepped in supine then positioned in prone.

(B) Surrounding area is prepped first and anus last.

(C) Anus is prepped first and surrounding area last.

(D) It is done before the buttock tape is placed.

26. During prepping and draping, if the STSR contaminates their hand, they should:

(A) finish draping and change

(B) change glove immediately

(C) remove all drapes and start over

(D) do nothing; it does not matter

27. Drapes that are self-adhering, transparent, and provide an impervious barrier over an incision are called:

(A) incise drapes

(B) nonwoven drapes

(C) fenestrated drapes

(D) woven drape

28. Arrange the following procedures of removing drapes at the end of the procedure in proper order:

1. Remove all instruments and equipment from sterile field.
2. Roll drapes from the head proceeding to the patient's feet.
3. Place dressings and hold dressings in place while removing drapes.
4. Dispose of drapes in garbage.

(A) 1, 3, 2, 4

(B) 1, 2, 3, 4

(C) 2, 3, 4, 1

(D) 2, 4, 1, 3

29. A sterile barrier between the face and head used in nose and throat procedures is a/an:

    (A) fenestrated drape
    (B) self-adherent drape
    (C) head drape
    (D) incise drape

30. What is the body's primary defense against infection?

    (A) Hair
    (B) Skin
    (C) Proper prepping and draping
    (D) Good hygiene

31. The word "fenestrated" refers to:

    (A) an opening
    (B) length of drape
    (C) width of drape
    (D) transparent

32. All prep solutions are different and should be used according to manufacturer's instructions; however, they all have one thing in common, which is:

    (A) they should not be used on the patient with allergies to iodine and shellfish
    (B) they have a residual effect for 5–6 hours following applications
    (C) they should be dry prior to placing the drape sheets
    (D) they should be placed in hot sterile water to warm them prior to prepping

33. Alcohol prep solutions should contain what percentage of isopropyl alcohol to be considered an effective prep solution?

    (A) 70%
    (B) 10%
    (C) 50%
    (D) None specific

34. If a shave prep is ordered, when is it performed?

    (A) Two days prior to surgery
    (B) As close to the time of the surgical procedure as possible
    (C) The morning of the procedure
    (D) They are no longer performed

35. All apply to hair removal prior to surgery EXCEPT:

    (A) the shave prep should be performed in the patient holding area not the OR
    (B) eyebrows should be shaved with an electric razor
    (C) when hair is removed for a craniotomy procedure, the patient's hair should go into a secure bag that is labeled with the patient's name and identification number. This is the property of the patient and should be kept with the chart
    (D) it is recommended that an electric clipper be used, not a razor, to prevent cutting the patient's skin

36. Preps that require two separate preps include:

    (A) abdominal perineal prep
    (B) donor and recipient sites
    (C) mastectomy with reconstruction surgery
    (D) all of the above

37. When performing the skin prep using an iodine solution, all apply EXCEPT:

    (A) it is safe to use on mucous membranes
    (B) the prep using an iodine solution is performed in a back-and-forth motion
    (C) burns can occur if the prep solution is allowed to pool where in contact with the patient's skin and also if preheated
    (D) a diluted betadine prep solution may be used on the face and eye

38. The prep that involves the anatomical boundaries from the nipple line to symphysis pubis and lateral to both sides of the bed is:

    (A) abdominal
    (B) shoulder
    (C) pelvic
    (D) uterus

39. When prepping for an abdominoperineal procedure:

    (A) the perineal area is prepped first and covered
    (B) the abdominal area is prepped last to prevent contamination from below
    (C) they are considered two separate preps
    (D) all are true regarding an abdominoperineal prep

40. The drape sheet that has a hole with adhesive that surrounds the opening to help secure the drape is termed:

    (A) fenestrated sheet
    (B) transverse sheet
    (C) aperture sheet
    (D) split sheet

41. When performing the skin prep using ChloraPrep, all are FALSE EXCEPT:

    (A) when using 2% chlorhexidine gluconate in 70% isopropyl alcohol, the skin wash may be omitted
    (B) it needs to be immediately washed off following the surgical procedure because it can be toxic to the patient
    (C) the prep begins at the incision site to the periphery in a circular motion and does not require drying time
    (D) it can be used on mucous membranes

42. When using utility drapes, what is the correct order of handing them to the surgeon: (1) drape is handed and placed superior, (2) drape is handed and placed inferior, (3) drape is handed on the same side as the surgeon, (4) drape is placed opposite the first drape.

    (A) 1, 2, 3, 4
    (B) 2, 1, 3, 4
    (C) 3, 1, 2, 4
    (D) 4, 3, 1, 2

43. All apply to the sterile technique of draping EXCEPT:

    (A) once a towel clip or clamp has been fastened to a drape and goes through the drape, it cannot be removed until the end of the case to avoid contamination
    (B) if a hair is found on the sterile drape, it should be removed with your hand and handed off the sterile field; the area should be covered with another drape sheet
    (C) if a hole is discovered, it should immediately be covered with another drape sheet
    (D) towel clips are handed with the towels

44. The general rule regarding prepping a contaminated area is:

    (A) contaminated areas, including draining sinus, anus, and vagina, are prepped last
    (B) a stoma is covered with an incise drape, and the surrounding area is prepped first
    (C) exceptions include that the umbilicus is prepped first and traumatic wounds are washed and can be prepped with diluted Betadine first and the surrounding area is prepped last
    (D) all of the above

45. When performing a skin prep for a graft, which is true?

(A) The donor site is prepped first.

(B) The recipient site is prepped first because the donor site is considered potentially contaminated.

(C) Examples of areas requiring a skin graft include burns, ulcers, and traumatic wounds where the skin is gone.

(D) When prepping the donor site, a color-less prep solution is preferred.

46. Prior to draping the patient, all must be per-formed EXCEPT:

(A) anesthesia is given

(B) dispersive electrode is placed

(C) active electrode is secured

(D) Foley catheter is inserted

47. When draping the perineum, what is the correct order of the following steps: (1) fenes-trated drape, (2) under the buttocks drape, (3) legging drape?

(A) 1, 2 ,3

(B) 2, 1 ,3

(C) 3, 2 ,1

(D) 2, 3 ,1

48. An intraoperative x-ray is requested by the surgeon during the case. What should the STSR do to protect the sterile field from contamination?

(A) The STSR should step out into the sub-sterile room.

(B) The x-ray cassette should be covered with a sterile drape.

(C) The STSR needs to wear a lead apron and thyroid collar.

(D) All should face the x-ray machine when in use.

49. What type of prep would require two people?

(A) Two-step prep requiring a wash

(B) Patient placed in lateral position

(C) Extremity

(D) Vaginal perineal procedure

50. All apply to the split sheet/U-drape EXCEPT:

(A) commonly used in orthopedics

(B) when draping, the tails are always posi-tioned downward

(C) the tails are draped around the limb and the rest of the drape covers the body

(D) all of the above

51. Which is correct when removing the drapes?

(A) Remove the top drape first.

(B) Remove the first layer of drape sheets first.

(C) Roll the drape sheets from the head to the feet.

(D) Roll the drape sheets from the feet to the head of the patient.

Answers and Explanations

1. **(B)** Methods of skin prep may vary, but the objectives are the same—to remove dirt, oil, and microbes from the skin so the incision can be made through the skin with a minimal danger of infection. It also reduces the resident microbial count and prevents the growth of microbes.

2. **(C)** The current trend is toward a surgical scrub of antiseptic solution containing povidone-iodine. This reduces the number of bacteria on the skin and inhibits the growth. This process is eliminated in some ORs.

3. **(B)** When a breast is prepped for suspected malignancy, it is done gently or not at all. Scrubbing the breast with the usual amount of pressure could cause cancer cells to break loose from the lesion and spread the disease.

4. **(A)** The ideal shave should be performed in the patient's room; if it is not able to be done there, the next best practice would be to perform the shave in the holding area. This should be done as close to the time of surgery as possible.

5. **(A)** Contaminated areas (which can include draining sinuses, skin ulcers, vagina, or anus) should be scrubbed last or with separate sponges. This prevents dragging pathogens into the incisional area and, thus, reduces the possibility of infection.

6. **(A)** When using Betadine as a skin prep, it should be performed from the incision site to the periphery in a circular motion.

7. **(A)** Patients may be advised to begin bathing with a 3% hexachlorophene solution before admission for an elective procedure. Patients should shower or be bathed before coming to the OR suite. This action is bacteriostatic and reduces microbial contamination.

8. **(B)** Most disposable drapes now offer Velcro straps to secure tubing/cords to the drapes. When this is not available or additional cords and/or tubing need to be secured, the best choice is to use a nonmetal, nonpenetrating clamp.

9. **(D)** A sterile person turns his or her back to a nonsterile person or area when passing.

10. **(B)** When draping a table, open the drape toward the front of the table first. This establishes a sterile area close to the scrub.

11. **(D)** Stockinette may be used to cover an extremity. It is a seamless, stretchable tubing material that contours snugly to skin. It may be covered with plastic. Some have vinyl on outside layer.

12. **(D)** Drapes are placed on a dry area. The scrub nurse takes towel clips and skin towels to the side of the OR table from which the surgeon will apply them. Folded drapes are carried to the OR table. Drapes are held high enough to avoid touching nonsterile areas. Once a drape is placed, it may not be adjusted.

13. **(A)** B, C, and D are acceptable techniques. Gloved hands should not touch the skin of the patient. Protect gloved hands by cuffing end of sheet over them.

14. **(A)** The surgeon places a drape under the head while the circulator holds up the head.

This drape consists of a towel placed on a medium sheet. Center of towel edge is 2 in. in from center of sheet edge. Towel is drawn up on each side of face, over forehead or at hairline, and fastened with a clip. Additional towels surround operative site.

15. **(D)** In draping a nonsterile table, the scrub nurse should cuff the drape over his or her gloved hand in preparation for opening it. The side of the drape toward him or her is done first to minimize the possibility of contaminating the front of the gown.

16. **(A)** A wide cuff is used on the Mayo cover to protect the gloved hands.

17. **(B)** The table and sterile field should be kept as dry as possible. However, extra towels may be spread if a solution has soaked through a sterile drape.

18. **(B)** Scrub persons should not reach behind a member of the sterile team. They may go around the person, passing back to back.

19. **(D)** Triclosan is an antiseptic agent safe for ophthalmic use and in a face prep. The other agents are not safe for use on these areas.

20. **(C)** The clean area is prepped first, and with clean sponges, the contaminated area is cleaned.

21. **(C)** Prep solutions should be dry prior to applying drapes in order to enhance the antiseptic effect.

22. **(D)** Chemical burns result when prep solution is allowed to pool under the patient. Pressure and contact with the chemical over time can cause severe blistering and skin loss.

23. **(C)** Betadine is categorized as an iodophor.

24. **(B)** Prep for a neck procedure includes the chin to the nipple line to the waist and around the side of the body to the OR table on each side.

25. **(B)** The area is prepped cleanest to dirtiest areas.

26. **(B)** The STSR should change glove immediately.

27. **(A)** Incise drapes are self-adhering and transparent and provide an impervious barrier over an incision.

28. **(A)** At the end of the procedure, the STSR should remove all instruments and equipment from sterile field, place dressings on incision, and hold with hand while removing drapes from head to toe and placing them in garbage.

29. **(C)** A head drape is the sterile barrier between the face and head used during nose and throat procedures.

30. **(B)** Skin is the body's primary defense against infection.

31. **(A)** The word "fenestrated" refers to an "opening" in a drape.

32. **(C)** All prep solutions should dry prior to placing drape sheets.

33. **(A)** 70% is the percentage of isopropyl alcohol to be considered an effective prep solution.

34. **(B)** If a shave prep is ordered, it should be performed as close to the time of surgery as possible in order to reduce the risk for microbial growth in the case of a break in the skin, which can cause an infection.

35. **(B)** Eyebrows should never be shaved.

36. **(D)** All of the above require two separate setups.

37. **(B)** The iodine prep should begin at the incision site to the periphery in a circular motion. It is safe to use on mucous membranes, but you should always be careful not to allow the solution to pool and come in contact with the patient's skin because it can cause burns.

38. **(A)** The abdominal prep involves the anatomical boundaries from the nipple line to the symphysis pubis and lateral to both sides of the bed.

39. **(D)** All are true.

40. **(C)** The aperture drape sheet is a fenestrated drape sheet with adhesive that surrounds the opening to help secure the drape.

41. **(A)** ChloraPrep solution contains 2% chlorhexidine gluconate in 70% isopropyl alcohol, and because it is a broad-spectrum antiseptic, the skin wash may be omitted. When prepping with ChloraPrep, you use a back-and-forth motion and apply pressure for 30 seconds before moving to the periphery. Before applying the drapes, ChloraPrep must thoroughly be dry. It is toxic to mucous membranes, so it should never be used there. It should not be washed off the skin because it provides a long-term antimicrobial effect for up to 48 hours following surgery.

42. **(C)** The order of handing the utility drapes to the surgeon is as follows. First drape is handed on the same side as the surgeon. Second drape is handed and placed superior. Third drape is handed and placed inferior. Fourth drape is placed opposite the first drape.

43. **(B)** If a hair is found on the sterile drape, it should be removed with a clamp and handed off the sterile field, and the area should be immediately covered with another drape sheet. You should not use your gloved hand.

44. **(D)** The general rule to prepping a contaminated area is that the clean area is prepped first and the contaminated area last. Exceptions to this rule are the umbilicus; even though the umbilicus is considered contaminated, it is washed first, Betadine is poured into the belly button, and the surrounding area is then prepped. Traumatic wounds are washed and can be prepped with diluted Betadine first, and the surrounding area is prepped last.

45. **(B)** Recipient site is prepped second/last because it is considered potentially contaminated. A skin graft is performed because the recipient site is usually an infected wound. It can be due to a traumatic injury where there is skin loss, a burn, and/or ulcers.

46. **(C)** The active electrode is the cautery handpiece. This is not secured until the patient is draped and then secured with a nonmetal, nonperforating clamp.

47. **(D)** The first drape is placed under the buttock, the second is the legging drape, and the final drape is the sheet with the hole, or the fenestrated/perineal drape.

48. **(B)** A sterile drape is required to cover the cassette and protect the sterile field from contamination. When an intraoperative x-ray is requested and the OR team is not prepared with lead aprons and thyroid collars, they should cover their hands with a sterile towel and step into the substerile room until the x-ray is taken.

49. **(C)** An extremity prep is a circumferential prep and requires two people to properly perform the prep. One person holds the limb while the other performs the wash and prep.

50. **(B)** Split sheet/U-drapes are commonly used in orthopedic cases. The two tails can be positioned tails up or down according to the surgical procedure and wrapped around the limb. The remainder of the drape goes over the body.

51. **(C)** All instruments should be removed from the sterile field including the cautery and suction tips and the clamps securing them. The incision is washed, dried, dressed, and covered with a clean cloth towel. The dressings are held in place, and the drapes are rolled from the head of the patient to the feet and disposed of.

CHAPTER 15

Instruments

Questions

1. A surgical treatment for scoliosis could employ the use of:

    (A) skeletal traction
    (B) external fixation
    (C) compression plate and screws
    (D) Harrington rods

2. During surgery, towel clips:

    (A) may be removed only by the circulator
    (B) may not be removed once fastened
    (C) may be removed and discarded as long as the area is covered with sterile linen
    (D) may be removed and discarded from the field

3. As grossly soiled instruments are returned to the scrub, they should be:

    (A) placed in a basin of sterile saline to soak off debris
    (B) wiped off with a sponge moistened with water or soaked in a basin of sterile distilled water
    (C) wiped off with a dry sponge
    (D) discarded so that the circulator can clean them thoroughly

4. The sterile component of the electrosurgical unit (ESU) is the:

    (A) grounding pad
    (B) generator
    (C) foot pedal
    (D) active electrode

5. Deaver and Richardson retractors have an advantage over the Balfour and O'Connor–O'Sullivan retractors in that they provide:

    (A) less exposure
    (B) less fatigue
    (C) greater adjustability
    (D) more fatigue

6. Which suction tip is meant to be used during abdominal surgery?

    (A) Poole
    (B) Yankauer
    (C) Frasier
    (D) Tonsil

7. What kind of retractor is generally used in areas near viable nerves or blood vessels?

    (A) Sharp rakes
    (B) Skin hooks
    (C) Dull rakes
    (D) Sharp Weitlaner

8. All of the following instruments have teeth EXCEPT:

    (A) Allis
    (B) Heaney
    (C) Kocher
    (D) Babcock

9. All of the following are self-retaining retractors EXCEPT:

(A) O'Connor–O'Sullivan
(B) Balfour
(C) Weitlaner
(D) Richardson

10. What is the term that refers to separating tissue layers on a vertical plane using dissecting scissors?

(A) Incision
(B) Undermining
(C) Transecting
(D) Blunt dissection

11. The following surgeries do not require the use of a trocar EXCEPT for:

(A) laparoscopy
(B) cystoscopy
(C) proctoscopy
(D) bronchoscopy

12. The safest method for loading a blade on a knife handle is to use:

(A) gloved hand
(B) needle holder
(C) Mixter
(D) Adson forceps

13. What is a Lebsche used for?

(A) To open the sternum
(B) To retract spinal nerves
(C) To elevate the periosteum
(D) To separate the ribs

14. A rongeur used extensively in surgery of the spine and in neurosurgery is the:

(A) Adson
(B) Cobb
(C) Kerrison
(D) Cloward

15. A rib retractor is a:

(A) Weitlaner
(B) Finochietto
(C) Harrington
(D) Beckman

16. A Doyen is a:

(A) rib shears
(B) rib cutter
(C) rib spreader
(D) rib raspatory

17. The instrument used to enlarge the burr hole made during a craniotomy is a:

(A) rongeur
(B) periosteal elevator
(C) Gigli saw
(D) Cloward punch

18. Westcott scissors are used in:

(A) plastic surgery
(B) ophthalmic surgery
(C) vascular surgery
(D) orthopedic surgery

19. The instrument used in a splenectomy is a:

(A) Doyen
(B) Allen
(C) Jacobs
(D) pedicle clamp

20. Bowman probes are used in:

(A) common bile duct surgery
(B) lacrimal surgery
(C) kidney surgery
(D) bladder surgery

21. A Hurd dissector and pillar retractor is used for:

(A) appendectomy
(B) plastic surgery
(C) nasal surgery
(D) tonsillectomy

22. The Lempert elevator is used in surgery of the:

    (A) eye
    (B) nose
    (C) ear
    (D) bones

23. A Scoville retractor is used in a:

    (A) total knee replacement
    (B) meniscectomy
    (C) laminectomy
    (D) carpal tunnel release

24. A Bailey is a:

    (A) clamp
    (B) rongeur
    (C) dissecting forceps
    (D) rib approximator

25. A Sauerbruch is a/an:

    (A) elevator
    (B) raspatory
    (C) retractor
    (D) rongeur

26. An Auvard is a:

    (A) forceps
    (B) dissector
    (C) speculum
    (D) sound

27. A Babcock is used to:

    (A) grasp bone
    (B) grasp delicate structures
    (C) clamp vessels
    (D) retract soft tissue

28. Nasal cartilage is incised with a:

    (A) Ballenger swivel knife
    (B) Freer elevator
    (C) Duckbill rongeur
    (D) Hurd dissector

29. A self-retaining retractor is a:

    (A) Weitlaner
    (B) Lincoln
    (C) Hibbs
    (D) Deaver

30. A rectal speculum is a:

    (A) Percy
    (B) Hirschmann
    (C) Pennington
    (D) Hill

31. A small fine-needle holder used in plastic surgery is a:

    (A) Ryder
    (B) Heaney
    (C) Webster
    (D) Castroviejo

32. A kidney pedicle clamp is a:

    (A) Lincoln
    (B) Herrick
    (C) Love
    (D) Little

33. Uterine dilators are:

    (A) Hanks
    (B) Van Buren
    (C) Bakes
    (D) Graves

34. A technique utilizing the insertion of a needle or wire through a needle in order to identify suspicious breast tissue is a/an:

    (A) incisional biopsy
    (B) wire localization
    (C) Silverman needle biopsy
    (D) magnetic resonance imaging (MRI)

35. A forceps used to remove stones in biliary surgery is a:

    (A) Mixter
    (B) Lahey gall duct
    (C) Potts–Smith
    (D) Randall

36. Right-angled pedicle clamps would be found on a setup for:

    (A) splenectomy
    (B) cholecystectomy
    (C) hemorrhoidectomy
    (D) thyroidectomy

37. Blunt nerve hooks are selected for a _____ setup.

    (A) vagotomy
    (B) colostomy
    (C) gastrojejunostomy
    (D) abdominal-perineal resection

38. In which procedural setup would a T-tube be found?

    (A) Exploration of the common bile duct
    (B) Cholecystectomy
    (C) Cholelithotripsy
    (D) Choledochoscopy

39. Stapedectomy requires all of the following items EXCEPT:

    (A) small microsuction
    (B) speculum
    (C) prosthesis
    (D) autograft

40. Cochlear implants utilize an electrode device:

    (A) to restore hearing
    (B) to aerate the mastoid
    (C) to allow drainage
    (D) to relieve vertigo

41. All of the following are required for repair of a nasal fracture EXCEPT:

    (A) bayonet forceps
    (B) Ballenger swivel knife
    (C) splint
    (D) Asch forceps

42. A forceps used in nasal surgery is a/an:

    (A) bayonet
    (B) Russian
    (C) rat-tooth
    (D) alligator

43. All of the following instruments can be found on a nasal setup EXCEPT:

    (A) Freer elevator
    (B) bayonet forceps
    (C) Potts forceps
    (D) Frazier suction tube

44. On which setup would bougies be found?

    (A) Tonsillectomy
    (B) Esophagoscopy
    (C) Radical neck
    (D) Parotidectomy

45. All of the following can be found on a tonsillectomy setup EXCEPT:

    (A) Yankauer suction
    (B) Hurd dissector and pillar retractor
    (C) tongue depressor
    (D) Jameson hook

46. Tissue expanders are used in:

    (A) augmentation mammoplasty
    (B) reduction for gynecomastia
    (C) transrectus myocutaneous flap
    (D) breast reconstruction

47. The fracture treated with arch bars is:

    (A) nasal
    (B) mandibular
    (C) zygomatic
    (D) orbital

48. Rib removal for surgical exposure of the kidney requires all of the following EXCEPT a/an:

    (A) Alexander periosteotome
    (B) Doyen raspatory
    (C) Heaney clamp
    (D) Stille shears

49. Stone forceps on a kidney set are:

    (A) Lewkowitz
    (B) Randall
    (C) Satinsky
    (D) Mayo

50. A Sarot is a:

    (A) bronchus clamp
    (B) scapula retractor
    (C) lung retractor
    (D) lung grasping clamp

51. Which item would not be included on a setup for a transvenous (endocardial) pacemaker?

    (A) Tunneling instrument
    (B) Intra-aortic balloon pump
    (C) Fluoroscopy
    (D) Defibrillator

52. The most frequent conditions requiring the use of a permanent pacemaker are:

    (A) coronary or mitral insufficiency
    (B) pulmonary artery or vein stenosis
    (C) heart block, bradyarrhythmia
    (D) pulmonary stenosis, ventricular septal defect

53. Which setup would include distraction and compression components?

    (A) Harrington rods
    (B) Intramedullary nail
    (C) Arthrodesis
    (D) Tibial shaft fracture

54. Traction applied directly on bone via pins, wires, or tongs is:

    (A) internal
    (B) closed
    (C) skeletal
    (D) counterpressure

55. Skeletal traction of a lower leg is accomplished with the use of a/an:

    (A) Kirschner wire
    (B) Knowles pin
    (C) Eggers plate
    (D) Smith–Peterson nail

56. In orthopedic surgery, the viewing of the progression of a procedure on a television screen is known as:

    (A) image intensification
    (B) radiography
    (C) portable filming
    (D) x-ray

57. A neurological study in which a radiopaque substance is injected into the subarachnoid space through a lumbar puncture is called a/an:

    (A) cerebral angiography
    (B) myelogram
    (C) encephalogram
    (D) diskogram

58. A neuro headrest skull clamp is called a/an:

    (A) Sachs
    (B) Frazier
    (C) Adson
    (D) Mayfield

59. Maintenance of acceptable blood pressure and prevention of the development of air emboli in the neurosurgical patient can be accomplished by preoperative utilization of:

    (A) an antigravity suit
    (B) ace bandages
    (C) thromboembolic device (TED) stockings
    (D) adequate body support

60. Specialized instruments for a cleft lip repair include:

    (A) Cupid's bow
    (B) Logan's bow
    (C) arch bar
    (D) wire scissors

61. Cloward instrumentation would be included for surgery of the:

    (A) hip
    (B) femur
    (C) cervical spine
    (D) lumbar spine

62. On which setup would a Beaver knife handle be found?

    (A) Orthopedic
    (B) Pediatric
    (C) Gynecological
    (D) Eye

63. Which procedure requires a sterile setup?

    (A) Manual skin traction
    (B) Skin traction
    (C) Skeletal traction
    (D) Closed reduction

64. A craniotomy may employ the use of a _____ for exposure.

    (A) Mayfield
    (B) Sugita
    (C) Heifetz
    (D) Leyla–Yasargil

65. On which setup would either a Pereyra or a Stamey needle be found?

    (A) Urological
    (B) Eye
    (C) Orthopedic
    (D) Thoracic

66. Disintegration of kidney stones through a liquid medium is accomplished with a/an:

    (A) nephroscope
    (B) extracorporeal shock wave lithotripter
    (C) laser
    (D) cystoscope

67. A urology perineal retractor system is called:

    (A) Bookwalter
    (B) O'Sullivan–O'Conner
    (C) Omni–Tract
    (D) Lowsley

68. A procedure on which structure would utilize a Mason–Judd retractor?

    (A) Bladder
    (B) Uterus
    (C) Hip
    (D) Nose

69. A Furlow inserter is used in:

    (A) penile implantation
    (B) femoral-popliteal bypass
    (C) total hip replacement
    (D) intraocular lens (IOL) implant

70. A Millin is a:

    (A) prostatic enucleator
    (B) urological needle holder
    (C) stone forceps
    (D) retropubic bladder retractor

71. Which setup would include a Gomco clamp?

    (A) Colostomy
    (B) Breast augmentation
    (C) Circumcision
    (D) Femoral popliteal bypass

72. In which surgical specialty would a Humi cannula be used?

    (A) Gynecological
    (B) Ophthalmic
    (C) Orthopedic
    (D) Vascular

73. An instrument used in laparoscopy to manipulate the uterus for increased structure visibility is the:

(A) Veress
(B) Pratt
(C) Mayo–Hegar
(D) Hulka

74. A central venous pressure (CVP) catheter insertion requires:

(A) a sterile setup
(B) a crash cart
(C) an IV technician
(D) none of the above

75. The purpose of a set of Bakes would be:

(A) anal dilation
(B) esophageal dilation
(C) common duct dilation
(D) cervical dilation

76. A Steffee plate is a:

(A) shoulder replacement
(B) knee joint replacement
(C) femoral implant
(D) spinal implant

77. Skeletal traction is accomplished with:

(A) Sayre sling
(B) Minerva jacket
(C) Crutchfield tongs
(D) Steffee system

78. The Bookwalter is a _____ instrument.

(A) clamping
(B) holding
(C) suturing
(D) retracting

79. Which instrument is a retractor?

(A) Harrington
(B) Doyen
(C) Crile
(D) Allen

80. A long thoracic forceps is a:

(A) Semb
(B) Debakey
(C) Sauerbruch
(D) Doyen

81. A bougie is a:

(A) clamp
(B) dilator
(C) retractor
(D) grasper

Questions 82 through 84: The following group of questions is preceded by a group of instrument images (Figure 15–1). For each question, select the one-lettered option that is the best answer.

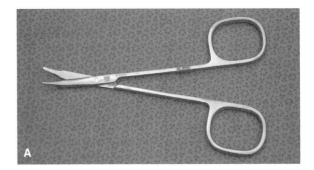

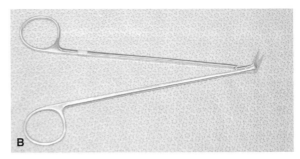

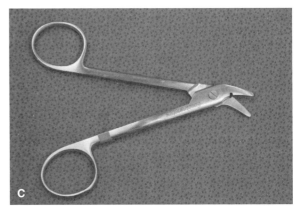

Figure 15–1.

82. If arch bars remain in the patient postoperatively, which instrument must accompany the patient to the postanesthesia care unit (PACU) in order to open the mouth in case of emergency?

(A) B

(B) A

(C) C

(D) None of the above

83. What instrument would be used to extend the incision on a carotid?

(A) A

(B) B

(C) C

(D) None of the above

84. Which instrument is used for a blepharoplasty?

(A) B

(B) C

(C) A

(D) None of the above

85. The name of the instrument below (Figure 15–2) is _____, which is also known as uterine dilators.

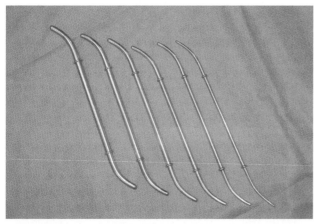

Figure 15–2.

(A) Bakes dilators

(B) Hanks dilators

(C) Hegar dilators

(D) Van Buren dilators

86. What are the instruments below (Figure 15–3) called?

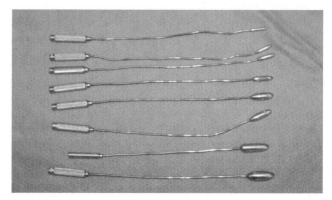

Figure 15–3.

(A) Van Buren sounds

(B) Bougies

(C) Bakes dilators

(D) Garrett dilators

Questions 87 through 90: The following group of questions is preceded by a group of instrument images (Figure 15–4). For each question, select the one-lettered option that is the best answer.

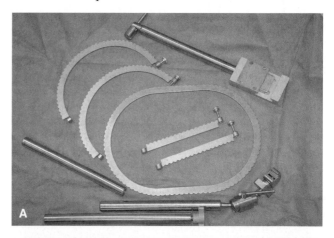

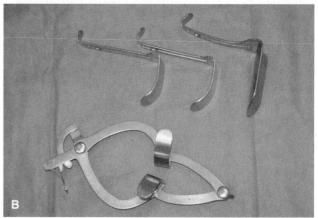

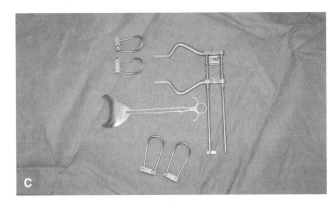

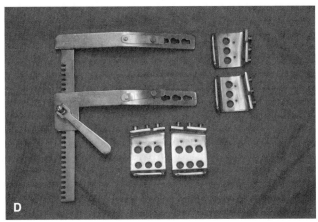

Figure 15–4.

87. Which instrument is the Bookwalter?

(A) A

(B) B

(C) C

(D) D

88. Which instrument is a chest spreader/rib spreader?

(A) B

(B) C

(C) D

(D) Both B and D

89. Which retractor is used in abdominal procedures and commonly used in pelvic procedures?

(A) A

(B) B

(C) D

(D) None of the above

90. Which instrument is the Balfour retractor?

(A) A

(B) B

(C) C

(D) D

91. The name of the instrument in Figure 15–5 is:

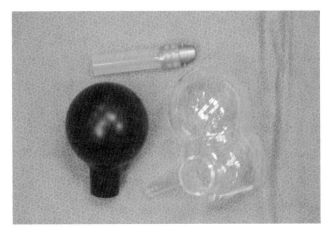

Figure 15–5.

(A) Toomey

(B) Microvasive evacuator

(C) Bulb

(D) Ellik

Questions 92 through 94: The following group of questions is preceded by a group of instrument images (Figure 15–6). For each question, select the one-lettered option that is the best answer.

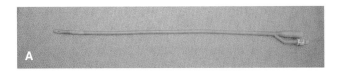

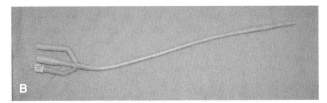

Figure 15–6.

92. Which catheter is used for intermittent or continuous bladder irrigation?

(A) A

(B) B

(C) Both A and B

(D) None of the above

93. Which catheter is also called a retention indwelling catheter?

(A) A

(B) B

(C) Both A and B

(D) None of the above

94. Figure 15–6A is a two-way Foley 5-cc balloon used for:

(A) urinary drainage

(B) tamponade

(C) irrigation and aspiration

(D) common nonretaining catheter

95. What is the name of the instrument in Figure 15–7?

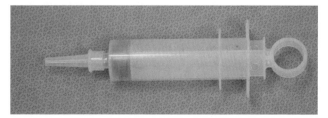

Figure 15–7.

(A) Luer-Lok syringe

(B) Toomey

(C) Asepto

(D) Ellik

Questions 96 through 101: The following group of questions is preceded by a group of instrument images (Figure 15–8). For each question, select the one-lettered option that is the best answer.

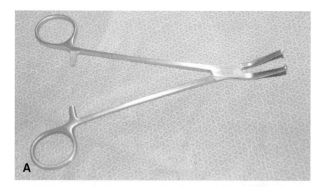

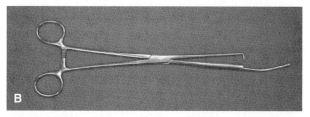

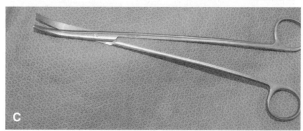

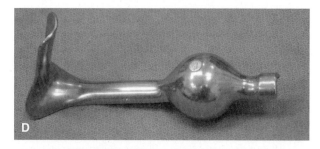

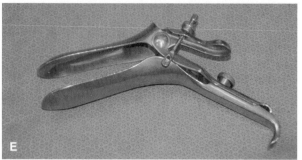

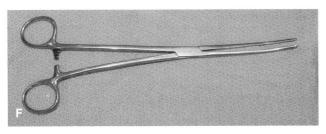

Figure 15–8.

96. What instrument provides retraction of the posterior vaginal wall?

(A) B
(B) D
(C) E
(D) F

97. What is the name of the instrument in Figure 15–8C?

(A) Jarit
(B) Heaney
(C) Jorgenson
(D) Westcott

98. What instrument is used as a uterine manipulator?

(A) A
(B) B
(C) E
(D) F

99. What is the name of the instrument in Figure 15–8F?

(A) Simpson
(B) Heaney
(C) Bozeman
(D) Ochsner

100. The name of the instrument in Figure 15–8A is called:

(A) Jacobs
(B) Schroeder
(C) Graves
(D) Phaneuf

101. Another name for the instrument in Figure 15–8E is the duckbill. What is the proper name for this instrument?

(A) Eastman
(B) Graves
(C) Young anterior
(D) Auvard

102. What is the name of the electrode in Figure 15–9?

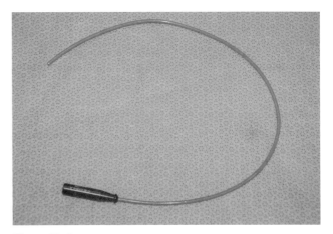

Figure 15–9.

(A) Ball loop
(B) Loop
(C) Bugbee
(D) The working element

103. What is the name of the electrode in Figure 15–10?

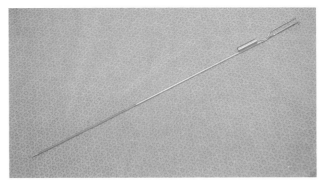

Figure 15–10.

(A) Ball loop
(B) Working element
(C) Randall
(D) Loop electrode

104. What is the name of the instrument in Figure 15–11?

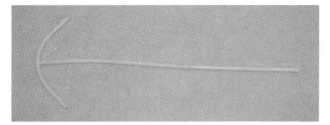

Figure 15–11.

(A)   Nephrostomy tube

(B)   Fogarty

(C)   T-tube

(D)   Cigarette drain

105. Instrument in Figure 15–12 would commonly be found on which setup?

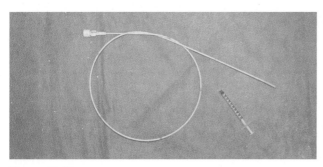

Figure 15–12.

(A)   Orthopedic

(B)   Vascular

(C)   Ophthalmology

(D)   Plastic

Questions 106 through 108: The following group of questions is preceded by a group of instrument images (Figure 15–13). For each question, select the one-lettered option that is the best answer.

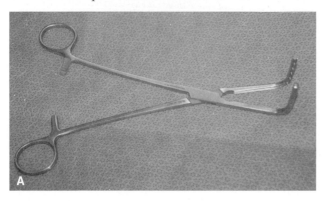

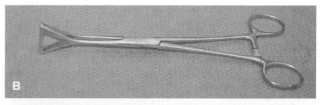

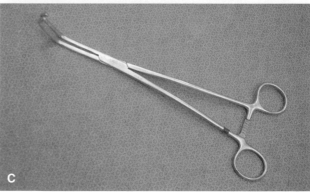

Figure 15–13.

106. What instrument is used to grasp the lung?

(A) A

(B) B

(C) C

(D) None of the above

107. What is the name of the instrument in Figure 15–13A?

(A) Sarot

(B) Cooley

(C) Potts–Smith

(D) Javid

108. What is the name of the instrument in Figure 15–13C?

(A) Glover

(B) Cooley

(C) Javid

(D) Statinsky

Questions 109 and 110: The following group of questions is preceded by a group of instrument images (Figure 15–14). For each question, select the one-lettered option that is the best answer.

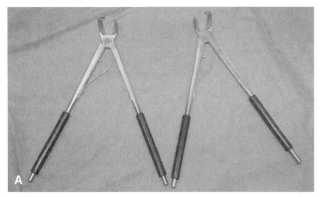

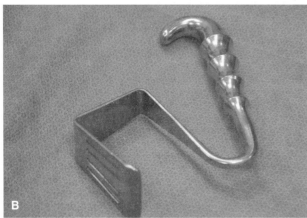

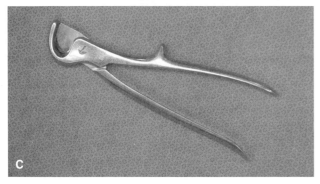

Figure 15–14.

109. The instrument used to cut rib bone is:

(A) A
(B) B
(C) C
(D) both A and C

110. The instrument in Figure 15–14B is:

(A) Allison lung retractor
(B) Cooley arterial retractor
(C) Davidson scapula retractor
(D) Finochietto retractor

111. The instrument in Figure 15–15 would commonly be found in what procedure?

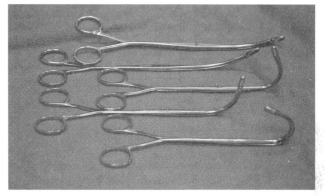

Figure 15–15.

(A) Colon resection
(B) Laparoscopic cholecystectomy
(C) Common duct exploration
(D) Hysterectomy

Questions 112 and 113: The following group of questions is preceded by Figure 15–16. For each question, select the one-lettered option that is the best answer.

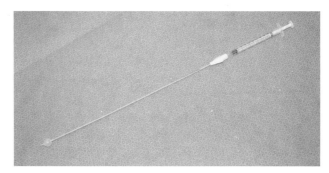

Figure 15–16.

112. The catheter in Figure 15–16 would be used on:

(A) common bile duct
(B) artery
(C) vein
(D) both B and C

113. The instrument in Figure 15–16 is called:

(A) Red Robinson catheter
(B) Fogarty embolectomy catheter
(C) Malecot
(D) Fogarty biliary catheter

114. The instruments in Figure 15–17 would commonly be found in what procedure?

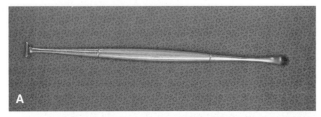

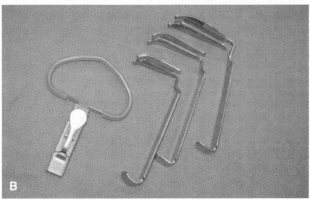

Figure 15–17.

(A) Arch bars
(B) Dental extraction
(C) Tracheostomy
(D) Tonsillectomy

Questions 115 through 118: The following group of questions is preceded by a group of instrument images (Figure 15–18). For each question, select the one-lettered option that is the best answer.

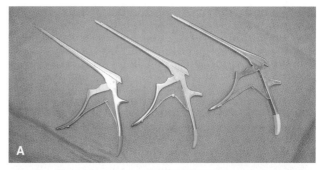

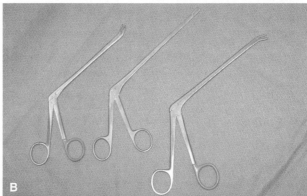

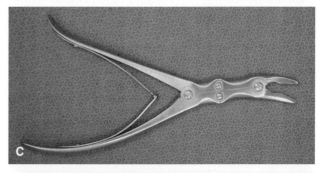

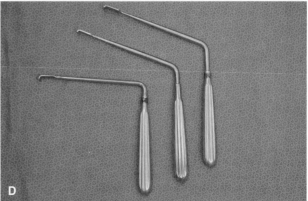

Figure 15–18.

115. The instrument in Figure 15–18A is called:

(A) Leksell

(B) Pituitary

(C) Scoville

(D) Kerrison

116. The instrument in Figure 15–18B is called:

(A) Leksell

(B) Pituitary

(C) Scoville

(D) Taylor

117. The instrument in Figure 15–18C is a Leksell rongeur. It is used:

(A) to remove pieces of bone and soft tissue surrounding the bone

(B) to remove the spinous processes

(C) to extract teeth

(D) both A and B

118. The instrument in Figure 15–18D is called:

(A) Scoville

(B) Cobb

(C) Pituitary

(D) Cloward

Questions 119 through 127: The following group of questions is preceded by a group of instrument images (Figure 15–19). For each question, select the one-lettered option that is the best answer.

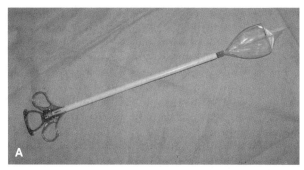

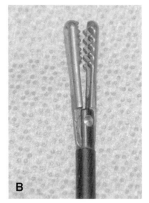
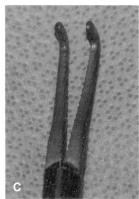

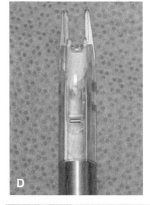
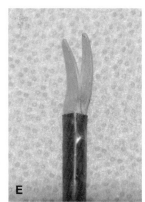

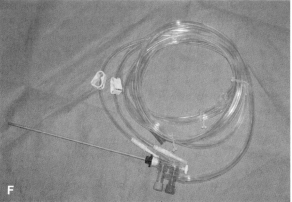

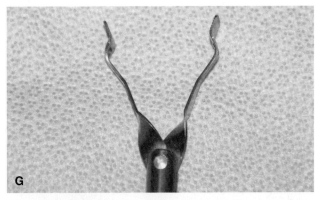

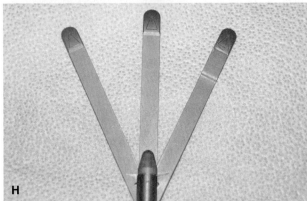

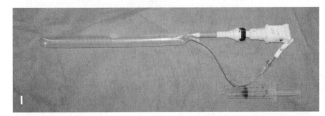

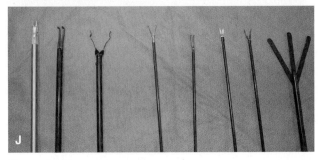

Figure 15–19.

119. Which instrument is used to put traction on the gallbladder?

(A) D
(B) B
(C) F
(D) E

120. Which instrument is used to peel adhesions to visualize the cystic duct and cystic artery?

(A) C
(B) E
(C) G
(D) H

121. Which instrument is used to ligate the cystic artery?

(A) C
(B) B
(C) D
(D) G

122. Which instrument is used to divide the cystic artery following the ligation?

(A) D
(B) E
(C) H
(D) G

123. Which instrument is used for hydrodissection?

(A) C
(B) D
(C) E
(D) F

124. Which instrument is used to cauterize fallopian tubes?

(A) B
(B) C
(C) G
(D) All of the above

125. Which instrument is used to retract the liver so that it does not obscure the view of the gallbladder?

(A) A

(B) H

(C) I

(D) F

126. Which instrument is used to expand the abdomen during a total extraperitoneal (TEP) inguinal hernia repair?

(A) I

(B) A

(C) G

(D) F

127. The instruments in Figure 15–19J are used for:

(A) laparoscopic hernia repair

(B) laparoscopic cholecystectomy

(C) laparoscopic bowel resection

(D) all of the above

Questions 128 through 130: The following group of questions is preceded by a group of instrument images (Figure 15–20). For each question, select the one-lettered option that is the best answer.

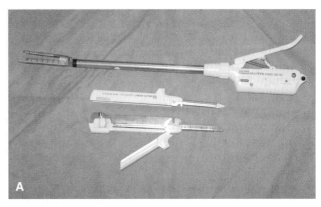

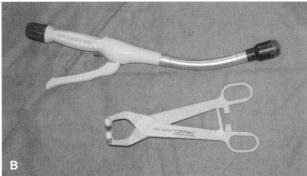

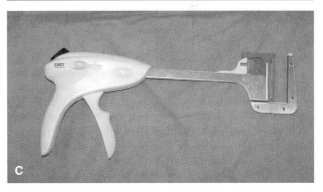

Figure 15–20.

128. What stapling instrument is used to join two arms of the intestines together, shown in Figure 15–20B?

(A) Thoracoabdominal (TA)

(B) Gastrointestinal intestinal anastomosis (GIA)

(C) End-to-end anastomosis (EEA)

(D) Ligate, divide, and staple (LDS)

129. The instrument in Figure 15–20C is used:

(A) to ligate and divide tubular structures and vessels

(B) to provide end-to-end or side-to-side anastomosis

(C) to provide the same function as a purse string suture

(D) for resection and transaction

130. The instrument in Figure 15–20A is used for:

(A) resection and transection

(B) resection and creation of an anastomosis

(C) resection of tubular structures and vessels

(D) performing the same function as a purse string suture

Answers and Explanations

1. **(D)** Harrington rods are internal splints that help maintain the spine as straight as possible until vertebral body fusion becomes solid.

2. **(C)** Once a clip has been fastened through a drape, do not remove it because the points are contaminated. If it is necessary to remove one during a case, discard it from the field and cover the area with a piece of sterile linen.

3. **(B)** Old blood and debris should be removed from instruments as soon as possible with water so that they do not dry on surfaces or in crevices. Saline can damage surfaces, causing corrosion and pitting.

4. **(D)** With the ESU, electrical energy flows from the generator through a sterile active electrode to the patient including both bipolar forceps and monopolar forceps.

5. **(C)** Self-retaining retractors, such as the Balfour, can cause bruising and nerve and muscle damage more than the handheld retractors.

6. **(A)** The Poole's suction tip has a guard that protects intestinal organs.

7. **(C)** Dull hooks and rakes are used in areas close to viable nerves and blood vessels, and sharp rakes are designed to grasp superficial tissue.

8. **(D)** Heaney, Allis, and Kocher contain teeth and/or serrations in order to grasp and facilitate in dissection and suturing.

9. **(D)** A Richardson retractor must be handheld, and self-retaining retractors use mechanical action; they have many attachments and hold tissue against the walls of the surgical wound.

10. **(B)** With this technique, scissors are inserted between the two tissue planes and opened. This separates the layers rather than cutting them.

11. **(A)** Trocars are used to create an opening in which endoscopic instruments can be exchanged where there is no natural opening.

12. **(B)** Blades must be loaded and removed from the handle with an instrument. Most commonly used is a needle holder; never use your hands.

13. **(A)** A Lebsche sternum knife is used in chest surgery to open the sternum.

14. **(C)** Kerrison refers to a rongeur. It is available in many angles and is used extensively in surgery of the spine and neurosurgery.

15. **(B)** A Finochietto is a rib retractor.

16. **(D)** A Doyen is a rib raspatory.

17. **(A)** An electric drill or a hand perforator is used to make the burr holes. A rongeur is used to enlarge the burr holes and increase exposure.

18. **(B)** Westcott tenotomy scissors are fine scissors with a spring action used in eye surgery.

19. **(D)** For splenectomy, prepare a basic laparotomy set plus two large right-angled pedicle clamps and long instruments and hemostatic materials.

20. **(B)** Bowman probes are used to probe the lacrimal duct in a dacryocystorhinostomy and in lacrimal probing to open a closed lacrimal drainage system.

21. **(D)** The tonsil lobe is freed from its attachments to the pillars with a Hurd dissector and pillar retractor.

22. **(C)** The Lempert elevator is used in delicate ear surgery.

23. **(C)** The Scoville is a retractor used in a laminectomy.

24. **(D)** The Bailey rib approximator is used to approximate the ribs for closure of a thoracic incision before closure of the chest with interrupted suture.

25. **(D)** A Sauerbruch is a rib rongeur used to resect a rib and is found in a thoracotomy rib instrument bone set.

26. **(C)** An Auvard is a speculum that is weighted for use in the vagina. It is placed in the posterior vagina.

27. **(B)** A Babcock forceps is a curved fenestrated blade clamp without teeth that grasps or encloses delicate structures such as the ureter, appendix, or fallopian tube.

28. **(A)** A Ballenger swivel knife is used in rhinologic surgery. The nasal cartilage is incised with a Ballenger knife.

29. **(A)** A Weitlaner is a self-retaining retractor.

30. **(D)** A Hill is a rectal retractor.

31. **(C)** A Webster needle holder is found in a basic plastic surgery instrument set.

32. **(B)** The kidney pedicle containing the major blood vessels is isolated and doubly clamped with a Herrick, Satinsky, or Mayo pedicle clamp.

33. **(A)** Uterine dilators are Hank uterine dilators.

34. **(B)** A lesion detected by a mammogram can be localized by the insertion of a needle(s) or a wire that is inserted through a needle. Once the suspected area is identified, the patient is sent to the operating room for a biopsy. After biopsy, the specimen can be sent back for mammography validation before pathological examination.

35. **(D)** Randall stone forceps are available in various angles and are used to remove stones from inaccessible areas.

36. **(A)** Instrumentation for splenectomy is a basic laparotomy plus two, large, right-angled pedicle clamps, long instruments, and hemostatic materials or devices.

37. **(A)** Two blunt nerve hooks are required on a vagotomy setup.

38. **(A)** In an exploration of the common bile duct, a drainage T-tube is placed into the common bile duct. It is used to confirm successful evacuation and patency of the ducts and stays in place as a drain.

39. **(D)** Prosthetic devices are made of stainless steel and Teflon. Microsuctions are used. A speculum provides view.

40. **(A)** Cochlear implantation is the placement of an electrode device in the cochlea in deaf people. Candidates should have a history of lingual skills before becoming deaf. The device receives sound and emits electrical impulses into the cochlea and along the acoustic nerve. Sound interpretations are taught to the patient postoperatively.

41. **(B)** A Ballenger swivel knife is used in nasal surgery. An anesthesia setup, a bayonet forceps, an

Asch septum-straightening forceps, a straight hemostat, impregnated gauze, packing, a splint, and adhesive tape are prepared for a nasal fracture, closed reduction.

42. **(A)** A bayonet forceps is used to introduce sponges into the nose.

43. **(C)** The Potts tissue forceps is a fine forceps associated with vascular and fine intestinal surgery. Nasal surgery requires, intranasally, an angled forceps such as the bayonet forceps, a Freer elevator, and a fine Frazier suction tube.

44. **(B)** Esophageal dilators (bougies) may be on an esophagoscopy setup.

45. **(D)** A Jameson hook is used in eye surgery. The Yankauer suction, Hurd dissector and pillar retractor, and tongue depressor are all found in a tonsil set.

46. **(D)** A tissue expander stretches normal tissue to accommodate a breast prosthesis, used postmastectomy. The expander is placed in a created pocket and exchanged for a permanent prosthesis after desired expansion has occurred.

47. **(B)** Mandibular and maxillary fracture reduction is most often accomplished by applying arch bars to the maxillary and mandibular teeth for immobilization in order to restore the patient's preinjury dental occlusion.

48. **(C)** The Alexander periosteotome, Doyen raspatory, and Stille shears are all instruments required to remove a rib. A Heaney clamp is a hemostatic clamp used in gynecological surgery.

49. **(B)** Randall stone forceps are part of a kidney instrument set.

50. **(A)** A Sarot is a bronchus clamp.

51. **(B)** An intra-aortic balloon pump (IPB) is not necessary. Fluoroscopy and a defibrillator are required plus vascular dissecting instruments, tunneling instrument, pacemaker and electrodes, introducer set, and an external pacemaker.

52. **(C)** A permanent pacemaker initiates atrial or ventricular contraction or both. The most common indications are complete heart block bradyarrhythmias.

53. **(A)** Harrington rods are internal splints—the distraction rods are placed concave to the curve and the compression rods on the convex side.

54. **(C)** Skeletal traction is the pulling force exerted to maintain proper alignment or position. It is applied directly on the bone following insertion of pins, wires, or tongs placed through or into the bone. Traction is applied by pulleys and weights to establish and maintain direction until fracture reunites.

55. **(A)** For a forearm or lower leg, a Kirschner wire or a Steinmann pin is drilled through the bone distal to the fracture site. Traction is applied.

56. **(A)** During orthopedic surgery, the mobile image intensification, also referred to as fluoroscopy or x-ray image, allows viewing of the case progression.

57. **(B)** The myelogram outlines the spinal subarachnoid space and shows distortions of the spinal cord or dura sac by means of an injection of contrast media.

58. **(D)** Sachs, Frazier, and Adson are metal suction tips that suck and also conduct coagulation. Gardner and Mayfield are skull clamps and part of a neuro headrest setup.

59. **(A)** An antigravity suit applied before positioning may help prevent air embolism and assist in maintaining blood pressure.

60. **(B)** After wound closure, a Logan's bow is applied to the cheeks with tape strips to relieve tension on the incision and to splint the lip. It is a curved metal frame.

61. **(C)** A Cloward is the removal of anterior cervical disk with fusion using Cloward instruments. It entails removal of disk fusion of the vertebral bodies and the use of bone dowels for the fusion obtained from the patient's iliac crest.

62. **(D)** A Beaver knife handle is found on the instrumentation for lens procedures in the eye.

63. **(C)** Skeletal traction requires the use of sterile supplies (traction bow, pins, and drills).

64. **(D)** A Leyla–Yasargil is a self-retaining retractor. The others are aneurysm clips.

65. **(A)** A Pereyra or a Stamey is used for bladder neck suspensions to correct urinary stress incontinence. It is a ligature carrier and is inserted through a suprapubic incision.

66. **(B)** Extracorporeal shock wave lithotripsy (ESWL), a noninvasive procedure, utilizes the lithotripter, which introduces shock waves through a liquid medium to disintegrate stones. Fluoroscopy and the image intensifier are used for visualization.

67. **(C)** The Omni–Tract is an adjustable urology perineal retractor system.

68. **(A)** A Mason–Judd is a bladder retractor.

69. **(A)** The Furlow inserter is used to place a penile implant.

70. **(D)** A Millin is a retropubic bladder retractor.

71. **(C)** The Gomco is a circumcision clamp used for infants. For adults, a plastic instrument set is used.

72. **(A)** A Humi cannula is used in gynecological surgery for placement into the uterine cavity via the cervix for intraoperative chromotubation with diluted methylene blue or indigo carmine solution.

73. **(D)** The Hulka forceps may be introduced into the cervix to manipulate the uterus for better visibility.

74. **(A)** A central venous pressure catheter insertion is a minor operative procedure requiring sterile gloves, drapes, and instruments.

75. **(C)** Bakes are a set of common duct dilators.

76. **(D)** A Steffee plate is an internal spinal implant fixation system used for treatment of fractures, spondylolisthesis, and idiopathic scoliosis of the thoracolumbar spine.

77. **(C)** Crutchfield tongs are used for skeletal traction.

78. **(D)** The Bookwalter is a self-retaining retractor system.

79. **(A)** A Harrington is a large retractor.

80. **(B)** A Debakey is a long thoracic forceps.

81. **(B)** Bougie dilators are available in graduated sizes for esophageal dilation.

82. **(C)** The wire cutter scissor needs to accompany the patient to PACU postoperatively in case of emergency, and the mouth needs to be opened.

83. **(B)** Potts–Smith scissors are used to extend the arteriotomy incision during a carotid endarterectomy.

84. **(C)** Figure 15–1A. A Stevens scissor is used for delicate plastic surgery such as a blepharoplasty.

85. **(B)** Hanks dilators are used on the uterus to dilate the cervix. Hegar dilators are also used to dilate the cervix (they are not pictured). Van Buren dilators are used to dilate the male urethra.

86. **(C)** Bakes dilators are used on the common bile duct to open and expand the duct to allow passage of bile from the live. Bougies are esophageal dilators, and Garrett dilators are used to dilate vessels.

87. **(A)** The Bookwalter is used to retract large abdominal wounds. It is a self-retaining retractor that attaches to the operating room table. All individual pieces need to be included in the count.

88. **(C)** Figure 15–4D is the Finochietto. It is a chest/rib spreader. Other chest spreaders include the Burford and the Ankeney. They are not pictured but look very similar.

89. **(B)** The retractor commonly used in abdominal surgery and mostly pelvic procedures (gynecological [GYN]) is the O'Connor–O'Sullivan retractor.

90. **(C)** The Balfour is a self-retaining retractor used for retraction of a large abdominal wound. It has multilateral blades and a wide center blade. The set also includes the frame and a wing nut.

91. **(D)** The Ellik evacuator is a double glass bowl and bulb with an adapter tip. It is used to remove tissue segments/blood clots from the bladder. A microvasive evacuator does the same thing but is disposable.

92. **(B)** The three-way Foley catheter is used for intermittent or continuous bladder irrigation.

93. **(C)** Both the two-way and the three-way Foley catheters are the most common indwelling catheters. The Foley has a balloon at one end and is used to hold the catheter in place. A large-mL Foley catheter would be used postoperatively for a tamponade (used to apply pressure against a tissue opening); an example would be following transurethral resection of the prostate (TURP).

94. **(A)** Two-way Foley 5 cc is used for urinary drainage. One port is used to inflate the balloon, and the other hooks to the drainage bag. A common nonretaining urinary catheter is a Robinson red rubber catheter.

95. **(B)** Figure 15–7 is a Toomey syringe. It aspirates specimens and blood clots from the bladder. It is often used to check for bleeding following a TURP. Fluid is injected into the bladder with a Toomey syringe and then aspirated out of the bladder with the Toomey syringe, checking the color of the fluid.

96. **(B)** The Auvard speculum provides retraction of the posterior vaginal wall. The blade is placed into the vaginal vault, and the weight of the speculum allows it to hang in place.

97. **(C)** The instrument in Figure 15–8C is a Jorgenson dissecting scissor commonly found on the GYN tray. A Jarit is a retractor used to retract small shallow wound edges.

98. **(B)** Figure 15–8B is the Hulka tenaculum. It is used for grasping and holding. It is used to manipulate the uterus during laparoscopic examination of pelvic structures. The probe is inserted into the cervical os, and the sharp prong penetrates the anterior cervical lip.

99. **(C)** The instrument in Figure 15–8F is a Bozeman uterine dressing forceps. It is used to place vaginal packing in the vagina following vaginal procedures. A Simpson forceps is used to facilitate the fetal decent when the fetus is lodged in the birth canal. The Ochsner is a curved Kocher, a grasping penetrating clamp.

100. **(D)** A Phaneuf is a hysterectomy instrument used to clamp vessels and uterine ligaments used during a hysterectomy. The Jacobs Vulsellum is used to grasp the anterior lip of the cervix for manipulation. The Schroeder is a single-toothed tenaculum used to grasp the cervix.

101. **(B)** The instrument in Figure 15–8E is the Graves vaginal speculum. It is used to retract the anterior and posterior walls. The Eastman is a lateral vaginal retractor, and the Young anterior retractor is a prostate retractor used in prostate surgery.

102. **(C)** A Bugbee electrode is used to coagulate small areas usually following a bladder biopsy. It is also the working element.

103. (D) Figure 15–10 is the loop electrode. It is used for resection and coagulation of the prostate and bladder tissue during transurethral procedures. The ball loop electrode is used for coagulation of a larger surface area. Example is the bladder. Randall forceps are used to grasp renal stones and common bile duct stones.

104. (C) A T-tube is inserted into the bile duct for drainage of bile. The T-tube is a type of passive drain.

105. (B) A Fogarty embolectomy catheter would commonly be found on a vascular setup. It is the method of removing thrombi.

106. (B) The instrument in Figure 15–13B is a Duval lung forceps. It is used to grasp and hold lung tissue.

107. (A) The instrument in Figure 15–13A is a Sarot bronchus clamp. Is used to hold and occlude the bronchus while stapling during a lung procedure. A Cooley is used to clamp deep anatomical vessels. The Javid carotid artery clamp is used to secure the Javid shunt in the carotid artery, and Potts–Smith are used to grasp and hold tissue.

108. (D) The Statinsky vena cava clamp has the jaws of the Debakey design. It is used to encircle the superior and the inferior vena cava before placement of umbilical tape around the vessel.

109. (D) Figure 15–14A is a Bethune rib cutter. This heavy shear has straight cutting blades. Figure 15–14C is the Gluck rib shear. The outside blade covers the rib, and the inside blade cuts down. Another common rib cutter is the Sauerbruch (not pictured). A patient's anatomy and which rib is being excised determine which rib cutter will be used.

110. (C) The instrument in Figure 15–14B is the Davidson scapula retractor. It is used to retract the scapula and expose the ribs during thoracic entry and closure. The Allison lung retractor looks like a whisk and is used to retract lung tissue (not pictured). The Cooley arterial retractor is used to retract the atrium during a mitral valve procedure.

111. (C) The forceps in Figure 15–15 are Randall stone forceps. They are used to grasp stones in the biliary system. They come in different intensities of curvature.

112. (A) This biliary catheter is used to retrieve stones from the common bile duct.

113. (B) A Fogarty embolectomy catheter is used to remove thrombus from vessels, and a Malecot is a self-retaining urethral catheter. Instead of using a balloon, the tip of the Malecot has either two or four wings that expand out to hold it in place.

114. (D) The instrument in Figure 15–17A is a Hurd dissector. It is used to retract the soft palate for oral procedures and to dissect tonsil tissue. Figure 15–17B is a mouth gag used to retract the mouth open for exposure of the oral cavity. Another commonly used mouth gag is the Jennings mouth gag.

115. (D) The instrument in Figure 15–18A is a Kerrison rongeur. It is used to excise the lamina and create access to the disc. It is used during a spine procedure. They come as up biting, straight, and down biting.

116. (B) The pituitary is used to remove the herniated disc. A Taylor spinal retractor is used for wound retraction during lumbar spine procedures.

117. (D) The Leksell rongeur is used to remove pieces of bone and soft tissue and is also used to remove the spinous process during a laminectomy.

118. (A) This instrument is called the Scoville nerve root retractor. It is used to retract the dura and the nerve root. The shaft can be straight or angled. Cobb curettes are used to scrape bone during spine surgery. Cobb ring curettes are used to strip muscle and peritoneum off the bone.

119. **(B)** Figure 15–19B is a blunt grasper that is used for grasping and manipulating organs causing minimal trauma; these graspers are often used on tissue that is going to be removed.

120. **(A)** The Maryland dissector is curved with fine tapered jaws with horizontal serrations running the length of its jaws. It is used for fine dissection and separation of thin adventitia.

121. **(C)** Figure 15–19D is the endoclip applier. It is used for occluding vessels or other tubular structures. It comes in various titanium clip sizes from 5 to 10 mm and in different-size lengths.

122. **(B)** Endoscopic scissors are used to cut and dissect tissues, ducts, vessels, and suture material. They have a rounded blunt tip with curved blades.

123. **(D)** Figure 15–19F is a suction irrigator, which is used to irrigate and aspirate fluid and debride from the surgical site. It is a hollow suction tube attached to a combination tubing that has a suction valve and an irrigation valve.

124. **(C)** The Kleppinger is a paddle tip forceps that attaches to a bipolar cord used to grasp tissues and vessels between the jaws and stepping on the foot pedal during laparoscopic procedures.

125. **(B)** The endo-fan retractor is used for elevation, retraction, and mobilization of organs and tissues and provides optimal visualization of the surgical field.

126. **(A)** During a repair of an inguinal hernia, using the TEP approach, the instrument used is a balloon expander. It is inserted into an incision and inflated with air or normal saline. The balloon dissector is then removed and is maintained with gas insufflations.

127. **(D)** Figure 15–19J shows common laparoscopic instruments that are commonly used on all laparoscopic surgeries.

128. **(C)** EEA or end-to-end stapler has a circular double row of staples and a knife blade within the instrument that resects excess tissue and creates a circular anastomosis. The LDS is used for ligation and division of blood vessels and other tissues during abdominal GYN and thoracic procedures. It is commonly used in gastrointestinal surgery to ligate and divide the greater omentum and mesentery (not pictured).

129. **(D)** The thoracoabdominal staple gun is used to transect and resect. It has a double or triple staggered row of staples commonly used in lung and abdominal surgery.

130. **(B)** The gastrointestinal anastomosis stapling device is used for resection and anastomosis. It provides two rows of double staggered staples and simultaneously divides tissue between them.

CHAPTER 16

Sutures, Stapling Devices, and Drains

SUTURES

- The choice of suture depends on the health of the patient, surgeon's preference, and preexisting conditions
- Types of suture material
  - Absorbable—absorbed by the body. Never used on vessels and arteries
  - Nonabsorbable—resists enzymatic breakdown and absorption by human tissue
  - Monofilament—one single strand that glides through tissue
  - Multifilament—several strands braided together
- When working with chromic and plain sutures, do not pull on the sutures to reduce their memory because handling weakens the sutures
- Nylon sutures are held between gloved hands to remove the memory. Suture is held on each end away from needle. Commonly used in neurosurgery
- Do not crush or clamp suture, including stainless steel, with an instrument as it can put a crimp in the suture, causing it to create a larger hole when going through tissue, which causes bleeding
- Keep silk suture dry—being wet decreases its tensile strength

Classification of Suture Material

1. Plain gut	• Absorbable natural • Monofilament • From cow or sheep intestines • Packaged in alcohol • Treated with a salt solution
2. Chromic	• Same as above • Not treated with a salt solution
3. Polydioxanone/ PDS	• Provides a long duration of wound support
4. Polyglactin 910/ Vicryl	• Also called Vicryl • Can be used in presence of infection
5. Nylon	• Commonly used in neuro
6. Polyethylene	• Commonly used for tendon repair (strong) • Also called Ethibond
7. Polypropylene	• Also called Prolene • Nonabsorbable • Inert in tissue • Suture of choice for vascular • Can be used in the presence of infection besides steel
8. Stainless steel	• The most inert in tissue • Can be used in the presence of infection • Has the highest tensile strength but the worst handling qualities
9. Surgical silk	• Commonly used on the serosa of the gastrointestinal tract • Must be used dry • Cannot be used in the presence of infection

- Sutures should be passed using the "neutral zone" technique
- Information on the suture pack includes:
  - Surgical application
  - Product code number
  - Suture length and color
  - Suture size
  - Diagram of the size and shape of the needle
  - Needle point
  - Lot number
  - Expiration date
- Gauge—refers to the diameter of the suture
  - The larger the suture gauge, the smaller the diameter of the thread.
  - The higher the number, the finer the suture
- Knot tensile strength
  - This is the amount of force or pull that a suture strand can withstand before breaking

- Ligatures/ties are used to occlude vessels and ducts and also to retract
- Free tie—this type of suture is handed as a single strand
  - Ligature reel—used on superficial bleeders
  - The ligareel is radiopaque; the suture material is wrapped around the reel
  - You pull the suture to make a 2-in tail prior to handing the reel with tail to surgeon
- Instrument tie/tie-on-a-passer—used to occlude deeper vessels
  - Single strands of suture are clamped to the tip of the instrument—Adson or a Mixter—and handed to the surgeon
  - Pass the instrument the same way as usual while holding the tip of the suture with your other hand
- Suture ligature/stick tie—this is used to occlude deeper vessels. There is a swaged needle attached
  - Figure-of-eight stick tie—this is used with a clamp. When the surgeon clamps off a bleeder, he may prefer to use a stick tie instead of a ligareel
- Loading the suture—the needle should be clamped one-third of the way from the swaged end of the needle

CUTTING SUTURE

- You should use your dominant hand for best control
- Your ring finger and thumb are placed in the rings and your index finger on the box lock/screw joint for control
- Use the tip of the scissors to cut the suture. Slightly open the scissors, slide the one blade down the suture, and cut above the knot unless otherwise instructed by the surgeon

NEEDLES

- Needles are made of steel
- Eye of the needle—the part of the needle where the suture is attached/swaged on. There are three types of needles including:
  - Closed eyed—the holes in the needle are round or square. These needles cause more damage to tissue than eyeless needles because the holes are larger
  - French eyed—this needle is easier to load than a closed needle because there is an opening on the top so the suture thread can be pulled through quicker

- Eyeless and double armed—the needle may be swaged on or can be control-release needles (pack contains eight needles—suture easily pulls off)

Needle Points

- Needles can be:
  - Cutting
    - Conventional cutting needle—has three razor sharp edges; they place a small cut in the tissue
    - Reverse cutting—opposite cutting edges as a conventional cutting needle. These are commonly used for skin
    - Side cutting/spatula—used for eye procedures
  - Tapered
    - Taper needle—do not have a cutting edge. The needle punctures the tissue. Commonly used on the gastrointestinal tract or delicate tissue
  - Blunt
    - It has a round shaft and a blunt tip. Commonly used on the kidney and liver and delicate friable tissue
  - Keith needle
    - Straight needle—comes free or swaged on

Suture Coding for Commonly Used Sutures	
BP	Blunt point
C/CV	Cardiovascular
CE	Cutting edge
CP	Cutting point
CT	Circle taper
CTB	Circle taper blunt
CTX	Circle taper extra large
DP	Double point
FS	For skin
KS	Keith straight
M	Muscle
MO	Mayo needle
OS	Orthopedic surgery
P	Plastic
PC	Plastic cosmetic
PS	Plastic surgery
RB	Renal artery bypass
SC	Straight cutting
ST	Straight taper
TN	Trocar needle
TP	Taper point
UR	Urology

HYPODERMIC NEEDLES

- These are used to inject medications into tissue and IV tubing
- They are also used to withdraw blood from the patient
- They come in various sizes and lengths

ARTERIAL OR VENOUS/CANNULA NEEDLES

- This needle is used to place an indwelling catheter for IV fluids or blood
- Angiocath is commonly used for IV fluids

Arterial Needles

- These needles are used to guide catheters used for angioplasty over guide wires into the arterial system; they include:
  - Potts
  - Cournand

Venous Needles

- With an aspirating syringe, these are used to puncture large veins to introduce monitoring catheters (Swan–Ganz)
- Swan–Ganz catheterization—the passing of a (catheter) into the right side of the heart and the arteries leading to the lungs. It is done to monitor the heart's function and blood flow

IRRIGATION NEEDLES

- Used for irrigating

VERESS NEEDLE

- Used for laparoscopic cases to introduce CO_2 into the abdomen to create a pneumoperitoneum

BIOPSY NEEDLES

- Dorsey cannulated needle for brain tissue biopsy
- Chiba—biopsy needle used for lung tissue
- Franklin–Silverman cannulated biopsy needle—used for liver and other internal organs
- Tru-Cut biopsy needle—commonly used for the liver
- Bone biopsy needles—used to retrieve bone marrow or for biopsy of the spine

- Spinal needles—used to introduce anesthetic medication into the epidural space and subdural space as well as to obtain spinal fluid

SUTURING TECHNIQUES

- Dr. Halsted developed the principles of suture technique
  - Continuous/running suture
    - Single strand of suture that runs the entire length of the wound
    - As the surgeon is suturing, the assistant follows by holding tension and keeping the suture out of the surgeon's line of sight
  - Continuous running locking/blanket stitch
    - Same as continuous except after each stitch a technique is used to lock the stitch in place
  - Subcuticular—stitches are hidden under the skin layer
    - The suture runs along the tissue below the skin. There is no visible suture
  - Steri-Strips and Dermabond are used to reinforce the wound
  - Purse string—this is a draw string suture around a tubular structure
    - Commonly used on an appendectomy
  - Interrupted suture—used on tissues under tension and infected tissue
    - There are many variations of the interrupted stitch
  - Buried suture—the knot of the suture is buried under the tissue layer and not sticking out
  - Traction sutures—used to retract tissue. Commonly used on the eye, heart, common bile duct (CBD), tongue
  - Retention sutures—large sutures that are nonabsorbable and interrupted that are placed through all layers of tissue for wound reinforcement when needed
  - Bridges/bolsters—used with the retention suture to prevent the heavy suture from cutting into the patient's skin
    - They are tubular pieces of plastic or rubber
  - Endoscopic sutures—used in laparoscopic procedures. There are two types of techniques used:
    - Extracorporeal—the knot is tied outside the body and slipped back in

- Intracorporeal—the suture is tied inside the body
  - Endoloop and Endo Stitch are two types of suture used

ALTERNATIVE SKIN CLOSURE METHODS

- Wound zipper—leaves no suture holes
- Dermabond—(cyanoacrylate)—liquid glue
- Fibrin glue—biologic adhesive that can be used on deep tissue. Approximates wounds and helps control bleeding
- Button suture—used on tendon repair—the button helps eliminate tissue damage
- Umbilical tape
  - Originally used to tie off the umbilical cord on an infant
- Vessel loops—elastic strips used for retraction. They come in different colors for identification
  - Red—arteries
  - Blue—veins
  - White and yellow—nerves or ducts
- Suture anchors—used in orthopedic surgery to attach ligaments to bone
- Suture boots—small silicone covers that go on the end of mosquito clamps
  - They are used to identify and hold suture material
  - They are clamped on one end of the suture where the needle is. Used to keep track of the second needle but also used for traction
  - Booties prevent the suture material from becoming kinked and causing a larger hole in the vessel
- Steri-Strips—used with tincture of benzoin so that they stick better
- Skin staples—can be stainless steel or titanium. They are quicker to place than suture, cause minimal scaring, and are a choice for skin. Not used in plastic surgery cases. Staples are never used in the presence of infection. Two people are required to place staples; one person places staples, and second person uses forceps to approximate the skin

DRAINS

- They are used to drain fluids and air from a wound
- Drains can be active or passive
- Passive drains—air and fluids drain from high pressure to low pressure. There is no suction involved. These drains include:

- Penrose drain
  - A type of latex tubing placed in the wound
  - They drain by capillary action
- Cigarette drain
  - It is a Penrose drain with a gauze strip inside
  - It works by wicking action
- T-tube
  - This tubing is placed in a tubular structure for drainage
  - Most commonly used in the CBD
  - One side is placed in the duct and the other brought out to the skin and connected to a bile bag
- Gastrostomy tube/feeding tube/PEG tube (percutaneous endoscopic gastrostomy feeding tube)
  - Inserted through the abdominal wall into the stomach for drainage and nutritional feeding
- Cystostomy tube
  - Inserted through the abdomen into the bladder for drainage
- Nephrostomy tube
  - *Inserted percutaneously into the kidney for drainage*
- Tympanostomy tube—myringotomy tubes—a small incision is made in the tympanic membrane, and the tiny tube is placed into the incision with alligator forceps. This procedure is performed to equalize pressure in the middle ear and for drainage from chronic otitis media
- Active drains—drainage occurs by suction, mechanically or manually. They include:
  - Hemovac—used when a moderate amount of drainage is expected. Commonly used in orthopedic surgery
  - Jackson–Pratt drain—commonly used on thyroid, breast, orthopedics, and abdominal procedures with minimal drainage. It uses a tube and a grenade
  - Stryker—works off a battery evacuation pump—mainly used in hips and knees. It is very effective in eliminating dead space
  - Gastrointestinal (GI) decompression—a plastic or rubber nasogastric (NG) tube—NG tube is inserted through a nostril down into the stomach or intestine to remove gas, fluids, and other contents to decompress the GI tract. Types of tubes used include:

- NG tubes are Levin tube (stomach)
- Miller–Abbott tube (intestines)
- Salem sump (NG suction)
  - Urinary drainage—urinary catheters provide constant drainage of the bladder and kidneys during surgical procedures to provide decompression of the bladder
  - Pleur-Evac chest drainage system—closed water-seal drainage system—consists of a chambered collection system and a connecting hose. One end attaches to the patient's chest tube, and the other end to the collection unit. This can be used as a gravity drain and vacuum
    - This provides drainage of the pleural cavity and expansion of the lungs after surgery.
    - You always want to maintain negative pressure in the pleural space or the lungs will collapse
    - When it is not attached to suction, the collection unit must be kept below the chest level of the patient because gravity will allow the fluid contents to go back into the plural space and collapse the lung
    - Chest tubes—clear plastic drains that are inserted into the chest cavity—the tubing from the Pleur-Evac is connected to the chest tube

STAPLING DEVICES

- Staples are made of various materials including:
  - Stainless steel
  - Titanium
  - Absorbable materials

Skin Stapler
- Used to approximate skin edges
- One staple is fired at a time
- Adson forceps are used to approximate the skin edges. The gun is lined up with the skin edges, and the staple is released
- Depending on the manufacturer, the average gun holds from 28–36 staples

Linear Stapler
- There are two basic types; they include:
  - GIA—GI anastomosis
  - TA—thoracoabdominal

- GIA
  - This gun places two double rows of staggered staples and has a blade that ligates and divides the tissue
  - This is commonly used to join tubular segments together side by side
  - Commonly used in the GI tract and the thoracic cavity
- TA
  - This gun places two double rows of staggered staples. Same as above but does not have a blade within the gun
  - The target tissue is placed in the jaws of the TA gun, which is closed and fired. The staples are released. The target tissue is sealed, and a free scalpel blade is used to ligate the tissue
  - Commonly used to close a side or end of bowel or lung tissue
- LDS—ligating and dividing stapler
  - A double row of staples are released side by side for a one-time staple and cut
  - This is commonly used to ligate small vessels and small tubular structures. An example would be the omentum
- EEA—end-to-end anastomosis/intraluminal staple gun
  - This is a circular staple gun with a double row of staggered staples and a blade attached
  - Commonly used on tubular structures of the lower GI tract, distal colon, or rectum
  - When the gun is fired, it staples and ligates tissue, leaving behind two pieces of tissue shaped like a doughnut. They are sent to pathology separately to determine that both pieces of tissue are intact and contain no cancerous margins and that a proper seal from the gun has been made
- Endoscopic stapler
  - These staple guns are endoscopically inserted through a trocar system
  - They are used to ligate and divide
  - Same principle as discussed above
- Ligating clip applier/Hemoclip applier
  - They are used to occlude small vessels, ducts, and tissue
  - Two clips are placed: one proximally and one distally on a structure. The structure can be divided with a blade or scissor

Questions

1. Which of the following is a monofilament suture?

   (A) Prolene
   (B) Silk
   (C) Polyester
   (D) Vicryl

2. The size of the suture is based on its diameter. An example of a suture with the same diameter is a 2-0 silk and:

   (A) 3-0 silk
   (B) 2-0 nylon
   (C) 4-0 silk
   (D) both A and C

3. Which term refers to the amount of force needed to break the suture?

   (A) Multifilament
   (B) An absorbable quality
   (C) Tensile
   (D) Nonabsorbable

4. Which needle would be used on a liver resection?

   (A) Cutting
   (B) Tapered
   (C) Keith
   (D) Blunt

5. Which suture needle is contraindicated for a repair of nerve tissue?

   (A) Taper
   (B) Cutting
   (C) Reverse cutting
   (D) Both B and C

6. Hemoclip staples are made from:

   (A) stainless steel
   (B) titanium
   (C) absorbable staples
   (D) all of the above

7. In an appendectomy, a purse string suture is used to:

   (A) tie off the appendix
   (B) invert the stump of the appendix
   (C) retract the appendiceal stump
   (D) all of the above

8. A cutting needle would not be used on:

   (A) the skin
   (B) the bowel
   (C) the tendon sheath
   (D) the eye

9. If the surgical technician in the scrub role receives a broken needle back from the surgeon, the technician should:

   (A) order an x-ray
   (B) report it to the circulator
   (C) remember to add to the final count
   (D) tell the surgeon immediately

10. All of the following are absorbable sutures EXCEPT:

    (A) polyglactin 910
    (B) chromic
    (C) nylon
    (D) plain gut

11. What suture would be used on a coronary artery bypass and an aortic valve replacement?

    (A) Polypropylene
    (B) Silk
    (C) Dexon
    (D) Vicryl

12. Which of the following sutures is treated with chromium salt solution to decrease the rate of absorption?

    (A) Vicryl
    (B) Plain gut
    (C) Chromic
    (D) Polypropylene

13. Which of the following sutures would commonly cause the least tissue reaction?

    (A) Chromic
    (B) Silk
    (C) Stainless steel
    (D) Vicryl

14. What term is used for a suture thread preattached to a needle?

    (A) Swaged
    (B) Tensile strength
    (C) French eye
    (D) Continuous

15. Retention sutures with bolsters would be used in what type of incision?

    (A) Pfannenstiel
    (B) Abdominal midline
    (C) Oblique
    (D) Transverse

16. What type of suture technique is used for a cosmetic surgery?

    (A) Purse string
    (B) Detach
    (C) Retention
    (D) Subcuticular

17. A Keith needle is:

    (A) a straight needle with a tapered point
    (B) a straight needle with a cutting point
    (C) another name for a spatula needle
    (D) an extremely large curved needle

18. The name given to suture material that is passed around a vessel or a duct for ligation is:

    (A) tie-on-a-passer
    (B) control release
    (C) swaged needle
    (D) ligareel

19. A strand of suture material attached to the top of an Adson clamp or a right angle is:

    (A) stick tie
    (B) Keith
    (C) tie-on-a-passer
    (D) ligareel

20. The technique used to reduce suture memory is:

    (A) hold needle in one hand with thread in the other and lightly tug on suture strand
    (B) hold suture thread between gloved hands and lightly tug on thread
    (C) either of the above will work but you must stretch the suture until the memory is gone
    (D) none are acceptable techniques to reduce memory

21. The reason for using suture boots on a suture thread instead of just a clamp is:

    (A) the clamp is part of the count and should not be used
    (B) once you clamp the suture, it should not be removed until the end of the case
    (C) if you use a clamp on suture, it will crimp suture, altering the integrity of the suture
    (D) they are yellow and easy to identify

22. Another name for polyglactin 910 is:

    (A) Vicryl
    (B) PDS
    (C) nylon
    (D) none of the above

23. Silk suture must be kept dry because moisture causes:

    (A) a crimp in the suture
    (B) contamination
    (C) decreased tensile strength
    (D) hardness of the suture

24. Which information is included on each suture packet?

    (A) Lot number
    (B) Product code number
    (C) Suture length and color
    (D) All of the above

25. The type of needle commonly used for skin:

    (A) is reverse cutting
    (B) is packaged in alcohol
    (C) gets absorbed within 70–90 days
    (D) is made from submucosa of horse intestines

26. All apply to chromic sutures EXCEPT:

    (A) treated with a salt solution
    (B) Cournand
    (C) Angiocath
    (D) both A and B

27. The needle used to obtain tissue from the brain for specimen is:

    (A) Dorsey cannulated needle
    (B) Pereyra needle
    (C) Spinal needle
    (D) Tru-Cut biopsy needle

28. Who developed the principle of suture technique?

    (A) Pasteur
    (B) Lister
    (C) Halstead
    (D) Debakey

29. Suture techniques include all EXCEPT:

    (A) Keith
    (B) continuous running locking
    (C) interrupted
    (D) subcuticular suture

30. Retention sutures:

    (A) are used to retract tissue
    (B) are used for tendon repair
    (C) were originally used to tie off the umbilical cord of infants
    (D) are large, nonabsorbable, interrupted sutures and placed through all layers to reinforce closure

31. All of the following pertain to drains EXCEPT:

    (A) drain fluids and air from a wound
    (B) can be active
    (C) can be passive
    (D) are never removed from the patient

32. The drain commonly used after thyroid surgery is:

    (A) Hemovac
    (B) Jackson–Pratt
    (C) Stryker
    (D) all of the above

33. When loading the suture, the needle should be placed:

    (A) one-third the distance from the swaged end
    (B) one-half the distance from the swaged end
    (C) one-fourth the distance from the swaged end
    (D) on the area of the needle that the swaged end attaches to the thread

34. The suture code RB on the package means:

    (A) renal artery bypass
    (B) retrobulbar
    (C) retinal blunt
    (D) reverse blunt

35. The CTX needle suture code stands for:

    (A) cardiac transplant
    (B) circle taper extra large
    (C) cutting
    (D) none of the above

36. Arterial needles used to guide angioplasty catheters over guide wires include:

    (A) Potts
    (B) Cournand
    (C) Dorsey
    (D) both A and B

37. The biopsy needle commonly used on the liver is:

    (A) Chiba
    (B) Franklin–Silverman
    (C) Tru-Cut
    (D) Both B and C

38. Suture techniques include:

    (A) continuous running
    (B) blanket stitch
    (C) subcuticular
    (D) all of the above

39. Which of the following sutures are nonabsorbable, placed interrupted, and placed through all layers of tissue for wound reinforcement?

    (A) Traction
    (B) Buried
    (C) Bridges
    (D) Retention

40. All apply to a Penrose drain EXCEPT:

    (A) it is a passive drain
    (B) it works by a wicking action
    (C) it drains by capillary action
    (D) it can be used for retraction

41. Where is a T-tube commonly placed for drainage purposes?

    (A) Cystic artery
    (B) Cystic duct
    (C) CBD
    (D) Hepatic artery

42. Active drains include:

    (A) Stryker
    (B) Hemovac
    (C) GI decompression
    (D) all of the above

43. GI decompression drainage tubes include:

    (A) Levin tube (stomach)
    (B) Miller–Abbott tube (intestines)
    (C) Salem sump (nasogastric suction)
    (D) All of the above

44. All apply to closed chest drainage system EXCEPT:

    (A) it provides drainage of the pleural cavity and expansion of the lungs after surgery
    (B) you always want to maintain a positive pressure in the pleural space or the lungs will collapse
    (C) when it is not attached to suction, the collection unit must be kept below the chest level of the patient because gravity will allow the fluid contents to go back into the plural space and collapse the lung
    (D) chest tubes are clear plastic drains that are inserted into the chest cavity, and the tubing from the Pleur-Evac is connected to the chest tube

45. All apply to the skin stapler EXCEPT:

    (A) it is used to approximate skin edges
    (B) one staple is fired at a time
    (C) Adson forceps are used to invert the skin edges, the gun is lined up with the skin edges, and the staple is released
    (D) depending on the manufacturer, the average gun holds 28–36 staples

46. All are false in regard to linear staple guns EXCEPT:

    (A) the GIA gun places two double rows of staggered staples and has a blade that ligates in between the staples and divides the tissue
    (B) they are commonly used to ligate small vessels and small tubular structures, for example, the omentum
    (C) they are commonly used on tubular structures of the lower GI tract, distal colon, or rectum
    (D) two clips are placed proximal and distal on a structure and can be cut with a blade or scissors to divide the structure

47. What are two basic types of abdominal/thoracic linear staple guns?

    (A) LDS and EEA staple guns
    (B) endoscopic staplers and Hemoclip appliers
    (C) skin stapler
    (D) GIA and TA

48. LDS is the acronym for:

    (A) ligating and dividing stapler device
    (B) used for ligating ducts and small vessels
    (C) lysis of duct structures
    (D) all of the above

49. In what type of surgical procedure are you most likely to use an EEA stapler device to create an end-to-end anastomosis?

    (A) Hysterectomy
    (B) Distal colon resection
    (C) Ovarian cystectomy
    (D) Hemorrhoidectomy

50. A Centers for Disease Control and Prevention (CDC) guideline that addresses the care of "sharps" includes all of the following EXCEPT:

    (A) needles should always be recapped
    (B) needles should not be bent or broken by hand
    (C) needles should not be removed from disposable syringes
    (D) needles should be discarded in puncture-resistant containers for disposal

51. In a GI closure, the mucosa of the intestinal tract is closed with:

    (A) chromic 4-0 or 3-0
    (B) silk 4-0 or 3-0
    (C) Dacron 3-0 or 2-0
    (D) Novafil 3-0 or 2-0

52. What type of suture is used in orthopedic surgery to secure tendons and ligaments to bone?

    (A) Mesh
    (B) Biological
    (C) Suture anchors
    (D) Stainless steel

53. All apply to sutures EXCEPT:

    (A) sutures should be passed by "neutral zone" technique
    (B) nylon sutures are held between gloved hands to remove the memory, not by pulling the suture when it is on the needle holder
    (C) pass the suture with the needle facing away from the surgeon's chest while holding the other end of the suture so it does not fall below the sterile field
    (D) suture packets are designed to remove the needle from the pack without touching it

54. When cutting with suture scissors, all apply EXCEPT:

    (A) open the scissors wide when entering the body to cut, slide the one blade down the suture, and cut above the knot unless instructed by the surgeon

    (B) if possible, you should use your dominant hand for best control

    (C) your ring finger and thumb are placed in the rings, and your index finger is placed on the screw joint for control

    (D) use the tip of the scissors to cut the suture

55. A closed-wound suction system works by:

    (A) positive pressure

    (B) negative-pressure vacuum

    (C) air displacement

    (D) constant gravity drainage

56. Mersilene is a/an:

    (A) wire mesh

    (B) absorbable suture

    (C) nonabsorbable suture

    (D) synthetic mesh

57. All the following drains are considered active postoperative drains that are attached to an external force EXCEPT:

    (A) sump

    (B) chest

    (C) Penrose

    (D) Hemovac

58. A continuous suture placed beneath the epidermal layer of the skin in short lateral stitches is called a:

    (A) mattress suture

    (B) transfixion suture

    (C) retention suture

    (D) subcuticular suture

59. Which procedure is followed if the scrub is pricked with a needle?

    (A) Change glove only

    (B) Discard needle, change glove

    (C) Place new glove over old

    (D) Change gown and gloves

60. Natural absorbable sutures are broken down in the body by:

    (A) capillarity

    (B) enzymatic digestion

    (C) granulation

    (D) metabolic factors

61. #1 and 4-0 sutures are the most commonly used sutures. 4-0 and 5-0 are used for anastomosis on the ____. 6-0 and 7-0 are used for ____. #1 and #0 are used for ____ because of their tensile strength. 8-0 to 11-0 you will find on a/an ____. A 4-0 is used to close the ____.

    1. eye
    2. aorta
    3. smaller vessels; femoral/popliteal.
    4. dura
    5. orthopedic cases

    (A) 2, 3, 5, 1, 4

    (B) 3, 2, 1, 4, 5

    (C) 1, 5, 2, 3, 4

    (D) 1, 5, 2, 3, 4

62. Abdominal wounds are closed in layers. They include, from the inner layer to the outer layer, peritoneum, fascia, muscle, subcutaneous, and skin. Which of these layers must be closed securely because it is the primary supportive tissue layer?

    (A) Skin/subcutaneous

    (B) Muscle

    (C) Fascia

    (D) Peritoneum

63. Alternative skin closure methods include:

    (A) Montgomery straps
    (B) wound zipper
    (C) polymethyl methacrylate
    (D) reconstituted thrombin

64. What is the term used when the STSR assists the surgeon when closing a wound using a continuous running method by keeping the suture secure and out of the surgeon's suture line?

    (A) Retention
    (B) Follows
    (C) Anchoring
    (D) Intention

65. What is the potential outcome of tissue that is approximated too tightly when suturing?

    (A) Dehiscence
    (B) Adhesions
    (C) Ischemia
    (D) Blood clot

66. Mesh is used to reinforce tissue. All are true regarding mesh EXCEPT:

    (A) polypropylene mesh can be used in the presence of infection
    (B) biological mesh can include tissue from the patient's thigh, from the muscle of cattle, and/or from porcine small intestines
    (C) porous mesh allows fibers to grow through the mesh and bond and strengthen the tissue
    (D) stainless steel should never be used as mesh because it is rigid and difficult to work with

67. Which of the following mesh types is considered absorbable?

    (A) Polypropylene
    (B) PTFE (polytetrafluoroethylene)
    (C) Polyglactin 910
    (D) All of the above

68. Dacron tape is also known as umbilical tape and:

    (A) is used to tie off the umbilical cord following the birth of a baby
    (B) can be used to retract the spermatic cord during an indirect hernia repair
    (C) can be wrapped around structures to identify them
    (D) all of the above

69. Barbed suture:

    (A) is used in cosmetic surgery
    (B) is a type of unidirectional suture
    (C) holds its position and locks in place as it goes through tissue without having to tie a knot
    (D) all of the above

70. All apply to myringotomy tubes/tympanostomy tubes EXCEPT:

    (A) used to facilitate drainage and equalize pressure of the eardrum between the inner ear and the middle ear
    (B) a small incision is made in the tympanic membrane
    (C) are placed with an instrument called an alligator forceps
    (D) commonly fall out on their own

71. Which staple gun requires a scalpel blade to divide the tissue?

    (A) Linear staple gun
    (B) GIA
    (C) TA
    (D) Both B and C

72. Which stapling device is commonly used to divide the mesentery and omentum during GI procedures?

    (A) Linear dissecting stapler
    (B) BIA
    (C) Liga-clip
    (D) Surgi-clip

Answers and Explanations

1. **(A)** Prolene is a single continuous fiber made of a polymer chemical (ie, chains of the same molecule strung together) that is extruded and stretched.

2. **(B)** A 2-0 silk has the same diameter as a 2-0 nylon suture. A numbering system indicates the suture's outside diameter and ensures that a stated size is the same regardless of the material.

3. **(C)** Tensile strength refers to the amount of force needed to break the suture.

4. **(D)** A blunt needle is the least traumatic and the safest needle point. It is used on friable tissue and organs that are soft and spongy.

5. **(D)** The taper needle has a round body that tapers to a sharp point. Its primary use is for suturing soft tissue such as the biliary tract, the dura, GI structures, muscle, and nerve.

6. **(D)** Hemoclip staples are made from stainless steel, titanium, and absorbable material.

7. **(B)** A purse string suture is used to invert the stump of the appendix into the cecum.

8. **(B)** A cutting needle is not used on the bowel because it lacerates the bowel.

9. **(D)** When the STSR receives a broken needle back from the surgeon, the STSR should immediately tell the surgeon. The STSR should also inform the circulating nurse because when they find the all of the broken needle, each piece needs to be added to the final count.

10. **(C)** All are absorbable except nylon, which is a nonabsorbable suture.

11. **(A)** Polypropylene is commonly used on soft tissue and in cardiovascular surgery.

12. **(C)** Chromic gut is an absorbable suture that is treated with a salt solution to aid in decreasing the absorption rate.

13. **(C)** Surgical stainless steel is the strongest of suture materials. It has no significant inflammatory properties. It is available in monofilament and twisted and is commonly used in the presence of infection.

14. **(A)** The suture is inserted into the eye end of the needle and is crimped and sealed. This is referred to as swaged on.

15. **(B)** Retention sutures provide additional support to wound edges in abdominal surgery.

16. **(D)** In subcuticular stitching, the needle is placed within the dermis from side to side. This technique brings the skin edges together, and no suture material is visible from the outside. This technique produces a very fine scar or no scar.

17. **(B)** A Keith needle is a straight needle with a cutting point frequently used in gynecological procedures and on superficial tissue.

18. **(A)** A tie-on-a-passer is a piece of suture attached to a clamp that is passed around a vessel or a duct for ligation and is commonly used in deeper cavities.

19. **(C)** A tie-on-a-passer is a strand of suture material attached to the top of an Adson or right-angle clamp.

20. **(B)** You can only hold the suture. If you grasp the needle, you may pull it off. You can never get all the memory out without causing damage to the suture.

21. **(C)** Suture boots are used to identify and hold one end of a double-armed suture but are ideally used to prevent a kink in the thread, which can lead to vessel damage.

22. **(A)** Another name for polyglactin 910 is Vicryl.

23. **(C)** When silk becomes wet, this compromises its tensile strength.

24. **(D)** All of the above are included on a suture package.

25. **(A)** A reverse cutting needle is commonly used for skin closure. A side cutting needle is commonly used for eye procedures. Tapered needles are used in the GI tract and for delicate tissue. Hypodermic needles are used to inject medications into tissue and IV fluids.

26. **(D)** Chromic sutures are made mainly from bovine intestines and also sheep intestines.

27. **(A)** The Dorsey cannulated needle is used to obtain tissue for a brain biopsy. A Pereyra needle is used for stress incontinence. A spinal needle is used to introduce anesthetic medication into the epidural space and subdural space and to obtain spinal fluid. A Tru-Cut needle is used for a liver biopsy.

28. **(C)** Dr. Halstead developed the principles of suture technique. Lister contributed to antiseptic technique. Debakey is known for his contributions to cardiac surgery.

29. **(A)** A Keith is a straight needle and has nothing to do with sewing technique.

30. **(D)** Retention sutures are large sutures. They are nonabsorbable and placed interrupted through all layers of tissue for wound reinforcement.

31. **(D)** Active drains are removed from the patient.

32. **(B)** Jackson–Pratt drain is commonly used following thyroid surgery. A Hemovac is used when a moderate amount of drainage is expected. They are commonly used in orthopedic surgery. A Stryker drain works off of a battery. It is an evacuation pump mainly used on hips and knees. It is very effective in eliminating dead space.

33. **(A)** When loading the suture, the needle should be placed one-third of the distance from the swaged end.

34. **(A)** The RB suture code stands for renal artery bypass.

35. **(B)** The CTX suture code stands for circle taper extra-large needle. C/CV is a cardiovascular needle.

36. **(D)** Potts and Cournand are two types of angioplasty catheters. A Dorsey needle is a cannulated needle used for brain biopsies.

37. **(D)** The Tru-Cut biopsy needle is commonly used for a liver biopsy. The Franklin–Silverman biopsy needle can be used for a liver biopsy along with other organs. The Chiba biopsy needle is commonly used for lung tissue.

38. **(D)** All of the above are suture techniques.

39. **(D)** Retention sutures are large, nonabsorbable, interrupted sutures that are placed through all layers of tissue for wound reinforcement. Traction sutures are used to retract tissue during eye, heart, CBD, or tongue surgery. Buried suture is when the knot of the suture is buried under the tissue layer and not sticking out. Bridges and bolsters are used with the retention suture to prevent the heavy suture from cutting into the patient's skin.

40. **(B)** All apply to the Penrose drain except it does not work by wicking action. The cigarette

drain is a Penrose drain with a gauze strip inside that works by wicking.

41. **(C)** The T-tube is commonly used for drainage of the CBD.

42. **(D)** The Stryker drain works off a battery evacuation pump and is mainly used in hips and knees; it is very effective in eliminating dead space. Hemovac is used when there is a moderate amount of drainage and is commonly used in orthopedic surgery. GI decompression tube is a plastic or rubber NG tube and is inserted through a nostril down into the stomach or intestine to remove gas, fluids, and other contents to decompress the GI tract.

43. **(D)** The Levin tube is used for stomach decompression. The Miller–Abbott is used to decompress the intestines, and the Salem sump is used for NG suction.

44. **(B)** You always want to maintain a negative pressure in the plural cavity or the lungs will collapse.

45. **(C)** Adson forceps are used to evert the skin edges, and the gun is lined up with the skin and the edges of the skin and the staple is released.

46. **(A)** The GIA gun places two double rows of staggered staples and has a blade that ligates in between the staples and divides the tissue. The LDS (ligating and dividing staple) gun is commonly used to ligate small vessels and small tubular structures, for example, the omentum. The EEA gun is used on tubular structures of the lower GI tract, distal colon, or rectum. Hemoclips are two clips placed proximal and distal on a structure and can be cut with a blade or scissors to divide the structure.

47. **(D)** GIA and TA linear staple guns are stapling devices that are commonly used to divide and join tubular segments back together side by side for intestinal (GI) or thoracic procedures. All other choices are NOT basic types of linear staple guns.

48. **(A)** Ligating and diving stapler is the acronym for an LDS stapler device. This device releases a double row of two staples side by side for a one-time staple and cuts between with a blade within the gun. It is also commonly used to ligate small vessels and small tubular structures.

49. **(B)** The EEA stapler device is a circular staple gun with a double row of staggered staples and a blade attached to cut around this circular lumen within the tissue. It is commonly used on tubular structures of the lower GI tract, such as distal colon or rectum surgical procedures.

50. **(A)** Precautions must be taken to prevent injuries. To prevent needle stick injuries, needles should not be recapped, purposely bent or broken by hand, removed from the disposable syringes, or otherwise manipulated by hand. Sharps should be place in a puncture-resistant container for disposal.

51. **(A)** In a GI closure, the mucosal layer is closed with chromic 4-0 or 3-0; the seromuscular layer is closed with chromic 3-0 or 2-0 and silk 4-0 or 3-0.

52. **(C)** Suture anchors are a type of fixation device used in orthopedic surgery to attach tendons and ligaments to bone. They consist of a type of an anchor/screw that is inserted into the bone, and suture material is attached to the anchor through the eye of the anchor. They are commonly used in shoulder surgery to repair the labrum.

53. **(C)** All apply to sutures except that when you properly pass the suture to the surgeon, the point of the needle is actually facing the surgeon. You can also tell if you have properly loaded a lefty or righty because the point of the needle should be facing the surgeon.

54. **(A)** It is always best to use your dominant hand for best control, but this is not always possible. Positioning at the sterile field can be a factor, which is why it is very important to master using both hands. Ring finger and

thumb are placed in the rings, and your index finger directs the position. Never proceed toward the target suture to be cut with the scissors in an open position as damage can be done to tissues. Always keep the scissors closed until the hand reaches the suture.

55. **(B)** This portable system is used to apply suction to a large closed-wound site postoperatively. A constant, negative vacuum evacuates tissue fluid and blood to promote healing by reducing edema and media for microbial growth.

56. **(D)** Synthetic meshes, such as Mersilene or Martex, are helpful in repair of recurrent hernias requiring a strong repair.

57. **(C)** Sump, chest, and Hemovac drains are all active drains attached to an external force of vacuum to create suction. The Penrose exits the wound and provides a path of least resistance for drainage into the dressing.

58. **(D)** A subcuticular suture is a continuous suture placed beneath the epithelial layer of the skin in short lateral stitches. It leaves a minimal scar.

59. **(B)** Change a glove at once and discard needle or instrument if a glove is pricked by a needle or snagged by an instrument.

60. **(B)** Natural absorbable sutures are broken down in the body by enzymes in the body that attack the suture strand and destroy it. The term capillarity refers to the suture being able to harbor bacteria and spread the bacteria. That is why multifilament sutures should not be used in the presence of infection. They can spread the infection through the length of the strand of suture.

61. **(A)** 4-0 and 5-0: aorta. 6-0 and 7-0: smaller vessels (polypropylene). #1 and #0: orthopedics (Vicryl/polyglactin 910). 8-0 to 11-0: eyes. 4-0: dura (Ethilon/nylon).

62. **(C)** The fascia layer is the tough connective layer and holds the majority of the wound closure. The peritoneal layer is thin and does not always need to be closed if the fascia is closed properly. Muscle is not commonly closed. Muscles are commonly retracted and not cut if it can be avoided so they do not always need to be closed. Subcutaneous tissue can be friable. It is made of fat cells and connective tissue and not very strong. Commonly, a few stiches may be used to secure the layer. Skin closure is the final step in wound closure and is performed using a variety of techniques.

63. **(B)** Alternative skin closure methods include a wound zipper. Adhesive strips are positioned alongside the wound, and the zipper is attached and closed. It is a noninvasive and atraumatic skin closure method. Another type of skin closure commonly used is Dermabond/fibrin glue. It is an adhesive placed directly on the wound. It takes a few minutes to dry and provides a strong flexible closure. Skin closure tapes are applied to the skin to reinforce a subcutaneous closure. They are commonly used for cosmetic closures. Prior to applying the tape, tincture of benzoin is placed on both sides of the incision so that the steri-strips/skin tape adheres better.

64. **(B)** The term for assisting the surgeon by holding the suture taut and out of the suture line when closing is *follows* or *runs*.

65. **(C)** Tissue that is approximated too tightly is compromised by a lack of blood flow to the target tissue, causing ischemia. Dehiscence is when there is wound disruption and the wound opens. Adhesions are bands of scar tissue commonly found in the intestines.

66. **(D)** All are true regarding mesh including using stainless steel. It is rigid and can be difficult to work with, but it is the most inert of the material and can be used in the presence of infection.

67. **(C)** Polyglactin 910 is an absorbable mesh.

68. **(D)** Dacron/umbilical tape is a cotton braided tape. It is not as commonly used today as it

was in the past. It can be used to tie off the umbilical cord and retract and identify structures in the body. It is also used as part of the Rumel peripheral vascular tourniquet for vascular occlusion.

69. **(D)** All of the above apply to a barbed suture. It actually resembles barbed wire.

70. **(A)** Myringotomy tubes are placed in the tympanic membrane with an alligator forceps to facilitate drainage and equalize pressure between the middle and outer ear. They do not require a second surgery to remove them because they commonly fall out on their own.

71. **(D)** A TA (thoracoabdominal) staple gun is a linear staple gun. It has two rows of parallel staples and a surgical blade that is used to divide the tissue. It is commonly used in the GI tract and for lung tissue.

72. **(A)** The LDS stapling device is commonly used to divide the mesentery and omentum during a bowel resection.

CHAPTER 17

Wound Healing and Dressings

Factors that affect wound healing include:

- Age
- Obesity
- Nutritional status
- Smoking
- Immunocompromise
- Radiation exposure

Types of Wound Closure	Phases of Wound Healing	Wound Classifications
• PRIMARY INTENTION—easy closure no infection, skin edges come together example would be a hernia • SECONDARY CLOSURE—a lot of tissue loss and can't close the incision—heals by GRANULATION • THIRD INTENTION—infected, not much tissue loss, closed within a few days of surgery	• FIRST INFLAMMATORY—clot formation • SECOND PROLIFERATION—new tissue is formed, fibroblasts • THIRD MATURATION—"mature" wound is closed, collagen	• CLASS 1—CLEAN CASE—no infection, no break in aseptic technique, good case • Example: Coronary artery bypass grafting or craniotomy • CLASS 2—CLEAN/CONTAMINATED—when there is no spillage of contents. An example is removing the gallbladder with no spillage of bile/appendix/vagina • CLASS 3—CONTAMINATED—open trauma case/gunshot wound/spillage from intestinal tract • CLASS 4—DIRTY—infected case, perforated bowel or resection of ruptured appendix

Complications of wound healing include:

- Infection
- Hemorrhage
- Dehiscence—the wound separates after it has been closed
- Evisceration—the contents of the abdomen protrude out from the wound
- Dead space—separation of wound layers where air and/or blood accumulate and cause infection
- Fistula—an abnormal tube-like passage from a normal cavity or tube to a free surface or to another cavity
- Sinus tract—a tract that is open at one end only. It runs between two epithelium-lined structures. It causes infection and drainage
- Suturing material and technique used

Types of wounds include:

- Contusion—bruise
- Laceration—tear or cut
- Thermal—can be caused by heat, cold, or chemicals
- Abrasion—scrape
- Closed wound—skin remains intact. Some damage to underlying tissue
- Open wound—skin is cut/open
- Clean wound—clean cut, skin edges can be approximated
- Contaminated wound—open wound with bacteria and infection
- Complicated wound—a foreign body may remain in the wound; the edges of the wound cannot be approximated because of tissue loss
- Chronic wound—a wound that takes an extended period of time to heal

Dressing is used to:

- Immobilize
- Apply even pressure over the wound
- Collect drainage
- Provide comfort for the patient
- Protect the wound

Biologic dressings include:

- Integra—a bilayer matrix wound dressing made of bovine tendon and collagen matrix

- Dermagraft—manufactured from human fibro-blast cells derived from newborn foreskin tissue

Skin grafts include:

- Autologous skin graft—taken from the patient's own body
- Homograft—taken from a cadaver donor
- Xenograft/heterograft—taken from another species
- Porcine—taken from pigs

One-Layer Dressing

This is used to cover:
- A small wound with minimal drainage
- Endoscopic incisions
- IV site

They are a transparent film with an adhesive backing. They include:
- Opsite/Tegaderm
- Bioclusive
- Collodion—liquid chemical dressing that forms a seal over the incision. Commonly used on pediatric patients. Applied with Q-tips dipped in the solution
- Aerosol adhesive sprays
- Steri-Strips—used with tincture of benzoin to help the Steri-Strips to stay in place
- Dermabond—liquid skin—used to close wounds

Three-Layer Dressing

A type of dressing used when there is drainage expected
Consists of three layers:
- Primary/inner/contact layer
- Secondary/intermediate/absorbent layer
- Tertiary/outer/securing layer

Three-Layer Dressing

THE PRIMARY/INNER LAYER—this type of dressing is in direct contact with the wound. It provides a wicking action to draw the fluid away from the wound. They include:

Nonpermeable/occlusive
- This will not stick to the wound. It creates an airtight and watertight seal. Examples include:
  ◦ Xeroform gauze
  ◦ Vaseline gauze
  ◦ Band-Aid

Semipermeable/semiocclusive
- When removed, it can take a small amount of tissue with it
- Water and air can pass through this dressing (it contains a layer of gel forming material)
  ◦ This is a type of a hydrocolloid dressing—commonly used on burns
  ◦ Aqua-Gel

- Permeable/nonocclusive
- Have a wicking action that allows air and fluid to pass
- This nonocclusive dressing should be painless when removed
- They include:
  ◦ Telfa
  ◦ Adaptic—this is a nonadherent dressing used to draw secretions from the wound

---

INTERMEDIATE/SECONDARY/ABSORBENT LAYER—this is placed over the contact layer
- This includes:
  ◦ 4 × 4's
  ◦ 2 × 2's
  ◦ Fluffs (4 × 4's opened and packed together)
  ◦ Kerlix
  ◦ ABDs—abdominal pads

TERTIARY/OUTER/SECURING LAYER—this layer is used to secure all the dressings
- This layer includes:
  ◦ Tape
  ◦ Wraps—ace bandages, Coban, and Kling
  ◦ Stockinette
  ◦ Tube gauze
  ◦ Montgomery straps—used for frequent dressing changes; look like a corset

Pressure   dressing/bolster   dressing/tie-over dressing

- This is a type of three-layer dressing
- Commonly used in plastic surgery following skin grafts
- It is applied tightly to:
  - Immobilize an area
  - Absorb excessive drainage
  - Provide even pressure
  - Eliminated dead space
  - Reduce edema
  - Reduce hematoma formation
- Stent dressing—a type of pressure dressing
  - The primary layer usually consists of Xeroform gauze
  - The secondary layer is fluffs
  - Tertiary layer consists of silk suture securing the dressing in place
- Wet-to-dry dressing
  - The dressing is soaked in saline, applied wet to the wound, and allowed to dry. The dressing is then removed with a layer of the wound tissue
- Wet-to-wet dressing
  - Wet sponges are applied to the wound and removed before they dry. This type of dressing also debrides the wound but with less pain than the wet-to-dry dressing
- Thyroid collar/Queen Anne collar—a circumferential wrap is used to secure dressing
- Ostomy bag—dressing applied over a stoma
- Drain dressing—surgical dressing cut in the shape of a "Y" to wrap around a drain
- Tracheostomy dressing—surgical dressing used to secure a tracheostomy
- Eye pad—oval-shaped gauze pad used to cover the eye and keep the eyelid closed
- Eye shield—rigid oval-shaped shield used to cover the eye pad and protect the eye from trauma
- Perineal/peri-pad—pad used to absorb vaginal and perineal drainage

Splints	Casts

• They are made of molded plastic, metal, and aluminum
• They are applied to one side of a body part to limit movement and to prevent flexion
	• They are made of fiberglass or plaster
	• They encircle a body part to provide support and prevent movement
	• Types of casts include:
	  ○ Body jacket—this cast immobilizes the lower thorax and lumbar area. It goes from the axilla to the hips
	  ○ Walking cast—cylindrical cast of the lower extremity
	  ○ Spica cast—used to support the torso to the hip or thigh. It includes the trunk and one or both legs
	  ○ Minerva jacket—immobilizes the body from the head to the hips, immobilizing the cervical and upper thoracic vertebrae

- Packing material—long strips of gauze used to:
  - Provide hemostasis
  - Provide pressure, eliminate dead space
  - Support a wound
  - Comes plain or impregnated with an antiseptic (iodoform) and a radiopaque mark

Burns—can be caused by:

- Heat
- Chemicals
- Electricity
- Gases
- Radiation

Burns are classified by four degrees:

First-Degree Burn	Second-Degree Burn	Third-Degree Burn	Fourth-Degree Burn
• Affects the epidermis • Redness to the skin causing inflammation and pain • An example—sunburn	• Affects the epidermis and part of the dermis • Blisters with slight thickening of the skin	• Full-thickness burn • Affects the epidermis and dermis • Thickness of the skin with a white pearly appearance • Because of the extensive damage to nerves, a third-degree burn is not always painful	• Affects the epidermis and dermis down to the bone

- Burns are assessed by:
  - The rule of nines—this is the method used to calculate the body surface area involved in burns using the value of 9
    - The head and neck = 9%
    - The front of the body trunk = 9%
    - The back of the body trunk = 9%
    - Arms—4.5% right arm/4.5% left arm = 9%
    - Legs—9% right leg/9% left leg = 18%
    - Perineal area = 1%
  - Lund and Browder—method used for estimating the extent of the burns to the body surface relating to different ages. Commonly used for children

Questions

1. A surgical wound that is sutured together heals by:

   (A) granulation
   (B) primary intention
   (C) inflammatory means
   (D) secondary intention

2. Which classification of wound healing is involved with perforated bowel?

   (A) Secondary intention
   (B) Primary intention
   (C) Third intention
   (D) Fourth intention

3. Which wound is assigned to tissue healing by granulation?

   (A) Secondary intention
   (B) Third intention
   (C) Fourth intention
   (D) Inflammatory intention

4. Which type of wound healing requires debridement and continuous irrigation?

   (A) Primary
   (B) Secondary
   (C) Third
   (D) Fourth

5. What is the correct order of the wound-healing process: (1) remodeling, (2) proliferation, and (3) inflammatory?

   (A) 1, 2, 3
   (B) 2, 3, 1
   (C) 3, 2, 1
   (D) 2, 1, 3

6. Which of the following is associated with secondary intention wound healing?

   (A) Wound that is sutured together
   (B) Infected contaminated wound
   (C) Wound space that is packed
   (D) Wound that is not sutured

7. During which phase of healing is a scab formed?

   (A) Inflammatory
   (B) Proliferation
   (C) Remodeling
   (D) Primary

8. Conditions that affect wound healing include:

   (A) surgical technique
   (B) obesity
   (C) age
   (D) all of the above

9. A sunburn is classified as a:

   (A) second-degree burn
   (B) first-degree burn
   (C) third-degree burn
   (D) not classified

10. Which of the following burns cause destruction of the entire thickness of skin?

    (A) First degree
    (B) Second degree
    (C) Third degree
    (D) Fourth degree

11. Which burn classification is characterized by dry white skin and generally little pain?

    (A) First degree
    (B) Second degree
    (C) Third degree
    (D) Fourth degree

12. Another name for a scar is:

    (A) infection
    (B) fibrin
    (C) cicatrix
    (D) eschar

13. Which nonadherent surgical dressing is used for a clean surgical wound and also care of specimens?

    (A) Sterile gauze
    (B) Telfa
    (C) ABD
    (D) Xeroform

14. What type of dressing is most often used on a skin graft?

    (A) Pressure
    (B) Stent
    (C) Flat
    (D) Both A and B

15. What type of pressure dressing is molded into a thick pad that fits into the graft area and is secured with sutures?

    (A) Supportive
    (B) Stent
    (C) Flat
    (D) Tegaderm

16. Gauze packing is used:

    (A) on a small incision
    (B) for wrapping a limb
    (C) in nose or open wound
    (D) when compression is needed

17. A strong, thin, transparent liquid useful in sealing certain wound edges is:

    (A) Dermabond
    (B) tincture of benzoin
    (C) collodion
    (D) both A and C

18. The main purpose of Webril is:

    (A) cast padding
    (B) under pneumatic tourniquet
    (C) pressure dressing
    (D) both A and B

19. What type of gauze dressing is used on a circumcision?

    (A) Sponge
    (B) Tegaderm
    (C) Vaseline gauze
    (D) Roll gauze

20. What is the correct order of dressing a surgical wound? (1) Place dressings, (2) wash the incision, (3) cover sterile dressing with a towel, and (4) remove drapes.

    (A) 1, 2, 3, 4
    (B) 2, 1, 3, 4
    (C) 3, 4, 1, 2
    (D) 3, 4, 2, 1

21. A circumferential bandage should be applied to an extremity:

    (A) distal to proximal
    (B) proximal to distal
    (C) anterior to lateral
    (D) medial to anterior

22. The classification of a wound without infection, including a hernia, coronary artery bypass graft (CABG), or craniotomy, is:

    (A) class I
    (B) clean wound
    (C) class II
    (D) both A and B

23. Dead space is a term that indicates:

    (A) separation of wound layers
    (B) the contents of the abdomen protrude outside the incision
    (C) the separation of the wound after healing
    (D) space where an organ has been removed

24. A tract that is open at both ends that runs between two epithelial line structures is:

    (A) a fissure
    (B) dead space
    (C) a fistula
    (D) both A and C

25. A one-layered dressing includes all EXCEPT:

    (A) Band-Aid
    (B) Steri-Strips
    (C) Tegaderm
    (D) ABD

26. Another name for a scrape is a/an:

    (A) laceration
    (B) contusion
    (C) abrasion
    (D) open wound

27. In a three-layer dressing, all are included EXCEPT:

    (A) Xeroform
    (B) fluffs
    (C) Coban
    (D) Steri-Strips

28. A circumferential wrap used to secure dressings commonly used after a thyroid procedure is a:

    (A) stockinette
    (B) Queen Ann collar
    (C) Coban
    (D) all of the above

29. The type of cast used to immobilize the hip or thigh, including the trunk and one or both legs, is a:

    (A) walking cast
    (B) spica cast
    (C) Minerva jacket
    (D) body jacket

30. An item used for padding that has smooth and clingy layers is called:

    (A) Webril
    (B) stockinette
    (C) Telfa
    (D) gypsum

31. A temporary biologic dressing is:

    (A) porcine
    (B) Telfa
    (C) collagen
    (D) mesh

32. Which of the following is NOT a reason for a pressure dressing?

    (A) Prevents edema
    (B) Conforms to body contour
    (C) Absorbs extensive drainage
    (D) Distributes pressure evenly

33. Adherent, occlusive dressings that are used when slight or no drainage is expected and are made of transparent polyurethane film are:

    (A) Telfa
    (B) Bioclusive
    (C) Opsite
    (D) both B and C

34. In a wet-to-dry dressing:

    (A) the primary layer consists of Xeroform gauze
    (B) the dressing is soaked in saline and applied wet to the wound and allowed to dry. The dressing is then removed with a layer of the wound tissue
    (C) moist sponges are applied to the wound and removed before it dries
    (D) the tertiary layer consists of a tubular gauze

35. Which type of dressing is used for frequent dressing changes on an abdominal incision?

    (A) Montgomery straps
    (B) ABD
    (C) Xeroform
    (D) All of the above

36. Wounds fit into which category?

    (A) Surgical
    (B) Traumatic
    (C) Chronic
    (D) All of the above

37. Place the wound classifications in the proper order:

    1. these wounds are created aseptically where there is minimal tissue damage
    2. the wound edges are intentionally delayed by 3 or more days
    3. these surgical wounds have extensive tissue loss

    (A) 1 = first intention/2 = second intention/ 3 = third intention
    (B) 3 = third intention/2 = second intention/ 1 = first intention
    (C) 1 = first intention/3 = third intention/ 2 = second intention
    (D) 2 = second intention/3 = third intention/ 1 = first intention

38. A direct inguinal hernia is considered a:

    (A) clean wound
    (B) clean/contaminated wound
    (C) contaminated wound
    (D) dirty wound

39. A cholecystectomy with no break in technique and no spillage from the gallbladder is considered a:

    (A) class I wound
    (B) class II wound
    (C) class III wound
    (D) class IV wound

40. A penetrating fractured tibia would be classified as what type of wound?

    (A) Clean wound/class I
    (B) Clean contaminated wound/class II
    (C) Contaminated wound/class III
    (D) Dirty wound/class IV

41. A negative-pressure wound dressing/vacuum-assisted closure apply to all EXCEPT:

    (A) removes wound drainage, provides a moist environment, and reduces edema
    (B) a closed system applies negative pressure over the wound
    (C) is commonly used on wounds where bones, blood vessels, and organs are exposed
    (D) is applied in the operating room following surgery

42. Tissue breakdown at the wound edges is:

    (A) dehiscence
    (B) evisceration
    (C) an adhesion
    (D) a keloid

43. Fourth-degree burns affect:

    (A) epidermis
    (B) epidermis and dermis
    (C) epidermis, dermis, and subcutaneous tissue
    (D) epidermis, dermis, and subcutaneous tissue down to bone

44. Pressure dressings added to the intermediate layer of a three-layer dressing are used to:

    (A) concentrate pressure in one area and help absorb drainage
    (B) eliminate dead space
    (C) immobilize a body part
    (D) all of the above

45. A scar that is hypertrophic and bulbous and usually does not reduce over time is a/an:

    (A) papilloma
    (B) keloid
    (C) eschar
    (D) nevus

46. A split-thickness skin graft is used to cover which type of burn?

    (A) First degree
    (B) Second degree
    (C) Third degree
    (D) Fourth degree

47. 47. What is the term for a birthmark or a mole on the skin, especially a birthmark in the form of a raised red patch?

    (A) Basal cell
    (B) Melanoma
    (C) Squamous cell
    (D) Nevus

48. 48. The rule of nines is used to determine:

    (A) body surface burned
    (B) depth of the tissue destruction
    (C) length of healing time
    (D) protocol for dressing changes

49. A wound is described as a _____ when there is a collection of pus around the incision.

    (A) hematoma
    (B) suppuration
    (C) granulation
    (D) dehiscence

50. Wound complications include:

    (A) hematoma
    (B) seroma
    (C) evisceration
    (D) all of the above

51. The most common area on the body where pressure ulcers develop is the:

    (A) sacrum
    (B) ischium
    (C) heel
    (D) all of the above

52. What is the wound classification that is indicated by a delayed closure?

    (A) Primary intention
    (B) Secondary intention
    (C) Third intention
    (D) Fourth intention

53. If a wound is approximated too tightly, it can cause:

    (A) ischemia
    (B) excessive scar tissue
    (C) keloids
    (D) adhesions

Answers and Explanations

1. **(B)** In a primary intention wound, the cut tissue edges are in direct contact. This is an aseptic wound with minimum tissue damage and reaction.

2. **(C)** Third intention or a delayed closure is a process in which an infected or a contaminated wound is treated. An example is perforated bowel.

3. **(A)** This type of wound heals from the base. The healing process involves filling the tissue gap with granulation tissue.

4. **(C)** A delayed closure may be performed when the wound is infected or requires continuous irrigation and debridement.

5. **(C)** The phases of wound healing are inflammatory, proliferation, and remodeling.

6. **(D)** A wound that is not sutured must heal by secondary intention.

7. **(A)** During the inflammatory phase, platelet aggregation and the formation of a scab are followed by the cellular phase.

8. **(D)** All of the above, including the immune system, chronic disease, and nutrition, are factors in wound healing.

9. **(B)** Burns are classified by the depth of the burn. First-degree burns involve only the outer layer of the epidermis, for example, sunburn.

10. **(C)** Burns that cause the destruction of the entire thickness of skin are third-degree burns.

11. **(C)** Third-degree burns are characterized by dry white skin and generally have little pain.

12. **(C)** Another name for a scar is cicatrix. An eschar is a dark thick scab that is devitalized, nonelastic tissue associated with severe burns.

13. **(B)** A Telfa is a nonadherent flat fabric pad used for clean surgical wounds and also used in surgery for the care of specimens.

14. **(D)** A stent dressing is a type of pressure dressing. They are used to apply slight pressure on the graft site. This prevents serous fluid from lifting the skin graft away from the recipient site.

15. **(B)** A stent dressing is molded into a thick pad that fits into the graft area. Sutures are placed around the graft site. The long suture ends are tied over the pad to secure it in place.

16. **(C)** Gauze packing is used in a cavity such as the nose or an open wound. It is available in long thin strips and packaged in a bottle or a similar container.

17. **(D)** Dermabond and collodion are liquid self-adhesives and occlusive dressings.

18. **(D)** Webril is a soft felt padding used under a pneumatic tourniquet and cast padding.

19. **(C)** Vaseline gauze is used to cover delicate incisions where tearing of tissue would disrupt repair. Examples are minor burns, skin grafts, and circumcisions.

20. **(B)** The correct order of dressing the surgical wound is wash the incision, place dressings, cover sterile dressing with a towel, and remove drapes.

21. **(A)** The bandage should be applied from distal to proximal as this prevents blood from pooling at the surgical site.

22. **(D)** A class I wound is also defined as a clean wound. There is no presence of infection or break in aseptic technique. A class II wound is a clean contaminated wound; there is no spillage of contents. Example is a gallbladder or appendix. A class III contaminated wound is an open trauma wound. Example would be a gunshot. Class IV is a dirty wound, which can include perforated bowel.

23. **(A)** Dead space is the separation of wound layers where air and/or blood accumulate causing infection. Evisceration is when the contents of the abdomen protrude out form the incision. Dehiscence is when the wound separates following closure.

24. **(C)** A fistula is defined as a tract open at both ends that runs between two epithelium-lined structures.

25. **(D)** An ABD is an example of a secondary type of dressing used in a three-layer dressing. This is the absorbent layer that is placed over the contact layer.

26. **(C)** Abrasion is the term used for a scrape. Laceration is a cut or tearing of the skin. A contusion is a bruise. An open wound is when the skin is cut.

27. **(D)** Steri-Strips are considered a one-layer dressing

28. **(B)** A Queen Anne collar is commonly used following thyroid surgery along with a Jackson–Pratt drain. A stockinette is a tubular elastic type of dressing commonly used in orthopedics. Coban is an elastic pressure wrap that adheres to itself and is also commonly used in orthopedics.

29. **(B)** A hip spica cast is used to immobilize the hip or thigh including the trunk and one or both legs. A walking cast is a cylindrical cast used for the lower extremity. The Minerva jacket is used to immobilize the body from the head to the hips. It immobilizes the cervical and upper thoracic vertebrae. The body jacket is used to immobilize the thorax and lumbar area from the axilla to the hips.

30. **(A)** Webril is a soft, lint-free cotton bandage. The surface is smooth but not glazed, so that each layer clings to the preceding one and the padding lies smoothly in place.

31. **(A)** Pigskin (porcine) is used as a temporary biologic dressing to cover large body surfaces denuded of skin.

32. **(C)** A pressure dressing does not absorb excessive drainage. A pressure dressing prevents edema, distributes pressure evenly, gives extra wound support, and provides comfort to the patient postoperatively.

33. **(D)** Sterile, transparent occlusive dressings, such as Bioclusive and Opsite, are made of transparent polyethylene and may be used when slight or no drainage is expected. They are usually removed after 24–48 hours.

34. **(B)** In a wet-to-dry dressing, the dressing is soaked in saline and applied wet to the wound and allowed to dry. The dressing is then removed with a layer of the wound tissue. In a wet-to-wet dressing, wet moist sponges are applied to the wound and removed before they dry. This type of dressing also debrides the wound but with less pain than the wet-to-dry dressing. Xeroform is used as a primary dressing material for a three-layer dressing.

35. **(A)** Montgomery straps can be a corset-type dressing or adhesive straps that allow for frequent dressing changes on an abdominal incision without having to change the tape used to secure the dressing material; they prevent the skin from being compromised and help to prevent skin irritation from frequent tape removal.

36. **(D)** Wounds are classified as surgical—caused by an incision; traumatic—caused by thermal,

mechanical, or chemical trauma; or chronic—caused by pathophysiological conditions.

37. **(C)** A first intention wound, also known as a primary intention wound, is created aseptically where there is minimal tissue damage and no tissue loss and is commonly closed with skin staples, sutures, and/or Steri-Strips. A secondary intention wound is also called a granulation wound. These have extensive tissue loss, heal from the inside out, and are known to leave an extensive scar. A third intention wound is when the wound edges are intentionally delayed by 3 or more days. They often require debridement, and retention sutures are commonly used.

38. **(A)** In a clean wound, there is no infection and no break in sterile technique and the wound has been closed with a primary suture line.

39. **(B)** A cholecystectomy procedure with no spillage from the gallbladder and no break in sterile technique is considered a class II wound, or a clean contaminated wound. These wounds have the potential to become contaminated even though there are no visible signs of infection or break in technique

40. **(C)** A fractured tibia where the bone broke through the skin is considered a contaminated wound/class III.

41. **(C)** This type of wound dressing is not used on injuries where the bone, blood vessels, and organs are exposed.

42. **(A)** Dehiscence is caused by poor wound healing as a result of infection, increased abdominal pressure, obesity, diabetes, or malnutrition.

43. **(D)** Fourth-degree burns affect the epidermis and dermis all the way down to the bone.

44. **(D)** Pressure dressings concentrate pressure in one area and help to absorb drainage, eliminate dead space, and immobilize a body part.

45. **(B)** A keloid scar is not harmful, just cosmetically unappealing. The scar is raised with ridges and becomes bigger and wider than the original incision. A papilloma is a wart-like growth usually found on the skin or on mucous membranes. An eschar is a dry, dark scab or falling away of dead skin typically caused by a burn. A nevus is a type of mole or birthmark that is usually red in color.

46. **(C)** A split-thickness skin graft is commonly used to cover a third-degree burn.

47. **(D)** A nevus is a type of mole or birthmark that is usually red in color. Basal cell, squamous cell, and melanoma are all types of skin cancers.

48. **(A)** The two ways to estimate body surface burns are the Lund–Browder method and the rule of nines. Lund–Browder uses a chart with variables according to age. The rule of nines estimates the total body surface burned using increments of 9%.

49. **(B)** A wound with accumulating pus surrounding the wound is known as a suppuration. A hematoma is when tissue under your skin is damaged and results in a bruise, blood pooling, and clots, which cause swelling. Granulation is when a wound heals from the inside out (second intention healing). Dehiscence is when a wound becomes compromised and the wound edges separate from each other.

50. **(D)** Hematoma, seroma, and evisceration are all complications of wound healing.

51. **(C)** The most common area on the body for a pressure ulcer to form is the heal.

52. **(C)** Third intention closure is a delayed closure. The patient is treated with systemic antibiotics, and the wound is left open, irrigated, and packed. It may be closed in a few days.

53. **(A)** If a wound is approximated too tightly, it can become ischemic due to lack of blood supply.

CHAPTER 18

General Surgery

GENERAL SURGERY: GASTROINTESTINAL TRACT/BILIARY/LIVER/PANCREAS/SPLEEN/HERNIA/BREAST/SURGICAL INCISIONS

Gastrointestinal Tract
- Gastrointestinal (GI) tract is also called the alimentary tract
- The GI tract includes:
  - Esophagus
  - Stomach
  - Small intestines
  - Large intestines
  - Rectum
- The basic functions of the GI tract include:
  - Ingestion
  - Secretion
  - Digestion
  - Absorption
- ESOPHAGUS—transports ingested material by peristalsis from the pharynx to the stomach
- ESOPHAGOGASTRODUODENOSCOPY—EGD—also referred to as GASTROSCOPY—scoping of the esophagus, stomach, and duodenum
  - Endoscopes are considered semi-critical and must undergo high-level disinfection before each use
  - Endoscopic accessories such as biopsy forceps, cytology brushes, and fine-needle aspiration instrumentation are considered critical devices because they enter the mucosa and must be sterile
- GASTROESOPHAGEAL REFLUX DISEASE (GERD)—a condition of backflow of gastric or duodenal contents into esophagus causing pain, heartburn, coughing, and respiratory distress
- BARRETT'S ESOPHAGUS—Barrett's esophagus is an abnormal growth or development of cells of the mucosal lining of the distal esophagus. This could be a precursor for cancer.
- ESOPHAGECTOMY—removal of a portion of the esophagus. This can be performed by several different approaches and procedures, including:
  - Transthoracic
  - Transhiatal
  - VATS—video-assisted thoracic surgery
- ZENKER'S DIVERTICULUM—a weakening in the wall of the esophagus that collects food and causes a feeling of fullness in the neck
- ESOPHAGEAL HIATAL HERNIA / DIAPHRAGMATIC HERNIA—a defect in the diaphragm where a part of the stomach protrudes up into the thoracic cavity
- LAPAROSCOPIC NISSEN FUNDOPLICATION—performed to restore the function of the lower esophageal sphincter (the valve between the esophagus and the stomach) by wrapping the stomach around the esophagus. This procedure prevents reflux of the acid and bile from the stomach into the esophagus.
- ESOPHAGEAL DILATION—performed to dilate the esophagus due to strictures caused by scaring of past surgeries, chemical or thermal burns, and anomalies
  - Instruments needed include a gastroscope, video equipment, MALONEY BOUGIE DILATORS AND SAVARY-GILLIARD DILATORS
- STOMACH—lies between the esophagus and the duodenum. It is located in the upper left abdominal cavity, beneath the diaphragm. The stomach is divided into:
  - Cardia (below the esophageal sphincter)
  - Fundus (upper portion)
  - Body
  - Pyloric antrum (above the pylorus)

- It is connected to the lower portion of the esophagus by the esophageal sphincter and to the duodenum by the pyloric sphincter
- The superior mesenteric artery supplies blood to the proximal large bowel
- The lower margin of the stomach is known as the "greater curvature" and the upper margin is the "lesser curvature"
- Attached to the greater curvature is the OMENTUM (it is a double fold of peritoneum containing fat that covers the intestines)
- The hepatogastric and hepatoduodenal
- The MESENTERY—connects the intestines with the posterior abdominal wall
  - Functions of the stomach include:
    - Storage of ingested material
    - Chemical and mechanical digestion (peristaltic waves, which mix and push stomach contents [chime—semifluid mass of partially digested food] into the duodenum)
- VAGOTOMY—a surgical procedure in which one or more branches of the vagus nerve are cut to reduce gastric secretions into the stomach
- PYLOROPLASTY/PYLOROMYOTOMY—a procedure performed to create a larger passageway between the pyloric area of the stomach and a portion of the duodenum
  - More common in infants—symptoms are projectile vomiting
- PERCUTANEOUS ENDOSCOPIC GASTROSTOMY (PEG)—PEG is the most common gastrostomy tube used. PEG uses a flexible gastroscope and a gastrostomy tube for placement through the abdominal wall
  - It is used for gastric decompression and external feedings
- GASTROJEJUNOSTOMY—performed to treat a benign obstruction in the pyloric end of the stomach, or an inoperable lesion of the pylorus of the stomach when a partial gastrectomy cannot be done. This provides a larger opening without sphincter obstruction. This procedure makes a permanent communication between the proximal jejunum and stomach, without removing any portion of the GI tract
- PARTIAL GASTRECTOMY—BILLROTH I and BILLROTH II
  - BILLROTH I is a gastrectomy resection of the diseased portion of the stomach, and an anastomosis between the stomach and duodenum

- BILLROTH II is a gastrectomy resection of the distal portion of the stomach, and an anastomosis between the stomach and the jejunum
- TOTAL GASTRECTOMY—complete removal of the stomach
- PARTIAL GASTRECTOMY—partial removal of the stomach
- BARIATRIC SURGERY—bariatric surgery is also known as weight loss surgery. This is performed for the surgical treatment of obesity
  - MORBID OBESITY—defined as a BODY MASS INDEX (BMI) of 40 kg (kilograms) or more
  - 45 kg = 100 lb
  - This procedure reduces the size of the stomach. Food is digested and absorbed normally, and because the stomach is smaller, it has a feeling of fullness, and the patient eats less. Examples include:
    - ADJUSTABLE GASTRIC BAND/LAP BAND
    - LAP BAND—a silicone strip and an elastic ring placed around the top of the stomach. A fold of stomach is wrapped around the band to secure it in place. The band has a port that is inflated with saline 4 weeks postoperatively. This procedure is adjustable and reversible
- LAPAROSCOPIC ROUX-EN-Y GASTRIC BYPASS—this procedure is a gastric bypass; it reroutes the passage of food from a small pouch created with surgical staples or sutures in the proximal stomach to a segment of the proximal small bowel. It is commonly performed laparoscopically
- SMALL INTESTINE—the longest part of the digestive tract. It begins at the pylorus of the stomach and ends at the ileocecal valve
- It is divided into three parts:
  - Duodenum
  - Jejunum
  - Ileum
- LIGAMENT OF TREITZ—the duodenojejunal flexure where the duodenum and jejunum connect
- MECKEL'S DIVERTICULUM—an outpouching from the small intestine. It is failure of a congenital duct to be eliminated. The diverticulum can become inflamed or ulcerated, bleed, perforate, or cause an obstruction

- INTUSSUSCEPTION—a telescoping of a part of the intestine; this can lead to intestinal obstruction
- LARGE INTESTINES—begin at the ileocecal valve and end at the anus. They are divided into the:
  - Cecum
  - Colon
  - Rectum
- CECUM—forms a pouch from which the APPENDIX projects
- COLON—the colon is divided into four parts:
  - Ascending colon
  - Transverse colon
  - Descending colon
  - Sigmoid colon
- RECTUM—begins at the sigmoid colon and ends in the anus
- ANUS—the anal canal is a narrow passage; it is controlled by two muscle groups that form the:
  - Internal anal sphincter
  - External anal sphincter
- LAYERS/WALL OF THE INTESTINE:
  - Serosa—outer layer
  - Muscularis
  - Submucosa
  - Mucosa—inner layer
- HAUSTRA—outpouchings on the intestines; they give them the bubble appearance
- The primary function of the large intestine is to:
  - Reabsorb water and electrolytes
  - Break down vitamin K and B complex vitamins
  - Help eliminate solid food and waste through defecation
- APPENDECTOMY—removal of the appendix. This procedure is performed to remove an acute inflamed appendix and prevent the spread of infection and peritonitis (inflammation of the peritoneum)
  - McBurney incision is used
  - Bowel technique is used here, and any instruments that come in contact with the appendix should be isolated
  - PURSE-STRING suture commonly used on an appendix
- INTESTINAL STOMA—a surgically created opening or stoma that extends from a portion of the bowel to the outside of the abdominal wall. This is performed for:

- Diverting intestinal contents so the bowel can heal
- Bypassing an obstruction or a tumor
- Stomas include:
  - Ileostomy—performed for removal of the colon
  - Cecostomy
  - Colostomy—creating an opening any-where along the colon
- POLYPECTOMY—polyps are small growths, typically benign; they protrude from a mucous membrane
- HEMICOLECTOMY/TRANSVERSE COL-ECTOMY/ANTERIOR RESECTION/AND TOTAL COLECTOMY. These procedures are performed for:
  - Colitis
  - Diverticulitis
  - A new and abnormal growth of tissue in some part of the body
- WHIPPLE PROCEDURE—PANCREATICO-DUODENECTOMY—removal of:
  - HEAD OF THE PANCREAS
  - DISTAL ONE-THIRD OF THE STOMACH
  - ENTIRE DUODENUM
  - PROXIMAL JEJUNUM
  - GALLBLADDER (GB)
  - CYSTIC AND COMMON BILE DUCTS
  - PANCREATIC LYMPH NODES
- BOWEL TECHNIQUE/ISOLATION TECHNIQUE
  - All items that come in contact with the GI tract are considered contaminated
  - There should be two setups. One for the clean part and one for the dirty
  - Instruments from the contaminated setup should be isolated from the clean
  - The STSR should not touch anything that is dirty and then go back to the clean part of the case until the case is over and their gown and gloves have been changed
  - Once the GI tract is closed, the STSR should replace the suction and cautery tips, contaminated instruments, and the sterile towels that were placed at the beginning of the case
  - All surgical team members should change gown/gloves
- ABDOMINAL PERINEAL RESECTION (APR)—performed to remove malignant lesions and to treat inflammation of the:
  - Sigmoid colon

○ Rectum

○ Anus

- ADHESIONS—fibrous bands of tissue that cause organs and tissues to adhere to one another
- HEMORRHOIDECTOMY—surgical removal of dilated veins or prolapsed mucosa of the anus and rectum. They can be external or internal or both. They can be ligated with:
  ○ Silastic band sutures
  ○ Bovie or laser
- FISTULOTOMY/FISTULECTOMY—an abnormal or surgically made passage between a hollow or tubular organ and the body surface, or between two hollow or tubular organs. The procedures performed include:
  ○ Fistulotomy—this is an opening into the tract for drainage. The wound heals from the inside out
  ○ Fistulectomy—the tract is excised
  ○ Procedure includes dye (methylene blue) injected into the fistula tract, and a probe and grove director are used to identify the tract, follow it, and open it using a blade
- PILONIDAL CYST—a cyst or abscess near or on the cleft of the buttocks that often contains hair and skin
- LAPAROTOMY—a surgical opening into the peritoneal cavity
- LAYERS OF THE ABDOMINAL WALL:
  ○ Skin
  ○ Subcutaneous
  ○ Fascia
  ○ External oblique
  ○ Internal oblique
  ○ Transverse abdominis
  ○ Fascia
  ○ Peritoneum
- LAPAROSCOPY
  ○ Also referred to as MIS—minimally invasive surgery
  ○ Laparoscopic gynecological (GYN) procedures were originally called: Band-Aid, keyhole, belly button procedures
- LAPAROSCOPIC-ASSISTED PROCEDURES—performed with a laparoscope. Additionally, one port site is enlarged in order for the surgeon to bring the tissue outside of the wound for repair. The surgeon may bring the operative tissue out of the body to repair (EXTRACORPOREAL REPAIR) or reach his hand into the opening and perform a (INTRACORPOREAL) repair

- SIL—SINGLE PORT LAPAROSCOPIC SURGERY—one port is used to gain access to the abdominal cavity. The port is placed through the umbilicus
  ○ HASSON CUT-DOWN TECHNIQUE—this is performed with a cut-down technique using a blade and blunt trocar instead of a sharp trocar system
  ○ EQUIPMENT and INSTRUMENTATION include:
    ■ Veress needle—provides access for CO_2 to create a pneumoperitoneum.
    ■ CO_2 intra-abdominal pressure is between 12 and 15 mm Hg and should not exceed 18 mm Hg
    ■ 10-, 11-, 12-, and 5-mm trocar and cannulas are introduced into the abdomen according to surgeon's preference

Biliary System

- GALLBLADDER-BILIARY SYSTEM
  ○ It is located in the right upper quadrant, under the right lobe of the liver
  ○ The main function of the GB is to store bile
  ○ Removal of the GB is performed for:
    ■ Cholecystitis—acute or chronic inflammation of the GB
    ■ Cholelithiasis—stones in the GB (gallstones are sent to pathology in a dry container)
  ○ In both open and laparoscopic cholecystectomies, the surgeon stands and operates from the patient's left side
- CHOLECYSTECTOMY—subcostal/Kocher incision
- LAPAROSCOPIC CHOLECYSTECTOMY—removal of the GB endoscopically
  ○ Biliary instruments include:
    ■ Randall Stone forceps—used to remove stones from the GB (look like polyp forceps and come in various angles)
    ■ Bakes dilators—used to dilate the common bile duct (CBD)
    ■ T-tube—a type of drain that is inserted into the CBD for additional drainage
    ■ Fogarty biliary catheter—this is used to remove stones in the CBD
    ■ Harrington—used to retract the liver

- Potts scissors—used to extend the incision in the CBD
- CHOLANGIOGRAM—an x-ray using fluoroscopy of the bile ducts (cystic/common bile ducts)
  - DIATRIZOATE SODIUM/HYPAQUE, RENOGRAFIN—types of dyes that are injected into the bile ducts through a catheter called a CHOLANGIOCATHETER and a picture is taken
  - It is also important to clear all bubbles from the cholangiocatheter tubing when doing a cholangiogram because the bubbles may show up as stones on the x-ray
- When removing the GB specimen from the abdomen, you can use these techniques:
  - The GB specimen is removed in an endocatch bag to prevent spillage
  - Kelly clamps are used to extend the port opening to remove the GB
  - The GB can also be decompressed with suction
- ERCP—ENDOSCOPIC RETROGRADE CHOLANGIOPANCREATOGRAPHY—an endoscopic procedure used to identify the presence of stones, tumors, or narrowing in the biliary and pancreatic ducts
- CHOLEDOCHODUODENOSTOMY— performed to bypass an obstruction in the distal end of the CBD. The anastomosis is between the CBD and the duodenum
- CHOLEDOCHOJEJUNOSTOMY—the anastomosis is between the CBD and the JEJUNUM
- CHOLEDOCHOTOMY—a T-tube is inserted into the CBD after stones have been removed from the duct to provide drainage
- TRANSDUODENAL SPHINCTEROPLASTY— performed because the SPHINCTER OF ODDI does not function properly; the sphincter of Oddi is the muscle that controls passage of pancreatic/gastric/bile juices into the ampulla of Vater, which empties into the duodenum

Liver

  - Located in the right upper abdominal quadrant of the abdominal cavity beneath the diaphragm and directly above the stomach
  - Divided into right and left lobes by the falciform ligament
  - Glisson's capsule—the outer covering of the liver
  - Bile is manufactured in the liver
- LIVER NEEDLE BIOPSY
  - Performed for liver disease
  - A Silverman or Tru-Cut needle is used for the biopsy
- SUBPHRENIC ABSCESS
  - This is an abscess in or around the liver
- LIVER RESECTION
  - This is performed for benign and metastatic primary tumors
  - The entire liver cannot be removed without a transplant
  - This procedure can be performed open/ laparoscopic/robot assisted
  - Instruments used are:
    - Laparotomy set
    - Biliary instruments
    - Vascular instruments
  - Blunt needles are always used on the liver
  - Self-retaining retractors—Bookwalter retractor
  - CUSA—Cavitron Ultrasonic Surgical Aspirator
  - Dissects tissue using ultrasonic waves incorporated with fluid and suction
  - The handpiece is similar to the electrosurgical unit (ESU) and cuts through the tissue, emulsifying it and thinning the tissue with fluid so it can be suctioned
  - Intraoperative ultrasonography—the ultrasonic probe is draped and used inside the body in conjunction with the surgery
  - Right subcostal incision
- LIVER TRANSPLANTATION
  - This is an implantation of a liver from a donor patient to a recipient patient
  - This procedure is performed only after the donor patient is pronounced brain dead and the family consent for organ donation has been obtained
  - The procedure:
    - Retrieving the liver from the donor patient
    - Performing a hepatectomy on the recipient patient
    - Implanting the donor liver
  - Instrumentation:
    - Basic laparotomy instruments
    - Cardiovascular instruments
    - Sternal saw
    - Nephrectomy instruments

- The procurement team provides special solutions to flush the organs to procure them. They include:
  - Collins solution
  - University of Wisconsin solution
- There are two operating rooms, one for each patient
- Supine position
- Bilateral subcostal incisions/midline incision

Spleen

- The spleen is located in the upper left abdominal cavity, protected by the 10th/11th/12th ribs, and directly beneath the dome of the diaphragm
- SPLENECTOMY—this is performed for:
  - HYPERSPLENISM—splenomegaly—an enlarged spleen with a decrease in red blood cells, white blood cells, and platelets
  - Also performed for tumors and trauma
  - HODGKIN'S DISEASE (a type of cancer that starts in the cells of lymphocytes); one of the places it can start is the spleen
  - SICKLE CELL DISEASE—in this inherited form of anemia, abnormal red blood cells block the flow of blood through vessels and can lead to organ damage, including damage to the spleen. People with sickle cell disease need immunizations to prevent illnesses their spleen helped fight
  - THROMBOCYTOPENIA—(low platelet count): an enlarged spleen sometimes stores excessive numbers of the body's platelets. Splenomegaly can result in abnormally few platelets circulating in the bloodstream where they belong
  - This procedure can be performed open or laparoscopic
  - Supine position
  - General anesthesia
  - Incisions include:
    - Left rectus paramedian
    - Midline
    - Subcostal
  - Hemorrhage is the main intraoperative complication

Pancreas

- The pancreas is located behind the stomach in the back of the abdomen. It is spongy and shaped like a fish

- The head of the pancreas is the largest part and lays on the right side of the abdomen where the stomach is attached to the first part of the duodenum
- The tail or the body of the pancreas is its narrowest part; it is next to the spleen
- The pancreatic duct is also known as the duct of Wirsung
- AMPULLA OF VATER—formed by the pancreatic duct and the common bile duct
- SPHINCTER OF ODDI—this is the muscular valve that controls the flow of gastric juices through the ampulla of Vater
- There are two main types of tissue found in the pancreas:
  - Exocrine—tissue that produces pancreatic enzymes to aid digestion
  - Endocrine—tissue that produces cells known as islets of Langerhans. These grape-like cell clusters produce important hormones that regulate pancreatic secretions and control blood sugar
    - Insulin
    - Glucagon
- PANCREATICOJEJUNOSTOMY—this procedure is performed for obstructed ducts and pseudocysts; this is associated with chronic alcoholic pancreatitis
  - Pancreatic pseudocyst—a collection of fluid around the pancreas. The fluid in the cyst is usually pancreatic juice that has leaked out of a damaged pancreatic duct
  - A loop of the jejunum is anastomosed to the pancreatic duct
- PANCREATICODUODENECTOMY/WHIPPLE procedure—this procedure is performed on patients with cancer on the head of the pancreas or the ampulla of Vater. Usually there is distant metastasis to the lymph nodes/liver/lungs, and the prognosis is usually poor
- Whipple—removal of:
  - Head of the pancreas
  - Entire duodenum
  - A portion of the jejunum
  - Distal third of the stomach
  - Gallbladder
  - Lower half of the common bile duct
- PANCREATECTOMY
  - This procedure is performed for:
    - Cancer of the pancreas
    - Benign tumors

- Chronic pancreatitis
- Trauma
  ○ This can be a total and partial removal of the pancreas
- TOTAL PANCREATECTOMY—a surgical procedure performed to treat chronic pancreatitis when other treatment methods are unsuccessful
  ○ This procedure involves the removal of the entire pancreas, as well as the gallbladder, common bile duct, and portions of the small intestine and stomach and, most often, the spleen
- PANCREATIC TRANSPLANTATION—this procedure is performed to replace a diseased pancreas with a healthy pancreas
  ○ The best candidates:
    - Are between 20 and 40 years old
    - Are able to regulate their glucose levels
    - Have few complications with diabetes
    - Are in good cardiovascular health

Hernia

- Hernia—Latin word for rupture
  ○ Hernia—a protrusion of viscus through an opening in the wall of a cavity
  ○ It can be a congenital defect or an acquired defect
- Hernia types
  ○ INGUINAL HERNIAS
  ○ DIRECT INGUINAL HERNIA
    - This hernia is acquired
    - Commonly found in men
    - It occurs in Hesselbach's triangle, which involves:
      □ Rectus abdominus muscle
      □ Inguinal ligament
      □ Deep epigastric vessels
- INDIRECT INGUINAL HERNIA
  ○ Congenital hernia
  ○ The main focus in this type of hernia is caused by a weakness or tear in the transversalis fascia
  ○ The defect is in the internal inguinal ring and protrudes into the scrotum
  ○ Femoral hernia
    - Most common in women
    - Can be misdiagnosed as a lymph node
- VENTRAL HERNIA
  ○ Occurs anywhere on the abdominal wall other than the groin

  ○ Incisional hernia
    - This occurs at a previous incision site (where previous surgery was performed)
- UMBILICAL HERNIA
  ○ Commonly found in children—congenital
  ○ In adults, usually acquired
  ○ Hernia protrudes through the umbilical ring
- DIAPHRAGMATIC/HIATAL HERNIA
  ○ Occurs more often in women, overweight people, and people over 50
  ○ Occurs at the level of the stomach where it joins the esophagus
  ○ Symptoms include heartburn and GERD (gastroesophageal reflux disease)
- PANTALOON HERNIA
  ○ Both direct and indirect hernias are present
  ○ French word meaning pants
- EPIGASTRIC HERNIA—above the umbilicus
- HYPOGASTRIC HERNIA—below the level of the umbilicus
- SPIGELIAN
  ○ Difficult to diagnose
  ○ The defect is usually between muscle layers, not between two muscles
  ○ Intestinal obstruction is associated with this hernia
  ○ It is usually diagnosed because of the obstructed intestines
  ○ Surgery is immediately required
  ○ Commonly found in the left lower quadrant

Classifications of Hernias

- REDUCIBLE HERNIA
  ○ The hernia sac can be manipulated back into its normal position in the abdomen
- IRREDUCIBLE/INCARCERATED
  ○ The hernia cannot be manipulated back into its normal position
  ○ The hernia contents (intestines) become trapped and cause an intestinal obstruction
  ○ Immediate surgery required
- STRANGULATED HERNIA
  ○ The hernia contents become trapped and the viscera becomes necrotic
  ○ This is a surgical emergency—the hernia cannot be repaired without a bowel resection
  ○ Richter's hernia is a type of strangulated hernia

OPEN HERNIA REPAIR

- MCVAY/COOPER REPAIR
  - Performed on an indirect inguinal hernia
  - Transversalis fascia involved
  - Penrose on a Kelly
  - Mesh graft
- MESH GRAFT
  - The hernia is reduced and mesh is placed on the weakened area; it is secured with sutures
  - Mesh comes in various sizes and shapes—surgeon's choice
  - Mesh material includes:
    - Gore-Tex
    - Teflon
    - Dacron
    - Marlex
    - Prolene
- BASSINI/SHOULDICE HERNIA REPAIR—not often used anymore
  - Tension repair—this type of repair involves reducing the hernia and pulling the muscles together and suturing them with heavy suture or wire
- LITTRE HERNIA REPAIR
  - This type of hernia involves a Meckel's diverticulum
  - A Meckel's diverticulum is a congenital defect in the distal ileum; it is a pouch on the wall of the ilium
- MAYDL HERNIA REPAIR
  - This type of hernia involves two loops of bowel
- LAPAROSCOPIC HERNIA REPAIR
  - Laparoscopy—a way of performing a surgery. Instead of making a large incision, 5- to 10-mm incisions are made and instruments are inserted, including a scope attached to a camera to view the internal organs and repair or remove tissue
- HASSON TROCAR AND CANNULA SYSTEM
  - Cut-down is used to insert this trocar and cannula (this is when they create a small incision using a blade/scissors/forceps, instead of a puncture)
- There are two basic techniques used for a laparoscopic hernia repair. The difference between these two approaches is the way the preperitoneal space is entered

- TEP—totally extraperitoneal patch—a dissecting balloon is used to enter the preperitoneal space without entering the peritoneal cavity
- TAPP—transabdominal preperitoneal patch—standard trocars, Veress needle, or a cut-down with the Hasson system is used

Breast

- BREAST
  - The nipples are at the level of the fifth rib
  - Areola—the pigmented skin around the nipple
  - There are no muscles in the breast, but muscles lie under each breast and cover the ribs
- ARTERIAL BLOOD SUPPLY to the breast includes:
  - Internal thoracic
  - Lateral mammary
  - Intercostal

LYMPH GLANDS AND THE LYMPHATIC SYSTEM

- LYMPH NODES
  - Are found in the area of breast tissue, under the skin that leads into the axilla. The armpits have many lymph glands, also known as lymph nodes
  - The lymph glands are part of the natural drainage system of the body called the lymphatic system. The lymphatic system is made up of a network of lymph glands that are connected throughout the body by tiny vessels called lymph vessels
  - Lymph is a yellow fluid that flows through the lymphatic system and drains into veins. This helps to get rid of waste products from the body and also is responsible for spreading malignant disease to other organs of the body
- Lymphatics drain into two main areas:
  - AXILLARY NODES
  - INTERNAL THORACIC NODES (there are very few of these but they drain the inner half of the breast)
- The most common forms of breast cancer are:
  - Intraductal carcinoma in situ—originating from the ducts
  - Lobular carcinoma—originating from the lobules

- There is an increased risk if your mother, sister, or aunt had breast cancer (two or more people on your mother's side)
- MAMMOGRAM
  - This is the most common screening tool used today
  - Mammography and ultrasound are used to detect breast masses that are too small to detect on a clinical examination
  - MAMMOGRAPHY is the study of the breast using x-ray. The actual test is called a mammogram
  - Mammograms detect:
    - Abnormal densities (lumps/masses)
    - MICROCALCIFICATIONS—commonly found in intraductal carcinoma in situ (they are course calcium deposits). They appear on a mammogram as bright white tiny spots. More common in the aged breast
- ULTRASOUND
  - Uses sound waves to make a picture of the tissue inside the breast. A breast ultrasound can show all areas of the breast, including the area closest to the chest wall, which is hard to study with a mammogram
  - A breast ultrasound is used to see whether a breast lump is filled with fluid (a cyst) or if it is a solid lump. An ultrasound does not replace the need for a mammogram, but it is often used additionally to check abnormal results from a mammogram
- DIGITAL STEREOTACTIC
  - This is performed after a mammogram/ultrasound to further diagnose a possible breast cancer
  - This is a minimally invasive procedure performed to locate and remove tissue from the tumor for diagnosis. A needle is passed into the suspicious area in the breast, and specimen is removed for the pathologist
- MRI—MAGNETIC RESONANCE IMAGING
  - A breast MRI captures multiple images of your breast. Breast MRI images are combined using a computer to generate detailed pictures
- POSITRON EMISSION TOMOGRAPHY (PET) SCAN
  - This is used to find out whether the cancer has spread to organs beyond the breast

- Terms used to describe the stages of breast cancer:
  - LOCAL—the cancer is confined within the breast
  - REGIONAL—the lymph nodes, primarily those in the armpit, are involved
  - DISTANT—the cancer is found in other areas of the body as well
- BRCA1, BRCA2 GENES—GENE TESTING
  - These are mutations in the genetic code of a gene that affect its function
- CORE BIOPSY—NEEDLE BIOPSY
  - A disposable cutting needle is introduced into the mass to core out a plug of tissue; the specimen is sent to pathology for a diagnosis
- NEEDLE ASPIRATION
  - This is performed to aspirate fluid for diagnosis
- BREAST BIOPSY
  - Incisional biopsy—a portion of the mass is excised and sent to pathology
  - Excisional biopsy—the entire portion of the mass and surrounding normal tissue is removed
- LUMPECTOMY
  - This is removal of a mass with a margin of normal tissue included to make sure all the potential cancerous margins are clear. Surgical clips are sometimes put in the spot where the specimen was removed
- NEEDLE-WIRE LOCALIZATION
  - This procedure is performed when a mass is detected on a mammogram and is too small to palpate or the breasts are too dense. A biopsy is recommended
  - The patient goes to radiology and a wire is inserted into the mass under x-ray
- SENTINEL LYMPH NODE BIOPSY
  - The sentinel node chain is the first set of nodes closest to the cancerous tumor site. It is believed that when cancer cells travel, they settle in the first set of nodes
  - The sentinel node is not the same in every patient (because cancer tumors are not the same in every patient)
  - Blue dye/isosulfan blue dye/Lymphazurin
  - Can be used alone to identify the sentinel nodes or can be used with technetium-99—(a radioactive dye). This is injected in the nuclear medicine department

- A gamma tracer probe is draped by the STSR and used like a Geiger counter to trace and follow the dye to the sentinel node
- LYMPHEDEMA following breast surgery is caused by the excision of lymph nodes followed by radiation therapy to the area. The lymphatic system works as a drainage system to drain fluid away from tissues back to the heart. If too many lymph nodes are removed, there is no drainage and the patient's arm may fill with fluid
- SUBCUTANEOUS MASTECTOMY
  - All breast tissue is removed and the skin and nipple are left intact
- SIMPLE MASTECTOMY
  - Removal of the entire breast without lymph node dissection
- MODIFIED RADICAL MASTECTOMY
  - The entire breast and axillary lymph nodes are removed
- RADICAL MASTECTOMY
  - Breast
  - Lymph nodes
  - Muscles—pectoralis major and minor

Incisions

- LAYERS OF THE ABDOMINAL WALL INCLUDE:
  - Skin
  - Fascia (Camper's and Scarpa's)
  - Muscle—linea alba
  - Transversalis fascia
  - Extraperitoneal fat
  - Peritoneum
- VERTICAL INCISIONS
- MIDLINE INCISIONS
  - Offers good exposure to any part of the abdominal cavity
  - The incision can be extended from just below the sternal notch, around the umbilicus, back

to the midline, and down to the symphysis pubis
- EPIGASTRIC INCISION
  - The incision is above the umbilicus to the xiphoid process at the midline
- SUBUMBILICAL INCISION
  - Below the umbilicus
- PARAMEDIAN INCISION
  - The paramedian is a vertical incision placed 2–4 cm laterally to the midline on either side of the upper and lower abdomen

TRANSVERSE INCISION

- UPPER TRANSVERSE is used for the pancreas
- LOWER TRANSVERSE/PFANNENSTIEL
  - Used for access to the pelvic organs
  - Maylard and Cherney are also two lower transverse incisions
  - Pfannenstiel/Maylard/Cherney—are slightly different but all are used for access to pelvic organs
- SUBCOSTAL/KOCHER INCISION—the subcostal incision starts at the midline about 2–5 cm below the xiphoid and can extend downward, outward, or parallel to the costal margin
  - RIGHT SUBCOSTAL—biliary tract
  - LEFT SUBCOSTAL—spleen
- OBLIQUE INCISIONS—NEAR THE GROIN.
  - Used for inguinal hernia repairs
  - The incision is through the external oblique muscle
- MCBURNEY
  - This is a type of oblique incision
  - Used for an appendectomy
- THORACOABDOMINAL INCISION
  - Access to the pleural cavity
  - Right can be used for a hepatic resection
  - Left can be used for the esophagus, stomach, and liver resection

Questions

1. A Nissen fundoplication procedure is done to correct:

   (A) repeated attacks of volvulus
   (B) antireflux disease
   (C) bladder prolapse
   (D) gastroesophageal stenosis

2. A dissecting sponge that is a small roll of heavy cotton tape is a:

   (A) Kittner
   (B) peanut
   (C) tonsil
   (D) both A and B

3. Peanuts and dissecting sponges are generally:

   (A) used dry
   (B) moistened with saline
   (C) moistened with water
   (D) moistened with antibiotic solution

4. Intra-abdominally, lap pads are most often used:

   (A) dry
   (B) moistened with saline
   (C) moistened with water
   (D) moistened with glycine solution

5. Specimens may be passed off the sterile field by the scrub person on all of the following items EXCEPT:

   (A) sponge
   (B) towel
   (C) basin
   (D) paper

6. A catheter commonly used in a gastrostomy is a:

   (A) mushroom
   (B) Rehfuss
   (C) Cantor
   (D) Sengstaken–Blakemore

7. Before handing a Penrose drain to the surgeon:

   (A) place it on an Allis clamp
   (B) attach a safety pin to it
   (C) cut it to the desired length
   (D) moisten it in saline

8. The disposable intraluminal staple designed to hold two tubular structures together after resection is known as:

   (A) TA linear
   (B) LDS
   (C) EEA
   (D) GIA

9. Transduodenal sphincterotomy refers to the incision made into the ____ to relieve stenosis.

   (A) cardiac sphincter
   (B) ileocecal sphincter
   (C) sphincter of Oddi
   (D) pyloric sphincter

10. In surgery, cancer technique refers to:

    (A) the administration of an anticancer drug directly into the cancer site
    (B) the discarding of instruments coming in contact with tumor after each use
    (C) the use of radiation therapy at the time of surgery
    (D) the identification of the lesion

11. Why are gowns, gloves, drapes, and instruments changed following a breast biopsy and before incision for a mastectomy?

    (A) To respect individual surgeon's choice
    (B) To follow aseptic principles
    (C) To accommodate two separate incisions
    (D) To protect margins of healthy tissue from tumor cells

12. A postoperative complication attributed to glove powder entering a wound is:

    (A) granulomata
    (B) infection
    (C) inflammation
    (D) keloid formation

13. The correct procedure for sterile dressing application is:

    (A) apply dressing after drape removal
    (B) apply dressing before drape removal
    (C) apply Raytec sponges in thick layer
    (D) apply dressing in recovery room

14. When bowel technique for an intestinal procedure is utilized:

    (A) two Mayo stands are used
    (B) drapes and gloves do not need to be changed
    (C) contaminated instruments are discarded, and gloves are changed
    (D) a separate setup is used for the closure

15. The Sengstaken–Blakemore tube is used for:

    (A) esophageal hemorrhage
    (B) tonsillar hemorrhage
    (C) uterine hemorrhage
    (D) nasal hemorrhage

16. Dark blood in the operative field may indicate that the patient is:

    (A) hyperkalemic
    (B) hypovolemic
    (C) hypotensive
    (D) hypoxic

17. The term transduodenal sphincterotomy indicates surgery of the:

    (A) hepatic duct
    (B) proximal end of the common bile duct
    (C) distal end of the common bile duct
    (D) pyloric sphincter

18. McBurney is an incision used for:

    (A) appendectomy
    (B) cholecystectomy
    (C) herniorrhaphy
    (D) pilonidal cystectomy

19. The simplest abdominal incision offering good exposure to any part of the abdominal cavity is the:

    (A) right subcostal
    (B) Kocher's
    (C) midabdominal transverse
    (D) vertical midline

20. During an appendectomy, a purse-string suture is placed around the appendix stump to:

    (A) amputate the appendiceal base
    (B) retract the appendix
    (C) tie off the appendix
    (D) invert the stump of the appendix

21. Gastrointestinal technique is required in all of the following procedures EXCEPT:

(A) cholecystectomy
(B) low anterior colon resection
(C) appendectomy
(D) hemicolectomy

22. A hernia occurring in Hesselbach's triangle is called:

(A) indirect
(B) spigelian
(C) direct
(D) femoral

23. Pathologic enlargement of the male breast is called:

(A) subcutaneous adenoma
(B) gynecomastia
(C) hypoplasia
(D) cystic mastitis

24. Sutures placed in a wound to prevent wound evisceration are called:

(A) stent
(B) fixation
(C) retention
(D) traction

25. Surgical enlargement of the passage between the prepylorus of the stomach and the duodenum is a:

(A) duodenectomy
(B) pyloroplasty
(C) Billroth I
(D) Billroth II

26. A Whipple operation is surgically termed a:

(A) pancreatectomy
(B) pancreaticoduodenectomy
(C) pancreatic cyst marsupialization
(D) transduodenal sphincterotomy

27. A left subcostal incision indicates surgery of the:

(A) gallbladder
(B) pancreas
(C) spleen
(D) common bile duct

28. A lower oblique incision is a/an:

(A) Pfannenstiel
(B) inguinal
(C) paramedian
(D) midabdominal

29. The curved transverse incision used for pelvic surgery is:

(A) midabdominal transverse
(B) Poupart
(C) Pfannenstiel
(D) McVay

30. Which breast procedure removes the entire breast and axillary contents but preserves the pectoral muscles?

(A) Lumpectomy
(B) Wedge resection
(C) Modified radical mastectomy
(D) Radical mastectomy

31. The breast procedure performed to remove extensive benign disease is a/an:

(A) axillary node dissection
(B) simple mastectomy
(C) radical mastectomy
(D) modified radical mastectomy

32. What incision is indicated for an esophagogastrectomy?

(A) Left paramedian
(B) Upper vertical midline
(C) Thoracoabdominal
(D) Full midabdominal

33. In which incision could retention sutures be used?

    (A) Vertical midline
    (B) McBurney
    (C) Transverse
    (D) Thoracoabdominal

34. In which hernia is the blood supply of the trapped sac contents compromised and in danger of necrotizing?

    (A) Direct
    (B) Indirect
    (C) Strangulated
    (D) Reducible

35. In which hernia does the herniation protrude into the inguinal canal but NOT the cord?

    (A) Incisional
    (B) Femoral
    (C) Direct
    (D) Indirect

36. Which hernia leaves the abdominal cavity at the internal inguinal ring and passes with the cord structures down the inguinal canal?

    (A) Direct
    (B) Umbilical
    (C) Spigelian
    (D) Indirect

37. In a cholecystectomy, which structures are ligated and divided?

    (A) Cystic duct and cystic artery
    (B) Common bile duct and hepatic duct
    (C) Cystic duct and common bile duct
    (D) Hepatic duct and cystic artery

38. All of the following statements refer to pilonidal cyst surgery EXCEPT:

    (A) it is performed with an elliptical incision
    (B) the wound frequently heals by granulation
    (C) probes are required on setup
    (D) the cyst is removed, but the tract remains

39. An important consideration during a cholangiogram is to:

    (A) irrigate with distilled water
    (B) remove all air bubbles from the cholangiocath
    (C) flash sterilize the choledocoscope
    (D) dip the catheter in lubricating jelly

40. The intestinal layers, in order from inside to outside, are:

    (A) serosa, mucosa, musculature
    (B) mucosa, submucosa, serosa
    (C) serosa, musculature, mucosa
    (D) mucosa, serosa, musculature

41. A common postoperative patient complaint following a laparoscopic procedure is:

    (A) headache
    (B) diarrhea
    (C) gastric upset
    (D) shoulder pain

42. A subphrenic abscess occurs in the:

    (A) pancreas
    (B) spleen
    (C) lung
    (D) liver

43. Portal pressure measurement is indicated in:

    (A) liver transplant
    (B) splenectomy
    (C) hepatic resection
    (D) Whipple operation

44. Which organ is removed because of trauma, a blood condition, or as a staging procedure for malignancy?

    (A) Adrenals
    (B) Spleen
    (C) Liver
    (D) Pancreas

45. Following a hemorrhoidectomy:

    (A) dry dressing of 4 × 4's is packed in the rectum

    (B) petroleum gauze packing is placed in the anal canal

    (C) stent dressing is applied

    (D) Steri-Strip dressing is used

46. Which term is used when requiring intraoperative x-rays during a cholecystectomy?

    (A) Choledochoscopy

    (B) Cholelithotripsy

    (C) Choledochoduodenostomy

    (D) Cholangiogram

47. In a pilonidal cystectomy, the defect frequently is too large to close and requires use of a/an:

    (A) skin graft

    (B) traction suture

    (C) implant

    (D) packing and pressure dressing

48. The instrument most commonly used to grasp the mesoappendix during an appendectomy is a/an:

    (A) Kelly

    (B) Kocher

    (C) Babcock

    (D) Allis

49. Vaporization and coagulation of hemorrhoidal tissue can be accomplished with:

    (A) cautery, bipolar

    (B) cautery, monopolar

    (C) CO_2 laser

    (D) cryosurgery

50. An entire breast tumor/mass removal is termed:

    (A) needle biopsy

    (B) staging biopsy

    (C) excisional biopsy

    (D) incisional biopsy

51. Thrombosed vessels of the rectum are known surgically as:

    (A) polyps

    (B) hemorrhoids

    (C) fistulas

    (D) anorectal tumors

52. A procedure done to give the colon a rest and that is then reversed is:

    (A) temporary colectomy

    (B) temporary colostomy

    (C) abdominoperineal resection

    (D) McVay procedure

53. A device that may obviate the need for an abdominoperineal resection because a low anterior anastomosis can be performed is a/an:

    (A) end-to-end anastomosis (EEA)

    (B) GIA

    (C) TA 55

    (D) LDS

54. Advanced inflammation of the bowel could be conservatively treated with which procedure?

    (A) Temporary colostomy

    (B) Anterior resection

    (C) Hemicolectomy

    (D) Abdominal perineal resection

55. Blunt dissection of the gallbladder from the sulcus of the liver requires the use of a:

    (A) Metzenbaum

    (B) Kelly

    (C) tampon

    (D) peanut

56. Direct visualization of the common bile duct is accomplished with a:

    (A) cholangiocath

    (B) cholangiogram

    (C) choledochoscope

    (D) trocar

57. Fogarty biliary catheters are used to:

    (A) drain the gallbladder
    (B) drain the common bile duct
    (C) instill contrast media
    (D) facilitate stone removal

58. Bariatric surgery treats:

    (A) ulcers
    (B) obesity
    (C) thyroid disease
    (D) carcinoma of the pancreas

59. Which incision would require cutting through Scarpa's fascia?

    (A) Subcostal
    (B) Inguinal
    (C) Pfannenstiel
    (D) McBurney

60. A gastroplasty:

    (A) reduces stomach size
    (B) corrects gastric junction stenosis
    (C) releases adhesions
    (D) provides an avenue for hyperalimentation

61. Which item retracts the spermatic cord structure in herniorrhaphy?

    (A) Army–Navy retractor
    (B) Penrose drain
    (C) Green retractor
    (D) Silk suture

62. An irreducible hernia whose abdominal contents have become trapped in the extraabdominal sac is called a/an:

    (A) incarcerated hernia
    (B) sliding hernia
    (C) spigelian hernia
    (D) strangulated hernia

63. A palliative invasive procedure done to prevent malnutrition or starvation is known as:

    (A) Roux-en-Y
    (B) gastrotomy
    (C) gastrostomy
    (D) gastrojejunostomy

64. The use of noninvasive high-energy shock waves to pulverize gallstones into small fragments for easy passage through the common bile duct and out of the body is called:

    (A) choledochoscopy
    (B) cholelithotripsy
    (C) choledochostomy
    (D) choledochotomy

65. Intraoperative cholangiograms can be performed either through open abdominal or laparoscopic procedures using administration of a contrast medium directly into the common bile duct through a:

    (A) cystocath
    (B) cholangiocath
    (C) T-tube
    (D) red rubber catheter

66. Intra-abdominal pressure during the instillation of CO_2 for creation of pneumoperitoneum is 10–15 mm Hg. A pressure reading higher than this may indicate that the needle may be:

    (A) buried in fatty tissue
    (B) buried in the omentum
    (C) in a lumen of intestines
    (D) all of the above

67. The proper method of removing the gallbladder specimen after complete dissection and irrigation of the operative site in a laparoscopic cholecystectomy is to:

    (A) utilize an Endobag
    (B) pull gallbladder through the largest port
    (C) decompress the gallbladder by suctioning bile before removal
    (D) all of the above

68. During a laparoscopic cholecystectomy, the surgeon generally stands:

    (A) at the right side of the patient
    (B) at the bottom of the patient's table
    (C) at the left side of the patient
    (D) in front of the first assistant

69. Gastrointestinal decompression during a general surgical procedure can be effected by the use of a:

    (A) Levine tube
    (B) Miller–Abbott tube
    (C) Vari-Dyne
    (D) Both A and B

70. A selected alternative to a conventional ileostomy that denies spontaneous stool exiting from the stoma and requires catheterization of the stoma daily to evacuate the contents is a/an:

    (A) cecostomy
    (B) ileoanal pull-through
    (C) ileal conduit
    (D) Kock pouch

71. When both direct and indirect hernias occur in the same inguinal area, the defect is termed:

    (A) sliding
    (B) pantaloon
    (C) femoral
    (D) spigelian

72. An inguinal hernia containing a Meckel's diverticulum is called a:

    (A) Richter
    (B) Littre
    (C) Maydl
    (D) spigelian

73. Drainage of an incision following a simple or modified radical mastectomy is accomplished by a:

    (A) Penrose
    (B) sump
    (C) closed-wound drainage
    (D) cigarette drain

74. During laparoscopic cholecystectomy, the camera operator usually stands

    (A) across from the surgeon
    (B) to the right of the surgeon
    (C) to the right of the first assistant
    (D) behind the Mayo stand

75. The maximum pressure allowed to prevent the possible intraoperative complications of bradycardia, blood pressure changes, or potential gas emboli during a laparoscopic procedure is:

    (A) 8 mm Hg
    (B) 10 mm Hg
    (C) 15 mm Hg
    (D) 20 mm Hg

76. Place tissue layers of the abdominal wall in their correct order from the outside in: (1) fascia, (2) skin, (3) peritoneum, (4) subcutaneous, (5) muscle.

    (A) 1, 2, 3, 4, 5
    (B) 2, 3, 4, 5, 1
    (C) 2, 4, 1, 5, 3
    (D) 3, 5, 1, 4, 2

77. What is the technique used on a laparoscopic direct inguinal hernia repair where the peritoneal space is inflated with a balloon dissector?

    (A) TEP (total extraperitoneal)
    (B) Hasson
    (C) TAPP (transabdominal preperitoneal laparoscopy)
    (D) Open

78. When viscera have protruded outside of the body, this condition is called:

    (A) dehiscence
    (B) evisceration
    (C) ischemia
    (D) fistula

79. The position that facilitates a symmetrical outcome during a mastopexy is:

    (A) supine
    (B) dorsal recumbent
    (C) Fowler's
    (D) lateral

80. Which breast reconstruction procedure reconstructs the breast without the use of implants?

    (A) TRAM
    (B) TEP
    (C) PPE
    (D) Augmentation

81. The procedure where a hooked wire is inserted under fluoroscopy into the suspicious tissue is called:

    (A) a hook wire
    (B) wire localization
    (C) staging
    (D) frozen section

82. What procedure involves injection of dye and/or a radioactive material into the breast mass to track the lymph nodes?

    (A) Stereotaxis
    (B) Excisional biopsy
    (C) Staging
    (D) Sentinel node biopsy

83. What is the correct order of the outermost to the innermost tissue layers that make up the wall of the stomach: (1) serosa, (2) mucosa, (3) muscularis, (4) submucosa?

    (A) 1, 2, 3, 4
    (B) 4, 3, 2, 1
    (C) 3, 2, 1, 4
    (D) 2, 3, 4, 1

84. The pancreatic duct (the duct of Wirsung) and the common bile duct from the liver drain their contents into which section of the intestine?

    (A) Jejunum
    (B) Ileum
    (C) Cecum
    (D) Duodenum

85. A sheet of vascular tissue that supplies blood and lymph to the lower section of the small intestines is:

    (A) omentum
    (B) stoma
    (C) mesentery
    (D) cecum

86. Arrange the large intestine in correct order from proximal to distal: (1) rectum, (2) transverse colon, (3) ascending, (4) sigmoid, (5) descending.

    (A) 1, 2, 3, 4, 5
    (B) 3, 2, 5, 4, 1
    (C) 2, 3, 4, 1, 5
    (D) 2, 3, 4, 5, 1

87. A condition that causes bowel obstruction when one section of intestine telescopes over another and that is most common in children is:

    (A) evisceration
    (B) Crohn's disease
    (C) gastroschisis
    (D) intussusceptions

88. What kind of tube is used to decompress the stomach or as a means of feeding the patient?

(A) Nasogastric tube
(B) Esophageal tube
(C) Gastrostomy tube
(D) T-tube

89. During a laparotomy, the surgeon packs the abdominal contents away from the diseased area with:

(A) Raytec 4 × 4's
(B) moist laps
(C) Gelfoam and thrombin
(D) Dry laps

90. During a laparotomy procedure, the duties of the STSR include:

(A) keep 4 × 4's and needles on the back table
(B) keep the ESU free of debris and in its holster
(C) keep surgical field free of instruments not in use
(D) all of the above

91. An esophageal diverticulum is also known as:

(A) hiatal hernia
(B) GERD
(C) Hirschsprung's disease
(D) Zenker's diverticulum

92. In what procedure is a portion of the stomach removed with an anastomosis created between the stomach and a jejunum?

(A) Billroth I
(B) Billroth II
(C) Jejunectomy
(D) Gastrectomy

93. The procedure traditionally performed to treat gastric ulcers and gastric carcinoma and that is currently used to treat morbid obesity is:

(A) Roux-en-Y
(B) band gastroplasty
(C) Billroth I
(D) none of the above

94. Morbid obesity is defined as a BMI (body mass index) greater than:

(A) 30
(B) 40
(C) 10
(D) 25

95. A common staple gun used to transect the stomach is _____, and the _____ gun is used to transect and anastomose the jejunum during a Billroth II procedure.

(A) EEA, LDS
(B) TA, GIA
(C) Hemaclip, GIA
(D) Purse-string, LDS

96. The portion of the small intestine where a Meckel's diverticulum arises is the:

(A) duodenum
(B) jejunum
(C) pylorus
(D) distal ileum

97. Twisting of the bowel is known as:

(A) strangulation
(B) intussusception
(C) volvulus
(D) paralytic ileus

98. The procedure to treat venous distention causing pain, bleeding, and a prolapse outside the anal canal is known as:

(A) anorectal fistulectomy
(B) pilonidal cystectomy
(C) hemorrhoidectomy
(D) proctoscopy

99. The pancreatic duct is also known as:

(A) ampulla of Vater
(B) duct of Wirsung
(C) sphincter of Oddi
(D) circle of Willis

100. Which tube may be inserted to produce a continuous postoperative drainage of the common bile duct?

(A) Nasogastric tube
(B) Levine tube
(C) T-tube
(D) Foley

101. A choledochoduodenostomy is an anastomosis between the:

(A) pancreas and common bile duct
(B) common bile duct and duodenum
(C) gallbladder and duodenum
(D) both B and C

102. A Whipple procedure consists of removal of:

(A) pancreas, duodenum, jejunum, stomach, and common bile duct
(B) head of pancreas, duodenum, portion of jejunum, gallbladder, distal stomach, cystic duct, and distal portion of common bile duct
(C) duodenum, jejunum, distal stomach, and gallbladder
(D) head of pancreas, portion of liver, gallbladder, and common bile duct

103. The passageway for foods and liquids into the digestive system and for air into the respiratory system is the:

(A) trachea
(B) larynx
(C) epiglottis
(D) pharynx

104. Which of the abdominal muscles originates at the pubic bone and ends in the ribs?

(A) Rectus abdominis
(B) Transversus abdominis
(C) External oblique
(D) Internal oblique

105. The spleen filters:

(A) antibodies
(B) tissue fluid
(C) lymph
(D) blood

106. The spleen is located:

(A) in the left hypochondriac region
(B) behind the liver
(C) behind the left kidney
(D) behind the right kidney

107. All of the following are parts of the lymphatic system EXCEPT the:

(A) thyroid
(B) tonsils
(C) spleen
(D) thymus

108. The S-shaped bend in the lower colon is called the:

(A) hepatic flexure
(B) splenic flexure
(C) rectum
(D) sigmoid

109. The reabsorption of water and electrolytes is the main function of the:

(A) sigmoid colon
(B) large intestine
(C) small intestine
(D) liver

110. The terminal portion of the large intestine is the:

   (A) sigmoid
   (B) rectum
   (C) anus
   (D) anal canal

111. Which structure lies retroperitoneally?

   (A) Sigmoid colon
   (B) Spleen
   (C) Liver
   (D) Kidney

112. The first portion of the large intestine is the:

   (A) sigmoid
   (B) cecum
   (C) colon
   (D) ileum

113. The appendix is attached to the:

   (A) ascending colon
   (B) transverse colon
   (C) cecum
   (D) descending colon

114. The primary function of the gallbladder is:

   (A) storage of bile
   (B) production of bile
   (C) digestion of fats
   (D) drainage of the liver

115. When the gallbladder contracts, bile is ejected into the:

   (A) liver
   (B) duodenum
   (C) jejunum
   (D) pancreas

116. The area in the duodenum where the common bile duct and the pancreatic duct empty is called:

   (A) the duct of Santorini
   (B) the ampulla of Vater
   (C) Wirsung duct
   (D) the islet of Langerhans

117. Which structure is also known as the "fatty apron"?

   (A) Greater omentum
   (B) Lesser omentum
   (C) Mesentery
   (D) Falciform ligament

118. The common bile duct is the union of the:

   (A) cystic duct and cystic artery
   (B) cystic duct and hepatic duct
   (C) cystic artery and hepatic duct
   (D) hepatic vein and cystic duct

119. The yellow tinge in the skin symptomatic of obstructive jaundice is caused by the accumulation of what substance in the blood and tissue?

   (A) Cholesterol
   (B) Bile salts
   (C) Enzymes
   (D) Bilirubin

120. The head of the pancreas is located:

   (A) in the curve of the duodenum
   (B) by the spleen
   (C) on the undersurface of the liver
   (D) in the curve of the descending colon

121. The sphincter at the junction of the small and large intestines is the:

   (A) sphincter of Oddi
   (B) ileocecal sphincter
   (C) pyloric sphincter
   (D) duodenal sphincter

122. The portion of the small intestine that receives secretions from the pancreas and the liver is the:

(A) ileum
(B) jejunum
(C) duodenum
(D) pylorus

123. The region of the stomach that connects to the duodenum is the:

(A) fundus
(B) body
(C) pylorus
(D) cardia

124. The mesentery is:

(A) a double-layered peritoneal structure shaped like a fan
(B) a word synonymous with "fatty apron"
(C) the membrane covering the surface of most abdominal organs
(D) a structure that supports the sigmoid colon

125. The large central portion of the stomach is called the:

(A) pylorus
(B) body
(C) fundus
(D) cardia

126. The muscle serving as a valve to prevent regurgitation of food from the intestine back into the stomach is known as the:

(A) sphincter of Oddi
(B) ileocecal sphincter
(C) cardiac sphincter
(D) pyloric sphincter

127. The digestive passageway that begins at the pharynx and terminates in the stomach is the:

(A) larynx
(B) trachea
(C) windpipe
(D) esophagus

128. The point at which the esophagus penetrates the diaphragm is called the:

(A) hiatus
(B) meatus
(C) sphincter
(D) fundus

129. The liver has:

(A) two lobes
(B) three lobes
(C) four lobes
(D) five lobes

130. The cell saver is contraindicated for:

(A) the cancer patient in whom the tumor is resected en bloc
(B) if Avitene is used
(C) orthopedic procedures
(D) diabetic patients

131. An enteroscopy is the scoping of the:

(A) large intestine
(B) small intestine
(C) sigmoid
(D) stomach

132. Chronic gastroesophageal reflux disease can cause:

(A) dysphasia
(B) aspiration
(C) Barrett's esophagus
(D) all of the above

133. Cellular changes of the mucosal lining of the distal esophagus that are known to be a precursor for esophageal cancer are termed:

(A) Meckel's diverticulum
(B) Zenker's diverticulum
(C) Barrett's esophagus
(D) GERD

134. The ligament of Treitz supports the:

(A) ascending colon and transverse colon

(B) duodenum and jejunum

(C) transverse colon and descending colon

(D) splenic flexure and hepatic flexure

135. A hiatal hernia is also termed:

(A) diaphragmatic

(B) pantaloon

(C) Meckel's

(D) direct

136. The procedure performed for an esophageal diaphragmatic hernia is termed:

(A) TAPP

(B) laparoscopic Nissen fundoplication

(C) McVay

(D) Bassini

137. A balloon catheter that is inserted into the esophagus and into the stomach and provides pressure to control bleeding from esophageal varices is termed:

(A) Bougie

(B) Bakes

(C) Sengstaken–Blakemore

(D) Hank

138. What procedure is performed to reduce gastric secretions?

(A) Total gastrectomy

(B) Percutaneous endoscopic gastrostomy

(C) Both A and B

(D) Vagotomy

139. All are true regarding a pyloromyotomy EXCEPT:

(A) it is more common in infants and the symptoms are projectile vomiting

(B) it is performed for treatment of peptic ulcers and removal of bands around the pyloric ring and relieves spasms and permits emptying of the stomach

(C) it establishes a permanent connection between the anterior and posterior portion of the stomach and the jejunum without removing any portion of the GI tract

(D) special equipment includes a nasogastric (NG) tube

140. All are true regarding placement of a PEG tube EXCEPT:

(A) a PEG tube uses a flexible gastroscope for placement through the abdominal wall

(B) it is used for internal feedings

(C) moderate sedation or local is used

(D) it can be performed in the endoscopy suite, in the operating room, or at the patient's bedside

141. Adhesions are caused by all EXCEPT:

(A) radiation

(B) previous surgeries

(C) foreign body reaction

(D) too much irrigation

142. Billroth I is a resection of the diseased portion of the:

(A) stomach with anastomosis between the stomach and duodenum

(B) stomach with anastomosis between the stomach and jejunum

(C) proximal duodenum with anastomosis between distal duodenum and jejunum

(D) stomach and distal esophagus

143. The common hepatic duct becomes the common bile duct when the common hepatic duct joins the:

    (A) hepatic artery
    (B) cystic artery
    (C) cystic duct
    (D) hepatic vein

144. The retractor used to lift the edge of the liver is:

    (A) Harrington
    (B) Senn
    (C) sweetheart
    (D) Both A and C

145. The instrument used to extend the CBD incision is the _____. _____ is used to remove stones from the CBD. _____ is used to dilate the common bile duct. And _____ is used to drain the CBD.

    (A) Potts, Randal, Bakes, T-tube
    (B) Potts, Bakes, Randal, T-tube
    (C) Metz, Pennington, Hagar, Red Robinson
    (D) Metz, Bakes, van Buren, T-tube

146. The procedure performed to drain the common bile duct is called a:

    (A) choledochotomy
    (B) cholecystectomy
    (C) choledochoduodenotomy
    (D) none of the above

147. All are true regarding bariatric surgery EXCEPT:

    (A) it is performed for obesity
    (B) the procedure reduces the size of the stomach
    (C) it is also called a lap band
    (D) it is performed for BMI below 25

148. All are true regarding the liver EXCEPT:

    (A) it is located in the left upper quadrant
    (B) it produces bile
    (C) it is encased by Glisson's capsule
    (D) right and left lobes are divided by falciform

149. What instrument is used to obtain a liver biopsy?

    (A) Silverman needle
    (B) Tru-Cut needle
    (C) Both A and B
    (D) Blunt needle

150. Hodgkin's disease and sickle cell disease patients may require:

    (A) hepatectomy
    (B) splenectomy
    (C) pancreatectomy
    (D) cholecystectomy

151. Which hernia occurs between the muscle layers of the abdomen and is difficult to diagnose?

    (A) Richter
    (B) Maydl
    (C) Bassini
    (D) Spigelian

152. Which type of hernia involves the stomach protruding through the diaphragm?

    (A) Hiatal
    (B) Diaphragmatic
    (C) Both A and B
    (D) Spigelian

153. The mesh used to repair a hernia is made of:

    (A) Gore-Tex
    (B) Prolene
    (C) Teflon
    (D) All of the above

154. When doing a cut-down procedure for laparoscopic surgery, which type of trocar and cannula system is used?

    (A) TEP
    (B) TAPP
    (C) Hasson
    (D) None of the above

155. Which of the following is the most proximal portion of the GI tract?

   (A) Esophagus
   (B) Stomach
   (C) Ileum
   (D) Rectum

156. Which of the following blood vessels supplies blood to the proximal large bowel?

   (A) Superior mesenteric artery
   (B) Middle colic artery
   (C) Celiac artery
   (D) Inferior mesenteric artery

157. Which of the following tasks can the circulator and the STSR both perform during the perioperative period?

   (A) Open sterile items
   (B) Assist with the surgical specimen
   (C) Maintain the sterile field
   (D) Both A and B

158. All are variations of the transverse incision EXCEPT:

   (A) Maylard
   (B) Cherney
   (C) Pfannenstiel
   (D) oblique

159. Which organ is considered to have the largest mass of lymphatic tissue?

   (A) Thyroid gland
   (B) Liver
   (C) Spleen
   (D) Gallbladder

160. The triangle of Calot, also known as the cystohepatic triangle, is associated with which body system?

   (A) Respiratory
   (B) Biliary
   (C) Lymphatic
   (D) Reproductive

161. A patient is diagnosed with portal hypertension. Common causes of this disease can include:

   (A) Blockage of the portal vein
   (B) Hepatitis
   (C) Cirrhosis of the liver
   (D) All of the above

162. A T-tube placed in the CBD following laparoscopic cholecystectomy would exit through:

   (A) an umbilical incision
   (B) a right subcostal incision
   (C) a 5-mm port site
   (D) any of the above

163. Alcohol abuse is a precursor to:

   (A) cholecystitis
   (B) Zenker's diverticulum
   (C) cirrhosis
   (D) rectal cancer

164. What is the fibrous covering of the liver?

   (A) Glisson's
   (B) Medulla
   (C) Galea
   (D) Sella turcica

165. What procedure is commonly performed with a hemorrhoidectomy?

   (A) Sigmoidoscopy
   (B) Proctoscopy
   (C) Anoscopy
   (D) All of the above

166. It is important to prevent damage to the long thoracic nerve during which surgical procedure?

   (A) Direct hernia repair
   (B) Radical mastectomy
   (C) Axillary lymph node dissection
   (D) Both B and C

Answers and Explanations

1. **(B)** A Nissen fundoplication is a procedure that prevents reflux of gastric juices back into the esophagus. The three most frequently performed procedures are Nissen, Hill, and Belsy Mark IV.

2. **(D)** Kittner and peanuts are dissecting sponges that are small rolls of heavy cotton tape that are held in forceps/clamps.

3. **(B)** Peanuts are moistened with saline.

4. **(B)** Normal saline is usually used to moisten sponges because it is an isotonic solution.

5. **(A)** Specimen may be passed from the field in a basin, on a piece of paper wrapper, or on a towel. Never place specimen on a sponge that may leave the operating room (OR) and disrupt the sponge count.

6. **(A)** Mushroom, Malecot, and Foley catheters are frequently used in the anterior gastric wall and are held in place by a purse-string suture.

7. **(D)** Moisten the drain in saline before handing it to the surgeon.

8. **(C)** The end-to-end anastomosis (EEA) stapler is designed to hold two tubular structures, to join the structures with staples, and to cut the structures internally so proper lumen is provided.

9. **(C)** The sphincter of Oddi is located at the junction of the common bile duct, main pancreatic duct, and the duodenum. It may become scarred because of biliary obstruction, stones, or disease. Transecting the duodenum at the site of the sphincter allows the surgeon to reduce the stenosis and encourage the flow of bile and pancreatic juices into the gastrointestinal system.

10. **(B)** To minimize the risk of disseminating malignant tumor cells outside the operative area, some surgeons follow a special technique in which instruments in contact with tumor cells are discarded after use.

11. **(D)** Gown, gloves, drapes, and instruments are changed. The tumor is incised during biopsy for diagnosis. However, margins of healthy tissue surrounding a radical resection must not be inoculated with tumor cells.

12. **(A)** The postoperative complication of powder granulomata can result from powder that is not properly removed from gloves before surgery. This can be avoided by rinsing gloves before approaching the operative site.

13. **(B)** Sterile dressings should be applied before drapes are removed to reduce risk of the incision being touched by contaminated hands or objects.

14. **(C)** In bowel technique, the contaminated instruments are discarded in a single basin. Gloves (and possibly gowns) are changed by the surgical team, and the incisional area is redraped with clean towels.

15. **(A)** A Sengstaken–Blakemore tube is used to control esophageal hemorrhage. Pressure is exerted on the cardiac portion of the stomach and against bleeding esophageal varices by a double balloon tamponade.

16. **(D)** Hypoxia is lack of adequate amounts of oxygen; if prolonged, it can result in cardiac

arrhythmia or irreversible brain, liver, kidney, and heart damage. The treatment is immediate adequate oxygen intake to stimulate the medullary centers and prevent respiratory system failure. Dark blood on the operative field is a symptom of hypoxia.

17. **(C)** The sphincter of Oddi is the smooth muscle where the CBD and the pancreatic duct meet and enter the duodenum. A transduodenal sphincterotomy is performed on the lower end of the CBD to remove impacted stones, spasms, or a stricture of the CBD and pancreatic ducts.

18. **(A)** The McBurney muscle-splitting incision is used for appendix removal. It is an 8-cm oblique incision that begins well below the umbilicus, goes through McBurney's point, and extends upward toward the right flank.

19. **(D)** The vertical midline is the simplest abdominal incision to perform. It is an excellent primary incision offering good exposure to any part of the abdominal cavity.

20. **(D)** A purse-string is a continuous suture placed around the lumen of the appendiceal stump to invert it. It is tightened, drawstring fashion, to close the lumen.

21. **(A)** Whenever a portion of the gastrointestinal tract is entered, gastrointestinal technique must be carried out. Any instrument used after the lumen of the stomach or intestines has been entered cannot be used after it is closed. A cholecystectomy does not enter the gastrointestinal tract. An appendectomy, hemicolectomy, and an anterior resection of the sigmoid all require bowel technique.

22. **(C)** Hesselbach's triangle is formed by the boundaries of the deep epigastric vessels laterally, the inguinal ligament inferiorly, and the rectus abdominis muscle medially. Hernias occurring here are direct.

23. **(B)** Gynecomastia is a relatively common pathologic lesion that consists of bilateral or unilateral enlargement of the male breast.

Surgery consists of removal of all subareolar fibroglandular tissue and surgical reconstruction of the resultant defect.

24. **(C)** Retention sutures may be used as a precautionary measure to prevent wound disruption and possible evisceration of the wound.

25. **(B)** Pyloroplasty is the formation of a larger passage between the pylorus of the stomach and the duodenum. It may include the removal of a peptic ulcer if one is present.

26. **(B)** A Whipple operation or pancreaticoduodenectomy is a radical surgical excision of the head of the pancreas, the entire duodenum, a portion of the jejunum, the distal third of the stomach, and the lower half of the common bile duct. There is then reestablishment of continuity of the biliary, pancreatic, and gastrointestinal systems. This is done for carcinoma of the head of the pancreas and is a hazardous procedure.

27. **(C)** A left subcostal incision is generally used for spleen surgery. The right subcostal is used for gallbladder, common bile duct, and pancreatic surgery.

28. **(B)** A lower oblique incision, either right or left, is an inguinal incision. This incision gives access to the inguinal canal and cord structures.

29. **(C)** The Pfannenstiel incision is frequently used for pelvic surgery. It is a curved transverse incision across the lower abdomen, 1.5 in above the symphysis pubis. It provides a strong closure.

30. **(C)** A modified radical mastectomy involves removal of the involved breast and all three levels of axillary contents. The underlying pectoral muscles are not removed.

31. **(B)** Simple mastectomy is removal of the entire breast without lymph node dissection, performed to remove extensive benign disease or a confined malignancy.

32. **(C)** The diseased portion of the esophagus and stomach are removed through a left thoracoabdominal incision, including a resection of the seventh, eighth, or ninth ribs. Here, an anastomosis is accomplished between the disease-free ends of the stomach and the esophagus.

33. **(A)** Retention or tension sutures may be used in a vertical midline incision to ensure strength of closure and support.

34. **(C)** The great danger of an incarcerated hernia is that it may become strangulated—the blood supply of the trapped sac contents becomes compromised, and eventually the sac contents necrose.

35. **(C)** Direct hernias protrude into the inguinal canal but not into the cord.

36. **(D)** Indirect hernias leave the abdominal cavity at the internal ring and pass with the cord structures down the inguinal canal; thus, the indirect hernia sac may be found in the scrotum.

37. **(A)** In cholecystectomy, there is exposure of the neck of the gallbladder, the cystic duct, and the cystic artery. The cystic artery and duct are doubly ligated and divided, facilitating gallbladder removal.

38. **(D)** In a pilonidal cystectomy, the cyst and sinus tract must be completely removed to prevent recurrence.

39. **(B)** A cholangiocatheter is prepared using a 20-cc syringe of saline and a 20-cc syringe of contrast medium using a stopcock and Luer-Lok ports. All air bubbles are removed because they may be misinterpreted as gallstones on x-ray. The cholangiocath is irrigated with saline before and during the catheter insertion into the cystic duct and CBD.

40. **(B)** The layers of the large intestine from inside to outside are mucosa, submucosa, and serosa. Mucosa suture closure is most frequently absorbable suture, while the serosa layer is closed with nonabsorbable silk.

41. **(D)** Postoperative shoulder pain may follow use of pneumoperitoneum. This is referred pain caused by pressure on the diaphragm, which is somewhat displaced by CO_2 during the procedure.

42. **(D)** A subphrenic abscess is a liver abscess that may require incision and drainage.

43. **(C)** For hepatic resection, supplies and equipment should be available for hypothermia, electrosurgery, measurement of portal pressure, thoracotomy drainage, and replacement of blood loss.

44. **(B)** Splenectomy is removal of the spleen, usually performed for trauma to the spleen, for specific conditions of the blood such as hemolytic jaundice or splenic anemia, or for tumors, cysts, or splenomegaly.

45. **(B)** Petroleum gauze packing is placed in the anal canal. A dressing and a T-binder are applied.

46. **(D)** An intraoperative cholangiogram is usually performed in conjunction with cholecystectomy to visualize the common bile duct and the hepatic ductal branches and to assess patency of the common bile duct.

47. **(D)** The defect resulting from recurrences may become too large for primary closure. In this case, the wound is left opened to heal by granulation. The wound is packed, and a pressure dressing is applied.

48. **(C)** After the abdomen is opened through a McBurney's incision, the mesoappendix is grasped with a Babcock and the appendix is gently dissected away from the cecum.

49. **(C)** The CO_2 laser may be used for vaporization and coagulation of hemorrhoidal tissue.

50. **(C)** In an excisional biopsy, the entire tumor mass is excised. In a needle biopsy, a plug of tissue is removed. In an incisional biopsy, a portion of the mass is excised.

51. **(B)** Varicosities of veins in the anus and rectum are called hemorrhoids. They may occur externally or internally. They must be ligated and ligatured after the sphincter of the anus is dilated.

52. **(B)** A temporary colostomy is performed to decompress the bowel or give the bowel a rest and time to heal after inflammation.

53. **(A)** A low colon lesion may require an abdominoperineal resection and colostomy. The EEA (end-to-end anastomosis) is a stapling device that allows a very low anastomosis and thus avoids a colostomy.

54. **(A)** Advanced inflammation of the colon is frequently treated with a temporary colostomy, often done to decompress the bowel or give the bowel a rest.

55. **(D)** Blunt dissection, using a Kittner or peanut, is employed when removing the gallbladder from the infundibulum up to the fundal region.

56. **(C)** Choledochoscopy is direct visualization of the common bile duct by means of an instrument (choledochoscope) introduced into the common bile duct. This takes the place of cholangiography in difficult cases.

57. **(D)** A Fogarty-type balloon-tipped catheter is used to facilitate the removal of small stones and debris as well as to demonstrate patency of the common bile duct through the duodenum.

58. **(B)** Morbid obesity and bariatric surgery have been developed for people who weigh more than 100 lb over ideal weight.

59. **(B)** The groin area contains the superficial group of muscles, the obliques, and Scarpa's fascia. An inguinal herniorrhaphy requires incision of Scarpa's fascia.

60. **(A)** A gastroplasty treats obesity by resecting the stomach to reduce its capacity.

61. **(B)** A Penrose drain is used to retract the spermatic cord structures for better exposure.

62. **(A)** An irreducible hernia is one in which the contents of the hernia sac are trapped in the extra-abdominal sac and is called incarcerated.

63. **(C)** Gastrostomy is a palliative procedure performed to prevent malnutrition or starvation. These may be caused by a lesion or stricture situated in the esophagus or cardia of the stomach.

64. **(B)** Cholelithotripsy is a noninvasive procedure done generally under intravenous (IV) sedation using spark-gap shockwaves generated by an electrode and passed on through the fluid medium into the body focused at the stone with an ultrasound probe until they reach the stone.

65. **(B)** T-tubes are used to stent a common bile duct after common duct exploration. Red rubber catheters can be used to irrigate postoperatively. Cholangiocaths are plastic catheters used to insert dye into the common bile duct before x-ray or fluoroscopy.

66. **(D)** Gas flow is initiated at 1–2 L/min. The intra-abdominal pressure is normally in the 10–14 mm Hg range and is used as an indicator for proper Veress needle placement. If the gauge indicates a higher pressure, the needle may be in a closed space such as fat, buried in omentum, or in a lumen of intestines.

67. **(D)** Facilitating removal of the gallbladder can be achieved by using a trocar and suction to decompress the gallbladder, expanding the largest port with a long Kelly clamp, and using an endobag.

68. **(C)** The surgeon performing the laparoscopic procedure stands at the patient's left, while his or her assistant stands at the patient's right.

69. **(D)** Both the Levine tube and the Miller–Abbott tube effect gastrointestinal decompression. The Levine tube is placed through the nasal passageway into the stomach, while the Miller–Abbott tube reaches into the small intestines.

70. **(D)** An alternative to a conventional ileostomy for selected patients is the Kock pouch, or continent ileostomy. The internal pouch is constructed of small intestine with an outlet to the skin. When it is functioning properly, no stool spontaneously exits from the stoma. A catheter is inserted several times a day to evacuate the contents.

71. **(B)** When both direct and indirect hernias are present in the same patient, the defect is called a pantaloon hernia after the French word for pants, which the situation suggests.

72. **(B)** An inguinal hernia containing Meckel's diverticulum is called a Littre hernia; one containing two loops of bowel is called a Maydl hernia. A special type of strangulated hernia is a Richter hernia. A spigelian hernia is usually located as a peritoneal sac that is between the different muscle layers of the abdominal wall.

73. **(C)** Following meticulous hemostasis of the operative site, the wound is irrigated with normal saline, and a closed wound drainage system (Jackson–Pratt drain) is inserted through a stab wound and secured to the skin with nonabsorbable suture and a cutting needle.

74. **(C)** The camera operator stands to the right of the first assistant, across from the scrub person. He or she must closely follow the surgeon's actions.

75. **(C)** During the procedure, the perioperative nurse should set the insufflation unit to a maximum pressure of 15 mm Hg. When intraabdominal pressure reaches 15 mm Hg, the flow will stop. Pressure higher than 15 mm Hg may result in bradycardia or a change in blood pressure or may force gas emboli into an exposed blood vessel during the procedure.

76. **(C)** The correct order from the outside in is the skin, subcutaneous tissue, fascia, muscle, and peritoneum.

77. **(A)** TEP approach to the peritoneal space is when a balloon dissector is used to expand tissue planes.

78. **(B)** Evisceration is when the viscera have protruded outside of the body. Dehiscence is separation of wound edges after closure. Ischemia is poor blood supply to body tissue or organs, and a fistula is an abnormal connection between two body parts caused by infection, injury, and/or surgery.

79. **(C)** The Fowler's position assists the physician with assuring symmetrical breasts.

80. **(A)** A transverse rectus abdominus myocutaneous (TRAM) flap is a tissue flap containing skin, subcutaneous, and muscle and is raised from the lower abdomen and transferred to the mastectomy site.

81. **(B)** A wire localization is a procedure where a hooked wire is inserted under fluoroscopy into the tissue suspected of being cancerous. The tissue surrounding the hook wire is removed.

82. **(D)** During a sentinel node biopsy, both materials, the dye and the gamma ray emission, may be used to track the lymph nodes. The technetium-99 is tracked with a device similar to a Geiger counter (gamma ray–detecting probe).

83. **(A)** The correct order from outermost to innermost layers of the stomach are the serosa, mucosa, muscularis, and submucosa.

84. **(D)** The duodenum is the first section of the small intestines, and the pancreatic and common bile ducts drain here from the liver.

85. **(C)** The sections of the duodenum and jejunum are suspended from the abdominal wall by a sheet of vascular tissue known as the mesentery.

86. **(B)** The large intestine from proximal to distal is ascending, transverse, descending, sigmoid, and rectum.

87. **(D)** Intussusception is a condition that causes bowl obstruction because one section of intestine telescopes another.

88. **(A)** A nasogastric tube is used to decompress the stomach or as a means of feeding the patient.

89. **(B)** Moist lap pads are used to pack the abdominal contents away from the diseased area of the bowel.

90. **(D)** All of the above are duties of the STSR.

91. **(D)** An esophageal diverticulum, sometimes called Zenker's diverticulum, is mucosa and submucosa that have herniated through the cricoid pharyngeal muscles. Food particles become temporarily trapped and cause problems.

92. **(B)** In a Billroth II, a portion of the stomach is removed and an anastomosis is created between the stomach and the jejunum.

93. **(A)** A Roux-en-Y is done to bypass the distal stomach and reestablish continuity from the stomach to the jejunum. A large portion of the stomach is bypassed and a gastric pouch is created.

94. **(B)** When the BMI is at least 40, this condition is known as morbid obesity. BMI is calculated using a specific formula of weight and height.

95. **(B)** The TA is used to staple the stomach, and the GIA is used to transect and anastomose the jejunum during the Billroth II.

96. **(D)** A Meckel's diverticulum occurs at the distal ileum. It arises from a congenital remnant of the umbilical duct.

97. **(C)** Twisting of the bowel is known as a volvulus.

98. **(C)** Hemorrhoids are defined as venous distention causing pain, bleeding, and a prolapse outside the anal canal.

99. **(B)** The duct of Wirsung is the central duct of the pancreas. It communicates with the duodenum at the ampulla of Vater, a location shared with the common bile duct.

100. **(C)** A T-tube is inserted to produce continuous drainage of bile following a common duct exploration.

101. **(B)** A choledochoduodenostomy is an anastomosis between the common bile duct and the duodenum.

102. **(B)** A Whipple involves removal of the head of the pancreas, duodenum, portion of jejunum, distal stomach, and the distal portion of the common bile duct.

103. **(D)** The muscular pharynx serves as a passageway for food and liquids into the digestive tract. It is also the path for air into the respiratory system. The throat runs from the nares and runs partway down the neck, where it opens into the esophagus (posterior) and the larynx (anterior).

104. **(A)** On the anterior portion of the abdominal wall, the rectus abdominis forms a strap-like mass of muscle. It runs from the pubic bone at the floor of the abdominal cavity straight up to the xiphoid process of the sternum and the lower margins of the rib cage.

105. **(D)** The spleen is an organ containing lymphoid tissue designed to filter blood. It is frequently damaged in abdominal trauma, causing it to rupture. This causes severe hemorrhage, which requires prompt splenectomy.

106. **(A)** The spleen is located in the upper left hypochondriac region of the abdomen and is normally protected by the rib cage. It is between the fundus of the stomach and the diaphragm.

107. **(A)** Lymph, lymph vessels, lymph nodes, tonsils, the thymus, and the spleen make up the lymphatic system. Its function is to drain protein-containing fluid that escapes from the blood capillaries from the tissue spaces. It also transports fats from the digestive tract to the blood.

108. **(D)** The S-shaped bend where the colon crosses the brim of the pelvis and enters the

pelvic cavity (where it becomes the rectum) is the sigmoid colon. It begins at the left iliac crest, projects toward the midline, and terminates at the rectum.

109. **(B)** The large intestine has little or no digestive function. It serves to absorb water and electrolytes. It also forms and stores feces until defecation occurs.

110. **(D)** The narrow, distal part of the large intestine is called the anal canal. The rectum is the last 8 in of the gastrointestinal tract. The terminal 2 in is the anal canal.

111. **(D)** Some organs lie on the posterior abdominal wall and are covered by peritoneum on the anterior surface only. Such organs, including the kidney and pancreas, are said to be retroperitoneal.

112. **(B)** The beginning (proximal) portion of the large intestine is the cecum. It hangs below the ileocecal valve. It is a blind pouch 2.5 in long.

113. **(C)** To the cecum is attached a small blind tube known as the appendix. It is a twisted, coiled tube, 3 in in length.

114. **(A)** The gallbladder stores bile between meals and releases it when stimulated by gastric juice, fatty foods, and the hormone cholecystokinin. Bile is produced in the liver. The gallbladder stores and concentrates bile.

115. **(B)** When the gallbladder contracts, it ejects concentrated bile into the duodenum. Bile is forced into the common bile duct when it is needed.

116. **(B)** Pancreatic juice leaves the pancreas through the pancreatic duct, the duct of Wirsung. The pancreatic duct unites with the common bile duct from the liver and gallbladder and enters the duodenum in a small raised area called the ampulla of Vater.

117. **(A)** The greater omentum is the largest peritoneal fold and hangs loosely like a "fatty apron" over the transverse colon and coils of the small intestine.

118. **(B)** The hepatic duct joins the slender cystic duct from the gallbladder to form the common bile duct. The common bile duct and the pancreatic duct enter the duodenum in a common duct, the hepatopancreatic.

119. **(D)** The bile pigments, bilirubin, are products of red blood cell breakdown and are normally excreted in bile. If their excretion is prevented, they accumulate in the blood and tissues, causing a yellowish tinge to the skin and other tissues. This condition is called obstructive jaundice.

120. **(A)** The pancreas is an oblong, fish-shaped gland that consists of a head, tail, and body. The head rests in the curve of the duodenum, and its tail touches the spleen. It is linked to the small intestine by a series of ducts.

121. **(B)** The ileocecal sphincter or valve joins the large intestine to the small intestine.

122. **(C)** The duodenum receives secretions from the pancreas and the liver. The duodenum originates at the pyloric sphincter and extends 10 in, where it merges with the jejunum.

123. **(C)** The pylorus is the region of the stomach that connects to the duodenum.

124. **(A)** A broad fan-shaped fold of peritoneum suspending the jejunum and the ileum from the dorsal wall of the abdomen is the mesentery.

125. **(B)** The stomach has four main regions: cardia, fundus, body, and pylorus. The large central portion is the body.

126. **(D)** At the end of the pyloric canal, the muscular wall is thickened, forming a circular muscle called the pyloric sphincter. Pyloric stenosis is a narrowing of the pyloric sphincter, which prevents food from passing through.

127. (D) The esophagus is a straight, collapsible tube about 10 in long. It lies behind the trachea. It pierces the diaphragm at the esophageal hiatus.

128. (A) The esophagus penetrates the diaphragm through an opening, the esophageal hiatus, which then empties into the stomach.

129. (A) The liver is the largest gland in the body. It is divided into left and right segments or lobes. It is located under the diaphragm. Bile is one of its chief products.

130. (B) The cell saver is not used on procedures where Avitene is used because it cannot always be washed out of the cells. This can cause disseminated intravascular coagulation or acute respiratory distress syndrome. It is beneficial to use with cancer patients but only when the cancer is resected en bloc. It can be used on orthopedic procedures and patients with diabetes.

131. (B) Enteroscopy is the scoping of the small intestines. A colonoscopy is scoping of the large intestines. A sigmoidoscopy is scoping of the sigmoid colon.

132. (D) Chronic GERD can cause dysphasia, aspiration, and Barrett's esophagus.

133. (C) Barrett's esophagus is a condition caused by GERD. It is cellular changes in the mucosal lining of the distal esophagus. A Meckel's diverticulum is an outpouching of the distal ileum, and a Zenker's diverticulum is an outpouching in the esophagus.

134. (B) The ligament of Treitz supports the duodenal jejunal flexure and is also used as a surgical landmark for the end of the duodenum and the beginning of the jejunum.

135. (A) Diaphragmatic hernia is also termed hiatal/esophageal hernia. A pantaloon hernia is both a direct and indirect hernia. A Meckel's is a diverticulum in the distal ileum. A direct hernia occurs in Hesselbach's triangle.

136. (B) Laparoscopic Nissen fundoplication is a procedure used to repair a diaphragmatic hernia. A TAPP hernia repair is a laparoscopic hernia repair. McVay and Bassini are also types of inguinal hernia repairs.

137. (C) Sengstaken–Blakemore tube is used to insert pressure in the esophagus. Bougie dilators are used to dilate the esophagus. Bakes dilators are used to dilate the common bile duct. Hank dilators are used to dilate the cervix.

138. (D) A vagotomy is performed to reduce gastric secretions in patients with duodenal ulcers. A gastrectomy is removal of the stomach. A PEG tube is used for gastric decompression and external feedings.

139. (C) A gastrojejunostomy is performed for a benign obstruction or an inoperable tumor. It creates a permanent connection between the stomach and jejunum without removing any part of the distal stomach or duodenum.

140. (B) A PEG tube is used for external feedings.

141. (D) Adhesions can be caused by radiation, pelvic inflammatory disease, Crohn's disease, abdominal surgeries, and a reaction to a foreign body.

142. (A) Billroth I is a resection for a diseased portion of the stomach, and the anastomosis is between the distal stomach and duodenum. A Billroth II is resection of the diseased portion of the distal stomach with anastomosis of stomach to jejunum.

143. (C) The hepatic duct joins with the cystic duct to form the common bile duct.

144. (D) The Harrington is also called the sweetheart. They are commonly used to retract the liver. A Senn retractor is a small rake retractor.

145. (A) A Potts scissor is used to extend the CBD incision, Randal stone forceps are used to remove stones from the CBD, Bakes dilators are used to dilate the CBD, and a T-tube is used to drain the CBD.

146. **(A)** The procedure performed to drain the CBD is called a choledochotomy. Cholecystectomy is removal of the gallbladder, and a choledochoduodenostomy is an anastomosis between the CBD and the duodenum.

147. **(D)** The patient must have a BMI of 40 or greater to be approved for the surgery. Bariatric surgery is performed for morbid obesity. The stomach is reduced in size. A lap band is an example of a procedure performed.

148. **(A)** The liver is located in the left upper quadrant. It produces bile and is covered by Glisson's capsule, and the right and left lobes are divided by the falciform ligament.

149. **(C)** A Silverman and a Tru-Cut needle can be used for liver biopsies. A blunt needle is used when suturing the liver.

150. **(B)** Splenectomy is performed for Hodgkin's disease and sickle cell anemia. A hepatectomy is removal of the liver. Pancreatectomy is removal of the pancreas, and a cholecystectomy is removal of the gallbladder.

151. **(D)** A spigelian hernia occurs between the muscles of the abdomen. A Maydl hernia involves two loops of bowel. A Bassini is a hernia repair. The Richter hernia is a strangulated hernia.

152. **(C)** A hernia where the stomach protrudes through the diaphragm is a hiatal hernia, which is also called a diaphragmatic hernia. A spigelian hernia occurs between two muscle layers in the abdomen.

153. **(D)** Mesh materials include Gore-Tex, Teflon, Dacron, Marlex, and Prolene.

154. **(C)** A cut-down procedure is used when using a Hasson trocar. A TEP is a laparoscopic hernia repair using the balloon preperitoneal dissector. A TAPP is a laparoscopic hernia repair.

155. **(A)** The esophagus is the most proximal portion of the GI tract; the rectum would be the most distal.

156. **(A)** The superior mesenteric artery supplies blood to the proximal large bowel. The middle colic artery is a branch of the superior mesenteric artery that mostly supplies the transverse colon. The celiac artery supplies blood to the liver, stomach, esophagus, spleen, and superior half of both the duodenum and the pancreas. The inferior mesenteric artery is a branch of the abdominal aorta. It supplies blood to part of the transverse colon, splenic flexure, descending colon, sigmoid colon, and rectum.

157. **(B)** The circulator and the STSR both assist in the proper care of the surgical specimen.

158. **(D)** The Pfannenstiel, Charney, Maylard, and Kutchner are all transverse incisions with slight variations in their curve, which is used to access the pelvic organs. An oblique incision is commonly made in the right lower quadrant and is used for an appendectomy.

159. **(C)** The spleen is the largest mass of lymphatic tissue.

160. **(B)** The triangle of Calot is an important landmark of the biliary system. It is made up of the common hepatic duct, cystic duct, and the inferior edge of the liver.

161. **(D)** Portal hypertension is increased pressure in the portal vein. This prevents blood flow through the liver. It can be caused by blockage of the portal vein, hepatitis, and cirrhosis of the liver.

162. **(C)** Following a laparoscopic cholecystectomy, a choledochostomy tube/T-tube can be placed for drainage in the CBD and brought out through one of the 5-mm ports used for instrumentation.

163. **(C)** Alcohol abuse and hepatitis are both diseases that are known to cause cirrhosis of the liver; Zenker's diverticulum is found in the

esophagus, and cholecystitis is the presence of stones in the gallbladder.

164. **(A)** Glisson's capsule is the fibrous tissue covering of the liver. The medulla oblongata is a portion of the brainstem. The galea aponeurotica is the fibrous connective tissue that covers the cranium, and the pituitary gland rests in the sella turcica.

165. **(D)** Anoscopy, proctoscopy, and sigmoidoscopy are procedures performed to look at the inner lining of the anus, rectum, and the lower part of the large intestine. They can get a clear vision of internal hemorrhoids and abnormal growths. An anoscope is the smallest of the three viewing instruments and does not allow viewing into the colon. The proctoscope is slightly longer but does not reach into the colon as the sigmoidoscope does.

166. **(D)** The long thoracic nerve helps to lift the shoulder and aid in respiration. The long thoracic nerve can be damaged during breast surgery, specifically on a radical mastectomy that involves axillary node dissection for breast cancer.

CHAPTER 19

Obstetrics and Gynecology

- Skene's glands/periurethral glands—located on the anterior wall of the vagina. They drain into the urethra
- Bartholin's glands—glands located at the lower end of the vagina that secrete a fluid that lubricates the vulva
- Marsupialization of Bartholin's cyst—performed for obstruction of the Bartholin's gland
- Marsupialization—refers to the type of closure used. The cyst is opened, an incision and drainage is performed, and the edges are sutured to the edges of the incision
- The uterus is lined with a membrane called the endometrium. When a woman does not become pregnant, the lining is shed, resulting in a woman's period (menstruation)
- The uterine tube (fallopian tube) carries an egg from the ovary to the uterus. At the end of the tube are fimbriae, which are finger-like projections that help guide the egg into the fallopian tube
- Ectopic pregnancy—pregnancy anywhere outside of the uterus
- Tubal pregnancy is a pregnancy that takes place within the fallopian tube
- Ovaries—a pair of reproductive glands in women. The ovaries are located in the pelvis, one on each side of the uterus. The ovaries produce eggs (ova) and female hormones estrogen and progesterone
- A female baby is born with all the eggs that she will ever have
- Cervix—a cylinder-shaped tissue that connects the vagina and uterus. The opening in the center of the cervix is known as the external os. It is the passage between the uterus and vagina
- Uterine ligaments include:
  - Broad
  - Round
  - Cardinal
  - Uterosacral
- Gynecological (GYN) procedures can be performed:
  - Vaginal approach—with the vaginal approach, the patient is in the lithotomy position; a major complication is thrombosis (blood clot)
  - Abdominal approach
  - Both—vaginal and abdominal
- Diagnostic procedures include:
  - Laparoscopy
  - Pelvic ultrasound
  - Magnetic resonance imaging (MRI)
  - Computed tomography (CT) scan
- Hysterosalpingogram—an x-ray of the uterus and fallopian tubes; usually performed for diagnosing infertility
- Colposcopy—a procedure to closely examine your cervix, vagina, and vulva for signs of disease. During colposcopy, your doctor uses a special instrument called a colposcope
- Hysteroscopy—performed endoscopically to visualize the uterus for diagnostic and operative procedures. The scope is inserted transvaginally/transcervically
- To distend the uterus, the medium used is a nonelectrolytic fluid; they include:
  - Sorbitol
  - Glycine
  - Dextrose
- Cone biopsy of the cervix—performed to rule out cervical cancer; instruments used include:
  - Laser
  - Scalpel
  - Cervitome (cold knife conization)
  - LEEP (loop electrosurgical excision procedure)

- Culdocentesis—a procedure to extract fluid from the rectouterine pouch posterior to the vagina with a needle that is inserted transvaginally. It is a diagnostic procedure used in identifying pelvic inflammatory disease and ectopic pregnancy
- PID—pelvic inflammatory disease—inflammation of the female genitalia. It can result in sterility and can be caused by several microorganisms including:
  - Chlamydia
  - Gonococci
- Dilation and curettage (D&C)/fractional curettage—performed for histological studies. Tissue may be taken from the cervix (endocervical) or the uterine lining (endometrial)
- Menorrhagia—an abnormally heavy and prolonged period monthly
- Menometrorrhagia—prolonged or excessive bleeding that occurs irregularly and more frequently than a normal period
- Dysmenorrhea—abnormally painful periods
- Amenorrhea—an abnormal absence of menstruation
- Chromopertubation—performed to test patency of the fallopian tubes. Methylene blue or indigo carmine dye is injected into the uterine cavity through a uterine manipulator (Zumi/Humi), and the patency of the tubes are confirmed by an abdominal laparoscope
- Laparoscopy—performed for direct visualization of the pelvic organs
- Tubal ligation—performed to prevent pregnancy. This can be done with:
  - Electrocoagulation (bipolar)
  - Electrosurgical unit (ESU) with partial resection
  - Falope ring
  - Filshie clip
- Salpingostomy for ectopic pregnancy—salpingostomy is an opening into the fallopian tube to remove the products of conception. Usually, the tube is not sutured but is left to close on its own. If reconstruction is required, fine sutures and Bowman's lacrimal probes are used
- Salpingectomy—removal of the fallopian tube
- Excision of condylomata—this is a type of wart caused by the human papillomavirus (HPV) virus. It can increase a woman's chance

of cancer. The warts can be removed by ESU/laser/excision
- You must always use suction/smoke evacuator when using the ESU/laser to remove genital warts because it is proven that the smoke plume that travels into the air still contains DNA from the virus, and prolonged exposure could cause the virus to travel to the throat and lungs
- Vulvectomy procedures are performed for carcinoma
  - Simple vulvectomy—removal of the labia majora, minora/clitoris
  - Total vulvectomy—wide excision is performed.
  - Radical vulvectomy—the vulva and, if the nodes are positive, vagina, urethra, and anus may be removed. Abdominal and perineal dissection is performed
- Vaginectomy/vaginoplasty—performed for cancer of the vagina
- An amnion graft (inner layer of a fetal membrane) or skin can be used for a vaginal graft
- Cystocele—a type of hernia. The bladder protrudes into the vaginal wall; symptoms include stress incontinence
- Marshall–Marchetti–Krantz—the Marshall–Marchetti-Krantz procedure surgically reinforces the bladder neck in order to prevent urinary incontinence
- Rectocele—performed for a herniation of the rectum into the vaginal wall
- Anterior and posterior repair—performed to treat a cystocele/rectocele
- Enterocele—a herniation involving a portion of the intestine
- Vesicovaginal fistula—a fistula is a small opening (tubular connection) that develops between the bladder and the vagina
- Urethrovaginal fistula—fistula between the urethra and the vagina
- Ureterovaginal fistula—fistula between the ureter and the vagina
- Rectovaginal fistula—fistula between the rectum and the vagina
- Trachelorrhaphy—performed for reconstruction of the cervix as a result of lacerations due to the trauma of childbirth
- Episiotomy—performed to extend the perineal area upon delivering the baby to prevent tearing of the perineum

- Uterine ablation—endometrial ablation is a procedure that burns the uterine lining to treat abnormal uterine bleeding. This can be performed by laser, radiofrequency ablation (balloon filled with saline solution that has been heated), and electricity (using a resectoscope with a loop or rolling ball electrode)
- Vaginal hysterectomy—removal of the uterus through an incision in the vaginal wall
- Suprapubic catheter—a catheter that is inserted into the bladder percutaneously or with a cutdown procedure. This is a urinary diversion catheter; it diverts the urine away from the vaginal area where the incision is
- Laparoscopic-assisted vaginal hysterectomy (LAVH)—a procedure using laparoscopic equipment to dissect the uterus and remove it through the vagina
- Total abdominal hysterectomy—removal of the uterus and cervix through an abdominal incision
- TAH BSO—total abdominal hysterectomy, bilateral salpingo-oophorectomy—this is removal of the uterus/fallopian tubes/ovaries. This is performed for malignant tumors
  - Uterus
  - Tubes
  - Ovaries
  - Ligaments
  - Upper part of the vagina
  - Bilateral pelvic lymph nodes
  - Some arteries and veins
- En bloc—removal of a tumor and/or organs involved without dissection of one; the entire tumor and organs are removed together in one piece
- Seeding—when removing cancerous tissue, you want to be extra careful not to drop tissue/cells into the abdominal cavity and prevent the spread of cancer
- Pelvic exenteration—performed for malignant cancer. The procedure is performed en bloc. The organs removed include:
  - All reproductive organs
  - Distal ureters
  - Bladder
  - Vagina
  - It can involve the rectum
  - Perineum
  - Pelvic lymph nodes

- Oophorectomy—removal of an ovary
- Oophorocystectomy—removal of an ovarian cyst on the ovary, not the ovary itself. The most common cysts include:
  - Dermoid cyst/teratoma—this cyst contains embryonic cells containing epidermis, hair follicles, and sebaceous glands
  - Follicular cyst
- Myomectomy—removal of fibroid tumors of the uterine lining
- Leiomyoma—a common tumor of the uterine lining
- Salpingo-oophorectomy—removal of the fallopian tube and part or the entire ovary
- Cervical cerclage—cervical cerclage is used for the treatment of cervical incompetency. This prevents the fetus from miscarrying when the fetus gets larger and weighs heavy on the cervix. A strong suture or Dacron tape is sutured around the cervix around weeks 12–14 and removed near the end of the third trimester. Two common procedures include:
  - Shirodkar
  - McDonald
- Abortion—an abortion is a pregnancy that ends before the baby can survive outside the womb because it has not yet reached viability
- Spontaneous abortion—the abortion occurs naturally
- Induced abortion—the pregnancy is terminated artificially or with medication
- Threatened abortion—this is when there is a problem with the pregnancy with symptoms that include bleeding and pelvic pain. The cervix remains closed, and under ultrasound, it shows the pregnancy is still viable
- Complete abortion—the pregnancy is terminated, and the uterus completely empties itself
- Incomplete abortion—miscarriage with some products of conception retained that must be removed with a D&C
- Missed abortion—the fetus is not viable but has not expelled itself from the uterus. A D&C is performed for complete elimination of retained products of conception
- Suction curettage—vacuum or suction with aspiration to remove uterine contents through the cervix
- Meconium—the first bowel movement of the fetus

- Amniotic fluid—the fluid surrounding the fetus in the womb
- Vernix—vernix caseosa—is the waxy white substance found on the skin of the newborn
- A common reason to perform a cesarean section (C-section) is cephalopelvic disproportion. The infant's head is too large to fit through the birth canal
- Placental abruption—placental abruption is when the placenta separates from the wall of the uterus prior to the birth of the baby
- Placenta previa—a condition in which the placenta blocks the opening of the uterus, interfering with normal delivery of a baby
- Pregnancy-induced hypertension—high blood pressure that occurs during pregnancy
- Eclampsia—can occur when the pregnant woman has high blood pressure, which could cause a convulsion, coma, and death if not treated
- Nuchal cord—when the umbilical cord is wrapped once or more around the baby's neck
- Cord prolapse—when the umbilical cord comes before the baby's head out into the vagina during birth
- Breech—occurs when the baby's feet/buttocks/knees come before the baby's head into the birth canal
- Gravida—the number of times that a woman has been pregnant
- Para gravida—the number of times that a woman has given birth to a fetus with a gestational age of 24 weeks or more
- Prima gravida—first pregnancy

- Oxytocin/Pitocin—medication used to induce labor, continue labor, and contract the uterus following the birth to help the uterus expel blood
- Hemabate—this medication is used to induce an abortion by dilating the cervix and producing uterine contractions that cause delivery
- Methergine—this medication is used to help control hemorrhage following birth
- Dextran—irrigation fluid left in abdomen to prevent adhesions
- Positioning for OB/GYN procedures includes supine and lithotomy position
- Complications of lithotomy position include peroneal nerve damage and an embolus
- Prep for OB/GYN procedures include:
  - Clean to dirty—prep the clean area with a Betadine prep stick, and then follow to the anal area and discard. Repeat the step
- Chloraprep should never be used on the mucous membranes, which include the vagina
- Draping for OB/GYN procedures includes:
  - A buttock drape is placed
  - Leggings
  - Fenestrated abdominal drape
- DeLee suction—this is attached to the fetal head and assists in delivery of the fetus
- Common incisions that allow access to the pelvic organs include Pfannenstiel, Cherney, and Maylard
- Radical hysterectomy/Wertheim—this is performed for cervical cancer and endometrial cancer. Organs removed include the vagina, uterus, cervix, Fallopian tubes, ovaries, bladder and rectum.

Questions

1. When handling uterine curettings:

   (A) never place them in preservative
   (B) keep the endometrial and the endocervical curettings separate
   (C) send the endometrial and the endocervical curettings to the laboratory in one container
   (D) send them on a 4 × 4 to the laboratory because it is too difficult to remove them

2. Labor can be induced using:

   (A) ergotrate
   (B) diazoxide
   (C) Pitocin
   (D) magnesium sulfate

3. Which radiological study might be ordered preoperatively for a patient scheduled for tuboplasty?

   (A) Angiography
   (B) Cholangiogram
   (C) Hysterosalpingogram
   (D) Retrograde urography

4. A Hulka uterine tenaculum forceps is commonly used in gynecological surgery to:

   (A) manipulate the uterus
   (B) stabilize the cervix
   (C) retract the vagina
   (D) both A and B

5. Which drug is given to aid in placental expulsion?

   (A) Oxytocic
   (B) Anticholinergic
   (C) Antihistamine
   (D) Hypoxic

6. Which is true of uterine manipulators?

   (A) Common uterine manipulators are the Humi and the Zumi.
   (B) They have a rounded smooth tip for easy entry into the cervix and uterus and prevent uterine perforation.
   (C) A balloon is inflated once inserted into the uterus in order to prevent leakage and manipulation.
   (D) All of the above

7. The aim of stress incontinence operations includes all of the following EXCEPT:

   (A) to improve performance of a dislodged or dysfunctional vesical neck
   (B) to restore normal urethral length
   (C) to tighten and restore the anterior urethral vesical angle
   (D) to repair a congenital defect

8. A procedure done on young women who have been diagnosed with benign uterine tumors but who wish to preserve fertility is a:

   (A) subtotal hysterectomy
   (B) Wertheim procedure
   (C) myomectomy
   (D) Le Fort procedure

9. A procedure to prevent cervical dilatation that results in release of uterine contents is a:

   (A) Shirodkar
   (B) Le Fort
   (C) Wertheim
   (D) marsupialization

10. An endoscopic investigation of the uterus and tubes is a:

    (A) Rubin's test
    (B) hysterogram
    (C) hysterosalpingogram
    (D) hysteroscopy

11. Sterility can be accomplished by all of the following procedures EXCEPT:

    (A) laparoscopy
    (B) minilaparotomy
    (C) posterior colpotomy
    (D) culdoscopy

12. The progress of the labor process is defined in how many stages?:

    (A) two
    (B) three
    (C) four
    (D) five

13. The role of the surgical technologist in a vaginal delivery includes all EXCEPT:

    (A) evaluate the progress of the patient during labor
    (B) assist the obstetrician and labor and delivery nurse
    (C) support the mother
    (D) assist with clamping and cutting the cord

14. An ectopic pregnancy may occur:

    (A) anywhere outside of the uterus
    (B) in the fallopian tube
    (C) in the oviduct
    (D) all of the above

15. What gynecological setup would include various sizes of sterile cannulas?

    (A) Cesarean
    (B) Hysterectomy
    (C) Oophorectomy
    (D) Suction curettage

16. A Foley catheter is placed into the presurgical hysterectomy patient to:

    (A) record accurate intake and output
    (B) distend the bladder during surgery
    (C) avoid injury to the bladder
    (D) maintain a dry perineum postoperatively

17. What would an anterior and posterior repair accomplish?

    (A) Repair of cystocele and rectocele
    (B) Repair of vesicovaginal fistula
    (C) Repair of vesicourethral fistula
    (D) Repair of labial hernia

18. An incision made during normal labor to facilitate delivery with less trauma to the mother is a/an:

    (A) colpotomy
    (B) colporrhaphy
    (C) episiotomy
    (D) celiotomy

19. Cervical carcinoma in situ can be classified as:

    (A) limited to the epithelial layer, noninvasive
    (B) microinvasive
    (C) clinically obvious
    (D) vaginal extension limitations

20. The fallopian tube is grasped with a:

    (A) Kocher
    (B) Babcock
    (C) Kelly
    (D) Lahey

21. Reconstruction of the fallopian tube setup would include:

   (A) Bowman lacrimal probes
   (B) Bakes dilators
   (C) Hegar dilators
   (D) Van Buren sounds

22. To confirm the diagnosis of ectopic pregnancy, it is sometimes necessary to perform a:

   (A) Rubin's test
   (B) culdocentesis
   (C) paracentesis
   (D) laparotomy

23. Cervical conization is accomplished using all of the following EXCEPT:

   (A) scalpel
   (B) cautery
   (C) laser
   (D) sclerosing solution

24. The most commonly identified ovarian cyst is the:

   (A) chocolate
   (B) follicle
   (C) serous cyst adenoma
   (D) dermoid

25. A herniation in the posterior cul-de-sac/pouch of Douglas/rectouterine pouch is a:

   (A) cystocele
   (B) hydrocele
   (C) enterocele
   (D) epiplocele

26. A vesicourethral abdominal suspension is known as a:

   (A) Le Fort
   (B) Wertheim
   (C) Marshall–Marchetti
   (D) Shirodkar

27. A condition causing leakage of urine into the vagina is a/an:

   (A) ureterovaginal fistula
   (B) cystocele
   (C) vesicovaginal fistula
   (D) rectovaginal fistula

28. What special technique is employed during a hysterectomy?

   (A) Discard instruments used on cervix and vagina
   (B) Use second set for closure
   (C) Redrape for closure
   (D) Remove Foley before uterus is removed

29. Papanicolaou indicates:

   (A) removal of small pieces of cervix for examination
   (B) cytological study of cervical smear
   (C) staining of the cervix for study
   (D) direct visualization of pelvic organs

30. A technique employed for cervical biopsy is:

   (A) random punches
   (B) multiple punches at 3, 6, 9, and 12 o'clock
   (C) one central punch at os
   (D) one inferior and one superior punch

31. In a cesarean birth, the uterus is opened with a knife and extended with a/an:

   (A) Metzenbaum
   (B) Heaney
   (C) iris scissor
   (D) bandage scissor

32. At which point in a cesarean is a bulb syringe used?

   (A) When the membranes are incised
   (B) When the fetal head is delivered
   (C) When the entire infant is delivered
   (D) After placental delivery

33. A medication used to control severe uterine hemorrhage following labor or an induced abortion is:

    (A) RhoGAM
    (B) Hemabate
    (C) oxytocin
    (D) epinephrine

34. When closing a uterus in a cesarean, the edges of the uterine incision are clamped with which of the following?

    (A) Allis
    (B) Kocher
    (C) Pennington
    (D) Babcock

35. Intraoperative chromotubation can be affected by all of the following surgical cannulae EXCEPT:

    (A) Humi
    (B) Rubin
    (C) Hui
    (D) Hulka

36. What suture would be placed into the wall of a large ovarian cyst before aspiration of its contents and final removal?

    (A) Mattress
    (B) Suture ligature
    (C) Purse-string
    (D) Figure-of-eight

37. What is the preferred procedure for recurrent or persistent carcinoma of the cervix after radiation therapy has been completed?

    (A) Wertheim's
    (B) Pelvic exenteration
    (C) Abdominal perineal resection
    (D) Low-anterior resection

38. Which of the following instruments would be used to grasp the anterior cervix of the uterus just before dissection from the vaginal vault during a total abdominal hysterectomy?

    (A) Allis
    (B) Heaney
    (C) Phaneuf
    (D) Kelly

39. Laparoscopic tubal occlusion may utilize all of the following methods of effecting sterilization EXCEPT:

    (A) bipolar coagulation
    (B) silastic bands
    (C) Surgitie ligating loop
    (D) spring clip

40. What is the term used to indicate the number of times a woman has given birth?:

    (A) Stages
    (B) Para
    (C) Descent
    (D) Gravida

41. What is the procedure performed to treat cervical cancer?

    (A) Episiotomy
    (B) Brachytherapy
    (C) Marsupialization
    (D) Abdominal perineal resection

42. Indications for a cesarean section include:

    (A) fetal distress
    (B) cephalopelvic disproportion
    (C) placenta abruption
    (D) all of the above

43. 43. Abnormal bending of the uterus is called:

    (A) cephalopelvic disproportion
    (B) retroverted
    (C) anteverted
    (D) both B and C

44. A Stamey endoscopic procedure is performed to:

    (A) suspend the vesicle neck
    (B) correct anterior wall prolapse
    (C) correct posterior wall prolapse
    (D) repair a bladder laceration

45. What is the name given to a radical vaginal hysterectomy?

    (A) Exenteration
    (B) Schauta
    (C) Wertheim's
    (D) Le Fort

46. What surgical procedure provides obliteration of the vagina by denuding and approximating the anterior and posterior walls of the vagina?

    (A) Vaginoplasty
    (B) Colpocleisis
    (C) Colpoperineorrhaphy
    (D) Colporrhaphy

47. The hysteroscope may be used to identify or remove all of the following EXCEPT:

    (A) fallopian adhesions
    (B) lost intrauterine devices (IUDs)
    (C) intrauterine adhesions
    (D) submucosa fibroids

48. Which of the following is an obstetric complication resulting from overstimulation of the clotting process:

    (A) spontaneous abortion
    (B) disseminated intravascular coagulation
    (C) eclampsia
    (D) placental abruption

49. All apply to the Rh factor EXCEPT:

    (A) Rh antibodies can be harmless until the mother's second or later pregnancies
    (B) this is a protein found inside of the red blood cell
    (C) if you have this protein, you are Rh positive
    (D) if the mother is Rh negative and the fetus is Rh positive, the mother's antibodies will pass into the fetal bloodstream and attack those cells. This causes severe anemia and possible death.

50. What is the term used for the area where two lateral openings in the uterus attach and where the fallopian tubes exit the uterus?

    (A) cornu
    (B) cervical os
    (C) uterine tube
    (D) ampulla

51. Endometrial ablation is performed to correct:

    (A) amenorrhea
    (B) metrorrhagia
    (C) menorrhagia
    (D) endometriosis

52. Endoscopic visualization of the uterine cavity is called:

    (A) pelviscopy
    (B) laparoscopy
    (C) hysteroscopy
    (D) colposcopy

53. Marsupialization of a Bartholin's cyst involves:

    (A) suturing the posterior wall of the cyst to the skin edges
    (B) removal of anterior wall of cyst
    (C) draining cyst contents
    (D) both A and B

54. What is the self-retaining retractor used in vaginal procedures?

    (A) O'Sullivan–O'Conner
    (B) Gelpi
    (C) Graves
    (D) Auvard

55. Extrauterine disease of the female reproductive system may utilize any of the following lasers via a colposcope or laparoscope EXCEPT:

    (A) CO_2
    (B) Nd:YAG
    (C) Candela
    (D) argon

56. A postoperative complication of the GYN patient in lithotomy position for an extended period of time is:

    (A) blood pressure changes
    (B) venous stasis
    (C) crushing injury to the hands
    (D) all of the above

57. A benign smooth muscle tumor of the uterus that causes abnormal uterine bleeding leading to anemia is:

    (A) dermoid
    (B) endometriosis
    (C) leiomyoma
    (D) cystocele

58. What incision is commonly used for a C-section?

    (A) McBurney
    (B) Upper midline
    (C) Lower paramedian
    (D) Pfannenstiel

59. Premature separation of the placenta from the uterine wall is:

    (A) placental prolapse
    (B) placenta previa
    (C) nuchal cord
    (D) placental abruption

60. The graft used for a vaginoplasty is:

    (A) full-thickness skin graft
    (B) biological skin graft
    (C) split-thickness skin graft
    (D) subcutaneous connective tissue

61. When all products of conception are expelled and surgical intervention is NOT necessary, it is a/an:

    (A) incomplete abortion
    (B) complete abortion
    (C) missed abortion
    (D) D&C

62. A cyst that is formed from the germ layer from the developing embryo is called a/an:

    (A) teratoma (dermoid)
    (B) leiomyoma
    (C) fibroid
    (D) endometrial cyst

63. Hypertension and seizure during pregnancy are known as:

    (A) preeclampsia
    (B) placenta abruption
    (C) malignant hypertension
    (D) eclampsia

64. Electrocoagulation, cryoablation, and radiofrequency ablation are procedures performed for:

    (A) dysfunctional uterine bleeding
    (B) malignant fibroids
    (C) benign fibroids
    (D) cervical cancer

65. LAVH is removal of the uterus by combined approach using:

    (A) laparoscopic and vaginal
    (B) abdominal and vaginal
    (C) Pfannenstiel and vaginal
    (D) lower midline and vaginal

66. The term describing specimen removal in one piece is:

    (A) in situ
    (B) en bloc
    (C) colon resection
    (D) none of the above

67. The umbilical cord preceding the fetal head is:

    (A) placenta abruption
    (B) placenta previa
    (C) cord prolapsed
    (D) nuchal cord

68. All of the following are uterine ligaments EXCEPT:

    (A) broad
    (B) round
    (C) cardinal
    (D) transcervical

Use the following information to answer Questions 69 and 70. A 29-year-old pregnant woman presents to the emergency room complaining of severe lower abdominal pain and slight vaginal bleeding. The ultrasound shows the products of conception are in the fallopian tube.

69. The tests show that the fertilized egg implanted itself outside the uterus. She is diagnosed with:

    (A) ectopic pregnancy
    (B) incompetent cervix
    (C) complete abortion
    (D) ovarian cyst

70. She is scheduled for:

    (A) laparoscopic removal of ectopic pregnancy
    (B) ovarian cystectomy
    (C) oophorectomy
    (D) hysteroscopy

71. The position when the surgeon chooses an open approach for emergent surgery for ectopic pregnancy is:

    (A) lithotomy
    (B) supine with a wedge under the affected side
    (C) supine
    (D) reverse Trendelenburg

72. The surgery performed to remove the embryo while preserving the tube is:

    (A) salpingo-oophorectomy
    (B) salpingectomy
    (C) salpingostomy
    (D) oophorectomy

73. The affected tube is grasped with:

    (A) Babcock
    (B) Allis
    (C) mixter
    (D) Kocher

74. Pathology of an ectopic pregnancy includes all EXCEPT:

    (A) a sexually transmitted disease
    (B) previous tubal surgery
    (C) exercising during first trimester
    (D) smoking

75. Tubal patency may be tested by the installation of _____ into the uterine cavity.

    (A) balanced salt solution
    (B) Chymar
    (C) methylene blue
    (D) gentian violet

76. Mrs. Jones had an abnormal Pap smear and was scheduled to have a cervical biopsy. When using an acetic acid, the abnormal cervical tissue will _____. When performing the Schiller's test, brown Lugol's solution is used. This has an iodine base. When applied to the cervix, the abnormal cells will _____.

    (A) turn white; turn white
    (B) turn white; turn brown
    (C) remain the same; turn brown
    (D) turn white; not pick up the stain. The tissue that turns brown with the stain is normal tissue.

77. After removal of the uterus in a hysterectomy:

    (A) cervical and vaginal instruments are isolated from the instrument set in a discard basin
    (B) the cervix is cauterized
    (C) new instruments are used on the cervical closure
    (D) cervical instruments are returned to the basket

Answers and Explanations

1. **(B)** The endometrial curettings should be kept separate from the endocervical curettings. Fractional curettage specimens differentiate between the endocervix and the endometrium of the corpus, which helps to locate a lesion more specifically.

2. **(C)** Pitocin is used to induce active labor or to increase the force or rate of existing contractions during delivery. It may be given postpartum to prevent or control hemorrhage. It acts on the uterus.

3. **(C)** A hysterosalpingogram is performed to show the internal shape of the uterus and patency of the fallopian tubes. A thin tube is inserted into the vagina and up into the uterus. Contrast media is infused into the tube and visualized on x-ray.

4. **(D)** The Hulka uterine forceps is commonly used in GYN procedures to stabilize the cervix and manipulate the uterus during a laparoscopic pelvic procedure.

5. **(A)** As soon as the shoulders are delivered, about 20 units of oxytocic per liter of fluid are given intravenously so the uterus contracts, aiding in expulsion of the placenta and membranes.

6. **(D)** Uterine manipulators are used to move the uterus during laparoscopic procedures. They are also used to inject dye into the uterus and tubes to test for tubal patency. They have a rounded smooth tip for entry into the uterine cavity and to prevent perforation. A balloon is used to hold the manipulator in place and prevent leakage.

7. **(D)** The aim of any operation for urinary stress incontinence is to improve the performance of a dislodged or dysfunctional vesical neck, to restore normal urethral length, and to tighten and restore the anterior urethral vesical angle.

8. **(C)** Myomectomy is usually done on young women with symptoms that indicate the presence of benign tumors who wish to preserve fertility.

9. **(A)** The postconceptional Shirodkar operation is placement of a collar-type ligature of Mersilene, Dacron tape, heavy nylon, or plastic-covered stainless steel at the internal os to close it when there is cervical incompetence characterized by habitual, spontaneous abortion.

10. **(D)** A hysteroscopy is an endoscopic visualization of the uterine cavity and tubal orifices for evaluation of uterine bleeding, location and removal of IUDs, diagnosis, and so forth.

11. **(D)** Laparoscopy, minilaparotomy, and posterior colpotomy are viable methods to create sterility. Culdoscopy cannot be used for this purpose.

12. **(C)** There are four stages to the labor process. In stage 1, labor begins; this stage ends when the cervix is fully dilated. In stage 2, the cervix is completely dilated, and the stage continues until the time the infant is born. Stage 3 begins when the infant is born and ends when the placenta is delivered. Stage 4 is when the mother is stabilized.

13. **(A)** The physician and labor and delivery nurse are responsible for evaluating the

progress of the mother. The surgical technologist is responsible for assisting the obstetrician and labor and delivery nurse, supporting the needs of the mother, assisting with clamping and cutting the umbilical cord, and collecting cord blood for blood gases.

14. **(D)** An ectopic pregnancy is a pregnancy where the fetus develops outside of the uterus. A tubal pregnancy is also an ectopic pregnancy when the fetus develops in the fallopian tube; the oviduct/uterine tube is another name for the fallopian tube.

15. **(D)** A suction curettage would require various-sized sterile suction cannulas for the termination of an early pregnancy, missed abortion, or incomplete abortion. The cannula is inserted into the uterus, and the suction is turned on to disrupt the products of conception.

16. **(C)** Because pelvic procedures involve manipulation of the ureters, bladder, and urethra, an indwelling Foley or suprapubic cystostomy catheter may be placed before or during operation to avoid injury to the bladder.

17. **(A)** Cystoceles (bulging bladder) and rectoceles (bulging rectum) occur because of weakened vaginal mucosa. Usually, the cause is traumatic childbirth, and the cure is an anterior and posterior vaginal repair.

18. **(C)** An episiotomy is an intentionally made perineal incision executed during a normal birth to facilitate delivery and prevent perineal laceration.

19. **(A)** Carcinoma in situ is limited to the epithelial layer with no evidence of invasion.

20. **(B)** The fallopian tube is grasped with either an Allis or Babcock forceps.

21. **(A)** Tuboplasty requires a basic gynecological instrument set plus iris scissors, Adson forceps, mosquitos, Bowman lacrimal probes, Webster needle holder, and Frazier suction. A microsurgical set and laser may also be used.

22. **(B)** Aspiration of fluid or blood from the cul-de-sac of Douglas (culdocentesis) confirms intraperitoneal bleeding caused by ectopic pregnancy.

23. **(D)** Cervical conization may be performed by scalpel resection and suturing, by application of the cutting of cautery, or by use of a laser.

24. **(B)** Functional cysts comprise the majority of ovarian enlargements. Follicle cysts are the most common.

25. **(C)** An enterocele is a herniation of small bowel that presses against the upper wall of the vagina. The cul-de-sac, pouch of Douglas, and the rectouterine pouch are all types of rectoceles. A hydrocele is fluid accumulation in the sheath surrounding the testicle. A cystocele is also known as a prolapsed bladder. The bladder bulges into the vaginal wall, and an epiplocele is a herniation that contains omentum.

26. **(C)** A Marshall–Marchetti procedure is an abdominal approach to repairing and elevating the fascial and pubococcygeal muscle surrounding the urethra and the bladder neck for the correction of stress incontinence.

27. **(C)** A vesicovaginal fistula may vary in size from a small opening that permits slight leakage of urine into the vagina to a large opening that permits all urine to pass to the vagina.

28. **(A)** Once the cervix is dissected away from and is amputated from the vagina, all of the potentially contaminated instruments used on the cervix and vagina are placed in a discard basin and removed from the field (includes sponge sticks and suction).

29. **(B)** Papanicolaou is a cytological study of smears of the cervical and endocervical tissue. Characteristic cellular changes can be identified.

30. **(B)** Multiple punch biopsies of the cervical circumference (at the 3, 6, 9, and 12 o'clock positions) may be taken with a Gaylor biopsy forceps.

31. (D) The uterus is opened with a knife and extended by cutting laterally with a large bandage scissor or by simply spreading with the fingers.

32. (B) As soon as the head is delivered, a bulb syringe is used to aspirate the infant's exposed nares and mouth to minimize aspiration of amniotic fluid and its contents.

33. (B) Hemabate is used to control severe uterine hemorrhage following labor or an induced abortion. It is also used for contraction of the uterus during and following childbirth and an induced abortion. RhoGAM is used to treat the Rh factor with an Rh-negative mother and an Rh-positive fetus. Oxytocin is used to stimulate contraction of the uterus during labor, and epinephrine is used to produce vasoconstriction/reduced blood flow and prolong the effects of local anesthesia.

34. (C) The edges of the uterine incision are promptly clamped with Pean forceps, ring forceps, or Pennington clamps.

35. (D) Once the vagina has been prepped and an indwelling catheter is placed into the bladder, chromotubation can be effected by placing a Kahn, Calvin, Hui, Humi, or Rubin cannula into the cervical opening using diluted methylene blue dye to identify a nonpatent fallopian tube as visualized through a laparoscope. Hulka forceps are used to grasp and stabilize the cervix and manipulate the uterus. They are not used for intraoperative chromotubation.

36. (C) For removal of a large ovarian cyst, a purse-string suture may be placed into the cyst wall, and a trocar is introduced into the center to aspirate its contents before the suture is tied.

37. (B) Pelvic exenteration is a preferred treatment for recurrent or persistent carcinoma of the cervix. It is considered the only surgical alternative after a thorough investigation of the patient and disease status to determine if there is a reasonable chance for a cure.

38. (A) After the vaginal vault is incised close to the cervix during the removal of the uterus, an Allis, Kocher, or tenaculum may be used to grasp the anterior lip of the cervix.

39. (C) Preknotted suture loops are used to ligate pedicle tissues. Bipolar coagulation, spring clips, and Silastic bands effect occlusion of fallopian tubes.

40. (B) Para is the term for the number of times a woman has given birth. Gravida is the term used for the number of times a woman has been pregnant. Descent is when the fetus moves through the pelvic canal, and stages refers to the four stages of the labor process.

41. (B) Brachytherapy is internal radiation therapy administered by placing radioactive seeds near the affected area of the cervix. Episiotomy is an incision in the perineal area between the vagina and the anus to prevent the perineal area from tearing during childbirth. Marsupialization is a surgical technique used to evert the edges of an infected cyst. An anterior and posterior repair is performed for anal or rectal cancer.

42. (D) Fetal distress, cephalopelvic disproportion is when the head of the fetus is too large to fit in the pelvis for a vaginal delivery. Placental abruption is when the placenta tears from the uterine wall causing hemorrhage.

43. (D) An anteverted uterus tilts forward, and a retroverted uterus tilts in a backward position. Cephalopelvic disproportion is when the head of the fetus is too large to fit in the pelvis for a vaginal delivery.

44. (A) Known as a Stamey procedure for female incontinence, the bladder neck is suspended by placing sutures on both sides of the vesico-urethral junction from the anterior rectus fascia into the vagina. This is aided by insertion of a cystoscope to ascertain correct needle placement through an incision into the rectus fascia.

45. **(B)** An operative approach to early carcinoma of the cervix is a radical vaginal hysterectomy called a Schauta operation. It is useful in obese patients and removes the uterus, upper third of the vagina, parametria, fallopian tubes, and ovaries.

46. **(B)** Colpocleisis is obliteration of the vagina by denuding and approximating the anterior and posterior walls of the vagina and is generally reserved for elderly high-risk patients with uterine prolapse.

47. **(A)** The hysteroscope is used most commonly for endometrial laser ablation. The hysteroscope also may be used to identify and remove polyps and submucous fibroids, retrieve lost uterine devices, or lyse intrauterine adhesions.

48. **(A)** Disseminated intravascular coagulation can be an obstetric complication resulting from the overstimulation of the clotting process. The body's clotting mechanisms do not work properly and spread throughout the body instead of to the specific area of the injury. This widespread coagulation in other parts of the body causes a depletion in the coagulation factor, and the blood does not clot properly; this causes bleeding in other parts of the body. This is a life-threatening disorder and can cause severe hemorrhage throughout the body. A spontaneous abortion is an abortion without any outside influence. It occurs naturally. Eclampsia is a condition of hypertension in the pregnant woman causing convulsions and serious health problems for the mother and fetus.

49. **(B)** All pertain to the Rh factor except that the protein is found on the surface of the red blood cell.

50. **(A)** The fallopian tubes are attached to and open into the uterus at the uterine os in the area called the cornu. The cervical os is the opening into the cervix from the vagina.

The uterine tube is another name for the fallopian tube.

51. **(C)** Endometrial ablation is done to treat abnormal uterine bleeding. The overall goal is to create amenorrhea or to reduce menstrual bleeding to normal. It may be an alternative to hysterectomy in some patients with chronic menorrhagia.

52. **(C)** Hysteroscopy is endoscopic visualization of the uterine cavity and tubal orifices. Laparoscopy may be done in association with hysteroscopy to assess the external contour of the uterus.

53. **(D)** True marsupialization of the Bartholin's cyst involves the removal of the anterior wall of the cyst and suturing the cut edges of the remaining cyst to adjacent sides of the skin.

54. **(C)** A Graves self-retaining speculum frequently is known as a duckbill speculum and is used for vaginal and cervical exposure.

55. **(C)** The Candela laser is valuable to disintegrate stones in the urinary tract because it is tunable, and the wavelength can be adjusted. The CO_2, argon, and Nd:YAG are used to treat pelvic endometriosis, cervical dysplasia, condylomata, and premalignant diseases of the vulva and the vagina.

56. **(D)** All of the above are injuries that can occur to a patient in lithotomy position including pressure injuries to the skin, blood vessels, and nerves. It can cause back, knee, and hip pain as well as cardiovascular and respiratory compromise.

57. **(C)** A leiomyoma is a benign smooth muscle tumor of the uterus.

58. **(D)** A low transverse, Pfannenstiel, or midline incision is used to perform a C-section.

59. **(D)** Placental abruption is premature separation of the placenta from the uterine wall after 20 weeks' gestation and before the fetus is delivered.

60. **(C)** During the first stage of the vaginoplasty, a split-thickness skin graft is taken from the buttocks or the thigh.

61. **(B)** A complete abortion is the expulsion of all products of conception. Surgical intervention is not necessary.

62. **(A)** A teratoma is a common ovarian tumor that arises from one of the germ layers of the developing embryo. It may contain hair, teeth, sebaceous material, and skin.

63. **(D)** Eclampsia is also referred to as toxemia. Hypertension can constrict blood flow to the placenta and the fetus.

64. **(A)** The goal of endometrial ablation is the destruction and scarification of the endometrium to render it nonfunctional.

65. **(A)** A laparoscopic-assisted vaginal hysterectomy is removal of the uterus by using a combined laparoscopic and vaginal approach.

66. **(B)** En bloc is a term meaning "in one piece." In surgery, it describes the technique of removing tissue usually performed in a radical hysterectomy.

67. **(D)** The umbilical cord is wrapped one or more times around the fetus's neck. This usually occurs with an active fetus and is seldom diagnosed before labor.

68. **(D)** The uterine ligaments are the broad, cardinal, uterosacral, and round.

69. **(A)** In an ectopic pregnancy, the fertilized egg implants itself outside the uterus. The fallopian tube is a common site of an ectopic pregnancy.

70. **(A)** A laparoscopic removal of the ectopic pregnancy would be performed.

71. **(C)** The patient is placed in supine position and prepped and draped for a laparotomy.

72. **(C)** A salpingostomy is an incision into the tube to remove the embryo while preserving the tube for future pregnancy.

73. **(A)** The tube is grasped with a Babcock, which is an atraumatic forceps.

74. **(C)** Risk factors of an ectopic pregnancy include a previous history of a PID, smoking, previous tubal surgery, and history of sexually transmitted disease.

75. **(C)** To test tubal patency, methylene blue or indigo carmine in a saline solution is introduced into the uterine cavity. The tubes are viewed through a laparoscope. Dye seen coming from one or both tubes indicates patency.

76. **(D)** The abnormal tissue coated with acetic acid will turn white. The abnormal tissue stained with Lugol's solution will not take on the brown color of the solution. It will remain unchanged.

77. **(A)** After the cervix is dissected and amputated from the vagina, the uterus is then removed. Potentially contaminated instruments used on the cervix and vagina are placed in a discard basin and removed from the field (sponge sticks and suction as well).

CHAPTER 20

Ophthalmology

- Conjunctiva—a thin transparent membrane that lines the surface of the eyelids and covers the sclera
- Globe—eyeball
- Cornea—a transparent window through which light passes to the retina; this is where images are focused
- Bony orbit—the two orbital cavities; they contain the globe (eyeball)
- Sclera—the white part of the external globe
- Lens—the lens changes shape and allows the eye to focus
- Retina—the photoreceptive layer of the eye
- Color blindness is caused by a defect in the retina
- There are six muscles that function to move the eye
- Block—retrobulbar (this block is performed directly into the base of the eyelids or into the back of the globe of the eye)
- Miotic drugs—constrict the pupil. Examples include:
  - Miochol—you must reconstitute immediately before using and must be used within 15 minutes
  - Pilocarpine
  - Miostat
- Mydriatics—dilate the pupil but allow the pupil to focus. Examples include:
  - Neo-Synephrine
  - Atropine
- Cycloplegics—dilate the pupil but inhibit focusing. Examples include:
  - Atropine (anticholinergic—nerve-blocking agent)
  - Epinephrine
- Topical anesthetics—a topical anesthetic is used to numb the surface of the eye. Examples include:
  - Tetracaine hydrochloride—Pontocaine
- Injectable anesthetics—an anesthetic that can be injected under/into the eye. Example includes:
  - Lidocaine
- Additives to local anesthesia—these medications combined with anesthetics can help to prolong the effects of the anesthesia, help to reduce bleeding, and increase diffusion. Examples include:
  - Epinephrine—prolongs the effect and reduces bleeding
  - Hyaluronidase—Wydase
    - Increases diffusion (the movement of particles from high concentration to low concentration (it spreads the medication quicker and more evenly)
    - Also used as a lubricant to help separate tissues before removal of the lens
- Viscoelastics—these drugs lubricate and maintain a separation between tissues. Examples include:
  - Healon
  - Provisc
  - Viscoat—used to coat the lens before implantation
- Irrigants—used to keep the cornea moist during surgery. Example includes:
  - BSS—balanced salt solution
- Anti-inflammatory agents—used to treat inflammatory and allergic conditions. Examples include:
  - Betamethasone—Celestone
  - Decadron
  - Depo-Medrol

- Antibiotics—infection treatment or prevention. Can be administered as ointments
  - Neomycin
  - Gentamicin
  - Tobramycin
- Anti-inflammatory—prevents swelling. Can be a steroid or a nonsteroidal anti-inflammatory drug (NSAID); controls postoperative inflammation
- Prednisone
- Decadron
- Celestone
- Evisceration—removal of the eye contents, leaving the sclera and attached muscles intact
- Enucleation—removal of the entire eyeball, with its muscle attachments and optic nerve
- Prosthetic implants are made of glass, silicone, and coralline
- Exenteration—removal of the entire orbital contents
- The lacrimal duct system helps to maintain moisture in the eye
- Lacrimal duct dilation—performed for excessive tearing caused by blockage of the duct
- Bowman lacrimal duct probes are used for dilatation; they come in graduated sizes
- Dacryocystorhinostomy—a procedure to relieve blockage of the nasolacrimal duct, which drains tears into the nose. This is performed for chronic dacryocystitis
- Chalazion—an obstruction of the meibomian gland
- Meibomian gland is a sebaceous gland that helps to lubricate the eyelids
- Blepharoplasty—a procedure to correct drooping skin and fat of the upper and lower eyelids (dermatochalasis)
- Pterygium—a benign growth on the nasal side of the conjunctiva
- Strabismus—a condition when eyes are not straight and do not focus on the same object because the muscles are either too long or too short
- Esotropia—cross eyes
- Exotropia—wall eyes
- Recession—this procedure is performed for esotropia (cross eyes)—it weakens the eye muscle by reattaching it further back on the eye
- Resection—this procedure is performed for exotropia (wall eyes)—it strengthens the muscle.

A portion of the muscle (lateral rectus muscle) is made shorter
- Keratoplasty—corneal transplant
- Trephine is an instrument used to make the cylindrical cut in the cornea for the transplant
- The corneal tissue is taken from a human cadaver
- Radical keratotomy—this is performed for myopia (nearsightedness)
- LASIK surgery—an excimer laser is used to reshape the cornea. This allows the patient to see well at a distance
- Argon/Nd:YAG lasers are commonly used in eye surgery because they are able to pass through clear tissue without heating it up
- Rods and cones are the two types of photoreceptor cells located in the fovea centralis in the macula located in the retina
- The macula is the distinct area of acute vision in the eye. Along with the macula, the fovea is a pit located in the macula. It provides the clearest vision. Rods are responsible for vision of shades of gray, black, and white
- Cones are responsible for distinguishing color
- Accommodation—ability of the lens to change its shape to maintain focus on an object
- Focal point—area where light rays converge after passing through the lens
- Refraction is the bending of light rays as they enter and pass through a transparent membrane in the front of the eye
- Zonules—fibrous strands that form a band. It connects the ciliary body with the lens of the eye
- A bridle suture is a traction suture used on the globe of the eye, specifically the superior rectus muscle to rotate the eye downward for ophthalmic procedures. It is called this because it resembles the reins of a horse's bridle
- There are six extrinsic muscles that control eye movement. They are referred to as extrinsic because they originate outside the eyeball on the surface. They include superior rectus, inferior rectus, lateral rectus, medial rectus, superior oblique, and inferior oblique.
- Cornea—the cornea refracts light (bends light) and allows images to be focused on the retina. It is avascular. It consists of five layers. They include corneal epithelium (outermost layer), Bowman's layer (second layer), corneal stroma

(third layer), Descemet's membrane (fourth layer), and corneal endothelium (innermost layer)

- Lacrimal canaliculus—the mucosal ducts through which tears drain from the eye into the nasolacrimal sac. They are located in the medial area of the eye where tears drain. Most eyelid lacerations are due to trauma
- Laceration of the lacrimal canaliculus—a Veirs rod is used to keep the eye open without obstructing the surgical field. Nonabsorbable suture is used for the repair

Questions

1. In cataract surgery, a viscoelastic drug sometimes used to occupy space in the posterior cavity of the eye is:

   (A) alpha-chymotrypsin
   (B) mannitol
   (C) Healon
   (D) Wydase

2. An example of a miotic drug is:

   (A) pilocarpine
   (B) homatropine
   (C) atropine
   (D) scopolamine

3. What topical anesthetic is used most frequently for preoperative ocular instillation?

   (A) Lidocaine
   (B) Tetracaine
   (C) Cocaine
   (D) Dorsacaine

4. The drug added to a local ophthalmic anesthetic to increase diffusion is:

   (A) alpha-chymotrypsin
   (B) hyaluronidase
   (C) epinephrine
   (D) varidase

5. A solution used for eye irrigation is:

   (A) phenylephrine HCl
   (B) normal saline
   (C) alpha-chymotrypsin
   (D) balanced salt solution

6. A synthetic local anesthetic that is effective on the mucous membrane and is used as a surface agent in ophthalmology is:

   (A) Miochol
   (B) Zolyse
   (C) dibucaine
   (D) tetracaine

7. Dilating eye drops are called:

   (A) mydriatics
   (B) miotics
   (C) myopics
   (D) oxytocics

8. Which of the following uses ultrasonic energy to fragment the lens in extracapsular cataract extraction?

   (A) Keratome
   (B) Ocutome
   (C) Cystotome
   (D) Phacoemulsifier

9. A chalazion is a chronic inflammation of the:

   (A) lacrimal gland
   (B) meibomian gland
   (C) eyelid
   (D) conjunctiva

10. What procedure is done for chronic dacryocystitis?

    (A) Extirpation
    (B) Lacrimal duct probing
    (C) Myomectomy
    (D) Dacryocystorhinostomy

11. A procedure to treat retinal detachment is:

    (A) scleral buckle
    (B) trabeculectomy
    (C) goniotomy
    (D) vitrectomy

12. Sagging and eversion of the lower lid is:

    (A) entropion
    (B) blepharitis
    (C) ectropion
    (D) ptosis

13. Removal of the entire eyeball is:

    (A) keratoplasty
    (B) exenteration
    (C) enucleation
    (D) evisceration

14. Which piece of equipment is used to treat glaucoma in addition to the slit lamp?

    (A) Argon or Nd:YAG laser
    (B) Cavitron
    (C) Phacoemulsifier
    (D) Cryoprobe

15. Removal of a portion of an ocular muscle with reattachment is called:

    (A) recession
    (B) resection
    (C) strabismus
    (D) myomectomy

16. Opacity of the vitreous humor is treated by performing a:

    (A) cataract removal
    (B) scleral buckling procedure
    (C) vitrectomy
    (D) goniotomy

17. Miochol solution is prepared for a cataract procedure no more than _____ minutes before the actual instillation.

    (A) 5
    (B) 15
    (C) 30
    (D) 60

18. A drug used as a lubricant and as viscoelastic support to maintain separation of tissues before removal of lens during cataract surgery is:

    (A) 5-fluorouracil
    (B) Healon
    (C) mitomycin
    (D) Miostat

19. A drug used to contract the sphincter of the iris during an intracapsular cataract extraction is:

    (A) Zolyse
    (B) Healon
    (C) Miochol
    (D) mitomycin

20. What procedure accomplishes correction of myopia?

    (A) Keratoplasty
    (B) Keratophakia
    (C) Radical keratotomy
    (D) Both B and C

21. An enzymatic drug commonly used with anesthetic solutions to increase tissue diffusion is:

    (A) Viscoat
    (B) epinephrine
    (C) Ophthaine
    (D) Wydase

22. Injection of anesthetic solution into the base of the eyelids or behind the eyeball to block the ciliary ganglion and nerves is known as:

    (A) retrobulbar
    (B) van Lint block
    (C) O'Brien akinesia
    (D) Bier block

23. A fleshy, triangular encroachment onto the cornea is surgically termed a/an:

    (A) pterygium
    (B) chalazion
    (C) ectropion
    (D) entropion

24. A procedure performed when the cornea is thickened or opacified is called a:

    (A) keratomileusis
    (B) keratotomy
    (C) corneal trephining
    (D) keratoplasty

25. What is the procedure used to correct accidental vitreous loss during a cataract extraction?

    (A) Posterior vitrectomy
    (B) Anterior vitrectomy
    (C) Pars plana vitrectomy
    (D) All of the above

26. A surgical treatment for chronic wide angle-closure glaucoma that reestablishes communication between the posterior and anterior chamber of the eye is:

    (A) iridectomy
    (B) Elliot trephination
    (C) cyclodialysis
    (D) posterior lid sclerectomies

27. What eye disease is treated using the argon slit lamp with a noninvasive procedure, which, if successful, prevents the need for more invasive surgery?

    (A) Cataract
    (B) Retinal detachment
    (C) Glaucoma
    (D) Pterygium

28. Removal of the entire contents of the orbit is:

    (A) exenteration
    (B) enucleation
    (C) evisceration
    (D) orbitectomy

29. A technique used for retinal detachment that involves a cold probe is:

    (A) nitro therapy
    (B) diathermy
    (C) cryothermy
    (D) cryodermy

30. Keratoplasty involves surgery of the:

    (A) eyelid
    (B) cornea
    (C) iris
    (D) retina

31. The photoreceptive layer of the eye is:

    (A) choroid
    (B) cornea
    (C) iris
    (D) retina

32. The gel-like substance that fills the posterior chamber and nourishes the tissue layers is:

    (A) vitreous humor
    (B) aqueous humor
    (C) conjunctiva
    (D) Healon

33. A condition caused by inadequate drainage of aqueous humor is:

    (A) retinal detachment
    (B) glaucoma
    (C) entropion
    (D) cataract

34. Inflammation or infection of the lacrimal sac is:

    (A) iritis
    (B) uveitis
    (C) conjunctivitis
    (D) dacryocystitis

35. When using an anticholinergic, such as atropine, during eye surgery, the pupils will:

    (A) dilate
    (B) constrict
    (C) not be affected
    (D) none of the above

36. Drugs that dilate the pupil but permit focusing are:

    (A) cycloplegics
    (B) mydriatics
    (C) anesthetics
    (D) viscoelastics

37. A transparent structure that permits the eye to focus rays to form an image on the retina is the:

    (A) sclera
    (B) retina
    (C) cornea
    (D) lens

38. The purpose of the iris is to:

    (A) regulate the amount of light entering the eye
    (B) protect the iris
    (C) supply the choroid with nourishment
    (D) receive images

39. The structure that is seen from the outside as the colored portion of the eye is the:

    (A) cornea
    (B) pupil
    (C) retina
    (D) iris

40. The nerve that carries visual impulses to the brain is the:

    (A) ophthalmic nerve
    (B) optic nerve
    (C) oculomotor nerve
    (D) trochlear nerve

41. The white outer layer of the eyeball is the:

    (A) conjunctiva
    (B) sclera
    (C) choroid
    (D) retina

42. A jelly-like substance in the eye's posterior cavity is called:

    (A) choroid
    (B) palpebra
    (C) vitreous humor
    (D) aqueous humor

43. The conjunctiva is the:

    (A) colored membrane of the eye
    (B) covering of the anterior globe except the cornea
    (C) gland that secretes tears
    (D) membrane lining the socket

44. Color blindness is caused by a defect in the:

    (A) cones in the retina
    (B) sclera
    (C) iris
    (D) lens

45. The function of the lacrimal duct system is to:

    (A) provide drainage of the meibomian gland
    (B) prevent pterygium
    (C) help the eyes to focus
    (D) help to maintain moisture in the eye

46. Bauman lacrimal duct probes are used:

    (A) for dilatation
    (B) to make a cylindrical cut on a keratoplasty
    (C) to measure intraocular pressure
    (D) none of the above

47. When the eyes do not focus on the same object, this condition is called:

    (A) extropia
    (B) recession
    (C) strabismus
    (D) astigmatism

48. Recession is performed for:

    (A) esotropia
    (B) extropia
    (C) obstruction of meibomian gland
    (D) obstruction of the nasolacrimal duct

49. During a resection, the muscle that is shortened to treat wall eyes is the:

    (A) inferior oblique
    (B) lateral rectus muscle
    (C) levator
    (D) superior oblique

50. All apply to a trephine EXCEPT:

    (A) used to measure intraocular pressure
    (B) used to make the cylindrical cut in the corner
    (C) used on a cadaver
    (D) used on a keratoplasty

51. What photoreceptive cells found in the retina are responsible for vision in dim light and for vision of shades of gray, black, and white?

    (A) cones
    (B) rods
    (C) lens
    (D) anterior chamber of the eye

52. What laser is commonly used for LASIK surgery?

    (A) Excimer
    (B) Argon
    (C) Nd:YAG
    (D) CO_2

53. Removal of the eye contents leaving the sclera and muscle intact is:

    (A) enucleation
    (B) evisceration
    (C) exenteration
    (D) corneal transplant

54. Removal of the entire eyeball including muscles and nerves is called:

    (A) enucleation
    (B) exenteration
    (C) evisceration
    (D) corneal transplant

55. All are true regarding exenteration EXCEPT:

    (A) removal of entire orbital contents
    (B) removal of external structures of the eye
    (C) removal of the globe only
    (D) performed for malignancy

56. The fluid that fills the anterior and posterior chamber of the eye is:

    (A) aqueous humor
    (B) vitreous humor
    (C) both A and B
    (D) none of the above

57. All are true of the canal of Schlemm EXCEPT:

    (A) it drains aqueous humor from the anterior chamber
    (B) if blocked, it can cause glaucoma
    (C) it is located between the lens and the retina
    (D) it is located in the anterior chamber

58. All are procedures to treat glaucoma EXCEPT:

    (A) goniotomy
    (B) cyclodialysis
    (C) iridectomy
    (D) scleral buckle

59. Following a vitrectomy, the vitreous humor is removed and replaced with:

    (A) saline
    (B) gas
    (C) both A and B
    (D) water

60. A mydriatic drug, Neo-Synephrine, is used to:

    (A) constrict the pupil
    (B) dilate the pupil
    (C) anesthetize the eye
    (D) lower intraocular pressure

61. Immobility of the eye and lowered intraocular pressure are facilitated by the use of:

    (A) Diprivan block
    (B) Versed block
    (C) xylocaine block
    (D) retrobulbar block

62. Miochol is a/an:

    (A) antihistamine
    (B) blood thinner
    (C) miotic
    (D) anti-inflammatory

63. An agent that keeps the cornea moist during surgery and is used for irrigation as well is:

    (A) mannitol
    (B) Miochol
    (C) Chymar
    (D) BSS

64. Perfluoropropane and sulfur hexafluoride are used in a scleral buckling procedure in conjunction with a vitrectomy to:

    (A) provide a retinal tamponade
    (B) maintain pressure on the retina
    (C) prevent adhesions in the retina
    (D) both A and B

65. The ability of the lens to change its shape to maintain focus on an object is termed:

    (A) focal point
    (B) refraction
    (C) accommodation
    (D) visual optic axis

66. The lens is a biconvex transparent capsule that is held in place by:

    (A) zonules
    (B) suspensory ligaments
    (C) eye muscles
    (D) both A and B

67. A triangular fleshy vascular growth on the nasal side of the conjunctiva is termed:

    (A) pterygium
    (B) chalazion
    (C) esotropia
    (D) ptosis

68. For a keratoplasty procedure, the cornea is harvested from:

    (A) live donor
    (B) cadaver donor
    (C) a portion of the cornea from the other eye
    (D) all of the above

69. The instrument used to make a cylindrical cut into the cornea for transplantation is termed:

    (A) phacoemulsifier
    (B) cryoprobe
    (C) trephine
    (D) tonometer

70. What is the name for the traction suture used on the globe of the eye, specifically, the superior rectus muscle to rotate the eye downward for ophthalmic procedures?

    (A) Retention
    (B) Bridle
    (C) Purse-string
    (D) Locking

71. What is the term for the condition caused by an irregular shaped cornea or lens?

    (A) Astigmatism
    (B) Cataract
    (C) Blindness
    (D) Strabismus

72. What instrument is used to measure the curve of the cornea?

    (A) Keratometer
    (B) Caliper
    (C) Trephine
    (D) Ruler

73. The area between the cornea and the iris that contains aqueous humor is termed:

    (A) vitreous body
    (B) anterior chamber
    (C) posterior chamber
    (D) posterior body

74. How many eye muscles control eye movement?

    (A) Two
    (B) Four
    (C) Five
    (D) Six

75. All apply to eye sutures except:

    (A) double-armed sutures are commonly used in eye surgery
    (B) a spatula and reversed cutting needle are commonly used in eye surgery
    (C) a 10-0 is a common suture size used in a corneal transplant
    (D) the sclera is always closed on an extra-capsular cataract

76. The cornea is composed of how many layers?

    (A) Two
    (B) Three
    (C) Five
    (D) Six

77. When performing an extracapsular cataract extraction with an intraocular lens implant, the lens is removed by using ultrasonic waves/vibration to fragment/emulsify the lens. This is called:

    (A) cryoprobe
    (B) phacoemulsification
    (C) hydrodissection
    (D) diathermy

78. At the end of a posterior capsulectomy, if the surgeon is having difficulty closing sclerotomies, which medication could the surgeon request?

    (A) Viscot
    (B) Hyaluronidase
    (C) Prednisolone
    (D) Mannitol

79. For laceration of the lacrimal canaliculus, what instrument is used to keep the eye open and not obstruct the surgical procedure?

    (A) Speculum
    (B) Retractor
    (C) Lid forceps
    (D) Veirs rod

80. What technique uses a laser to treat diabetic retinopathy?

    (A) Slit lamp
    (B) Endophotocoagulation
    (C) Photoemulsification
    (D) Cryotherapy

81. What diagnostic testing is performed for the evaluation of orbital and intracranial abnormalities?

    (A) Magnetic resonance imaging (MRI)
    (B) Computed tomography (CT)
    (C) Ultrasound
    (D) Both A and B

82. When performing microsurgery, the STSR must use the proper techniques when assisting the surgeon. They include:

    (A) prevent any movement of the microscope during surgery
    (B) use proper method of passing instruments by gently placing them in the surgeon's hands
    (C) have knowledge of the surgical procedure and the microscope
    (D) all of the above

83. All are proper techniques of handling the microscope EXCEPT:

    (A) move the microscope by holding the head with two hands
    (B) cover the microscope and its attachments at the end of the day to prevent dust from accumulating
    (C) check the brake and make sure it is locked before surgery
    (D) the microscope must be adjusted to the surgeon's and assistant's eyesight before surgery

Answers and Explanations

1. **(C)** Sodium hyaluronate (Healon) is a viscous jelly sometimes used to occupy space and prevent damage when opening the anterior capsule.

2. **(A)** Pilocarpine is a miotic. A miotic causes the pupil to contract.

3. **(B)** Tetracaine provides rapid, brief, and superficial anesthesia. It is widely used as a local ocular anesthetic. It is the generic name for Pontocaine.

4. **(B)** Hyaluronidase is commonly added to an anesthetic solution. This enzyme increases diffusion of the anesthetic through the tissue, thereby improving the effectiveness of the block.

5. **(D)** Balanced salt solution is an eye irrigant. It is used to keep the eye moist during surgery. It is supplied in a sterile solution.

6. **(D)** Tetracaine produces surface anesthesia in eye surgery and is available in a 0.5% concentration for this use. Pontocaine is the trade name for this topical solution.

7. **(A)** Mydriatics dilate the pupil while allowing the patient to focus. A cycloplegic drug also can dilate the pupil, but it disturbs focusing ability.

8. **(D)** In extracapsular extraction, the phacoemulsifier is used in a microsurgical technique to remove the lens. Ultrasonic energy fragments the hard lens, which can then be aspirated from the eye.

9. **(B)** Removal of a chalazion is the incision and curettage of a chronic granulomatous inflammation of one or more of the meibomian glands of the eyelid.

10. **(D)** Chronic dacryocystitis in adults requires dacryocystorhinostomy to establish a new tear passageway for drainage directly into the nasal cavity to correct deficient drainage with overflow of tears.

11. **(A)** A scleral buckling is the operative treatment for retinal detachment. The procedure is aimed at preventing permanent vision loss by sealing off the area in which a hole or tear is located.

12. **(C)** Ectropion is the sagging and eversion of the lower lid. It is common in older patients and is corrected by a plastic surgery procedure that shortens the lower lid in a horizontal direction.

13. **(C)** Enucleation is removal of the eyeball/globe. Evisceration is removal of the eye contents, leaving the sclera and muscles intact. Exenteration is an extensive surgical procedure requiring removal of the entire contents of the orbit. This includes the eyeball, eyelids, muscles, nerves, and surrounding tissue. Keratoplasty is performed for corneal transplantation.

14. **(A)** Argon or Nd:YAG laser therapy is used to treat acute (angle-closure) glaucoma and open-angle glaucoma. It is uncomplicated and utilizes a slit lamp for laser beam delivery. It is noninvasive and a fairly uncomplicated outpatient procedure.

15. **(B)** Resection of part of the ocular muscle rotates the eye toward the functional muscle and is reattached. This strengthens it.

16. **(C)** In its normal state, the vitreous gel of the eye is transparent. In certain disease states, it becomes opaque and must be removed.

17. **(B)** Miochol solution is used to constrict the pupil to prevent vitreous loss during a cataract extraction. The Miochol solution must be used within 15 minutes after preparation. If complications arise, new solution should be prepared.

18. **(B)** Healon functions as a lubricant and as a viscoelastic support maintaining a separation of tissues. It is used in intraocular procedures to protect the corneal epithelium and as a tamponade.

19. **(C)** After the lens is removed slowly from the eye, the pupil is constricted with Miochol or Miostat if an intraocular lens (IOL) is to be inserted.

20. **(C)** Radial keratotomy is the procedure used to correct myopia. Keratoplasty and keratophakia are procedures used to reshape the cornea with the use of donor corneal tissue.

21. **(D)** Wydase, also referred to as hyaluronidase, is an enzyme that increases tissue diffusion and effectiveness of nerve blocks during ophthalmology procedures.

22. **(A)** Retrobulbar anesthesia is an injection of anesthetic solution into the base of the orbital margins or behind the eyeball to block the ciliary ganglion and nerves.

23. **(A)** Pterygium is a fleshy, triangular encroachment onto the cornea and tends to be bilateral. When a pterygium encroaches on the visual axis, it is removed surgically.

24. **(D)** A corneal transplant is grafting of corneal tissue from one human eye to another. This is known as keratoplasty and is performed when one's cornea is thickened or opaque because of disease or injury.

25. **(B)** Vitreous humor may accidentally enter the anterior cavity of the eye if a miotic drug is not used during surgery. A vitreous catheter is placed through the cataract wound to remove vitreous humor and not allow it to fill the anterior chamber. It is then constricted with acetylcholine.

26. **(A)** All of the procedures treat glaucoma. Iridectomy provides a communication between the anterior and posterior chambers to relieve intraocular pressure.

27. **(C)** Argon or Nd:YAG laser therapy is being used to treat acute and open angle glaucoma. It is a noninvasive procedure and may, if successful, prevent more invasive procedures.

28. **(A)** Exenteration is an extensive surgical procedure requiring removal of the entire contents of the orbit. This includes the eyeball, eyelids, muscles, nerves, and surrounding tissue. Enucleation is removal of the eyeball/ globe. Evisceration is removal of the eye contents, leaving the sclera and muscles intact.

29. **(C)** Cryothermy is a technique in which a cold probe is used to freeze tissue such as sclera, ciliary body, or retinal detachment.

30. **(B)** Keratoplasty is surgery of the cornea. The term penetrating keratoplasty refers to corneal transplantation.

31. **(D)** The innermost layer of the posterior globe is called the retina. The retina is the posterior receptive layer of the eye. It records and transmits images to the brain via the optic nerve.

32. **(B)** Aqueous humor fills the anterior and posterior chambers of the eye.

33. **(B)** Glaucoma is a disease characterized by optic nerve and visual field damage usually caused by inadequate drainage of aqueous humor.

34. **(D)** Dacryocystitis is an infection of the lacrimal sac in the inner corner of the eye. Iritis is an infection of the iris (colored portion of the eye). Uveitis is an infection of the uvea (middle layer of the eye beneath the sclera), and conjunctivitis is an infection of the conjunctiva (clear membrane that covers the front surface of the eye).

35. **(A)** Anticholinergics dilate the pupil and inhibit focusing.

36. **(B)** Mydriatics are drugs that dilate the pupil and permit focusing.

37. **(D)** The lens is a transparent, colorless structure in the eye that is biconvex in shape. It is enclosed in a capsule. It is capable of focusing rays so that they form a perfect image on the retina.

38. **(A)** The purpose of the iris is to regulate the amount of light entering the eye. The pupil is the contractile opening in the center of the eye.

39. **(D)** The iris is a thin, muscular diaphragm that is seen from the outside as the colored portion of the eye.

40. **(B)** The optic nerve carries visual impulses received by the rods and cones in the retina to the brain. This is the second cranial nerve.

41. **(B)** The eyeball has three separate coats or tunics. The outermost layer is called the sclera and is made of firm, tough connective tissue. It is known as the white of the eye.

42. **(C)** Vitreous humor helps maintain the eye's conical shape and assists in focusing light rays. The posterior cavity lies between the lens and the retina and contains a jelly-like substance called vitreous humor, which helps prevent the eyeball from collapsing.

43. **(B)** Conjunctiva is the mucous membrane that lines the eyelids and covers the anterior surface of the globe, except for the cornea. It is reflected onto the eyeball.

44. **(A)** Color blindness is caused by a defect in the cones of the retina. Sclera is the white part of the eye. The iris contains the color of the eye. The lens allows the eye to focus.

45. **(D)** The lacrimal duct system moistens the eye. The meibomian gland is a sebaceous gland at the rim of the eyelids. The lens helps the eye to focus.

46. **(A)** These probes are used for dilatation. The instrument used to make the cylindrical cut in the keratoplasty is a trephine. The instrument used to measure intraocular pressure is a tonometer.

47. **(C)** Strabismus is when the eyes are not straight and cannot focus on the same object because the muscles are either too long or too short. Extropia is wall eyes. Recession is when the muscle is detached from the surface of the eye and reattached further back. Astigmatism is an irregularly shaped cornea and causes blurred and distorted vision.

48. **(A)** Esotropia requires a resection to fix crossed eyes. Extropia is wall eyes and requires a resection. Obstruction of meibomian gland is a chalazion. Obstruction of the nasolacrimal duct is a blockage of the duct.

49. **(B)** The lateral rectus muscle is shortened to treat wall eyes. The inferior oblique muscle pulls the eye upward and laterally. The levator is the muscle of the upper eyelid. The superior oblique muscle internally rotates the eye.

50. **(A)** A tonometer is used to measure intraocular pressure. A trephine is used to make a cylindrical cut on a cadaver for a keratoplasty.

51. **(B)** The rods and cones are the photoreceptive cells found in the retina responsible for vision at low levels of light. Rods are responsible for vision of shades of gray, black, and white. Cones are responsible for distinguishing color.

52. **(A)** The excimer laser is used for LASIK surgery. The argon laser is used for glaucoma.

The Nd:YAG is commonly used in cataract surgery and acute angles glaucoma. The CO_2 laser is used in other specialties.

53. **(B)** Evisceration is removal of the eye contents, leaving the sclera and muscles intact. Enucleation is removal of the eyeball/globe. Exenteration is an extensive surgical procedure requiring removal of the entire contents of the orbit. This includes the eyeball, eyelids, muscles, nerves, and surrounding tissue. The correct terminology for a corneal transplant is a keratoplasty.

54. **(C)** Evisceration is removal of the eye contents, leaving the sclera and muscles intact. Enucleation is removal of the eyeball/globe. Exenteration is an extensive surgical procedure requiring removal of the entire contents of the orbit. This includes the eyeball, eyelids, muscles, nerves, and surrounding tissue. The correct terminology for a corneal transplant is a keratoplasty.

55. **(C)** Exenteration is performed for malignancy. It is an extensive surgical procedure requiring removal of the entire contents of the orbit including the external structures of the eyeball (eyelids, muscles, nerves, and surrounding tissue). Enucleation is the procedure performed for removal of the globe only.

56. **(A)** Aqueous humor fills the anterior and posterior chamber of the eye. Vitreous humor is in the vitreous body.

57. **(C)** The canal of Schlemm is a circular channel and is located at the base of the cornea. It drains aqueous humor from the anterior chamber of the eye and can cause glaucoma when blocked. The vitreous body is located between the lens and the retina.

58. **(D)** A scleral buckle is performed to treat a detached retina.

59. **(C)** The vitreous body can be filled only with saline solution and/or gas to help retain the shape of the eyeball.

60. **(B)** Neo-Synephrine dilates the pupil.

61. **(D)** A retrobulbar block results in a quiet eye and also immobility of the eye and lowered intraocular pressure.

62. **(C)** Miochol is a miotic used to constrict the pupil. It reduces intraocular pressure and, in cataract surgery, helps prevent the loss of the vitreous.

63. **(D)** Balanced salt solution is used to keep the cornea moist during surgery and also is an irrigant for the anterior or posterior segment.

64. **(D)** Perfluoropropane and sulfur hexafluoride are two types of gas used in a scleral buckle procedure in conjunction with a vitrectomy to provide a tamponade (pressure on the retina). This provides traction on the retina and prevents further tearing.

65. **(C)** Accommodation is the ability of the lens to change its shape to maintain focus on an object. Focal point is the area where light rays converge after passing through the lens. Refraction is the bending of light rays as they enter and pass through a transparent membrane in the front of the eye.

66. **(D)** The lens is a biconvex transparent capsule held in place by the suspensory ligaments called zonules. They are fibrous strands that form a band. The band connects the ciliary body with the lens of the eye.

67. **(A)** Pterygium is a triangular fleshy vascular growth on the nasal side of the conjunctiva. Chalazion is an inflammatory lump on the eyelid caused by a blocked meibomian gland (sebaceous gland/oil gland). Esotropia is the term used for crossed eyes. Ptosis is a drooping of the upper eyelid commonly found in children.

68. **(B)** The corneal transplant tissue for a keratoplasty procedure is harvested from a cadaver donor. It is considered allograft tissue.

69. **(C)** A trephine is an instrument used to make a cylindrical cut in the cornea. A cryoprobe is

an instrument used to destroy or remove tissue by using extreme cold temperatures by applying a probe to the tissue. A tonometer measures intraocular pressure.

70. **(B)** A bridle suture is a traction suture used on the globe of the eye, specifically the superior rectus muscle to rotate the eye downward for ophthalmic procedures. It is called this because it resembles the reins of a horse's bridle. Retention sutures are heavy sutures used with bolsters to prevent tension on a primary suture line. A purse-string suture is commonly used for the appendix, and a locking suture is a type of running suture technique where each stitch is locked for increased strength.

71. **(A)** Astigmatism is the inability of the cornea to properly focus an image onto the retina. This is caused by an improperly shaped cornea or lens. The cornea is normally spherically shaped like a baseball, but with astigmatism, the shape can be elliptical like a football, causing blurred vision. Eyeglasses usually correct the vision problem. A cataract is an opacified lens of the eye. Strabismus is the term used for eyes that are not straight and do not focus on the same object. Eyes can turn in or out if the muscles that move the eyes do not work right or if the eyes are not able to focus properly. Blindness is the inability to see.

72. **(A)** A keratometer is an instrument used to measure the curve of the cornea. A caliper is an instrument used for measuring two opposite sides of an object. The Townley caliper is used to measure the acetabular head in hip surgery. The trephine is used to make a cylindrical cut for a corneal transplant. A ruler is used to draw straight lines and to measure distances.

73. **(B)** The area between the cornea and the iris is the anterior chamber. This contains aqueous humor. The posterior chamber of the eye is between the iris and the lens. This contains aqueous humor. The vitreous body is between the lens and the retina; it contains vitreous humor. Both the anterior and posterior chambers are located in the anterior cavity of the eye, and they contain aqueous humor.

74. **(D)** There are six extrinsic muscles that control eye movement. They are referred to as extrinsic because they originate outside the eyeball on the surface. They include superior rectus, inferior rectus, lateral rectus, medial rectus, superior oblique, and inferior oblique.

75. **(D)** Double-armed sutures are commonly used to close circumferential incisions. A spatula and reversed cutting needle are commonly used in eye surgery. A 10-0 is a common suture size used in a corneal transplant. Suture is not always required to close an incision following cataract surgery. It can be left to heal on its own.

76. **(C)** The cornea refracts light (bends light) and allows images to be focused on the retina. It is avascular and consists of five layers. They include corneal epithelium (outermost layer), Bowman's layer (second layer), corneal stroma (third layer), Descemet's membrane (fourth layer), and corneal endothelium (innermost layer).

77. **(B)** Phacoemulsification is the procedure where the lens is fragmented/emulsified by ultrasonic waves, irrigated, and aspirated for an extracapsular cataract extraction. Cryoprobe uses freezing temperatures to destroy or remove tissue. Hydrodissection is performed to mobilize and free up the lens by instilling BSS into the eye with a small cannula and syringe. Diathermy is performed for medical and surgical purposes. It uses electrical current to heat tissue and destroy abnormal cells, and it can also be used for therapeutic purposes.

78. **(D)** Mannitol decreases fluid volume, which will assist in closure following a posterior capsulectomy.

79. **(D)** A Veirs rod is a 10-mm stainless steel rod used to keep the eyelid open when repairing

an eyelid laceration involving the lacrimal canaliculus.

80. **(B)** Endophotocoagulation is a laser technique used to treat diabetic retinopathy. Diabetic retinopathy is a complication of diabetes. This causes damage to the blood vessels in the tissues in the back of the eye. Diabetic retinopathy can cause vision problems and blindness. Endophotocoagulation prevents the growth of new blood vessels that are weak and leak blood.

81. **(D)** MRI and CT scan are used to diagnose abnormalities of the orbital and intracranial structures. Ophthalmic ultrasound is used to measure the density of the eye tissue and detect abnormalities.

82. **(D)** The surgeon must never take his eyes off the surgical field during an eye case to prevent patient injury. The field of vision is magnified and very small, so the STSR must be aware of the procedure, properly passing instruments and the use of the microscope.

83. **(A)** When moving and positioning the microscope for surgery, the STSR must use both hands and hold the vertical column, not the head, of the microscope because holding the head can cause it to tip over. Always make sure it is positioned properly at the height of the surgeon's eyesight, and make sure it is always locked before surgery for patient safety. At the end of the day, the microscope should be covered to prevent any dust and/or debris from accumulating on it.

CHAPTER 21

Otorhinolaryngology

UPPER FACIAL FRACTURES

- The frontal bone is formed by the forehead and the upper part of the orbits and also contains the frontal sinus. A fracture in this area is called displaced frontal fracture—dent in the forehead
  - Orbital floor fracture is also called a blowout fracture. A Le Fort III procedure is performed to correct this type of fracture
  - Corneal eye protectors are used as a covering on the eye
  - Two incisions performed for this procedure include:
    - Subciliary—under the eyelashes
    - Transconjunctival—in the conjunctiva of the inferior eyelid
  - Instruments used for this procedure include:
    - Maxillofacial instruments
    - Small malleable retractors—brain spatula retractors
    - Periosteal elevators
    - #15 blades
- Zygomatic bone is also called the malar bone and cheek bone
  - A zygomatic fracture is commonly repaired with plates and screws and K-wires

MIDFACE FRACTURES

- LE FORT I—this fracture includes the nasal floor, septum, and teeth. It is also called a mustache fracture
- This fracture is repaired with ARCH BARS—MAXILLOMANDIBULAR FIXATION (MMF):
  - Arch bars are used to realign the teeth, mandible, and maxilla

- The arch bars can be left for a few weeks or removed immediately after the procedure as long as the face is stabilized with plates and screws
- A thin metal strip is wired to the teeth and then to each other with stainless steel
- The wire gauge used is 24–26
- The hooks on the arch bars are placed upward on the upper jaw and downward on the lower jaw
- The steel wires are passed and threaded with heavy needle holders
- Standard protocol is to insert the wires clockwise and remove them counterclockwise. In the event of an emergency, where they need to be removed immediately, protocol can be followed
- Wire cutters are kept with the patient at all times in the hospital and when they go home in the case of an emergency
- The STSR should remain sterile and be prepared to perform an emergency tracheostomy if the patient experiences respiratory difficulty
- Instruments used:
  - Arch bars
  - Maxillofacial instruments
  - Small malleable retractors—brain spatula retractors
  - Periosteal elevators
  - #15 blades
- The orbital floor defect is repaired with:
  - Bone grafts (autogenous or synthetic)
  - Nylon sheeting
  - Silastic sheeting
  - Molded metal implants

- LE FORT II—PYRAMID MAXILLARY FRACTURE—(frontal sinus fracture) involves the nasal cavity, hard palate, and orbital rim
  - This fracture can be associated with cerebrospinal fluid leakage and herniation of brain tissue into the nasal sinus
  - Neurosurgeon must be present
- Instruments include:
  - ENT
  - Maxillofacial power equipment
  - Neuro instruments
  - Raney clips are special neuro clips almost like a barrette but that provide a form of retraction and hemostasis
  - The frontal sinuses are checked to see if there is damage to them. Shattered pieces of bone are removed with mosquito clamps. Bone may be gently shaved with a power burr
  - The surgeon will try to enter through existing wounds instead of creating a new incision
- LE FORT III—ORBITAL FLOOR FRACTURE—BLOWOUT FRACTURE—CRANIOFACIAL FRACTURE—discussed above
- MANDIBULAR FRACTURES—repair of facial fractures of the lower jaw
  - Plates, screws, K-wires, power equipment, maxillofacial instruments, and ENT/plastic instruments
  - MMF fixation—arch bars
  - Incision for the open reduction internal fixation (ORIF) can include:
    - Gingival-buccal mucosa
    - Skin over fracture site
  - Periosteal elevators are used to repair the depressed fracture
- MAXILLOMANDIBULAR ADVANCEMENT (MMA)—this is performed to correct deformities of the upper jaw (maxilla) and the lower jaw (mandible) by moving them forward. It is also used to correct:
  - Malocclusion—the upper jaw and lower jaw do not line up properly and cause the teeth to be misaligned
  - It is also used for sleep apnea
- ODONTECTOMY—tooth extraction
  - LABIAL—the side of the mouth/teeth closest to the lips
  - LINGUAL—the tongue
  - BUCCAL—refers to the cheek

- THROAT PACKING—used during an extraction to prevent aspiration and any debris from being swallowed. This packing is part of the surgical count
- TEMPOROMANDIBULAR JOINT (TMJ)—this procedure is performed to reduce pain and increase mobility of the joint, which can cause:
  - Muscle tension
  - Grinding of the teeth
  - Malocclusion
  - Trauma

ENT

- The ear is divided into three parts: the external ear, middle ear, and inner ear
- Hearing is the last sense to disappear when you fall asleep and the first to return when you awaken
- INNER EAR—the inner ear is made up of a series of tunnels called LABYRINTHS. These are responsible for the body's equilibrium. The bony labyrinth consists of the:
  - Cochlea—snail-shaped structure that contains the organ of Corti
- THE MIDDLE EAR—extends from the tympanic membrane to the middle ear. It includes the OSSICLES:
  - Malleus—hammer bone
  - Stapes—stirrup
  - Incus—anvil
  - These bones extend across the middle ear and conduct vibrations from the tympanic membrane through the oval window
- EXTERNAL EAR—the external ear includes:
  - The outer surface of the tympanic membrane
  - AURICLE OR PINNA—outer cartilage of the ear covered by skin
  - The external auditory canal is lined with glands that produce a waxy substance called CERUMEN. It terminates at the tympanic membrane
- The Eustachian tube connects the nasopharynx to the middle ear
- Diagnostic testing for the ear includes:
  - Tuning fork
  - Audiometry
  - Otoscope—lighted instrument used to view the ear canal
  - Computed tomography (CT) scan
  - Magnetic resonance imaging (MRI)

- NASAL ANATOMY—the nose is covered by skin and is made up of bone and cartilage
  - The external nares are the opening into the nose for the passage of air
  - The nostrils and the tip of the nose are made up of ALAR CARTILAGE
  - The SEPTUM separates the two nostrils
  - The roof of the nose is formed by the NASAL BONE
  - The floor is formed by the maxilla and palatine bones
  - The nasal cavity is lined with mucous membranes that aid in warming and humidifying air. The cavity also contains small hairs that help filter out large particles
  - The nasal cavity is connected to the ear by the EUSTACHIAN TUBES
- CHOANAL ATRESIA—a congenital disorder where the passageway between the nose and pharynx is blocked by an abnormal bony tissue that closed during fetal development
  - The procedure performed to repair this defect is CHOANAL ATRESIA REPAIR
  - Instruments include:
    - SMR instrumentation
    - Power drills
    - Microdebrider
    - 30-degree scope
- PARANASAL SINUSES—include:
  - MAXILLARY—paired sinuses below the orbits where the roots of teeth are located
  - FRONTAL—lie behind the lower forehead
  - ETHMOID—are in the roof of the nasal cavity between the lateral wall and the turbinates (on the side of the nose by the eyes)
  - SPHENOID—lie above the ethmoid sinus and below the frontal sinuses
- ANTRUM—opening or a cavity
- ANTROSTOMY—surgical opening into the maxillary sinus performed to drain the sinus due to chronic infection (SINUSITIS)
- ORAL CAVITY—composed of the mouth and the salivary glands
  - The mouth is formed by the cheeks, hard palate, mandible, and tongue
  - The HARD PALATE forms the top of the mouth. It is formed by the maxilla and palatine bones
  - The MANDIBLE AND FLOOR OF THE MOUTH form the lower boundary of the oral cavity

- SALIVARY GLANDS—include:
  - SUBLINGUAL—these glands lie underneath the tongue beneath the mucous membrane on the floor of the mouth and the side of the tongue
  - SUBMANDIBULAR—these glands lie slightly above and slightly below the posterior half of the mandible
    - The submandibular duct is known as WHARTON'S DUCT
- PAROTID—the largest of the salivary glands. It lies below the cheek bone in front of the mastoid process and behind the ramus of the mandible
  - The PAROTID DUCT is known as STENSEN'S DUCT
  - During parotid surgery, it is important to preserve the seventh cranial nerve (facial nerve) and its branches
- PAROTIDECTOMY—this procedure is performed to remove a tumor, treat recurrent parotiditis, and/or treat obstruction of saliva from the parotid gland
  - The incision is made in the upper neck in front of the earlobe
  - You must be careful not to damage the seventh cranial nerve—facial nerve
- PHARYNX—a tubular structure that extends from the nose to the esophagus and is separated into three areas:
  - NASOPHARYNX
  - OROPHARYNX—tonsils are situated on each side of the oropharynx
  - HYPOPHARYNX—LARYNGOPHARYNX
- LARYNX—the larynx has three main functions; these include:
  - Passageway for respiration
  - Prevents aspiration
  - Vibratory source for vocalization
- It is divided into three portions; these are:
  - SUPRAGLOTTIS—upper portion above the true vocal cords
  - GLOTTIS—level of the true vocal cords
  - SUBGLOTTIS—below the true vocal cords
- The larynx consists of nine separate cartilages. Three are stand alone, and six are arranged in pairs; they include:
  - CRICOID
  - THYROID—ADAM'S APPLE
  - EPIGLOTTIS
  - TWO ARYTENOID

- ○ TWO CORNICULATE
- ○ TWO CUNEIFORM
- LARYNGEAL SURGERY—this surgery is performed for diagnostic purposes and/or treatment for malignant/benign tumors
  - ○ It can be performed endoscopically or open
  - ○ The larynx is also called the ADAM'S APPLE
  - ○ Laryngitis is an inflammation of the vocal cords
- LARYNGOSCOPY—this procedure is performed for direct visual examination of the larynx
  - ○ A rigid lighted scope is used (laryngoscope)
- LARYNGECTOMY—performed for partial/total removal of the larynx caused by malignant tumors and trauma to the larynx
  - ○ Once the larynx is removed, the person will breathe out of a permanent opening called a STOMA
  - ○ TOTAL LARYNGECTOMY includes:
    - Complete removal of the larynx
    - Hyoid
    - Strap muscle
  - ○ PARTIAL LARYNGECTOMY includes:
    - Partial removal of the larynx
- LASER SURGERY OF THE LARYNX—CO_2 LASERS, HELIUM, and NITROGEN are used to treat lesions of the larynx and vocal cords
  - ○ The combination of these lasers is used to destroy target tissue at the precise point without damaging surrounding tissue
  - ○ STAINLESS STEEL and COPPER ENDOTRACHEAL TUBES are wrapped with adhesive tape to prevent a fire
  - ○ Wet gauze is placed above the cuff
  - ○ Cloth towels are placed around the surrounding tissue to prevent damaging healthy tissue
- NASOPHARYNGOSCOPE—this is performed with a fiberoptic scope used for visualization of the vocal cords for nodules or polyps, for removal of a foreign body, or to obtain a diagnosis
- TRACHEA—composed of incomplete C-shaped rings of hyaline cartilage
- TRACHEOSTOMY—an opening into the trachea through a midline incision at a point below the cricoid cartilage. It can be temporary or permanent. A cannula is inserted and used to treat upper respiratory obstruction
  - ○ This includes:
    - Chronic lung disease
    - Radical neck procedures
    - Severe edema
    - Vocal cord paralysis
    - Trauma
    - Allergic reactions
- Procedure:
  - ○ Supine position with the neck hyperextended
  - ○ Local—lidocaine with epinephrine
  - ○ #15 blade, blunt dissection with a clamp through the platysma, and strap muscle
  - ○ The trachea is lifted with the trach hook
  - ○ Once the trachea is identified, an #11 blade is used to make a puncture through the second and third tracheal rings
  - ○ 1% lidocaine is injected into the trachea to reduce the coughing reflex as the tube is being inserted. A trach spreader is used to open the incision for visualization
  - ○ The tracheostomy tube is placed
  - ○ The obturator/cannula is removed and the balloon is inflated
  - ○ The tracheostomy tube is immediately suctioned with a catheter
    - The mouth is suctioned with a Yankauer suction
    - The trach is suctioned with a thin flexible catheter
  - ○ Patient is connected to ventilator
- BRONCHOSCOPY—performed to visualize the trachea, bronchi, and lungs. It is also performed for removal of a foreign body and for diagnosis. This procedure can be performed with:
  - ○ FLEXIBLE BRONCHOSCOPE—the patient is given topical anesthesia and is placed in a sitting position
  - ○ RIGID BRONCHOSCOPE—the patient is given general anesthesia and is placed in supine position
- ESOPHAGOSCOPY—direct visualization of the esophagus and stomach
  - ○ This is performed to remove tissue, secretions, tumors, and foreign bodies
  - ○ A RIGID ESOPHAGOSCOPE or GASTROSCOPE is used
- TONSILLECTOMY AND ADENOIDECTOMY (T&A)—this procedure is performed for enlarged infected tonsils. They are made up of lymphoid tissue
  - ○ PHARYNGEAL TONSILS—also known as the ADENOIDS
  - ○ PALATINE TONSILS—known as the TONSILS

- TONSILITIS can be acute or chronic
- Tonsils become infected by the STREPTOCCAL MICROORGANISM
- Procedural instrumentation includes:
  - Davis Mouth Gag or Jennings Mouth Gag—used to hold the mouth open
  - Wieder tongue depressor
  - Robinson catheter—used to retract the uvula. It is inserted through the nose to the throat
  - Tonsils are grasped with a long, curved Allis and extracted with a scalpel, tonsil snare, cautery, scissors, or the COBLATOR
  - COBLATOR—an instrument that uses radiofrequency energy combined with saline to remove the target tissue
  - Adenoids are removed with an adenotome, curettes, and Hurd dissector
  - Yankauer suction tip
  - Hurd dissector
  - Pilar retractor
- The position of the patient following a T&A is lateral with the head of the bed slightly raised
- FACIAL NERVE MONITORING—used during head and neck surgery to identify nerves and prevent damage to them. Important nerves of the head and neck include:
  - FIFTH CRANIAL NERVE—TRIGEMINAL—supplies sensory innervation to the face, oral cavity, nose, nasal cavity, and maxillary sinus
  - SEVENTH CRANIAL NERVE—RIGHT/LEFT FACIAL NERVE—responsible for all the movements of the facial muscles
  - EIGHTH CRANIAL NERVE—VESTIBULOCOCHLEAR—connects the inner ear to the brain
  - TENTH CRANIAL NERVE—VAGUS—important motor nerve of the pharynx and larynx
- MYRINGOTOMY—this procedure is performed for EFFUSION
  - EFFUSION—an abnormal accumulation of fluid between membranes causing ACUTE OTITIS MEDIA
  - OTITIS MEDIA—inflammation of the middle ear with fluid and infection
  - This can also be caused by congenital anomalies that include enlarged adenoids
- An incision is made in the pars tensa of the tympanic membrane with a myringotomy knife
- Fluid is suctioned with a Frazier suction tip, and small hollow tubes are placed
- These tubes are called:
  - PETs—PRESSURE EQUALIZATION TUBES
  - MYRINGOTOMY TUBES
  - TYMPANOSTOMY TUBE
- If left untreated, it can cause hearing loss, delayed language development, and MASTOIDITIS
- MASTOIDITIS—inflammation of the mastoid process of the temporal bone
- PROCEDURE:
  - Microscope and surgeon's loops are used
  - Supine position, head turned and placed in a donut headrest
  - No prep/drape
  - Farrier speculum is inserted into the ear
  - Wax is removed with a cerumen curette
  - Incision with myringotomy blade/knife
  - Tube is placed with an alligator forceps
  - Rosen needle facilitates placement of the tube
  - Antibiotics/steroid drops placed into the ear
  - External ear is packed with cotton
- TYMPANOPLASTY—this procedure is performed to repair the tympanic membrane
  - Membrane commonly injured by trauma
  - Graft is usually taken from the temporalis fascia
  - Drills/microcurettes are used
  - Drills are irrigated with sterile water to prevent heat from the burrs, which can cause damage to surrounding tissues
  - The graft is inserted with alligator forceps
  - Gelfoam packing is used to secure the graft
  - The external ear is packed with gelatin sponge pledgets, which are soaked in epinephrine and antibiotic ointment
- MASTOIDECTOMY—this is performed to remove a diseased portion of the mastoid bone
  - This procedure is performed for the treatment of CHOLESTEATOMA
  - CHOLESTEATOMA—a crystal-encrusted accumulation of squamous epithelium that forms a mass in the cells of the mastoid process
- STAPEDECTOMY—performed to restore the ossicular chain
  - The stapes bone becomes fused which prevents it from vibrating and carrying impulse. One of the main causes of this is OTOSCLEROSIS
  - OTOSCLEROSIS—an abnormal bone growth/hardening of bone that holds the stapes in place

- After a stapedectomy, the patient is instructed to avoid blowing the nose, coughing, sneezing, swimming, and air travel
- Various materials used as prostheses for the stapes include:
  - Stainless steel
  - Platinum
  - Teflon
- Fine hooks in different angles are used to dissect during a stapedectomy
- MENIERE'S DISEASE—a disease of the inner ear with dizziness and TINNITIS
- TINNITUS—buzzing or ringing in one or both ears with progressive hearing loss
- Procedures performed for Meniere's disease include:
  - LABYRINTHECTOMY
  - ENDOLYMPHATIC SAC PROCEDURE
    - VESTIBULAR NEURECTOMY
- LABYRINTH—made up of three compartments; they include:
  - Vestibule
  - Semicircular canals
  - Cochlea
- The principal organs that control equilibrium are the vestibule and semicircular canal
- BELL'S PALSY—an unknown virus that affects the seventh cranial nerve. The seventh cranial nerve controls facial muscles where one side becomes swollen or inflamed. The face feels stiff and can droop, causing your smile to be one sided and preventing your eye from closing properly
  - The procedure performed for the treatment of severe cases of Bell's palsy is FACIAL NERVE DECOMPRESSION—this procedure is performed to relieve compression of the facial nerve (seventh cranial nerve)
    - Trauma
    - Infection
    - Tumors
    - Bell's palsy
- MICROVASCULAR DECOMPRESSION SURGERY—this is performed to prevent a blood vessel from compressing the trigeminal nerve
- ACOUSTIC NEUROMA—VESTIBULAR SCHWANNOMA—slow-growing nonmalignant tumors of the eighth cranial nerve. Treatment includes:
  - Radiation therapy

- Surgery—there are three approaches used:
  - Translabyrinthine approach
  - Suboccipital approach
  - Middle fossa approach
- TRIGEMINAL NEURALGIA—a condition with episodes of facial pain that last from a few seconds to several minutes or hours
- Pain runs along the trigeminal nerve
- This is controlled with medication. Severe cases may require surgery
- COCHLEAR IMPLANTS—this procedure is performed for sensory neural deafness to restore sound perception and to treat deafness
  - Deafness can be either congenital or acquired
  - The primary reason for placing a cochlear implant in a child is to treat congenital deafness
  - The device is implanted in the cochlea with the receiver placed in the mastoid process
  - As the device receives sound through the receiver, it gives off electrical impulses into the cochlea and along the acoustic nerve
  - These impulses are interpreted as sound in the brain. The patient must be taught to interpret these sounds, which requires training
- SUBMUCOUS RESECTION (SMR)—NASOSEPTOPLASTY
  - This procedure is performed when the nasal septum is damaged, deformed, or fractured, causing an obstruction of the sinus opening
  - COCAINE is a topical medication commonly used before nasal surgery and most commonly used in ENT surgery
- A MOUSTACHE DRESSING—used following nasal surgery
  - The nose is packed using bayonet forceps and packing. Tape is placed on the nose and under the nose to block the nasal opening like a moustache
  - Instruments include:
    - BAYONET FORCEPS
    - FREER ELEVATOR
    - COTTLE SPECULUM
    - RASP
    - CHISELS and MALLOT
    - JENSEN–MIDDLETON FORCEPS
- TURBINECTOMY—this procedure is performed to improve nasal air flow. Enlargement of the turbinate causes congestion and rhinorrhea

- RHINORRHEA—persistent discharge of the nose
- CLOSED REDUCTION OF A NASAL FRACTURE—caused by trauma to the midface; usually, both nasal bones are fractured
  - Simple nasal fractures are repaired with local and topical anesthesia
  - A Joseph elevator and the surgeon's hands are used to repair the fracture
  - Nasal packing and a splint are used to stabilize the reduction
- EPISTAXIS—(nose bleed) treatment includes:
  - Direct pressure by squeezing the nasal openings for about 15 minutes
  - For more severe nose bleeds where the patient needs to go to the emergency room, the nose is packed using packing soaked in epinephrine
  - A balloon catheter can also be used to apply pressure to the bleeder
  - In serious cases, the patient may require endoscopic surgery to cauterize and control the bleeding and perhaps to have artery ligation surgery
- FUNCTIONAL ENDOSCOPIC SINUS SURGERY (FESS)
  - This procedure is performed to treat diseases of the paranasal sinuses, nasal cavity, and skull base and to improve nasal air flow
  - Lidocaine with epinephrine is injected
  - Packing with decongestant is inserted in the nose for a few minutes and then removed
  - Scopes used are 0, 30, 70, 90, and 120 degrees
  - Most commonly used scope is the 0 degree
  - Nasal drills
  - Cautery
- FUNCTIONAL ENDOSCOPIC SINUS SURGERY (FESS)—this procedure becomes more difficult if it needs to be repeated a second time because the surgical landmarks have been altered with the first surgery
- ENDOSCOPIC POLYPECTOMY—polyps are benign tumors that grow on a stalk and can be found on mucous membranes
  - The surgeon uses a nasal polyp snare or microdebriders. A morcellator breaks up the polyps into tiny pieces and suctions at the same time
- FRONTAL SINUS TREPHINATION—a small opening is made in the frontal sinus to drain pus and fluid. A drain may be placed for additional drainage
  - The word TREPHINATION indicates a surgical procedure where a hole is drilled or scraped into the skull bone
  - Symptoms are severe headache and fever
- CALDWELL–LUC—WITH RADICAL ANTROSTOMY—this procedure is performed to create an opening into the maxillary sinus for gravity drainage due to infection, polyps, or disease of the maxillary sinus
  - The CALDWELL–LUC is the approach used. The incision is in the CANINE FOSSA
  - CANINE FOSSA—under the upper lip into the gum
- RADICAL NECK DISSECTION—this is performed for squamous cell carcinoma and/or metastatic lesions of the mouth and jaw
  - The structures removed include:
    - Cervical lymph nodes
    - Jugular vein
    - Sternocleidomastoid muscle
  - A trifurcate neck incision is performed
  - This procedure is performed en bloc
  - A Hemovac drain is placed in the wound
  - To repair the mandible, a bone graft can be taken from the fibula
  - Pectoralis major and other muscles are also used for reconstruction

THYROID AND PARATHYROID

- THYROID GLAND—a highly vascular, butterfly/H-shaped GLAND that lies in the anterior portion of the neck at the midline of the trachea
  - It consists of a right and left lobe that are connected by a middle portion called the ISTHMUS
  - The thyroid produces two hormones; these are:
    - Thyroxine—T4
    - Triiodothyronine—T3
  - Thyroid function is controlled by the PITUITARY gland located beneath the brain
  - The PITUITARY GLAND produces a hormone called THYROID-STIMULATING HORMONE (TSH), which stimulates the thyroid to produce T3 and T4
- THYROID ASSESSMENT includes:
  - Palpation of the thyroid

- ○ CT, MRI, ultrasound
- ○ Thyroid scan
- ○ Fine-needle aspiration
- THYROID SCAN—determines the size/shape/position of the gland
  - ○ This procedure is performed in nuclear medicine
  - ○ Radioactive materials called RADIOTRACERS are used, which include:
    - RADIOACTIVE IODINE
    - TECHNETIUM-99M
    - The radiotracers are injected into a vein or ingested and go directly to the thyroid cells
    - The radioactive iodine is given, and a butterfly image appears on the screen showing the outline of the thyroid gland and can determine whether a nodule is considered hot or cold
- NODULE—abnormal growth of thyroid cells that form a mass. They can be hot or cold
  - ○ Hot nodule—shows up darker (absorbs more iodine)
  - ○ Cold nodule—shows up lighter (does not absorb as much iodine)
- HOT NODULES—these nodules absorb the radiotracer and will show up darker on the screen. These are considered to be HOT nodules and function independently. They overproduce the TSH hormone, which can lead to hyperthyroidism
- COLD NODULES—they are hypofunctional or nonfunctional. These nodules appear lighter because they do not absorb the iodine
- GOITER—refers to an enlarged thyroid gland. These can contain nodules, both benign and malignant. It looks like a large lump in the front of the neck
- ULTRASONIC SCAN—this test determines the size, shape, and number of nodules. This procedure also helps when needle placement is required for the FINE-NEEDLE ASPIRATION procedure
- FINE-NEEDLE ASPIRATION—this is the only true diagnostic test currently available to determine thyroid cancer. The procedure is performed under ultrasound guidance. Several samples are taken from the nodule
- HEMITHYROIDECTOMY/UNILATERAL THYROIDECTOMY—removal of one thyroid lobe with excision of the isthmus

- TOTAL THYROIDECTOMY—removal of both lobes of the thyroid and all thyroid tissue. This is performed for thyroid cancer. It is extremely important during thyroid surgery NOT to remove the parathyroid glands
  - ○ If there are lymph nodes present, they are also excised
- GRAVES' DISEASE—this is the most common form of HYPERTHYROIDISM. This is an autoimmune disease that causes the thyroid to secrete excessive amounts of the thyroid hormones. This can result in:
  - ○ A goiter
  - ○ Protruding eyes
  - ○ Palpations
  - ○ Excessive sweating
  - ○ Diarrhea
  - ○ Weight loss
  - ○ Muscle weakness
  - ○ Sensitivity to heat
- HASHIMOTO'S DISEASE—this is a disease caused by HYPOTHYROIDISM causing obstruction of the trachea. Symptoms include:
  - ○ Fatigue and sluggishness
  - ○ Increased sensitivity to cold
  - ○ Constipation
  - ○ Unexplained weight gain
  - ○ Muscle aches
- PARATHYROID GLAND—consists of four small endocrine glands located on the rear surface of the thyroid gland
  - ○ The parathyroid gland produces a hormone called the PARATHYROID HORMONE. This hormone controls the amount of CALCIUM in the blood and the bones
  - ○ Because the parathyroid controls calcium production and absorption, the surgeon must be very careful during thyroid surgery not to accidentally remove any of the parathyroid
- PARATHYROID ASSESSMENT—one of the biggest concerns with parathyroid malfunction is HYPOCALCEMIA
  - ○ HYPOCALCEMIA—lower than normal calcium levels in the blood causing a number of symptoms, including:
    - Muscle weakness/atrophy
    - Back/joint pain
    - Nausea/vomiting/constipation
    - Ulcers
    - Cardiac issues

- TETANY—a disease caused by hypocalcemia
- Laryngeal spasms—a complication the patient having neck procedures may experience. Laryngeal spasms cause respiratory problems. A TRACH SET should always be available and accompany the patient to the postanesthesia care unit (PACU) in the event of an emergency
- THYROID STORM—refers to an acute hyperthyroid period. The thyroid levels have changed drastically for the worse and can be life threatening
- Positioning for thyroid/parathyroid surgery includes:
  - Patient is in supine position
  - Neck is hyperextended
  - Arms are tucked at the side and a shoulder roll is placed
  - Transverse incision/COLLAR INCISION is used
- INSTRUMENTATION/PROCEDURE:
  - The skin flaps are retracted with stay sutures, which are usually silk
  - THE STRAP AND PLATYSMA MUSCLES ARE INCISED WITH A KNIFE
  - THE STERNOCLEIDOMASTOID MUSCLES ARE RETRACTED with a loop retractor or a self-retaining retractor
  - Allis/Lahey clamps are used to grasp the thyroid
  - Moist peanuts are used for blunt dissection
  - Dressings include: Queen Anne's collar, thyroid dressing, and a Jackson–Pratt drain
- It is extremely important to preserve the RECURRENT LARYNGEAL NERVE during thyroid surgery
- NERVE STIMULATOR—this device delivers mild shocks to a part of tissue identifying the nerves before cutting. The recurrent laryngeal nerve is identified using the nerve stimulator

- RECURRENT LARYNGEAL NERVE—this is a branch of the vagus nerve, which is the 10th cranial nerve
  - If there is UNILATERAL damage, the patient will be hoarse
  - If there is BILATERAL damage, the patient may not be able to speak and have difficulty breathing
- THYROGLOSSAL DUCT CYST—congenital cyst found in the neck. The thyroglossal duct is an embryonic structure arising from the thyroid gland into the anterior portion of the neck and forming a cystic pouch
- NECK DISSECTION—this is performed for lymph node metastasis, head and neck cancers, malignant melanoma, or metastasis of the cervical lymph nodes
- Procedure includes:
  - Use of the trifurcate neck incision
  - Patient in supine position
- The classical radical neck dissection encompasses removal of the following structures on one side of the neck:
  - The lymph nodes
  - Carotid artery
  - Vagus nerve.
  - Phrenic nerve
  - Brachial plexus
  - Internal jugular vein
  - Anterior scalene muscle
  - External jugular vein, inferior aspect cut and ligated
  - Hypoglossal nerve
  - Sternocleidomastoid muscle
- GLOSSECTOMY—performed to treat cancer of the tongue, which can be a partial or hemi removal

Questions

1. Which dressing is used after nasal surgery?

   (A) Collodion
   (B) Moustache
   (C) Pressure
   (D) Telfa

2. What combination of lasers is particularly useful in surgery of the larynx and vocal cords?

   (A) CO_2 and argon
   (B) CO_2 and helium–neon
   (C) CO_2 and Nd:YAG
   (D) Argon and helium–neon

3. The most common topical anesthetic agent used in ENT surgery is:

   (A) Xylocaine
   (B) procaine
   (C) cocaine
   (D) Surfacaine

4. Irrigation is used with the ear drill:

   (A) to remove bone fragments
   (B) to minimize transfer of heat from burr to surrounding structures
   (C) to add moisture
   (D) to control bleeding

5. A surgical schedule would describe the procedure to treat acute otitis media as a:

   (A) myringotomy
   (B) stapes mobilization
   (C) fenestration operation
   (D) Wullstein procedure

6. In myringotomy, the tube to facilitate drainage is placed into the tympanic membrane with a/an:

   (A) alligator forceps
   (B) Castroviejo
   (C) wire loop curette
   (D) Tobey forceps

7. A perforated eardrum is corrected by:

   (A) myringotomy
   (B) stapedectomy
   (C) stapedotomy
   (D) tympanoplasty

8. All surgical procedures can be used to treat vertigo associated with Meniere's disease EXCEPT:

   (A) labyrinthectomy
   (B) stapedectomy
   (C) endolymphatic shunt
   (D) vestibular neurectomy

9. Middle ear ventilation is facilitated by:

   (A) antrostomy
   (B) myringotomy
   (C) stapedectomy
   (D) turbinectomy

10. Cholesteatoma is treated by doing a:

    (A) tympanoplasty
    (B) myringotomy
    (C) stapedectomy
    (D) mastoidectomy

11. A benign tumor arising from the eighth cranial nerve, which may grow to a size that produces neurological symptoms, is a/an:

 (A) myoma
 (B) acoustic neuroma
 (C) teratoma
 (D) fibroma

12. Facial nerve trauma can be decreased by use of:

 (A) computerized nerve monitor
 (B) fluoroscopy
 (C) Berman locator
 (D) Doppler

13. Another name for submucous resection is:

 (A) septoplasty
 (B) rhinoplasty
 (C) antrostomy
 (D) trephination

14. Surgical correction of a deviated septum is known as a/an:

 (A) antrostomy
 (B) submucous resection
 (C) rhinoplasty
 (D) turbinectomy

15. A forceps used in nasal surgery is a/an:

 (A) bayonet
 (B) Russian
 (C) rat-tooth
 (D) alligator

16. Which sinus is entered during an intranasal antrostomy (antral window)?

 (A) Ethmoid
 (B) Sphenoid
 (C) Maxillary
 (D) Frontal

17. Nasal polyps are removed with either a polyp forceps or a/an:

 (A) antrum rasp
 (B) Coakley curette
 (C) Freer elevator
 (D) nasal snare

18. Which of the following medications would be used as a topical anesthetic before nasal surgery?

 (A) Numorphan
 (B) Codeine
 (C) Cocaine
 (D) Marcaine

19. Which surgery requires an incision under the upper lip above the teeth?

 (A) Caldwell–Luc
 (B) Submucous resection
 (C) Frontal sinus operation
 (D) Frontal sinus trephination

20. To establish a tracheostomy, a midline incision is created in the neck, below the:

 (A) suprasternal notch
 (B) hyoid bone
 (C) cricoid cartilage
 (D) corniculate cartilage

21. Which medication is found on a tracheostomy setup to reduce the coughing reflex at tube insertion?

 (A) Cocaine 4%
 (B) Lidocaine 1%
 (C) Cocaine 10%
 (D) Lidocaine 10%

22. When a tracheostomy tube is inserted, the obturator is quickly removed and the trachea is suctioned with a:

 (A) catheter
 (B) Frazier
 (C) Poole
 (D) Yankauer

23. The majority of benign salivary gland tumors occur in which gland?

    (A) Sublingual
    (B) Submaxillary
    (C) Parotid
    (D) Submandibular

24. Which position is used following a tonsillectomy?

    (A) Dorsal recumbent
    (B) On side, horizontally
    (C) Reverse Trendelenburg
    (D) Supine

25. Total laryngectomy includes all of the following EXCEPT:

    (A) soft palate
    (B) strap muscles
    (C) hyoid bone
    (D) larynx

26. What type of drain is used for a radical neck dissection?

    (A) T-tube
    (B) Jackson–Pratt drain
    (C) Hemovac drain
    (D) Both B and C

27. A trifurcate neck incision is done for a/an:

    (A) parotidectomy
    (B) submaxillary gland excision
    (C) uvulopalatopharyngoplasty
    (D) radical neck dissection

28. During ear surgery, pledgets generally used to control bleeding are soaked in:

    (A) saline
    (B) heparin
    (C) thrombin
    (D) epinephrine

29. In cochlear implantation, the receiver is placed into which bone of the skull to gather impulses and send it along to the cerebral cortex?

    (A) Parietal
    (B) Mastoid
    (C) Occipital
    (D) Frontal

30. Which of the following endotracheal tubes can prevent a fire?

    (A) Stainless steel
    (B) Silicone
    (C) Latex
    (D) Red rubber

31. Lesions of the larynx and vocal cords can be addressed surgically using which laser?

    (A) Nd:YAG
    (B) Holmium
    (C) CO_2
    (D) Argon

32. Which of the following surgical procedures would require the use of a microscope?

    (A) SMR
    (B) Tracheostomy
    (C) Stapedectomy
    (D) Turbinectomy

33. What is the instrument used to effect removal of the septal cartilage in a rhinoplasty?

    (A) Knight nasal scissor
    (B) Joseph nasal scissor
    (C) Jansen–Middleton forceps
    (D) Freer septum knife

34. After the anterior pillar of a tonsil is incised with a #12 blade, the tonsil is freed from its attachments with a:

    (A) Sluder guillotine
    (B) La Force guillotine
    (C) Hurd dissector
    (D) Boettcher scissors

35. A blockage in Wharton's duct involves the:

(A) parotid gland

(B) submandibular gland

(C) tongue

(D) palatine tonsils

36. What cartilage is commonly known as the Adam's apple?

(A) Thyroid

(B) Cricoid

(C) Hyoid

(D) Auricular

37. What is the visible external portion of the ear?

(A) Auricle

(B) Pinna

(C) Septum

(D) Both A and B

38. Maxillomandibular fixation (MMF) is a procedure used to realign the teeth or to maintain the patient's normal bite position. Which of the following is used during MMF?

(A) Arch bars

(B) Bicoronal plate

(C) Bicortical screw

(D) Plates and screws

39. If arch bars remain in the patient postoperatively, what must be kept with the patient at all times to access the airway in case of emergency?

(A) Endotracheal tube

(B) Nasoendotracheal tube

(C) Wire cutter

(D) Tracheostomy tray

40. What type of facial fracture is associated with the leakage of cerebrospinal fluid into the nasal sinus?

(A) Le Fort I

(B) Le Fort II

(C) Le Fort III

(D) Le Fort IV

41. What is the facial bone that makes up the chin?

(A) Frontal

(B) Zygomatic

(C) Maxilla

(D) Mandible

42. Temporomandibular joint (TMJ) arthroplasty is performed for all of these disorders EXCEPT:

(A) grinding of the teeth

(B) trauma

(C) wisdom teeth

(D) arthritis

43. During a thyroidectomy, the surgeon identifies and preserves which of the following structures?

(A) Recurrent laryngeal

(B) Parathyroid glands

(C) Superior laryngeal

(D) All of the above

44. What is the primary reason for performing a thyroplasty?

(A) Facial nerve paralysis

(B) Unilateral vocal cord paralysis

(C) Goiter

(D) Tumor in the lymph nodes

45. During a parotidectomy, what cranial nerve is carefully elevated and retracted in order to preserve it?

(A) Vagus

(B) Optic

(C) Oculomotor

(D) Facial

46. Epistaxis can be defined as:

(A) gene interaction

(B) bleeding from the nose

(C) congenital urethral defect

(D) extrachromosomal replication

47. The vocal cords are located in the:

    (A) larynx
    (B) pharynx
    (C) windpipe
    (D) trachea

48. The function of the trachea is to:

    (A) conduct air into the larynx
    (B) serve as a pathway for food into the esophagus
    (C) serve as a resonating chamber for speech
    (D) conduct air to and from the lungs

49. The nasal cavity is divided into two portions by the:

    (A) concha
    (B) septum
    (C) ethmoid
    (D) vomer

50. When repairing a simple nasal fracture closed reduction, the surgeon uses:

    (A) his hands and a Boies elevator
    (B) no manipulation just a dressing
    (C) Freer elevator
    (D) Jensen–Middleton

51. The bone located in the neck between the mandible and the larynx that supports the tongue and provides attachment for some of its muscles is the:

    (A) palatine bone
    (B) vomer
    (C) pterygoid hamulus
    (D) hyoid bone

52. The structure that connects the middle ear and the throat, allowing the eardrum to vibrate freely, is the:

    (A) membranous canal
    (B) external auditory canal
    (C) Eustachian tube
    (D) semicircular canal

53. All are treatments for epistaxis EXCEPT:

    (A) direct pressure
    (B) epinephrine and packing
    (C) artery ligation
    (D) Fogarty arterial balloon catheter

54. Which of the following structures transmits sound vibrations from the middle ear to the inner ear?

    (A) Pinna
    (B) Semicircular canal
    (C) Mastoid process
    (D) Ossicles

55. The winding, cone-shaped tube of the inner ear is the:

    (A) vestibule
    (B) semicircular canal
    (C) labyrinth
    (D) cochlea

56. Which of the following is not an auditory ossicle?

    (A) Cochlea
    (B) Stapes
    (C) Incus
    (D) Malleus

57. Why would an aspirated foreign body be more likely to enter the right bronchus rather than the left bronchus?

    (A) The right bronchus is more vertical, shorter, and wider than the left.
    (B) The division of the right bronchus is wider.
    (C) The right bronchus is longer.
    (D) The left bronchus is not in line with the trachea.

58. Adenoids are also called:

    (A) palatine tonsils
    (B) pharyngeal tonsils
    (C) lingual tonsils
    (D) uvula

59. The function of the molar teeth is to:

    (A) tear and crush food
    (B) manipulate food
    (C) help you smile
    (D) There is no function. They are often removed.

60. Mumps occur in the:

    (A) sublingual glands
    (B) submandibular glands
    (C) parotid glands
    (D) thyroid gland

61. All apply to a glossectomy EXCEPT:

    (A) it is performed for cancerous lesions of the tongue
    (B) it is partial or total removal of the tongue
    (C) the tongue can regenerate and partially grow back
    (D) you can still speak without the tongue

62. An orbital floor fracture is also called a:

    (A) blowout fracture
    (B) Le Fort III
    (C) Le Fort II
    (D) both A and B

63. The zygomatic bone is also called the:

    (A) orbit bone
    (B) cheek bone
    (C) chin bone
    (D) jawbone

64. All are true facts regarding MMF EXCEPT:

    (A) the wire gauge commonly used is 24–26
    (B) the steel wires are threaded and twisted with a heavy needle holder
    (C) standard protocol is to insert the wires counterclockwise and remove them clockwise
    (D) the hooks on the arch bars are placed upward on the upper jaw and downward on the lower jaw

65. Maxillomandibular advancement is performed:

    (A) to correct deformities of the upper and lower jaw
    (B) for malocclusion
    (C) for sleep apnea
    (D) all of the above

66. The inside of the mouth is termed _____. The area under the tongue is termed _____. And the space between your teeth and lips and sides of the mouth are _____.

    1. Buccal
    2. Labial
    3. Lingual
    (A) 1, 2, 3
    (B) 3, 2, 1
    (C) 1, 3, 2
    (D) 2, 3, 1

67. The bony labyrinths in the inner ear are responsible for:

    (A) equilibrium
    (B) vibration
    (C) TMJ
    (D) the production of cerumen

68. The external ear terminates at the:

    (A) pars tensa
    (B) ossicles
    (C) tympanic membrane
    (D) cochlea

69. The congenital disorder where the passage between the nose and pharynx is blocked by an abnormal bony tissue that failed to rupture during fetal development is termed:

    (A) dacryocystorhinostomy
    (B) choanal atresia
    (C) SMR
    (D) septoplasty

70. All are paranasal sinuses EXCEPT:

    (A) maxillary
    (B) ethmoid
    (C) nasopharynx
    (D) sphenoid

71. The submandibular duct is also known as:

    (A) Stensen's duct
    (B) parotid duct
    (C) Wharton's duct
    (D) duct of Wirsung

72. The tubular structure that extends from the nose to the esophagus and is separated into three divisions is termed:

    (A) larynx
    (B) pharynx
    (C) esophagus
    (D) epiglottis

73. The part of the larynx where the true vocal cords are located is the:

    (A) supraglottis
    (B) glottis
    (C) subglottis
    (D) cricoid

74. The three incisions or approaches that can be used to remove an acoustic neuroma/vestibular schwannoma are:

    (A) translabyrinthine/middle fossa/suboccipital
    (B) translabyrinthine/suboccipital/mastoid
    (C) transversalis fascia/trifurcate/transsphenoidal
    (D) through ear/under tongue/through back of throat

75. During a T&A, the uvula is retracted with:

    (A) Davis
    (B) Jennings
    (C) Robinson
    (D) coblator

76. The graft used for a tympanoplasty procedure is taken from the:

    (A) middle ear
    (B) pina
    (C) temporalis fascia
    (D) pars tensa

77. All apply to the stapedectomy procedure EXCEPT:

    (A) the stapes bone becomes fused and prevents it from vibrating and carrying an impulse
    (B) otosclerosis is the cause for a stapedectomy
    (C) the prosthesis used for a stapedectomy includes silicone and plastic; stainless steel is contraindicated for use
    (D) fine hooks in various angles are used

78. All are true regarding Meniere's disease EXCEPT:

    (A) it is a disease of the inner ear
    (B) it is a disease of the middle ear
    (C) symptoms include dizziness
    (D) symptoms include tinnitus

79. The virus that affects the seventh cranial nerve and causes stiffness and drooping of one side of the face is termed:

    (A) Bell's palsy
    (B) Meniere's disease
    (C) vestibulitis
    (D) ptosis

80. Slow-growing tumors of the eighth cranial nerve are:

    (A) acoustic neuromas
    (B) vestibular schwannomas
    (C) both A and B
    (D) glioblastoma

81. The procedure performed for sensory neural deafness is:

    (A) trigeminal neuralgia
    (B) cochlear implants
    (C) microvascular decompression
    (D) both A and C

82. The procedure performed to improve nasal airflow caused by congestion and rhinorrhea is:

    (A) rhinoplasty
    (B) SMR
    (C) closed reduction of a nasal fracture
    (D) turbinectomy

83. When performing a functional endoscopic sinus surgery (FESS), it becomes more difficult if a second surgery is needed because:

    (A) you cannot pass the scope through the nose
    (B) hemorrhage is a major consideration
    (C) the surgical landmarks have been altered by performing the first procedure
    (D) the nose can be easily broken by the endoscope the second time

84. The right and left lobes of the thyroid gland are connected by the:

    (A) isthmus
    (B) septum
    (C) parathyroids
    (D) goiter

85. The thyroid gland produces:

    (A) thyroxine
    (B) T3
    (C) TSH
    (D) both A and B

86. When performing a thyroid scan, _____ is used to determine the size, shape, and position of the gland.

    (A) radioactive iodine
    (B) technetium-99m
    (C) Lymphazurin
    (D) both A and B

87. The condition associated with hyperthyroidism is:

    (A) thyroid storm
    (B) Graves' disease
    (C) hypocalcemia
    (D) tetany

88. One of the most common complications of head and neck surgery is:

    (A) back pain from positioning
    (B) laryngeal spasms
    (C) hemorrhage
    (D) malignant hyperthermia

89. During a thyroid procedure, the _____ and _____ muscles are incised, and the _____ muscle is retracted.

    (A) platysma and strap/sternocleidomastoid
    (B) platysma and sternocleidomastoid/strap
    (C) pectoralis and strap/platysma
    (D) pectoralis and platysma/strap

90. A congenital cyst found in the neck formed from an embryonic structure arising from the thyroid gland is termed:

    (A) goiter
    (B) thyroglossal cyst
    (C) cervical lymph node
    (D) scalene node

91. An instrument used to elevate the thyroid lobe during surgical excision is a:

    (A) Babcock
    (B) Lahey
    (C) Green
    (D) Jackson

92. In a thyroidectomy, a loop retractor retracts the:

    (A) platysma muscle
    (B) cervical fascia
    (C) thyroid veins
    (D) sternocleidomastoid muscle

93. Which structure(s) is/are identified and preserved in thyroid surgery?

    (A) Parathyroid glands
    (B) Hyoid bone
    (C) Thyroglossal duct
    (D) Thyroid lobe

94. Indications for a tracheotomy include:

    (A) upper airway obstruction
    (B) prolonged intubation
    (C) thyroid nodules
    (D) inability to intubate

95. Which bone is transected with bone-cutting forceps before removal of a thyroglossal cyst?

    (A) Ethmoid
    (B) Hyoid
    (C) Pterygoid
    (D) Zygomatic process

96. Place the procedural steps of inserting a tracheostomy tube in the correct order.

    1. Remove the obturator
    2. Place the trach tube
    3. Place the inner cannula
    (A) 1, 2, 3
    (B) 2, 1, 3
    (C) 3, 2, 1
    (D) 2, 3, 1

97. A biopsy performed for diagnosis of disease of the intrathoracic cavity by removing the cervical lymph node is:

    (A) mediastinoscopy
    (B) scalene
    (C) thyroglossal
    (D) axillary

98. Frontal sinus trephination includes all EXCEPT:

    (A) a small opening is made in the maxillary sinus
    (B) a small catheter is placed for drainage
    (C) trephination pertains to creating a circular opening
    (D) this is performed for infection and drainage

99. Following a radical neck dissection in which a portion of the mandible is removed, the bone graft is commonly taken from the:

    (A) clavicle
    (B) sixth/seventh rib
    (C) iliac crest
    (D) fibula

100. A stone in the palatine tonsils is termed:

    (A) tonsillitis
    (B) abscess
    (C) tonsillolith
    (D) tonsilitis

Answers and Explanations

1. **(B)** A moustache dressing may be applied under the nose (nares) to absorb any bleeding.

2. **(B)** The CO_2 laser is efficient and has a high-power output. It uses a combination of CO_2, nitrogen, and helium. As energy levels subside, light beams are produced that form a single beam of light in the ultraviolet range that is invisible. For this reason, a red beam from a helium–neon laser is added so that it may be properly aimed at the affected tissue.

3. **(C)** Cocaine is unrivaled in its power to penetrate the mucous membrane to produce surface anesthesia. Onset is immediate. It also causes vasoconstriction to reduce bleeding. Administration is only topical because of its high toxicity.

4. **(B)** The scrub cleans the burrs during the procedure. Continuous irrigation is necessary to minimize the transfer of heat from the burr to surrounding bone and structures. A suction irrigation may be used.

5. **(A)** Incision of the tympanic membrane, known as myringotomy, is done to treat otitis media. By releasing the fluid behind the membrane, hearing is restored and infection controlled. Frequently, tubes are inserted through the tympanic membrane.

6. **(A)** An alligator forceps is used to insert the tube into the incision.

7. **(D)** Perforation of the eardrum (tympanic membrane) is the most common serious ear injury. Tympanoplasty using grafted tissue improves hearing and prevents recurrent infection.

8. **(B)** A labyrinthectomy, endolymphatic shunt, and vestibular neurectomy are all surgical procedures used to treat vertigo associated with Meniere's disease. A stapedectomy is performed to restore the ossicular chain.

9. **(B)** Myringotomy is an incision into the tympanic membrane to ventilate the middle ear.

10. **(D)** Mastoidectomy is the removal of the diseased bone of the mastoid, along with cholesteatoma that results from an accumulation of squamous epithelium and its products. This putty-like mass destroys the middle ear and mastoid, so diseased bone must be removed.

11. **(B)** An acoustic neuroma arises in the eighth cranial nerve (acoustic). These tumors are benign but may grow to a size that produces neurological symptoms. The main patient complaint is hearing loss.

12. **(A)** Computerized facial nerve monitoring is used intraoperatively to decrease trauma during tumor dissection and to assess facial nerve status.

13. **(A)** Submucous resection is also known as septoplasty—removal of either cartilage or bone portions of the septum that obstruct the sinus opening and prevent a clear airway.

14. **(B)** A submucous resection is done for nasal septum deformity, fracture, or injury that has impaired normal respiratory function and has impaired drainage.

15. **(A)** A bayonet forceps is used to introduce sponges into the nose.

16. **(C)** This surgery is done to relieve edema or infection of the membrane lining the sinuses and resultant headaches. An opening is made into the maxillary sinus.

17. **(D)** Polyps are removed with a snare, polyp forceps, and suction.

18. **(C)** Frequently, a topical anesthetic is used before nasal surgery. The drug of choice is cocaine, 10% or 4%, and would be administered by means of soaked applicators introduced into the nasal cavity and absorbed by the mucous membrane.

19. **(A)** A Caldwell–Luc procedure is performed by using an incision under the upper lip above the teeth in the canine fossa. This is performed for diseases in the maxillary sinus.

20. **(C)** Tracheostomy is the opening of the trachea and establishment of a new airway through a midline incision in the neck, below the cricoid cartilage. A cannula is put in place to maintain the airway. This is an emergency procedure.

21. **(B)** Lidocaine 1% (1 or 2 mL) may be instilled into the trachea to reduce the coughing reflex when the tube is inserted.

22. **(A)** A catheter is used to suction the trachea at tube insertion.

23. **(C)** Most neoplasms of the salivary glands are benign mixed tumors; most of these affect the parotid gland.

24. **(B)** The patient is placed in the semi-recumbent (Fowler's) position or on one side, horizontally, to prevent aspiration of blood and venous engorgement postoperatively.

25. **(A)** Total laryngectomy is complete removal of the larynx, hyoid bone, and the strap muscles.

26. **(D)** Depending on the extent of the surgery and surgeon's preference, a Jackson–Pratt or Hemovac can be used for drainage on a radical neck procedure.

27. **(D)** For radical neck dissection, a Y-shaped or trifurcate incision is used on the affected side of the neck. A parotid incision is also a Y-shaped incision but on both sides of the ear and below the angle of the mandible.

28. **(D)** During ear surgery, a local anesthetic with epinephrine is often the surgeon's choice because the epinephrine acts as a vasoconstrictor and prevents oozing in the wound. Epinephrine-soaked pledgets are also used to control bleeding.

29. **(B)** The device is implanted in the cochlea, with the receiver resting in the mastoid bone. As the device receives sound through the receiver, it emits electrical impulses through the transmitter into the cochlea and along the acoustic nerve. These impulses are interpreted as a sound in the temporal cortex of the cerebrum.

30. **(A)** Stainless steel and copper endotracheal tubes are the choice when using lasers. They are wrapped with adhesive tape, and wet gauze is placed above the tube to prevent fires. Moist cloth towels are placed around the surrounding tissue to prevent damage from the laser energy to this healthy tissue.

31. **(C)** The advent of the CO_2 laser added a new dimension to the laryngologist's treatment of lesions of the larynx and vocal cords. The laser is efficient and has a high-power output. It uses a combination of CO_2, nitrogen, and helium gas.

32. **(C)** A microscope is required for a stapedectomy procedure.

33. **(C)** During a rhinoplasty, the dorsal hump can be taken down with an osteotome. A cartilaginous hump can be removed by means of a cutting forceps, such as a Jansen–Middleton forceps.

34. **(C)** During a tonsillectomy, the tonsil is grasped with a tonsil-grasping forceps, the

mucous membrane of the anterior pillar is incised with a knife, and the tonsil lobe is freed from its attachments to the pillar with a tonsil dissector.

35. **(B)** The submandibular glands are paired salivary glands. Their main ducts that drain saliva are known as Wharton's ducts. They are located at the floor of the mouth under the tongue. The parotid gland is also known as Stenson's duct.

36. **(A)** The thyroid cartilage is also known as the Adam's apple. It protects the larynx. The Adam's apple is commonly found in men.

37. **(D)** Both the auricle and the pinna are terms used for the portion of the outer ear. The septum is the term used for the cartilage that separates the nostrils in the nose.

38. **(A)** Arch bars are thin metal straps. They are wired to each row of teeth. The bars are then wired together with stainless steel suture performed to occlude the jaw.

39. **(C)** Wire cutters are kept with the patient at all times in case of airway emergency.

40. **(B)** Le Fort II is associated with leakage of cerebrospinal fluid into the nasal sinuses.

41. **(D)** The lower face is composed of the mandible (chin).

42. **(C)** TMJ is characterized by persistent pain due to stress-related muscle tension, grinding of teeth, malocclusion, trauma, and arthritis.

43. **(D)** As the surgeon dissects the thyroid gland from the surrounding tissues, the parathyroid glands, the superior laryngeal nerve, and the recurrent laryngeal nerves are identified and preserved.

44. **(B)** A thyroplasty is performed for a unilateral vocal cord paralysis due to surgical trauma of the laryngeal nerve or prolonged intubation.

45. **(D)** If the deep lobe of the parotid must be excised, the facial nerve is elevated and retracted with vessel loops during a parotidectomy.

46. **(B)** Epistaxis is bleeding from the nose caused by local irritation of mucous membranes, violent sneezing, and a variety of other reasons. It is also known as nose bleed.

47. **(A)** The vocal cords lie in the upper end of the larynx. They are responsible for voice production.

48. **(D)** The windpipe, or trachea, conducts air to and from the lungs. It is a tubular passageway located anterior to the esophagus. It further divides into the right and left bronchi.

49. **(B)** The nasal cavity is a hollow area behind the nose. It is divided into right and left portions by the nasal septum. The anterior septum is made of cartilage.

50. **(A)** A simple nasal fracture closed reduction is performed with the surgeon's hands and a Boies elevator.

51. **(D)** The hyoid bone is located in the neck between the mandible and the larynx. It supports the tongue and provides an attachment for its muscles. It does not articulate with any other bone.

52. **(C)** Normally the air pressure on the two sides of the eardrum is equalized by means of the Eustachian tube. This connects the middle ear cavity and the throat. This allows the eardrum to vibrate freely with the incoming sound waves.

53. **(D)** All are treatments used for a nose bleed except using a Fogarty arterial embolectomy catheter. Direct pressure is the first step. In more severe cases, endoscopic cauterization, arterial ligation, laser, or balloon catheter may be used. A Fogarty embolectomy catheter is used in vascular surgery to dilate a vessel and remove clots.

54. **(D)** The ossicles include the stapes, incus, and malleus. They are responsible for conducting

vibrations from the tympanic membrane to the oval window and then to the inner ear to the cochlea.

55. **(D)** The cochlea looks like a small spiral-shaped shell. It is a tube coiled for about two and a half turns into a spiral, around a central axis of the bone.

56. **(A)** Expanding across the middle ear area are three exceedingly small bones called the auditory ossicles: the malleus, the incus, and the stapes.

57. **(A)** The right primary bronchus is more vertical, shorter, and wider than the left. As a result, foreign objects in the air passageways are more likely to enter it than the left and frequently lodge in it.

58. **(B)** Adenoids are also known as pharyngeal tonsils. They have a glandular appearance, particularly lymphoid like.

59. **(A)** Molars function to crush, tear, and grind your food so you can swallow it.

60. **(C)** Mumps typically attacks the parotid glands. It is an inflammation and enlargement (swelling).

61. **(C)** A glossectomy is partial or total removal of the tongue performed for cancerous lesions or oral cancer of the mouth. The tongue does not have the ability to regenerate and grow back.

62. **(D)** An orbital floor fracture is also called a blowout fracture and a Le Fort III.

63. **(B)** The zygomatic bone is also referred to as the cheek bone and the malar bone.

64. **(C)** Standard protocol is to insert the wires clockwise and remove them counterclockwise.

65. **(D)** MMA is performed for deformities of the upper and lower jaw, malocclusion, and sleep apnea.

66. **(C)** The inside of the mouth is termed the buccal cavity. Under the tongue is the labial cavity, which contains the frenulum between the upper teeth and gum. The lingual cavity is under the tongue and contains the inferior labial frenulum.

67. **(A)** The bony labyrinths in the inner ear are responsible for equilibrium, the ossicles in the middle ear are responsible for conduct vibrations, TMJ stands for temporomandibular joint, and cerumen is the wax in the external ear.

68. **(C)** The external ear terminates at the tympanic membrane.

69. **(B)** Choanal atresia is the congenital disorder where the passage between the nose and pharynx is blocked by an abnormal bony tissue that failed to rupture during fetal development. Dacryocystorhinostomy is performed to restore the flow of tears into the nose from the lacrimal sac. SMR is a submucous resection/septoplasty procedure to repair a deviated septum.

70. **(C)** The nasopharynx is a division of the pharynx.

71. **(C)** The submandibular duct is also known as Wharton's duct, and the parotid duct is known as Stensen's duct.

72. **(B)** The pharynx is a tubular structure that extends from the nose to the esophagus and is separated into three divisions: the nasopharynx, oropharynx, and hypopharynx (laryngopharynx).

73. **(B)** The part of the larynx where the true vocal cords are located is the glottis.

74. **(A)** The approach used to remove an acoustic neuroma, which is a slow-growing tumor of the eighth cranial nerve, is translabyrinthine, middle fossa, and suboccipital.

75. **(C)** The Robinson catheter is used to retract the uvula during a tonsillectomy, the Davis

and Jennings are types of mouth gags, and the coblator uses radiofrequency energy combined with saline to remove the tonsils.

76. **(C)** The graft used for a tympanoplasty procedure is taken from the temporalis fascia on the side of the head. The pinna is the outer cartilage of the ear covered by skin. The pars tensa is part of the tympanic membrane.

77. **(C)** The prostheses used on a stapedectomy include stainless steel, platinum, and Teflon.

78. **(B)** Meniere's disease is not a disease of the middle ear; it affects the inner ear with symptoms of dizziness and ringing in the ears.

79. **(A)** Bell's palsy is a virus that affects the seventh cranial nerve and causes stiffness and drooping of one side of the face.

80. **(C)** Slow-growing tumors of the eighth cranial nerve are acoustic neuromas, also known as vestibular schwannomas. Glioblastomas are an aggressive malignant brain tumor.

81. **(B)** The procedure performed for sensory neural deafness is cochlear implants. Trigeminal neuralgia is a condition of the trigeminal nerve causing facial pain, and microvascular decompression is performed to prevent a vessel from compressing the trigeminal nerve.

82. **(D)** Turbinectomy is the procedure performed to improve nasal airflow caused by congestion and rhinorrhea. A rhinoplasty is performed for cosmetic surgery, closed reduction of a nasal fracture is performed for fractured nasal bones, and an SMR is performed for a deviated septum.

83. **(C)** When performing an FESS (functional endoscopic sinus surgery), it becomes more difficult if a second surgery is needed because the surgical landmarks have been altered by performing the first procedure.

84. **(A)** The right and left lobes of the thyroid gland are connected by the isthmus.

85. **(D)** The thyroid gland produces thyroxine (T4) and triiodothyronine (T3); the pituitary produces thyroid-stimulating hormone (TSH).

86. **(D)** This procedure is performed in nuclear medicine. Radiotracers are administered for diagnostic imaging of the thyroid gland. The radiotracers commonly used are radioactive iodine and technetium-99m.

87. **(B)** The disease associated with hyperthyroidism is Graves' disease. Hypocalcemia is when the calcium level is lower than normal. Tetany is a disease caused by hypocalcemia, and a thyroid storm is an acute hyperthyroid episode.

88. **(B)** Laryngeal surgery is one of the most common complications of head and neck surgery.

89. **(A)** During a thyroid procedure, the platysma and strap muscles are incised, and the sternocleidomastoid muscle is retracted.

90. **(B)** A congenital cyst found in the neck formed from an embryonic structure arising from the thyroid gland is a thyroglossal duct cyst.

91. **(B)** A Lahey vulsellum forceps is used to grasp and elevate the thyroid lobe so that sharp dissection of the lobe away from the trachea can be accomplished.

92. **(D)** The sternocleidomastoid muscle is retracted with loop retractors.

93. **(A)** Care is taken throughout thyroid surgery to identify and preserve parathyroid glands. Removal of all parathyroid tissue results in severe tetany or death.

94. **(C)** The most common reasons for performing a tracheostomy are upper airway obstruction, prolonged intubation, inability to intubate, and complications from previous head and neck surgery. Thyroid nodules are not an indication for a tracheostomy.

95. (B) After the head is extended, the incision is made between the hyoid bone and the thyroid cartilage through the subcutaneous tissue. Sharp and blunt dissection is used to mobilize the cyst and duct, the hyoid bone is transected twice with bone-cutting forceps, and the cyst is freed from adjacent structures.

96. (B) The trach tube is placed, the obturator is removed, and the inner cannula is inserted

97. (B) Biopsy of the supraclavicular lymph node is a scalene node biopsy that provides a diagnosis of diseases of the thoracic cavity and lung and brain cancer screening.

98. (A) A small opening is made in the frontal sinus, and a drain is placed for irrigation and drainage of a frontal sinus infection. Trephination refers to a small circular hole.

99. (D) An autograft is commonly taken from the fibula for grafting of the mandible for a radical neck dissection.

100. (C) Although a calculus is a stone, the correct term for a tiny calculus/stone found in the tonsil is a tonsillolith.

CHAPTER 22

Plastic and Reconstructive Surgery

PLASTIC AND RECONSTRUCTIVE SURGERY

- Treats abnormal structures of the body caused by birth defects, developmental problems, disease, tumors, infections, or injury
- Intact skin is the most effective barrier to protect the body from harmful microorganisms
- Epidermis—the outermost protective nonvascular layer of the skin
- Dermis—the layer of skin below the epidermis. It consists of vascular connective tissue, nerve endings, hair roots, and sebaceous glands
- Langer's lines—these are natural lines in the skin. The plastic surgeon follows these lines for the surgical procedure to provide a better cosmetic appearance postoperatively

TISSUE LAYERS UNDER THE SKIN

- Subcutaneous layer/sub-q—a fatty layer of tissue below the dermis
- Fascia—a fibrous tissue that adds support the superficial skin layers and muscle
- Peritoneum—a thin two-layered membrane that lines the interior abdominal cavity and viscera
- From most superficial layer to deep layer:
  - Skin
  - Subcutaneous fat
  - Muscle
  - Fascia
- Cicatrix—a scar
- Keloid—a type of a scar that is raised, reddish, and can be nodular; they develop at the site of an injury

- Hypertrophic scar—similar to a keloid but not as pronounced
- Burns
  - Rule of nines—the body surface is divided into equal parts by using multiples of 9% of total body surface. This is used for adults. The breakdown includes:
    - 4.5% front of head
    - 4.5% back of head
    - 18% front of body
    - 18% back of body
    - 4.5% each arm front and back
    - 9% each leg front and back
  - Lund–Browder chart
    - The percentage of the burn is estimated on the basis of age in addition to the anatomic location of the burn. Most accurate for use with children
- Classification of burns
  - First-degree burn—superficial—only the outer layer of the epidermis is involved. The skin is red. A sunburn is considered a first-degree burn
  - Second-degree burn—partial thickness—all of the epidermis and some of the dermis are affected. The skin is blistered, painful, moist, and red
  - Third-degree burn—full thickness—all of the epidermis/dermis and subcutaneous tissue. The skin is dry, pearly white, or charred in appearance. No grafts are required
  - Fourth-degree burn—these burns damage down to the bone, muscle, tendons, blood vessels, and nerves

- Dressings—goal of dressings:
  - Immobilize
  - Apply even pressure over the wound
  - Collect drainage
  - Provide comfort for the patient
  - Protect the wound

One-Layer Dressing

- This is used on a clean incision that has been closed with sutures, staples, or skin closure tapes (Steri-Strips)
  - Cotton gauze
  - Telfa
  - Adaptic

Three-Layer Dressings

CONTACT LAYER—this layer uses a wicking action to help remove secretion and exudate; they include:

- Nonocclusive—does not stick to the wound
  - Telfa (the material used on a band aid)
  - Adaptic
  - Gauze 4 × 4's (primary dressing)
- Semiocclusive—these are types of dressings that contain hydroactive materials to help seal a wound
  - Hydrasorb
  - Hydrogel
- Occlusive—this dressing provides an air-tight seal, prevents the wound from drying, and allows drainage. This dressing is infused with a lubricant such as:
  - Petroleum
  - Xeroform

INTERMEDIATE LAYER—this is the layer of 4 × 4's that is placed over the contact layer dressing

OUTER LAYER—this layer of dressings holds the contact and intermediate layers of dressings in place. It consists of:

- Nonallergic tape
- Elastoplast
- Stockinette
- Kerlix
- Kling
- Ace

Wet to Dry Dressing

- Commonly used on burn wounds
- Dressing 4 × 4's are soaked in saline and applied to the wound; the dressings dry and are removed from the wound. When pulling them from the wound, it debrides the wound.
  - This procedure is very painful

Wet to Wet Dressing

- Commonly used on burn wounds
- Dressing 4 × 4's are soaked in saline, applied wet, and changed often

- Pressure dressings
  - Prevent edema
  - Absorb extensive drainage
  - Distribute pressure evenly
  - Eliminate dead space
- Stent dressing—type of pressure dressing; uses Xeroform, fluffs, 4 × 4's, and silk suture to criss-cross and tie
- Negative wound pressure dressing—type of dressing technique that provides negative pressure to the wound with a vacuum and special dressing. This dressing helps to pull the wound edges together and remove bacteria
- Skin grafts
  - STSG (split-thickness skin graft)
    - Contains epidermis and only a portion of dermis

  - Grafts may be meshed; this allows the skin graft to become stretched larger than its original size
  - FTSG (full-thickness skin graft)
    - Contains epidermis and dermis
- Types of grafts
  - Autograft—tissue taken from a patient's own body and transferred to a different part of their body
  - Heterograft/xenograft—tissue transplanted from a donor of a different species (pig to human/heart valve)
  - Allograft—transplantation of tissue from one person to another (of same species/human to human)
- When prepping the donor site, it should be done with a colorless solution

○ The proper technique when prepping for the graft is donor site first

○ There should be two different setups

- One donor and one recipient table

- Dermatome—a surgical instrument used to cut thin slices of skin from a donor area to use them as skin grafts

    ○ Dermatomes can be operated either manually or electrically

    - Brown dermatome—uses an oscillating blade and is electrically operated. This is commonly used today

    - Padgett dermatome and Reese dermatome—manual dermatome—hand controlled

    - Ferris–Smith/Watson/Weck—handheld knife dermatomes

    - Mesh device—Dermacarrier—this is used to stretch/expand the donor skin and provide skin that covers a larger surface area. Split-thickness skin graft is commonly used with this device

    ○ Procedure:

    - Mineral oil is used to lubricate the donor graft, and a tongue depressor is used to provide smooth traction

- Pedicle flap/graft—a full-thickness skin graft that remains attached at some point on the body; this is where it continues to receive its blood supply

- Basal cell skin cancer—grows on the skin surface; the cancer is in the basal cells. It is the least risky skin cancer

- Squamous cell skin cancer—squamous cells make up the main part of the epidermis layer of the skin. This cancer is a major form of skin cancer and can be considered aggressive

- Melanoma skin cancer—the most serious type of skin cancer; it is very aggressive and can spread to other organs

- Mohs surgery—technique used to remove a skin lesion; it is performed by removing thin layers of skin for examination under the microscope

- Pressure ulcers—a pressure ulcer usually occurs over a bony prominence. It begins with a reddened area that spreads to deeper tissue, causing a severe breakdown of tissue until it becomes an ulcer. Common sites include:

    ○ Sacrum

    ○ Ischium

    ○ Heel

BREAST SURGERY

- Reconstructive breast surgery following a mastectomy—surgery using tissue expanders—when a mastectomy is performed, it leaves a shortage of skin, and tissue expanders are introduced into a submuscular pocket of the breast and are used to stretch the skin by filling the expander with NaCl. Repeated office visits are made, and the tissue expanders are gradually filled with NaCl until the expander is the desired size

    ○ Implants are handled as little as possible

    ○ They are soaked in antibiotic solution prior to insertion

    ○ Drain is placed to prevent hematoma and seroma formation

    ○ Fiberoptic-lighted breast retractors are used to facilitate insertion

- Second stage of tissue expander breast reconstruction—the tissue expander is deflated, removed, and replaced with the permanent prosthesis

Breast Reconstruction Using a Myocutaneous Flap

- TRAM flap—transverse rectus abdominis muscle—this procedure is performed to reconstruct a breast from the muscle in the lower abdomen between the waist and the pubic bone "rectus abdominis." A flap of this skin, fat, and muscle is used. The muscle is severed distally and tunneled subcutaneously to form the breast

    ○ This is a type of pedicle flap

    ○ Blood supply to maintain this flap is:

    - Superior epigastric artery and vein

    ○ A Doppler is used to preserve the artery

    ○ An abdominoplasty is performed to close the defect in the abdomen

- Nipple reconstruction—a skin graft is taken to reconstruct the nipple after this reconstruction of the breast has healed. The technique of tattooing is used to recreate the areola

- Augmentation mammoplasty—this procedure is performed to increase the size of the breasts with implants

    ○ Breast implants are filled with silicone or saline

    ○ Incisions used for an augmentation include:

    - Inframammary

    - Periareolar

- Transaxillary
- Transumbilical
- Four different placement options for breast implants include:
  - Subglandular placement of the implant is below the mammary glands and above the muscle
  - Subfascial—above the muscle under the facia
  - Subpectoral—placement of the implant is below the pectoralis major muscle
  - Submuscular—placement is actually under the pectoralis major muscle
- When handling implants, the STSR should know:
  - Powder should be wiped off gloves before handling
  - There should be no oil on gloves
  - Implants should be placed on lint-free surface
  - Prosthetics usually are wet prior to insertion (soaked in an antibiotic solution)
- Capsulotomy/capsulectomy—this procedure is performed to remove scar tissue that has formed around the breast implant. This scar tissue can distort the symmetry of the implant and harden the area
  - The tissue can be removed and/or released
- Reduction mammoplasty—this procedure is performed to reduce the size of extremely large breasts. Extremely large breasts can cause:
  - Back and shoulder pain
  - Neck pain
  - Impaired breathing
  - Skin irritation and other health problems
  - Performed on men who suffer from gynecomastia
- Mastopexy—performed for breast ptosis (drooping of the breasts). It is a breast lift. Breast ptosis is caused by:
  - Gravity/aging skin
  - Breastfeeding
  - Hormonal changes
- When performing microsurgery, a microscope and/or loupes are needed

OTHER RECONSTRUCTIVE SURGERY

- Reimplantation of amputated finger
  - Needs to be performed within 4–6 hours after injury. Steps of the procedure include:
    - Debridement
    - Bone-to-bone fixation

- Tendon repair
- Nerve repair
- Arteries and vein repair
- Skin
- Scar revision—performed to reshape a scar for cosmetic results
  - Subcuticular suture technique is used
- Z-plasty—performed for a scar revision or closure of wound to get the best cosmetic results. Most common techniques used:
  - One or more Z-shaped incisions are made within the skin lines
  - It elongates the scar and gives a smaller appearance
  - Other techniques include:
    - W-plasty
    - M-plasty
    - Y–V-plasty
- Mentoplasty—performed for reconstruction of a deformity of the chin
- Otoplasty—performed to reconstruct and/or repair the ear. It can change the shape, size, and position of the ear
- Microtia—this is a congenital deformity of the pinna (outer portion of the ear). These babies are born with small deformed ears
- Rhytidectomy (facelift)—performed to improve sagging and aging in the middle face and neck
- Mini facelift—performed for severe drooping of the upper neck and jowl
  - Jowl—skin of the lower cheeks and jaw
- SMAS (superficial muscular aponeurotic system)—this muscular system is continuous with the platysma muscle in the neck. This muscle is tightened to provide a cosmetic effect of the jowl and midface
- Brow lift—this is also called a forehead lift; this is performed to reduce the wrinkle lines across the forehead; it raises the sagging eyebrows and the bridge of the nose
- Endoscopic brow lift—this is a minimally invasive procedure performed to reduce the wrinkle lines across the forehead and raise sagging eyebrows
  - Three tiny incisions are made in the hairline
- Blepharoplasty—this procedure is performed to remove fat deposits and excess skin from the eyelids to improve the cosmetic appearance of

the eyes. In some cases, severe sagging could impair vision
- Dermatochalasis—excessive sagging of the upper and lower eyelids. A blepharoplasty is performed for this
- Incisions include:
  - Subciliary incision
  - Transconjunctival incision
- Laser surgery
  - CO_2 laser—most popular for skin resurfacing
- Laser resurfacing is a treatment to reduce facial wrinkles and acne scars
- Tattoo removal
  - Candela dye laser and Q-switched laser are used
- Liposuction—the surgical removal of fat from parts of the body, including the abdomen, buttocks, hips, thighs, and knees. The fat is sucked out through a cannula that is inserted under the skin and attached to a high-pressure vacuum
  - A tumescent solution of lidocaine and epinephrine diluted mixture helps to swell and break up the fat while producing an anesthetic effect
  - Cannulas of various sizes are used to suck out the fat
  - Hemostasis is achieved, and a compression dressing is applied
- Gynecomastia/macromastia—the term used for large breasts in the male
  - The procedure to correct this condition can be performed by liposuction techniques or by an open procedure. With an open procedure, the incision is made under the armpit or around the areola
- Malar implants—a cosmetic procedure performed to emphasize a person's cheek bones. The implants are placed over the cheek bones; the patient's own fat can also be injected to add contour
  - The incision is in the canine fossa (gum line)
  - Sizers are used to determine the correct size and symmetry; they are removed, and the implants are placed
- Submalar implants—this procedure is performed for soft tissue reconstruction
- Rhinoplasty—this procedure is also called a "nose job"; it is performed for cosmetic correction of the nose and to put it in proportion with the face

- Straightening the internal septum
- Corrects sinuses/breathing
- Bone
- Skin
- Reduces the size of the nose
- Plastic instruments:
  - Iris scissors
  - Stevens tenotomy scissors
  - Skin hooks
  - Adson tissue forceps
  - Bishop–Harmon forceps
  - Webster needle holder
  - Frazier suctions
  - Blepharoplasty calipers
  - Castroviejo needle holder
- Epidermis layers—the epidermis contains five layers. They are listed from deepest to most superficial:
  - Stratum basale—forms the attachment of the epidermis to the dermis.
  - Stratum spinosum
  - Stratum granulosum—this layer of the epidermis acts as a barrier to prevent fluid loss from the body
  - Stratum lucidum—found on the palm of the hand and the sole of the feet
  - Stratum corneum—the barrier between the environment and body
- Panniculectomy—a surgical procedure performed to remove excess skin and fat from the abdomen. An abdominoplasty and tummy tuck are performed to remove excess skin and fat but also involve tightening the muscles of the abdominal wall
- DIEP flap—deep inferior epigastric perforator artery. It is a flap of skin, fat, and blood vessels (inferior epigastric perforators) removed from the lower abdomen to the chest for reconstruction following a mastectomy. Muscle is not utilized in this procedure. It is a long procedure and requires a microscope for reanastomosis of the vessels to reestablish blood flow. The latissimus dorsi flap utilizes skin, fat, and muscle from the back and is for breast reconstruction
- TRAM flap—transverse rectus abdominis; takes skin, fat, and muscles from the lower abdomen to reconstruct the breast.
- Radial dysplasia—also called club hand. This is a deformity of the radial bone causing the hand

and wrist to turn inward toward the thumb aspect of the hand. Splints can be used to secure the wrist straight. Surgery is the last resort

- Mesher—a mesher is used to expand the split-thickness skin graft (STSG) by placing small slits in the donor skin. It consists of a mesher device and clear graft plates. The skin is placed on the plate and fed through the mesher, and cuts are made into the STSG

- Doppler—an instrument (handheld transducer) used to measure the amount of blood flow through the veins. The probe can be used preoperatively, intraoperatively with a sterile drape, and postoperatively

- Apocrine glands—a type of sweat gland found in the skin

- Ceruminous glands—are round and found in the external auditory canal

- Merocrine glands—primary function is thermoregulation

- Sebaceous glands—the oil glands of the body

- Papillomas—growths that can be found on the skin or mucous membranes

- Cleft lip—an abnormality of the upper lip that occurs in the fetus around the second trimester during pregnancy. The repair is done so the infant can perform normal functions such as feeding and talking and to reduce dental problems. Cupid's bow is used as the guideline for cosmetic results of the repair

Questions

1. A dressing that is held in place by long suture ends crisscrossed and tied is called a:

   (A) passive dressing
   (B) strip closure
   (C) Proxi-Strip
   (D) stent

2. All of the following statements regarding the preparation for a skin graft are true EXCEPT:

   (A) the dermatome is placed on the recipient table
   (B) the donor site is prepared with a colorless antiseptic agent
   (C) separate setups are necessary for skin preparation of recipient and donor sites
   (D) items used in preparation of the recipient site must not be permitted to contaminate the donor site

3. How many layers does the epidermis contain?

   (A) Two
   (B) Three
   (C) Four
   (D) Five

4. Colorless prep solution may be indicated for:

   (A) orthopedic surgery
   (B) vascular surgery
   (C) plastic surgery
   (D) urological surgery

5. A graft containing epidermis and only a portion of the dermis is called a:

   (A) split-thickness graft
   (B) full-thickness Wolfe graft
   (C) composite graft
   (D) full-thickness pinch graft

6. A progressive disease of the palmar fascia is termed:

   (A) Dupuytren's contracture
   (B) tendinitis
   (C) carpal tunnel syndrome
   (D) synovitis

7. Microtia refers to:

   (A) protrusion of the external ear
   (B) underdeveloped external ear
   (C) total absence of the external ear
   (D) large external ear

8. Good contact between a skin graft and the recipient site is facilitated by use of a/an:

   (A) stent dressing
   (B) Elastoplast
   (C) splint–Ace bandage dressing
   (D) biological dressing

9. Syndactyly refers to:

   (A) an extra digit
   (B) an absent digit
   (C) webbing of the digits
   (D) an ear protrusion

10. A facelift is termed a:

    (A) blepharoplasty
    (B) mentoplasty
    (C) rhytidectomy
    (D) lipectomy

11. The intraoperative use of bone allografts requires all of the following responses from the scrub team EXCEPT:

    (A) culture before implant
    (B) wash with an antibiotic solution
    (C) completely thaw
    (D) both A and B

12. Bulky dressings added to the intermediate layer of a three-layer dressing are used to:

    (A) eliminate dead space
    (B) concentrate pressure in one area
    (C) immobilize a body part
    (D) both A and C

13. All of the following rules cover handling of prosthetic devices during plastic surgery procedures EXCEPT:

    (A) powder must be wiped from gloves before handling
    (B) prosthesis must be dried completely before implanting it
    (C) gloves must be used to prevent skin oils from causing inflammatory response
    (D) prosthesis must be placed on lint-free surface to sterilize

14. Free jejunal tissue transfers are frequently successful as adjunct surgical revisions following:

    (A) laryngectomy
    (B) esophagectomy
    (C) ileectomy
    (D) both A and B

15. What bandage affects the process of exsanguination of a limb prior to the use of a tourniquet?

    (A) Kling
    (B) Elastoplast
    (C) Esmarch
    (D) Ace

16. Which muscle is utilized to effect a TRAM flap in breast reconstruction?

    (A) Latissimus dorsi
    (B) Transverse rectus abdominis
    (C) Pectoralis major
    (D) Pectoralis minor

17. The most widely used method of scar revision next to scar removal is:

    (A) chemical peel
    (B) sanding
    (C) Z-plasty
    (D) planing

18. A scar that is hypertrophic and bulbous and usually does not reduce over time is a/an:

    (A) papilloma
    (B) keloid
    (C) eschar
    (D) nevus

19. Burned tissue that is nonelastic and may constrict underlying structures is:

    (A) eschar
    (B) split-thickness skin graft
    (C) keloid
    (D) none of the above

20. Which graft is derived from pig tissue?

    (A) Feline
    (B) Bovine
    (C) Porcine
    (D) Allograft

21. The skin provides which of the following vital functions?

    (A) Protects underlying tissues and organs
    (B) Excretes organic waste and stores nutrients
    (C) Excretes water and dissipates heat as a means of thermoregulation
    (D) All of the above

22. The most common type of skin cancer is:

    (A) basal cell
    (B) melanoma
    (C) squamous cell
    (D) nevi

23. A graft transferred from one individual to another is a/an:

    (A) hemograft
    (B) porcine
    (C) autograft
    (D) allograft

24. A graft made up of tissue taken from one species and grafted to another species is:

    (A) homograft
    (B) autograft
    (C) xenograft
    (D) allograft

25. Removal of nonviable tissue from a nonhealing or traumatic wound is known as:

    (A) debridement
    (B) undermining
    (C) grafting
    (D) Mohs surgery

26. A mentoplasty involves augmentation of:

    (A) chin
    (B) lips
    (C) ears
    (D) nose

27. Macromastia in males is referred to as:

    (A) accessory
    (B) gynecomastia
    (C) small breasts
    (D) none of the above

28. A panniculectomy is:

    (A) a surgical procedure performed to remove excess skin and fat from the lower abdomen
    (B) also known as an abdominoplasty
    (C) a surgical procedure performed to remove excess skin and fat and to tighten the muscles in the abdominal wall
    (D) also known as a tummy tuck

29. In order to reduce friction between the skin and the blade of the dermatome, the site is prepped with:

    (A) methylene blue
    (B) Betadine
    (C) Chloraprep
    (D) mineral oil

30. What are natural lines in the skin that are used as landmarks for plastic surgeons to provide optimum cosmetic results?

    (A) Keloids
    (B) Langer's
    (C) Lund
    (D) Browder

31. Place the following layers in the correct order from most superficial to deepest layer:

    (1) subcutaneous, (2) muscle, (3) fascia, and (4) skin.

    (A) 4, 1, 3, 2
    (B) 1, 2, 3, 4
    (C) 3, 1, 2, 4
    (D) 2, 3, 1, 4

32. The large scar with a raised, nodular, and reddish appearance is termed:

(A) cicatrix

(B) keloid

(C) hypertrophic

(D) eschar

33. When using the rule of nines burn assessment chart, what percentage is given to both legs together front and back?

(A) 9%

(B) 18%

(C) 27%

(D) 36%

34. What burn is characterized by a white pearly skin appearance and includes all of the epidermis, dermis, and subcutaneous tissue?

(A) First degree

(B) Second degree

(C) Third degree

(D) Fourth degree

35. What burn is characterized by destruction of skin, muscles, tendons, vessels, and bone?

(A) First degree

(B) Second degree

(C) Third degree

(D) Fourth degree

36. What is the manual instrument used to harvest thin slices of skin from a donor area for use in skin grafting?

(A) Brown

(B) Padgett

(C) Weck

(D) Watson

37. Which dermatome is commonly used to retrieve skin for a graft and contains an oscillating blade?

(A) Ferris–Smith

(B) Brown

(C) Reese

(D) Padgett

38. Which of the following is a handheld knife dermatome?

(A) Ferris–Smith

(B) Watson

(C) Weck

(D) All of the above

39. A pedicle flap is:

(A) a graft that includes the epidermis and part of the dermis

(B) a full-thickness graft that does not remain attached for the blood supply

(C) a full-thickness skin graft that remains attached to an area where it continues to receive blood supply

(D) a graft that only removes the epidermis

40. The most aggressive skin cancer that can spread to other organs is:

(A) basal cell

(B) melanoma

(C) squamous cell

(D) nevus

41. Sites of pressure ulcers include:

(A) sacrum

(B) ischium

(C) heel

(D) all of the above

42. The blood supply that maintains the TRAM flap is:

(A) iliac artery

(B) subclavian artery

(C) femoral artery

(D) superior epigastric artery and vein

43. A DIEP (deep inferior epigastric perforator artery) flap procedure involves all EXCEPT:

    (A) it is a flap of skin, fat, and blood vessels (inferior epigastric perforators) removed from the lower abdomen

    (B) it is a procedure performed for breast reconstruction following a mastectomy

    (C) it involves the latissimus dorsi muscle

    (D) a microscope is used for the intricate vessel repair to reestablish blood flow

44. What procedure is performed to increase the size of the breasts?

    (A) Augmentation mammoplasty

    (B) Mastopexy

    (C) Transverse rectus abdominis myocutaneous flap

    (D) Both A and B

45. The procedure performed to reduce the size of extremely large breasts is termed:

    (A) mastopexy

    (B) simple mastectomy

    (C) reduction mammoplasty

    (D) modified radical mastectomy

46. When performing the procedure for reimplantation of a finger, the order of repair is:

    (1) nerve repair, (2) bone-to-bone fixation, (3) debridement, (4) artery and vein repair, (5) skin, and (6) tendon.

    (A) 3, 2, 1, 4, 5, 6

    (B) 3, 2, 6, 1, 4, 5

    (C) 2, 3, 1, 4, 6, 5

    (D) 6, 5, 4, 3, 2, 1

47. A congenital deformity of the pinna is termed:

    (A) otitis media

    (B) mentoplasty

    (C) microtia

    (D) cheiloplasty

48. What procedure is performed to reduce the wrinkle lines across the forehead and raise the sagging eyebrows and the bridge of the nose?

    (A) Brow lift

    (B) Forehead lift

    (C) Endoscopic brow lift

    (D) All of the above

49. A blepharoplasty is performed to remove fat deposits and excess skin from the eyelids. Incisions used include:

    (A) subciliary

    (B) transconjunctival

    (C) both A and B

    (D) limbus

50. Dermatochalasis is the diagnosis for what procedure?

    (A) Rhytidectomy

    (B) Microtia repair

    (C) Blepharoplasty

    (D) Mastopexy

51. Tattoo removal is performed with which laser?

    (A) Candela dye laser

    (B) Q-switched laser

    (C) YAG

    (D) Both A and B

52. Which of the following pertain(s) to liposuction?

    (A) Tumescent solution is used.

    (B) It can be performed on the abdomen, buttocks, hips, and thighs.

    (C) Compression dressings are applied.

    (D) All of the above

53. The term used for large breasts is:

    (A) gynecomastia

    (B) macromastia

    (C) ptosis

    (D) microtia

54. Malar implants are inserted into:

    (A) chin
    (B) cheeks
    (C) eyelids
    (D) forehead

55. A rhinoplasty is:

    (A) nose job
    (B) facelift
    (C) cheek implants
    (D) brow lift

56. The burn classification that is characterized by a dry, pearly white, or charred-appearing surface is:

    (A) first degree
    (B) second degree
    (C) third degree
    (D) fourth degree

57. The Occupational Safety and Health Administration (OSHA) is a governmental regulating agency whose aim is to:

    (A) provide guidelines to prevent transmission of blood-borne infections
    (B) execute requirements designed to prevent transmission of blood-borne pathogens in the work environment
    (C) require that communicable diseases be reported to a public health agency
    (D) train employees how to recognize and execute safe practices

58. Inflammation is characterized by pain, redness, heat, swelling, and loss of function. The redness can be attributed to:

    (A) serum brought into the area
    (B) constriction of capillaries
    (C) vasodilation bringing more blood to the area
    (D) heat from metabolic reaction

59. The congenital deformity of radial dysplasia:

    (A) is also called club hand
    (B) occurs when the radial bone is not formed properly or not present at all
    (C) occurs when the hand and the wrist bend inward toward the thumb side of the hand
    (D) all of the above

60. If tissue is approximated too tightly, it can cause:

    (A) ischemia
    (B) excessive scar tissue
    (C) keloids
    (D) adhesions

61. Tensile strength of a wound refers to:

    (A) the suture strength
    (B) the ability of tissue to resist rupture
    (C) wound contraction
    (D) tissue approximation

62. The substance that unites with thrombin to form fibrin, the basic structural material of blood clots, is:

    (A) fibrinogen
    (B) prothrombin
    (C) fibrin
    (D) thrombin

63. A cicatrix is:

    (A) an abscess
    (B) a scar
    (C) pus
    (D) a wound

64. Why is a mesh device used on a skin graft?

    (A) It attaches skin to the donor site.
    (B) It expands the size of the skin graft by making small cuts in the graft.
    (C) It prevents scaring.
    (D) It makes the skin graft thicker.

65. A wound that is infected or in which there is excessive loss of tissue heals by:

    (A) primary intention
    (B) secondary intention
    (C) third intention
    (D) fourth intention

66. The type of wound healing that requires debridement is:

    (A) primary intention
    (B) secondary intention
    (C) third intention
    (D) fourth intention

67. To promote healing, a surgical wound must have all of the following requisites EXCEPT:

    (A) suture closure of dead space
    (B) drains to remove fluid or air
    (C) a moderately tight dressing
    (D) loose sutures

68. Wound healing that employs a technique allowing the wound to heal from the INSIDE OUT is called:

    (A) interrupted intention
    (B) first intention
    (C) second intention
    (D) third intention

69. A band of scar tissue that binds together two anatomical surfaces that are normally separate from each other is called:

    (A) keloid
    (B) adhesion
    (C) cicatrix
    (D) dehiscence

70. What is the classification of a wound that is indicated by a delayed closure?

    (A) Primary intention
    (B) Secondary intention
    (C) Third intention
    (D) Fourth intention

71. A complication of wound closure when the organs protrude through the edges of the wound is called:

    (A) adhesions
    (B) dehiscence
    (C) evisceration
    (D) hemorrhage

72. Arrange the three phases of wound healing in the correct order: (1) proliferation, (2) inflammatory, and (3) remodeling.

    (A) 1, 2, 3
    (B) 3, 2, 1
    (C) 2, 3, 1
    (D) 2, 1, 3

73. Tissue breakdown at the wound margin is:

    (A) adhesion
    (B) hematoma
    (C) debridement
    (D) dehiscence

74. Wound complications include:

    (A) hematoma
    (B) seroma
    (C) evisceration
    (D) all of the above

75. A wound is described as _____ when there is a collection of pus around the incision.

    (A) hematoma
    (B) suppurative
    (C) granulation
    (D) dehiscence

76. Which of the following statements regarding routine prepping for skin graft procedures is correct?

    (A) Donor site is prepped first and considered clean.

    (B) Donor site is prepped last and considered contaminated.

    (C) Recipient site is prepped first and considered contaminated.

    (D) Recipient site is prepped last and considered clean.

77. What would be used to confirm adequate blood supply to the pedicle flap during the TRAM flap procedure?

    (A) Nerve stimulator

    (B) Doppler

    (C) Pulse oximeter

    (D) Stethoscope

78. Which type of skin graft/flap would preserve skin sensation?

    (A) Porcine graft

    (B) Full thickness

    (C) Pedicle

    (D) STSG

79. All are glands found in the body EXCEPT:

    (A) apocrine

    (B) ceruminous

    (C) papilloma

    (D) sebaceous

80. For which procedure would the surgeon require a sterile tattoo machine?

    (A) Cleft lip repair

    (B) Endoscopic brow list

    (C) Nipple reconstruction

    (D) Reduction mammoplasty

81. The natural outline of the upper lip is known as Cupid's bow because of the obvious curve of the border of the upper lip. What surgical procedure would use this as a guideline?

    (A) Cleft lip

    (B) Ptosis

    (C) Chin procedures

    (D) Meatoplasty

Answers and Explanations

1. **(D)** A stent dressing or fixation is a method of applying pressure and stabilizing tissues when it is impossible to dress an area. In the case of the nose, for example, long suture ends are crisscrossed over a small dressing and tied.

2. **(A)** Separate setups are used in skin preparation of the recipient and donor sites. Items used in preparation of the recipient site must not be permitted to contaminate the donor site. The donor site should be scrubbed with a colorless antiseptic agent so the surgeon can evaluate the vascularity of the graft postoperatively. Always place the dermatome separately, never on the recipient table.

3. **(D)** The epidermis contains five layers. They are, from deepest to most superficial, as follows: stratum basale (this forms the attachment of the epidermis to the dermis), stratum spinosum, stratum granulosum (this layer of the epidermis acts as a barrier to prevent fluid loss from the body), stratum lucidum (this is found on the palm of the hand and the sole of the feet), and stratum corneum (this is the barrier between the environment and body).

4. **(C)** A colorless prep solution may be used in plastic surgery to facilitate observation of the true color of the skin.

5. **(A)** A split-thickness graft, or partial-thickness graft, contains epidermis and only a portion of the dermis.

6. **(A)** Dupuytren's contracture is a progressive disease involving the palmar fascia and the digital extensions of the palmar fascia. The surgery required is a palmar fasciectomy.

7. **(B)** Microtia is a congenital deformity where the pinna (external ear) is small and not properly formed. Anotia refers to when the external ear is completely missing. These can affect one or both ears.

8. **(A)** A stent or tie-over dressing exerts even pressure, ensuring good contact between graft and recipient site.

9. **(C)** Syndactyly refers to webbing of the digits of the hand or foot.

10. **(C)** A rhytidectomy is a facelift designed to improve appearance by removing excess skin and sometimes excess fat of the neck.

11. **(C)** Frozen allografts are stored in plastic or cloth wraps to ensure sterility and prevent grafts from drying out. When requested for a procedure, the allograft is delivered to the field slightly thawed. It is then cultured and washed with an antibiotic solution.

12. **(D)** Pressure dressings are used mainly in general surgery or plastic procedures to eliminate dead space, absorb extensive drainage, distribute pressure evenly, and immobilize a body part when muscles are moved.

13. **(B)** Breast prostheses and tissue expanders should be placed in a container with sterile saline or antibiotic solution on the sterile field.

14. **(D)** Reconstructive problems in patients undergoing laryngectomy and upper cervical esophagectomy can be adequately solved by a free jejunal transfer. Modern microscopic techniques greatly improve the success rate.

15. **(C)** An Esmarch bandage is used to exsanguinate the extremity before institution of a pneumatic tourniquet.

16. **(B)** The TRAM flap is a single-stage reconstruction of a postmastectomy breast with the transverse rectus abdominis muscle of the lower abdomen.

17. **(C)** The simplest form of scar revision is excision of an existing scar and simple resuturing of the wound. The Z-plasty is the most widely used method of scar revision. It breaks up linear scars, rearranging them so that all tissue lies in the same direction.

18. **(B)** A keloid is a hypertrophic scar usually occurring in dark-skinned individuals and does not reduce over time.

19. **(A)** Eschar consists of tissue that has been burned but remains adherent to the wound. Eschar is nonelastic and may constrict underlying structures and impair vital functions.

20. **(C)** Porcine is derived from pig tissue.

21. **(D)** The skin or the integumentary system performs a number of vital functions; one role is as a sensory organ that transmits touch, pressure, pain, and temperature, which alert the body to personal injury.

22. **(A)** Basal cell carcinoma is the most common cancer and arises from the basal layer of the epidermis.

23. **(D)** A graft that is transferred from one individual to another is known as an allograft or a homograft. The grafts are harvested from donors and preserved by the tissue bank until needed.

24. **(C)** A graft made up of tissue taken from one species and grafted to another species is a xenograft.

25. **(A)** Removal of tissue and burn wounds requires repeated debridement to remove dying and dead tissue so that healing can continue.

26. **(A)** Another name for a mentoplasty is a chin augmentation.

27. **(B)** Macromastia in males is referred to as gynecomastia.

28. **(A)** A panniculectomy is a surgical procedure performed to remove excess skin and fat from the abdomen. An abdominoplasty and tummy tuck are performed to remove excess skin and fat but also involve tightening the muscles of the abdominal wall.

29. **(D)** Mineral oil is applied to the donor graft site to reduce friction prior to using the dermatome.

30. **(B)** Langer's lines are the natural lines in the skin used for a landmark. Keloids are a type of scar. Lund–Browder is the chart used for burn assessment.

31. **(A)** The correct order is skin, subcutaneous, fascia, and muscle.

32. **(B)** A keloid is a raised, nodular scar. Cicatrix is a flattened scar. Hypertrophic is similar to a keloid but not as pronounced. An eschar is the debrided tissue from a burn.

33. **(D)** When using the burn assessment chart for "the rule of nines," the percentage given for both legs front and back is 36%. The front of each leg is 9%, and the back of each leg is 9%. Thus, the correct answer for the front and back of both legs together is 36%.

34. **(C)** A third-degree burn is appears as pearly white skin and includes the epidermis, dermis, and subcutaneous tissue. First degree is only the epidermis. Second degree is blistered, painful, moist, and red. Fourth-degree burns are deep into the muscles.

35. **(D)** Fourth-degree burns involve destruction of skin, muscles, tendons, vessels, and bone.

36. **(B)** The Padgett dermatome is manual. The Brown is electric with an oscillating saw. The Weck and Watson are dermatome knives.

37. **(B)** The Brown dermatome uses an oscillating blade. The Ferris–Smith is a dermatome knife. Reese and Padgett are manually used.

38. **(D)** Ferris–Smith, Watson, and Weck are all handheld knife dermatomes.

39. **(C)** A pedicle flap is a full-thickness skin graft that remains attached to a blood supply. STSG includes epidermis and dermis. A full-thickness skin graft does not remain attached to a blood supply.

40. **(B)** Melanoma is the most aggressive skin cancer that can metastasize to other organs. Basal and squamous cell carcinoma are less aggressive.

41. **(D)** Pressure ulcers can form on the sacrum, ischium, and heel, as those tissues remain touching the sheets for long periods of time without being rotated.

42. **(D)** The blood supply that feeds the TRAM flap comes from the superior epigastric artery and vein.

43. **(C)** The DIEP (deep inferior epigastric perforator artery) flap is a flap of skin, fat, and muscle from the back and is used for breast reconstruction. The TRAM (transverse rectus abdominis) flap takes skin, fat, and muscles from the lower abdomen to reconstruct the breast.

44. **(A)** Augmentation mammoplasty increases the size of the breast. A mastopexy is performed for breast ptosis. A TRAM flap is performed for breast reconstruction.

45. **(C)** A reduction mammoplasty reduces the size of extremely large breasts. A mastopexy is done for a breast ptosis. A simple mastectomy removes breast tissue.

46. **(B)** The order of repairs done for reimplantation of a finger are debridement, bone-to-bone fixation, tendon repair, nerve repair, artery and vein repair, and skin.

47. **(C)** Microtia is a congenital deformity of the pinna. Otitis media is inflammation of fluid in the inner ear. Mentoplasty is for reconstruction of a deformity of the chin. Cheiloplasty is repair of the lip.

48. **(D)** A brow lift, forehead lift, and endoscopic brow lift are all procedures that reduce wrinkles across the forehead and raise the sagging eyebrows and bridge of nose.

49. **(C)** A blepharoplasty can be performed through a subciliary or transconjunctival incision. A limbus incision is used for a cataract removal.

50. **(C)** A blepharoplasty is done for dermatochalasis. Rhytidectomy is a facelift. Microtia repair is done for small ears, and a mastopexy is performed for ptosis of breast.

51. **(B)** The candela dye laser and the Q-switched laser are used to remove tattoos.

52. **(D)** Liposuction is a surgical procedure done to remove fat from the abdomen, buttocks, hips, thighs, and knees. A tumescent solution of diluted lidocaine and epinephrine is injected into that area prior to the procedure to produce an anesthetic effect. Compression dressings are applied.

53. **(B)** Macromastia is the term used for large breasts. Gynecomastia is enlarged breast tissue in males due to hormones. Ptosis is a drooping of the breast, and microtia is small ears.

54. **(B)** Malar implants are inserted into the cheeks.

55. **(A)** A rhinoplasty is a nose job. A rhytidectomy is a facelift. Cheek implants are called malar.

56. **(C)** A third-degree burn includes the skin with all its epithelial structures and

subcutaneous tissue destroyed. It is characterized by a dry, pearly white, or charred-appearing surface void of sensation. The destroyed skin forms a parchment-like eschar over the burned area.

57. **(B)** In 1991, OSHA adopted requirements designed to prevent transmission of blood-borne pathogens in the work environment. It can fine health care facilities for noncompliance with regulations.

58. **(C)** The inflammatory response is the body's attempt to neutralize and destroy toxic agents at the site of injury and prevent their spread. After injury, the metabolic rate increases, quickening heartbeat. More blood circulates to the area, causing dilation of vessels. The large amount of blood in the area is responsible for redness.

59. **(D)** Radial dysplasia is also called club hand. This is a deformity of the radial bone causing the hand and wrist to turn inward toward the thumb aspect of the hand. Splints can be used to secure the wrist straight. Surgery is the last resort.

60. **(A)** Closure that is too tight or under tension causes ischemia, a decrease in blood supply to the tissues, and eventually tissue necrosis.

61. **(B)** When the collagen in the tissue remains constant, the fiber pattern reforms crosslinks to increase tensile strength in the tissue. Tensile strength is the ability of the tissues to resist rupture.

62. **(A)** Fibrinogen unites with thrombin (a product of prothrombin and thromboplastin) to form fibrin, which is the basic structural material of blood clots. It is essential for the clotting of blood.

63. **(B)** A cicatrix or scar is formed by the intertwining of cells surrounding the capillaries and binding together in final closure of a wound. It is a scar left by a healing wound.

64. **(B)** A mesher is used to expand the split-thickness skin graft by placing small slits in the donor skin. It consists of a mesher device and clear graft plates. The skin is placed on the plate and fed through the mesher, and cuts are made into the STSG.

65. **(B)** Healing by granulation (second intention) involves a wound that is either infected or one in which there is excessive loss of tissue. The skin edges cannot be adequately approximated. Generally, there is suppuration (pus formation), abscess, or necrosis.

66. **(C)** Healing by third intention implies that suturing is delayed for the purpose of walling off an area of gross infection involving much tissue removal, as in debridement of a burn when suturing is done later. Third intention of healing means that two opposing granulation surfaces are brought together. Granulation usually forms a wide, fibrous scar.

67. **(D)** Loose sutures prevent the wound edges from meeting and create dead spaces, which discourage healing. Tight sutures or closure under tension causes ischemia.

68. **(C)** Second-intention healing is commonly referred to as granulation healing. This form of wound healing takes longer than first intention, but is equally as strong once healed. It heals from the inside to the outside surface.

69. **(B)** A band of scar tissue that binds together two anatomical surfaces that are normally separate from each other is an adhesion. They are not commonly found in the abdomen, where they form after abdominal surgery, inflammation, or injury.

70. **(C)** Third intention is employed when the wound is infected or contaminated. There is a delayed primary closure.

71. **(C)** Evisceration is the protrusion of viscera through the edges of a totally separated wound.

72. **(D)** The three phases of wound healing are inflammatory, proliferation, and remodeling.

73. **(D)** Dehiscence is the tissue breakdown at the wound margin.

74. **(D)** All are wound complications.

75. **(B)** When a wound exudates a collection such as pus, serum, or dead cells around the incision, the wound is described as suppurative.

76. **(A)** The donor site is prepped first with a clear prep solution and considered clean. The recipient site is prepped last with a new set of prep sticks.

77. **(B)** The Doppler is an instrument (handheld transducer) used to measure the amount of blood flow through veins. The probe can be used preoperatively, intraoperatively with a sterile drape, and postoperatively.

78. **(C)** The pedicle flap would best provide sensation to the skin because of its attachments to skin, fat, and muscle.

79. **(C)** Apocrine is a type of sweat gland found in the skin. Ceruminous glands are found in the external auditory canal. Merocrine glands primary function is thermoregulation, and sebaceous glands are the oil glands of the body. Papillomas are growths that can be found on the skin or mucous membranes.

80. **(C)** A tattoo machine is used to reconstruct the areola during a breast reconstruction surgery.

81. **(A)** A cleft lip is an abnormality of the upper lip that occurs in the fetus around the second trimester during pregnancy. The repair is done so the infant can perform normal functions such as feeding and talking and to reduce dental problems. Cupid's bow is used as a guideline for cosmetic results from the repair.

CHAPTER 23

Genitourinary

GENITOURINARY

- Surgical anatomy includes—two kidneys, two ureters, bladder, urethra, prostate gland, two adrenal glands, male reproductive organs, and female reproductive system
- Kidneys—are located in the retroperitoneal space, one on each side of the vertebral column at the level of the 12th thoracic rib to the 3rd lumbar vertebra
  - Gerota's fascia—tissue and fat surrounding the fascia of the kidney, also called Gerota's capsule; helps keep the kidney in its normal position
  - Hilum—located on the medial side of the kidney; the renal vein/artery enters and exits the kidney
  - Renal pelvis—a funnel-shaped structure within the kidney, it divides into branches called the renal calyces
  - The major blood supply to the kidneys is from the renal artery
  - Glomerulus—a capillary network of blood vessels within the renal cortex that functions as a filter. It is surrounded by Bowman's capsule
  - Glomerular filtration—the first step of urine production where fluids are dissolved and forced through the membrane
  - The loop of Henle—helps to reabsorb filtered water and sodium, calcium, chlorine, and potassium in a normal kidney. The loop of Henle is found in the medulla of the kidney
- Nephron—the functional unit of the kidney responsible for removing waste and regulating fluid
  - Adrenal glands—each adrenal gland has a medulla that secretes epinephrine/adrenaline

- Adrenal cortex—makes cortisol and aldosterone. The medulla produces epinephrine and norepinephrine. These hormones are influenced by the pituitary gland
- ACTH—adrenocorticotropic hormone—the hormone secreted by the pituitary to the adrenals
- Ureters—each ureter is a continuation of the renal pelvis. It extends from the renal pelvis to the bladder
  - Peristaltic contractions in the ureters help transport urine from the kidney to the bladder
- Urinary bladder—the bladder acts as a reservoir for urine until micturition/voiding
  - Trigone area includes:
    - Two ureter openings
    - One urethral opening
- Urethra
  - The urethra in the male extends from the bladder to the penis
  - The urethra in the female lies beneath and behind the symphysis pubis anterior to the vagina
    - Because the female urethra is short and close to the anus and vagina, microorganisms have easy access to the bladder and can cause urinary tract infections (UTIs)
- The prostate gland—a donut-shaped gland located at the base of the bladder neck and completely surrounds the urethra
  - It is responsible for providing fluid for sperm
- Benign prostatic hyperplasia (BPH)—a noncancerous overgrowth of prostatic tissue that pushes against the bladder/urethra causing a blockage of urine flow
- KUB—an x-ray of the kidneys, ureters, and bladder. It shows the size, shape, and location of the organs

- IVU—intravenous urogram/pyelogram—x-ray with contrast media that shows the entire urological system

MALE REPRODUCTIVE ORGANS

- Scrotum—located behind and below the base of the penis and in front of the anus
  - The scrotum has two sacs lined with smooth glistening tissue called the tunica vaginalis
  - The tunica vaginalis has clear fluid within the sacs that also contain the testicles, epididymis, and some of the spermatic cord
  - The scrotum is separated by a septum called the median raphe
- Epididymis—this is where sperm are stored and mature. It secretes a seminal fluid that helps sperm to migrate
- Vas deferens—carries sperm from the testes to the urethra
- Ejaculatory duct—formed by the vas deferens and seminal vesicle duct. Semen passes through the prostate gland, enters the urethra, and exits the body via the tip of the penis through ejaculation
- Spermatic cord—contains veins, arteries, lymphatics, nerves, and vas deferens
  - The spermatic cord begins in inguinal ring and passes through the inguinal canal and ends at the superficial inguinal ring in the scrotum
- Cowper's glands/bulbourethral glands located on both sides of the bulbar urethras
  - Each gland secretes mucus into the urethra to aid in the ejaculation process
- Penis—contains a sponge-like body surrounding the urethra. It contains erectile tissue and an exit route for urine
  - Right corpus cavernosum and left corpus cavernosum—the two outer bodies
  - Corpus spongiosum urethra—the inner body, surrounds the urethra
  - These tissues are vascular channels that fill the penis with blood during an erection
- Prepuce/foreskin—located at the distal end of the penis; covers the glans penis
- Glans penis—head of the penis that contains the urethral orifice
- Special care must be taken when prepping for a genitourinary (GU) procedure; you must be careful of the perineal area to avoid contamination from the rectum to the urethra. The prep should be done in a downward motion and the sponge discarded once it has contacted the vagina or anal area
- Irrigation fluids are used to:
  - Distend the bladder for visualization
  - They should be warmed to meet the patient's body temperature to prevent hypothermia
  - They come in collapsible bags and provide continuous irrigation
  - You must know sterile technique because the sterile parts of the tubing and IV bag need to be kept sterile to prevent infection
- Distilled water—used for a simple cystoscopy, retrograde pyelogram, and bladder tumor fulguration
- Nonelectrolytic and nonhemolytic solution—these solutions do not conduct electricity
  - When using the electrosurgical unit (ESU), you cannot use saline solution because it can conduct electricity
  - They are used for transurethral resection of the prostate (TURP). They include:
    - Glycine
    - Mannitol
    - Sorbitol
- These solutions prevent:
  - Extravasation—entry of too much fluid into the blood
  - Hemolysis—rupturing of red blood cells (RBCs) and releasing their contents into the surrounding bloodstream due to extravasation
  - It is the STSR's/circulator's responsibility to keep track of the amount of irrigating solutions to be used to prevent extravasation from occurring
- Ureteral catheters
  - Used to identify the ureters during pelvic or intestinal surgery
  - To perform a retrograde pyelogram
  - Retrograde pyelogram—an x-ray of the kidney and ureter
- Contrast media is injected into the ureters to visualize the ureter and the kidney to see if there is a blockage in the urinary tract
- Used to bypass an obstruction in the ureter such as a tumor, stone, or stricture
- The most commonly used ureteral catheters are:
  - Whistle tip
  - Cone tip

○ Olive tip

○ Garceau tip

• Stents are specially designed hollow tubes made of a flexible plastic material that are placed in the ureter. They are used to:

○ Bypass an obstruction—commonly placed in the ureter, between the kidney and the bladder. They remain in the ureter following surgery or an obstruction—hence the name indwelling

○ Indwelling urethral stents include:

▪ Double pigtail

▪ Double J

• Urethral catheters function as stents and drainage tubes; they include:

○ Plain—temporarily inserted to:

▪ Drain urine from the bladder

▪ Decompress the bladder

▪ Obtain a urine specimen; example is a red Robinson and a Coude. These catheters do not require a drainage bag

▪ Commonly used to evacuate the bladder before a dilation and curettage (D&C)

○ Indwelling—used to measure urinary output and provide bladder decompression

▪ Examples include Foley catheters

▪ Most Foley catheters use gravity drainage bags (urimeter—measures the urine output). These gravity drainage bags must be kept below the level of the bladder to promote drainage and prevent reflux

▪ To fill the balloon on the Foley catheter, you use water not saline because it can erode the balloon

▪ To fill a 5-cc balloon, approximately 8–10 cc of water is used

○ A two-way Foley has two ports, one to fill the balloon and the second for urine drainage. This catheter is used on most operative procedures

○ The three-way Foley has three ports: one to fill the balloon, one for drainage, and the third for irrigation

○ Suprapubic—this catheter is placed in the bladder through a surgical opening in the abdomen. Examples of these catheters include:

▪ Foley

▪ Pezzer (mushroom)

▪ Malecot

○ The Pezzer and Malecot rely on their tip to hold the catheter in place, unlike the Foley, which uses a balloon

• Foley Goalie is a traction device used to prevent a Foley catheter from being pulled out of the male penis; if there is too much traction being forced on the catheter, the traction device tightens and prevents the catheter from coming out

• Nephrostomy tubes are inserted percutaneously into the kidneys to remove urine. The nephrostomy tube drains urine from your kidney into a collecting bag outside your body

• Interventional radiology—a separate department from the operating room (OR) and radiology where procedures are performed. Many OR procedures are now being done in interventional radiology. They place catheters and/or stents to introduce contrast media for fluoroscopy procedures

• Cystoscopy—an examination of the lower urinary tract including the urethra, bladder, and ureteral orifices. Indications for a cystoscopy include:

○ Hematuria—blood in the urine

○ Urinary retention

○ UTI

○ Cystitis

○ Tumors

○ Fistulas

○ Stones

○ Urinary incontinence

• Cysto table—stationary table that allows the patient to be positioned in supine, lithotomy, and various positions. It provides x-rays and fluoroscopy during the procedures. It has a mesh attachment for catching specimens and a drainage attachment built into the floor

• The most common stirrups used are Allen and Yellofin—they relieve pressure on the popliteal space

• Prep includes the entire pubic area, scrotum, and perineum

• Special cysto drape used; it has a sterile screen portion to allow irrigation/fluids to drain and catch specimens

• Basic cysto setup includes:

○ Light source

○ Cystoscope

○ Cystourethroscope

○ Bridge

- ○ Stopcock
- ○ Irrigation fluid and tubing
- ○ Rubber catheter nipples/adaptor
- Extra equipment sometimes needed for a cysto procedure includes:
  - ○ Randall Stone forceps
  - ○ Bladder biopsy forceps
  - ○ Instruments for crushing stones
  - ○ Instruments—general surgery/vascular/ thoracic, rib/long instruments
  - ○ Herrick pedicle clamp
- Flexible cystoscope—used on patients who have a rigid prostatic urethra and patients who cannot be placed lithotomy position. This procedure can be performed at the patient's bedside
- Litho-La-Paxy/litholapaxy—a procedure where large bladder stones are crushed in the bladder with a lithotrite (a special instrument used to crush stones) and removed through irrigation
- Endoscopy of the genitourinary tract is considered a class II clean contaminated case
- This requires high-level disinfection cleaning
- Glutaraldehyde is the choice of disinfectant; it is also called Cidex
  - ○ The level of disinfection is based on the time, temperature, and concentration of the disinfectant
  - ○ Once activated, the shelf life is 14 days
  - ○ Rinse with sterile water, and make sure all surfaces are rinsed including all ports and channels
  - ○ It is effective for (10 minutes/68–86°F/ 2.0–2.4%):
    - Bacteria
    - Fungi
    - Viruses—HIV/hepatitis B virus
    - Tuberculosis (45–90 minutes/77–86°F/ 2.0%)
    - Spores (10 hours/room temperature)
- Laser ablation of condylomata and penile carcinoma—these procedures are being performed with the laser more often than the ESU because the heat from the laser is distributed more evenly and can also target the underlying tissue
  - ○ Smoke evacuator must be used to prevent inhaling the plume because it is a carcinogen. The lasers used include:
    - Argon
    - CO_2

- KTP—potassium
- Nd—neodymium
- YAG
- Circumcision—procedure to excise the foreskin (prepuce) of the glans penis
  - ○ In males, it is performed for the relief of phimosis
  - ○ Phimosis—the foreskin becomes stenosed over the tip of the penis and is difficult to retract. This can cause infection because it is difficult to clean
  - ○ Basic instruments, ESU, and have available straight hemostats
  - ○ Dressings used are nonadherent allowing for urination, such as Xeroform and a 4 × 4
- Urethral meatotomy—an incisional enlargement of the urethral meatus performed for congenital/acquired stenosis or a stricture at the external urethral meatus
  - ○ This procedure is done to provide relief of a urethral stricture
  - ○ Van Buren sounds—urethral dilators
  - ○ Phillips filiforms and followers—plastic/ woven dilators that can pass through a stricture. The followers are then passed over the filiform to dilate the stricture. They come in graduated sizes
    - Filiforms are used to get past difficult strictures, and followers are used for dilation and drainage
- Urethroplasty—this is reconstructive surgery of the urethra due to:
  - ○ Strictures
  - ○ Infection
  - ○ Trauma or a congenital anomaly
- Penectomy—the partial or total removal of a cancerous penis
- Penile implant—performed for organic sexual impotence. Sexual impotence may be caused by:
  - ○ Diabetes
  - ○ Priapism (persistent and painful erection)
  - ○ Peyronie's disease (distorted/bent penis)
  - ○ Penile trauma
  - ○ Neurological/vascular problems
- The cylinders are implanted into the penis, the pump is implanted into the scrotum, and the reservoir is implanted in the abdomen
- Bacitracin antibiotic irrigation is used during the procedure and to soak the implants prior to implanting in the body

- Hydrocelectomy—a hydrocele is an abnormal accumulation of fluid in the tunica vaginalis layer of the scrotum. It is usually the result of trauma or infection
  - Procedure includes a scrotal incision where the fluid is suctioned out and the sac is inverted and sutured
- Vasectomy—this procedure is performed to sterilize males
  - Allis clamp is used to grasp the vas deferens
  - The vas deferens are separated and then tied/cauterized to prevent sperm from entering the seminal stream
- Vasovasostomy—this procedure is performed to correct obstructions of the vas deferens caused by:
  - Congenital anomalies
  - Inflammation
  - Trauma
  - It is also performed for reversal of a vasectomy
  - Microscope is used
- Epididymectomy—this procedure is performed to remove an inflamed portion of the epididymis. Fluid and sperm are prevented from passing through the epididymis
- Spermatocelectomy—an abnormal cyst/sac filled with fluid that may contain sperm
- Varicocelectomy—a varicocele is an abnormal dilatation of the spermatic veins in the spermatic cord that drain the testicles. This causes a painful swelling of the scrotum
  - Varicocelectomy is ligation of the spermatic vein performed to prevent a rise in temperature in the scrotum to preserve the sperm and increase sperm count
- Prostatectomy—the surgical removal of part or all of the prostate gland. The procedure can be performed:
  - Transurethral—through the urethra (TURP)
  - Suprapubic—through the bladder
  - Retropubic—around the bladder
- Symptoms of BPH are similar to that of prostate cancer. There are two screening tests to determine prostate disease; they include:
  - PSA—prostate-specific antigen
  - DRE—digital rectal examination
- The PSA is used to screen for prostate cancer
  - It measures the amount of PSA in the blood
- Another test used for screening of the prostate is the DRE (digital rectal examination). The prostate lies in the front of the rectum, and the physician can feel the gland by using a gloved/lubricated finger inserted into the rectum
- Gleason score—a system used to grade prostate cancer. Two cell types are tested and combined to give you a score
- Needle biopsy—once prostate cancer is clinically suspected, a needle biopsy of the prostate is indicated
  - Tru-Cut biopsy needle is used to obtain a prostate specimen
  - This procedure is performed in the urologist's office, and a 22-g needle is used transrectally or transperineally
- TURP—transurethral resection of the prostate—the endoscopic surgical removal of the prostate; part of or all of the prostate can be removed
  - This can be done transurethrally or open
  - TURP for BPH is done by direct visualization of the prostate with the cystoscope through the urethra
  - The tissue is removed with electrocautery/resectoscope—these are used for performing a resection with electrical current
  - The surgeon passes a resectoscope into the bladder through the urethra, and resects pieces of tissue from around the bladder neck and lobes of the prostate, leaving the capsule intact
  - Ellik evacuator/Toomey syringe—used to evacuate prostatic chips and clots following a TURP
  - A triple-lumen catheter is inserted at the end of the case for drainage and irrigation; it is a Foley triple-lumen catheter 30-cc balloon
    - One lumen is to fill the balloon
    - The second is for irrigation
    - The third is for drainage and aspiration
- Laser—light amplification by the simulated emission of radiation/laser procedures of the prostate
  - KTP laser—potassium-titanyl phosphate—also known as the GREEN LIGHT LASER—used for vaporization of benign prostatic disease
- Laser safety includes:
  - Eyewear
  - Fiberoptic beam must not be directly placed on the drapes
  - Proper suction equipment must be used for smoke plume
  - Laser signs should be posted on all doors/windows in the room to alert outside personnel

- Retropubic prostatectomy—removal of the hypertrophic prostate tissue with an extravesical approach (around the bladder)
- Suprapubic prostatectomy—removal of the prostate through a transvesical approach (through the bladder)
- Simple perineal prostatectomy—removal of a prostate through a perineal approach. This is done when there is suspicion of cancer
- Radical retropubic prostatectomy with pelvic lymphadenectomy—a radical prostatectomy is performed to remove the cancerous prostate gland
  - The entire gland, capsule, and seminal vesicles are removed
  - The posterolateral neurovascular bundles are spared to preserve erectile function
  - The second part of the procedure is to remove the lymph nodes en bloc to prevent seeding
- Laparoscopic radical prostatectomy—a minimally invasive procedure
- Robot-assisted laparoscopic radical prostatectomy—robotic equipment is used to perform this procedure, allowing the robot to imitate the surgeon's movement. Same advantages as a laparoscopic radical prostatectomy
  - The robotic system consists of:
    - Surgeon's console
    - Cart with interactive robotic arms and jointed instruments that simulate the human hand and wrist
    - A high-resolution three-dimensional image
- Transrectal seed implantation—performed for cancer that is contained within the prostate
  - For this procedure, there are many different physicians involved in a collaborative effort to treat the patient; they include:
    - Radiation oncologist
    - Medical physicist
    - GU surgeon
    - Oncologist
- Surgery of the bladder—surgeries of the bladder can be performed with an open abdominal incision or transurethrally
  - For most open bladder procedures, supine position/Trendelenburg (this position is used to displace abdominal organs for better visualization of the bladder)
- Suprapubic cystostomy—a cystostomy catheter is placed into the urinary bladder through a low abdominal incision

- When a drainage tube is inserted into the bladder through an abdominal incision, the procedure is called a cystostomy
- Transurethral resection of bladder tumors—TURB—bladder tumors are removed with:
  - Resectoscope working element, loop electrode, and biopsy forceps
  - The scope is inserted transurethrally into the bladder
- As with the TURP procedure, you must be aware of the irrigating solution you use and the amount used. With bladder tumors, sterile water is recommended
- Transurethral laser ablation—the YAG laser is used to destroy small recurrent bladder tumors and large bladder tumors
- Suprapubic cystolithotomy—removal of bladder stones with special instruments. Electrohydraulic lithotripter is used to crush the stones with an electric current
  - YAG laser can also be used to pulverize the stones

VESICO-FISTULAS

- They are an abnormal hollow or tubular connection between two organs
  - Vesicointestinal fistula—enterovesical fistula—fistula between the bladder and intestines
  - Vesicovaginal fistula—fistula between the bladder and vagina
- Vesicourethral suspension—Marshall–Marchetti–Krantz—this procedure is performed to treat urinary stress incontinence in women
  - The objective is to bring the bladder and the urethra back up into the pelvis; sutures are used to correct this
  - Everyone must be double gloved and change gloves every time they go into the vagina; they should change their gloves because the vagina is considered dirty
  - Pereyra needle—this is a surgical technique for the correction of stress incontinence
- TVT sling—tension-free vaginal tape—this is performed on women who have urinary stress incontinence or sphincter deficiency
  - The tape used is made of polypropylene mesh encased in plastic and is attached to two large trocar needles at each end of the tape

- The mesh is passed through the pelvic tissue and positioned under the urethra, creating a supportive sling
- A cystoscopy is performed at the beginning of the case to confirm the integrity of the bladder. This is performed after the first needle is inserted and again at the end to make sure the bladder was not perforated
- Radical cystectomy—total removal of the bladder and adjacent structures along with pelvic lymph node dissection
  - This procedure is done en bloc to prevent any further seeding
- Ileal conduit—this is an exterior urinary diversion where the bladder is removed with a radical cystectomy and the ureters are rerouted to a loop in the bowel, and it is brought out to the skin (ileostomy) and drains into a urinary drainage bag
- Bladder augmentation/neobladder—this is surgically performed to create a new bladder. Interior urinary diversion within the intestines is done, and a new bladder is created with the intestine
  - Names of the urinary diversion procedures include:
    - Knock pouch
    - Indiana pouch
    - Le bag
- Cutaneous ureterostomy—another type of urinary diversion where the ureters are brought out to the skin when bowel cannot be used
- Surgery of the ureters and kidneys—surgery is performed to prevent urine obstruction and subsequent renal failure
  - The most common causes of urinary tract obstructions include:
    - Stones
    - Infections
    - Tumors
    - Congenital malformations
    - Previous surgery
  - When surgery of these stones is performed, they are sent to pathology for chemical analysis and should always be sent dry
  - Staghorn calculus—a stone that lodges itself in the renal calyx and continues to grow large. Surgical intervention is required
  - Stones are sent to pathology in a dry container
  - The incision used for ureter and/or kidney surgery may require removal of the 11th and 12th ribs

- Urethrectomy—nephroureterectomy—complete removal of the ureter; usually involves removing the kidney due to tumors involving the kidney and ureter
- Ureteroenterostomy—diversion of the ureter into a portion of the intestines
  - Ureterocolostomy—rerouting the ureters into the colon
  - Ileal conduit—the entire procedure of removing the bladder and rerouting the ureters into a portion of the ileum
- Ureteroureterostomy—removal of the diseased portion of the ureter and then reconnecting it to another portion of the same ureter
- Ureterocystostomy—rerouting of the ureters into another part of the bladder. Even though the bladder is not removed in this procedure, a urinary diversion is still created
- Ureteropyeloscopy—removal of a stone or stricture in the ureter or kidney by way of transurethral approach—through the urethra to the bladder and into the ureter
- Nephrostomy—creating an opening into the kidney for temporary or permanent drainage of urine when there is an obstruction in the urinary tract to preserve the renal tissue. If urine does not flow out of the kidney, infection, renal failure, and destruction of the renal tissue will occur
- Nephrotomy—incision into the kidney usually due to a blockage from a calculus
- Percutaneous nephrolithotomy—this procedure is performed to remove stones from the patient's urinary tract by means of a flexible nephroscope passed into the kidney percutaneously (through the skin)
- ESWL—extracorporeal shock wave lithotripsy—uses shock waves to break a kidney stone into small pieces that can more easily travel through the ureter
  - High-energy sound waves pass through your body without injuring it and break the stone into small pieces
- Pyelolithotomy—removal of a calculus from the renal pelvis (part of the kidney that connects to the ureter)
- Pyelostomy—making an opening into the renal pelvis for temporary/permanent diversion of urine flow

- Pyelotomy—incision into the renal pelvis as an access to stones in the renal pelvis
- Laser lithotripsy—the laser is used to destroy stones, and there is no damage to the surrounding tissue. The YAG laser is used
- Nephroureterectomy—open approach—removal of the kidney and its entire ureter
  - This is performed for hydroureteronephrosis (distension and dilation of the renal pelvis and ureter)
  - This is caused by an obstruction in the renal pelvis and ureter
- Nephrectomy—open approach—surgical removal of the kidney. It is performed for:
  - Congenital hydronephrosis (distension/dilation of the kidney). Kidney becomes very large
  - Renal tumor
  - Renal trauma
  - Stones causing severe infection
- The 11th and 12th ribs may be removed for a nephrectomy
- Heminephrectomy—removal of a portion of the kidney
- Lateral kidney position:
  - The patient position is lateral with the operative kidney up and the dependent side placed on the kidney rest
    - Left lateral kidney—right side up
    - Right lateral kidney—left side up
  - The upper arm is supported on padded Mayo stand, and the lower arm is on a padded arm board
  - The patient's legs are positioned with a pillow between the legs, the lower leg is bent, and the upper leg is straight
  - The kidney rest is then raised, and heavy 2-in tape or a bean bag is used to stabilize the patient
  - The purpose of the kidney rest is to increase the space between the lower ribs and iliac crest
  - Before closing on a kidney case, the kidney rest is lowered and the table is straightened to help create better approximation of tissues
- Laparoscopic nephrectomy—the most common approach used for a laparoscopic nephrectomy is the transabdominal
  - You must always be prepared to open
- Radical nephrectomy—removal of the kidney, fatty tissue, adrenal gland, Gerota's capsule, and the lymph nodes

- Kidney transplant—a kidney transplant is the transplantation of a living related or a cadaver donor kidney into the recipient's iliac fossa. Common diagnosis for a kidney transplant is polycystic kidneys
  - The ideal donor is a twin or an immediate family member, usually a parent or sibling, or a cadaveric donor, which is the most common
  - Different IV solutions are used before, during, and after the procedure. Mannitol is given on the morning prior to surgery to the living donor to ensure diuresis before, during, and after the procedure
    - Mannitol—the drug of choice given to the donor patient to reduce swelling and increase urine output
      - Osmosis—when molecules of water go from where there are plenty of them to where there are few of them (high concentration to lower concentration)
    - Ringer's lactate IV solution—used to perfuse the harvested kidney (this solution is chilled)
- Collins or Sachs solution—used to perfuse the harvested kidney from a cadaver donor but should never be used to perfuse a kidney from a living donor. This solution is chilled
  - Two adjacent OR rooms are prepared for the surgery because the procedure is performed simultaneously
  - The right kidney is usually taken because it is the smaller one. The larger kidney is left in the donor
  - Gibson incision—commonly used for a transplant
  - The position for the recipient is left lateral decubitus
  - The cadaver donor is placed in supine position
- Adrenalectomy—the adrenal glands lie above each kidney; they produce hormones such as epinephrine, norepinephrine, androgens, estrogens, aldosterone, and cortisol. This procedure is performed to excise part or all of one or both adrenal glands
- This is performed for hypersecretion of the adrenal hormones
- Wilms tumor/nephroblastoma—congenital malignant tumor of the kidney found in children

Questions

1. The Pereyra needle is used in which specialty area of surgery?

   (A) Neurology
   (B) Urology
   (C) Orthopedics
   (D) Ophthalmology

2. The use of distilled water during a highly invasive genitourinary procedure such as a transurethral resection of the prostate (TURP) is prohibited for irrigation because of the potential for:

   (A) hemolysis of RBC
   (B) electrolytic dissipation of current
   (C) increase of blood pressure
   (D) body fluid shift

3. Why is a 30-cc balloon Foley used after a TURP?

   (A) Hemostasis
   (B) Decompression
   (C) Creation of negative pressure
   (D) Aspiration

4. The three lumens of a Foley are used for inflation, drainage, and:

   (A) prevention of urine reflux
   (B) access for sterile urine specimens
   (C) continuous irrigation
   (D) additional hemostasis

5. The purpose of the kidney bar or kidney lift is to:

   (A) increase the space between the lower ribs and iliac crest
   (B) increase the space between the ribs
   (C) stabilize the patient
   (D) support the body in the flexed position

6. Why is the table straightened before closing a kidney incision?

   (A) To facilitate easier respirations
   (B) To create better approximation of tissues
   (C) To facilitate better circulation
   (D) To prevent nerve damage

7. Nonmalignant enlargement of the prostate is termed:

   (A) prostatitis
   (B) benign prostatic hyperplasia (BPH)
   (C) balanitis
   (D) prostatism

8. Urethral strictures can be dilated by use of each of the following EXCEPT:

   (A) Philips filiform and followers
   (B) Van Buren sounds
   (C) Braasch bulb
   (D) McCarthy dilators

9. A staghorn stone is one that lodges and continues to grow in the:

   (A) renal calyx
   (B) space of Retzius
   (C) ureter
   (D) hilum

10. In cystoscopy, the irrigating solution is:

    (A) distilled water
    (B) glycine
    (C) mannitol
    (D) sorbitol

11. Rib removal for surgical exposure of the kidney requires all of the following EXCEPT a/an:

    (A) Alexander periosteotome
    (B) Doyen raspatory
    (C) Heaney clamp
    (D) Stille shears

12. Penile condylomata are most successfully removed by:

    (A) dermabrasion
    (B) laser
    (C) cautery
    (D) ultrasound

13. Removal of a testis or the testes is called:

    (A) orchiopexy
    (B) orchiectomy
    (C) epididymectomy
    (D) vasectomy

14. Which solution is NOT used during a transurethral prostatectomy?

    (A) Normal saline
    (B) Sorbitol
    (C) Mannitol
    (D) Glycine

15. Temporary diversion of urinary drainage by means of an external catheter that drains the renal pelvis is called:

    (A) vesicostomy
    (B) nephrostomy
    (C) pyelostomy
    (D) cystostomy

16. The procedure to treat organic sexual impotence is:

    (A) spermatocelectomy
    (B) varicocelectomy
    (C) testicular implant
    (D) penile implant

17. Microscopic reversal of the male sterilization procedure is termed:

    (A) spermatogenesis
    (B) orchiopexy
    (C) vasovasostomy
    (D) vasectomy

18. A needle biopsy of the prostate may be accomplished with a/an:

    (A) butterfly needle
    (B) angiocatheter
    (C) Tru-Cut needle
    (D) taper needle

19. A congenital condition in the male in which the urethra ends on the ventral side of the glans penis anywhere along the penile shaft, on the corona, or on the perineum is termed:

    (A) paraphimosis
    (B) phimosis
    (C) epispadias
    (D) chordee

20. Continuous irrigation following TURP is accomplished by use of a:

    (A) suprapubic cystotomy tube
    (B) 30-cc three-way Foley catheter
    (C) 5-cc three-way Foley catheter
    (D) 30-cc two-way Foley catheter

21. When the prostate gland is removed through an abdominal incision into the anterior prostatic capsule, it is called a ____ prostatectomy.

    (A) perineal
    (B) suprapubic
    (C) retropubic
    (D) transurethral

22. Kidney stones are sent to the laboratory in:

    (A) saline
    (B) water
    (C) dry state
    (D) formalin

23. A Pereyra procedure is done for:

    (A) stress incontinence
    (B) chronic bladder infection
    (C) drainage of the bladder
    (D) impotence

24. A percutaneous nephrolithotomy utilizes all of the following EXCEPT:

    (A) ultrasound wand
    (B) flexible nephroscope
    (C) lithotripter
    (D) lithotripter tub

25. Orchiopexy can be defined as:

    (A) fixation of an ovary
    (B) uterine suspension
    (C) testicle removal
    (D) fixation of a testicle

26. Abdominal resection of the prostate gland through an incision into the bladder is known surgically as a:

    (A) retropubic prostatectomy
    (B) suprapubic prostatectomy
    (C) transurethral prostatectomy
    (D) suprapubic cystostomy

27. A lumbar or simple flank incision for ureter or kidney surgery may include removal of which ribs?

    (A) 5 and 6
    (B) 7 and 8
    (C) 9 and 10
    (D) 11 and 12

28. An abnormal accumulation of fluid in the scrotum is a/an:

    (A) hydrocele
    (B) enterocele
    (C) varicocele
    (D) hydronephrosis

29. Bladder stones are crushed with a:

    (A) basket catheter
    (B) lithotrite
    (C) cautery
    (D) resectoscope

30. Urethral meatal stenosis is corrected by a/an:

    (A) frenulotomy
    (B) meatotomy
    (C) urethral dilation
    (D) extirpation of the penis

31. In a penile implant, the inflation pump is located in the:

    (A) distal penis
    (B) proximal penis
    (C) scrotum
    (D) groin

32. Excision of the tunica vaginalis is a:

    (A) vagotomy
    (B) vasectomy
    (C) varicocelectomy
    (D) hydrocelectomy

33. Circumcision refers to:

    (A) removal of the foreskin
    (B) removal of the glans
    (C) widening of the urethral opening
    (D) lengthening of the foreskin

34. An alternative approach to surgical TURP utilizing a basic cystoscopic setup is:

   (A) suprapubic prostatectomy
   (B) transcystoscopic urethroplasty
   (C) perineal prostatectomy
   (D) retropubic prostatectomy

35. The laser used to destroy small recurrent bladder tumors is the:

   (A) CO_2
   (B) argon
   (C) Nd:YAG
   (D) both A and B

36. Following anastomosis of a ureter during a ureteral reimplantation procedure, a _____ is left in place to ensure free drainage of the kidney postoperatively.

   (A) Foley catheter
   (B) ureteral catheter
   (C) T-tube
   (D) soft stent

37. A reverse sterilization procedure in the male is called a/an:

   (A) vasostomy
   (B) vasovasostomy
   (C) epididymovasostomy
   (D) both B and C

38. Before insertion of a penile implant, the insertion site, as well as the implant itself, is irrigated with:

   (A) normal saline
   (B) Betadine
   (C) sterile water
   (D) kanamycin and bacitracin

39. To prevent thrombi from forming in the walls of the renal vein during transfer from the donor to the recipient, _____ is given just before clamping of the renal vessels.

   (A) furosemide
   (B) protamine sulfate
   (C) heparin
   (D) mannitol

40. The drug of choice for adequate diuresis of a living donor before, during, and after removal of the kidney is:

   (A) urea
   (B) protamine sulfate
   (C) Ringer's lactate solution
   (D) mannitol

41. All of the following are ideal requirements of cadaver donors EXCEPT:

   (A) any age
   (B) free of infection or malignancy
   (C) normotensive up until death
   (D) under hospital observation before death

42. Cooling and flushing of pancreas, liver, and kidneys of cadaver donors are accomplished by cannulation of the organ and infusion of large amounts of cold:

   (A) saline solution
   (B) Ringer's lactate solution
   (C) sterile water
   (D) Sack's solution

43. Nonconducting, isosmotic glycine irrigating solution must be used in the surgical presence of a:

   (A) cystoscope
   (B) ureteroscope
   (C) resectoscope
   (D) nephroscope

44. All of the following procedures may be completed through a cystoscope EXCEPT:

    (A) biopsy of bladder tumor
    (B) removal of foreign body in bladder
    (C) total removal of bladder tumor
    (D) cystogram for diagnostic studies

45. After incision is made into the scrotum during a vasectomy, the forceps used to grasp the vas and bring it to the surface for surgery is the:

    (A) Allis
    (B) Babcock
    (C) Kelly
    (D) mosquito

46. Extracorporeal shock wave lithotripsy (ESWL) disintegrates stones by introducing shock waves into the body through the medium of:

    (A) water
    (B) air
    (C) gas
    (D) saline

47. Laser lithotripsy utilizes the tunable pulse-dyed laser known as:

    (A) diode
    (B) Nd:YAG
    (C) Candela
    (D) argon

48. The inability to control urination is:

    (A) reflux
    (B) urinary incontinence
    (C) hydrocele
    (D) chronic bladder infection

49. The radiographic diagnostic test used to outline the structures of the kidney, ureters, and bladder is known as:

    (A) MRI
    (B) retrograde pyelogram
    (C) GU radiograph
    (D) KUB

50. Overabsorption of irrigation fluid that may result in vascular overload is known as:

    (A) extravasation
    (B) intravasation
    (C) hemolysis
    (D) hydronephrosis

51. All are urethral catheters EXCEPT:

    (A) whistle tip
    (B) spiral tip
    (C) Braasch bulb
    (D) three-way Foley

52. When performing an ileal conduit for urinary diversion, the ureters are implanted into:

    (A) bladder
    (B) ileum
    (C) trigone
    (D) large intestine

53. If a patient is undergoing a right nephrectomy for a right renal tumor, the position is:

    (A) a right lateral kidney
    (B) a left lateral kidney
    (C) supine
    (D) prone

54. What syringe is used to evacuate bladder, prostate, or stone fragments?

    (A) Cystoscope
    (B) Ellik
    (C) Toomey
    (D) Both B and C

55. Which of the following dilators is used to dilate the urethra?

    (A) Hanks
    (B) Hagar
    (C) Cysto
    (D) Van Buren

56. Which incision is used when doing a TURP?

    (A) Suprapubic
    (B) Retropubic
    (C) Pfannenstiel
    (D) None of the above

57. Insertion of a suprapubic catheter into the bladder for drainage away from the vaginal and urethral area is:

    (A) Foley catheter
    (B) ileal conduit
    (C) cystostomy
    (D) Stamey procedure

58. Discharge of urine from the urinary bladder is called:

    (A) plasma flow
    (B) albumen urea
    (C) renal clearance
    (D) micturition

59. What is the condition in which the urethral meatus is located on the top side of the penis?

    (A) Penile implant
    (B) Hypospadias
    (C) Epispadias
    (D) Meatotomy

60. This procedure is performed on a patient with chronic and end-stage renal disease to aid in filtering the blood and removing ingested toxins.

    (A) Arteriovenous (AV) fistula
    (B) AV shunt
    (C) Peritoneal dialysis
    (D) All of the above

61. The tissue covering of the kidney that keeps it in its normal position is:

    (A) glomerulus
    (B) renal pelvis
    (C) Gerota's capsule
    (D) loop of Henley

62. Which of the following instruments is used to dilate the urethra?

    (A) Hank
    (B) Hagar
    (C) Bakes
    (D) Van Buren

63. The first step of urine production where fluids are dissolved and forced through the membrane is:

    (A) glomerular filtration
    (B) peritoneal dialysis
    (C) hemolysis
    (D) osmosis

64. The functional unit of the kidney responsible for removing waste and regulating fluid is:

    (A) renal pelvis
    (B) nephron
    (C) renal calyx
    (D) Gerota's capsule

65. A procedure to remove urinary calculus is:

    (A) ileal conduit
    (B) laparoscopic nephrectomy
    (C) ESWL
    (D) TURP

66. The trigone includes:

    (A) openings of both ureters
    (B) urethral opening in the bladder
    (C) Both A and B
    (D) connection of the kidney to ureter, ureter to bladder, and bladder to urethral meatus

67. Rupturing of RBCs and releasing their contents into the surrounding bloodstream is caused by:

    (A) hemolysis
    (B) extravasation
    (C) hydronephrosis
    (D) distribution

68. The catheter placed in the bladder through a surgical opening in the abdomen for urinary diversion is:

    (A) Coude
    (B) Robinson
    (C) suprapubic
    (D) none of the above

69. How many cubic centimeters (cc) of sterile water is used to fill a 16-Fr 5-cc Foley catheter?

    (A) 1–5
    (B) 5–6
    (C) 8–10
    (D) 10–12

70. When performing a penile implant, the reservoir is placed in the _____, the cylinders in the _____, and the pump in the _____.

    (A) scrotum, penis, abdomen
    (B) penis, scrotum, abdomen
    (C) abdomen, penis, scrotum
    (D) abdomen, scrotum, penis

71. Transrectal seed implantation is performed for cancer within the prostate. The physicians involved with the treatment include all EXCEPT:

    (A) radiation oncologist
    (B) OB/GYN
    (C) GU
    (D) medical physicist

72. A vesicovaginal fistula is a fistula between the:

    (A) vagina and intestines
    (B) vagina and anus
    (C) vagina and bladder
    (D) vagina and rectum

73. A TVT sling is used for:

    (A) urinary stress incontinence
    (B) kidney stones
    (C) kidney tumor
    (D) both B and C

74. All are true regarding a kidney transplant EXCEPT:

    (A) the right kidney is usually taken because it is the smaller one, and the larger kidney is left for the donor patient
    (B) Gibson incision is used
    (C) mannitol is used
    (D) a kidney transplant is the transplantation of only a cadaver donor kidney into the recipient's iliac fossa

75. The most common tumor of the kidney in children is:

    (A) Wilms tumor
    (B) neuroblastoma
    (C) nephrosarcoma
    (D) glioblastoma

76. The incision used in a simple open nephrectomy is:

    (A) Gibson
    (B) low transverse
    (C) subcostal flank
    (D) McBurney's

77. When placing a patient in lithotomy position, which of the following is the MOST acceptable technique?

    (A) Arms placed on arm boards placed at 110 degrees
    (B) Legs placed in stirrups one at a time
    (C) Both legs placed in stirrups simultaneously
    (D) Hips placed above the lower break of the table

78. Which prostatic approach requires the need of a resectoscope?

    (A) Perineal
    (B) Suprapubic
    (C) Retropubic
    (D) Transurethral

79. Which type of laser is typically used for stone fragmentation in the ureter?

    (A) Argon
    (B) Krypton
    (C) Carbon dioxide
    (D) Holmium:YAG

80. Necrotizing fasciitis confined to the perineum and scrotum is known as:

    (A) cellulitis
    (B) Gerota's fasciitis
    (C) boil
    (D) Fournier's gangrene

81. A cystectomy with ileal conduit was performed. The surgical technologist anticipates the need for a stoma:

    (A) pouch to collect body fluids
    (B) flange to create an artificial orifice
    (C) pouch to heal the wound
    (D) collar to provide suction for drainage

Answers and Explanations

1. **(B)** A Pereyra needle suspension is used to treat stress incontinence, a urinary condition.

2. **(A)** When water is used for irrigation on an invasive surgical procedure, the pressure of the water against the exposed vessels creates a hemolytic reaction and therefore destroys RBCs.

3. **(A)** Pressure from a 30-cc catheter balloon inserted after closure of the urethra helps obtain hemostasis by controlling venous bleeding.

4. **(C)** The third lumen provides a means for continuous irrigation of the bladder for a time postoperatively to prevent formation of clots in the bladder.

5. **(A)** The OR table is flexed so that the kidney elevator can be raised the desired amount to increase the space between the lower ribs and iliac crest.

6. **(B)** When the kidney position is being used, the table is straightened before closure to afford better approximation of tissues. It is used for procedures on kidneys and ureters. This is done by the anesthesiologist.

7. **(B)** As the male ages, the prostate gland may enlarge and gradually obstruct the urethra. This condition is known as benign prostatic hyperplasia (BPH).

8. **(C)** A Braasch bulb is a ureteral catheter used to occlude the ureteral orifice during x-ray study. Urethral dilatation is accomplished using McCarthy dilators, Philips filiform and followers, and Van Buren sounds.

9. **(A)** A stone may lodge in a renal calyx and continue to enlarge, eventually filling the entire renal collecting system. It is known as a staghorn stone.

10. **(A)** For simple observation cystoscopy or retrograde pyelogram, sterile distilled water may be used.

11. **(C)** The Alexander periosteotome, Doyen raspatory, and Stille shears are all instruments required to remove a rib. A Heaney clamp is a hemostatic clamp used in gynecological surgery.

12. **(B)** Laser ablation of condylomata is the eradication of diseased tissue by means of a laser beam. The recurrence rate with this technique is low.

13. **(B)** Removal of the testes (orchiectomy) renders the patient both sterile and hormone deficient. Bilateral orchiectomy usually denotes carcinoma. Unilateral orchiectomy may be indicated for cancer, infection, or trauma.

14. **(A)** Sorbitol, mannitol, and glycine do not produce hemolysis. They are nonelectrolytic and do not cause dispersion of high-frequency current with loss of cutting power as occurs with normal saline.

15. **(C)** Pyelostomy is entering the pelvis of the kidney with a small blade. A catheter is placed through the incision into the renal pelvis to create a short-term urinary diversion.

16. **(D)** A penile prosthesis is implanted for treatment of organic sexual impotence.

17. **(C)** Vasovasostomy is the surgical reanastomosis of the vas deferens, utilizing the operative microscope.

18. **(C)** The Tru-Cut or Vim–Silverman biopsy needle is used to retrieve a prostate biopsy.

19. **(D)** Chordee is when the male penis is curved ventrally with the meatus and the glans within close proximity to each other. Epispadias is when the urethral opening is on the dorsum of the penis. Phimosis is a congenital narrowing of the foreskin on the head of the penis. Paraphimosis is when the foreskin cannot be retracted from an uncircumcised penis, which can result in gangrene and amputation of the penis.

20. **(B)** Following a TURP, the urologist may insert a 30-cc three-way Foley catheter. The third lumen provides a means of continuous irrigation of the bladder for a period after surgery to prevent the formation of clots. The large balloon aids in hemostasis.

21. **(C)** Retropubic prostatectomy is the enucleation of hypertrophied prostate tissue through an incision into the anterior prostatic capsule. Good exposure and excellent hemostasis are obtained.

22. **(C)** Stones removed during surgery are subjected to chemical analysis and thus are submitted in a dry state. Fixative agents invalidate the results of the analysis.

23. **(A)** A Pereyra procedure is a bladder neck suspension involving ureterovesical suspension with vaginourethroplasty.

24. **(D)** A percutaneous nephrolithotomy facilitates the removal of stones using a rigid or flexible nephroscope. Accessory instrumentation includes an ultrasonic wand (sonotrode), lithotripter probe, stone basket, and stone grasper. A lithotripter tub is used in extracorporeal shock wave lithotripsy.

25. **(D)** Orchiopexy is regarded as the transfer or fixation of an imperfectly descended testicle into the scrotum and suturing it in place.

26. **(B)** After a suprapubic incision is made abdominally, an opening is made into the bladder, and the prostate is removed from above.

27. **(D)** The lumbar or simple flank incision may include removal of the 11th or 12th rib; thus, a rib set should be available.

28. **(A)** A hydrocele is an abnormal accumulation of fluid within the scrotum, contained in the tunica vaginalis.

29. **(B)** A lithotrite is used to crush large bladder calculi.

30. **(B)** Urethral meatotomy is an incisional enlargement of the external urethral meatus to relieve stenosis or stricture, either congenital or acquired.

31. **(C)** The pump is placed in the most dependent portion of the scrotum.

32. **(D)** A hydrocelectomy is the excision of the tunica vaginalis of the testis to remove the enlarged fluid-filled sac.

33. **(A)** Surgical removal of the foreskin of the penis is frequently performed immediately after birth. At times, the condition known as phimosis (stricture of the foreskin) causes a circumcision to be done on an adult male who was not circumcised at birth.

34. **(B)** Balloon dilatation of the prostatic urethra, also known as transcystoscopic urethroplasty, is an advanced alternative to transurethral prostatectomy. It is nonsurgical, and with a cystoscopic setup and balloon dilatation catheters, the urethra is stretched for a better urinary flow.

35. **(C)** The advantages of the Nd:YAG laser in the eradication of bladder tumors are that bleeding is minimized, only sedation is required, operating time is short, and there is minimal damage to healthy tissue.

36. **(D)** The proximal stoma is transferred to the site of the anastomosis for reimplantation.

Following anastomosis with fine atraumatic sutures, a stent is left in place until healing occurs.

37. (D) Both vasovasostomy and epididymovasostomy are microscopic reanastomosis options for sterilization reversal in the male. Success rates vary from 40% to 70%.

38. (D) A serious complication of a penile implant is infection. Meticulous aseptic technique and careful draping are essential. Intraoperatively and before insertion of the implant components, a prophylactic antibiotic irrigant of bacitracin is used on the implants and in the insertion sites.

39. (C) Heparin is given intravenously to the donor just before clamping the renal vessels before removal of the kidney. Immediately after the kidney is removed (and only in a live donor), 50 mg of protamine sulfate is given to reverse the action of the heparin in the donor.

40. (D) Forty-five minutes before surgery, 12.5 g of mannitol is given to the kidney donor to ensure diuresis during anesthesia induction. The dose is repeated 5 minutes before the renal vessel is clamped to maximize diuresis and once again at the end of the procedure.

41. (A) The ideal cadaver donor should be young, free of infection or cancer, and normotensive until just before death. There must also be family permission, and the medical examiner must unequivocally establish brain death.

42. (B) Just before completion of full dissection of the donor liver, the donor is heparinized and systemically cooled. Further cooling and flushing of the pancreas, liver, and kidneys is achieved by cannulation and infusion of cold Ringer's lactate solution via the inferior vena cava until properly cooled.

43. (C) The use of the resectoscope requires that irrigation be accomplished with a nonconducting, isosmotic solution to prevent conduction of current into the bladder, as well as to prevent hemolysis attributable to electroresection of tissue.

44. (C) All of the following procedures can be accomplished through a cystoscope: bladder biopsy, removal of a foreign body, insertion of radionuclide seeds, coagulation of a hemangioma with argon laser, and cystographic studies. Excision of a bladder tumor requires the use of a resectoscope.

45. (A) The vas is located by digital palpation of the upper part of the scrotum. A small incision is made over the vas. An Allis forceps is inserted into the scrotal incision to grasp the vas.

46. (A) A noninvasive approach to urolithiasis management is the use of ESWL. This device disintegrates stones by introducing shock waves into the body, utilizing a specially treated water as a medium.

47. (C) The Candela laser, a tunable dye laser, allows the operator to dial the desired wavelength within a limited range. It has the ability to disintegrate stones without damaging surrounding tissue. The technique may be used during an ureteropyeloscopy or nephroscopy.

48. (B) Urinary incontinence is the inability to control urination most commonly caused by loss of sphincter control at the bladder neck.

49. (D) KUB is a radiograph of the kidneys, ureters, and bladder.

50. (A) Extravasation is the absorption of irrigation fluids into the vascular system, which results in fluid overload and can result in cardiac arrest.

51. (D) A three-way Foley is used for irrigation and hemostasis.

52. (B) An ileal conduit is urinary diversion away from the bladder before or after a radical cystectomy, in which the bladder and surrounding tissue have been removed as a treatment for cancer.

53. **(B)** The patient is placed in a right lateral position with the flank over the table break with the operative side up.

54. **(D)** Small pieces of tissue or stones are released into the irrigation fluid in the bladder and evacuated with the Ellik evacuator or Toomey syringe.

55. **(D)** The Van Buren is the dilator commonly used to dilate the urethra.

56. **(D)** A TURP is done transurethrally with a resectoscope, and therefore, no incision is required.

57. **(C)** Cystostomy is an opening made into the urinary bladder through a low abdominal incision with insertion of a suprapubic catheter.

58. **(D)** Micturition refers to urination.

59. **(C)** Epispadias is a rare condition in which the urethral meatus is located on the top side of the penis.

60. **(D)** AV shunt and AV fistula are used to access the vascular system for hemodialysis. During peritoneal dialysis, a silastic tube is implanted in the suprapubic peritoneal space.

61. **(C)** Gerota's capsule is the tissue covering of the kidney. The glomerulus is a network of capillaries that help filter the kidney. The renal pelvis is the funnel-shaped structure within the kidney, and the loop of Henley helps to reabsorb filtered water, sodium, calcium, chlorine, and potassium in a normal kidney.

62. **(D)** Van Buren dilators are used to dilate the urethra. Hank and Hagar dilators are used on a D&C. Bakes dilators are used for common duct exploration.

63. **(A)** Glomerular filtration is the first step of urine production. Peritoneal dialysis is used for renal failure. Hemolysis is rupturing

of RBCs, and osmosis is the movement of fluid from a higher concentration to a lower concentration.

64. **(B)** The nephron is the functional unit of the kidney. The renal pelvis is the funnel-shaped structure within the kidney. The renal calyces are the chambers of the kidney where urine passes, and Gerota's capsule covers the kidney.

65. **(C)** ESWL is used to remove kidney stones. An ileal conduit follows a total cystectomy. A laparoscopic nephrectomy removes the kidney, and a TURP is a transurethral resection of the prostate.

66. **(C)** The trigone includes the openings of both ureters and the urethral opening in the bladder.

67. **(A)** Hemolysis is the rupturing of RBCs, which releases their contents into the bloodstream. Extravasation is too much fluid entering the bloodstream. Hydronephrosis is enlargement of the kidney due to failure. Distribution involves dividing and spreading.

68. **(C)** A suprapubic catheter is placed in the bladder through an opening in the abdomen. A Coude is an indwelling catheter with a curved tip. A Robinson is a straight catheter.

69. **(C)** 8–10 cc of sterile water are used to fill a 5-cc Foley.

70. **(C)** The reservoir of the penile implant is placed in the abdomen. The cylinders are placed in the penis and the pump in the scrotum.

71. **(B)** An OB/GYN surgeon is not needed during a transrectal seed implantation.

72. **(C)** A vesicovaginal fistula is a fistula between the vagina and the bladder.

73. **(A)** A TVT sling is used for urinary stress incontinence.

74. **(D)** A live donor's kidney can also be transplanted. It is not only a cadaver donor.

75. **(A)** Wilms tumor is the most common tumor of the kidney in children.

76. **(C)** A subcostal flank incision is made in a simple open nephrectomy. A Gibson incision is used for renal transplantation or as an extraperitoneal approach for distal ureters. A low transverse or Pfannenstiel incision is used for a cesarean section or a suprapubic prostatectomy. A McBurney's incision is used for an open appendectomy.

77. **(C)** Both legs should be placed simultaneously to prevent hip and back pain, blood pressure changes, and pressure injuries to the skin, nerves, and blood vessels. Arms are placed on arm boards at 90 decrees or less. Legs should not be placed one at a time due to potential for back, knee, and/or hip pain. Hips are placed at the break in the table so they are in the correct position when the lower portion of the table is removed.

78. **(D)** A resectoscope is used through the urethra (TURP). Perineal, suprapubic, and retropubic approaches do not require a scope.

79. **(D)** The holmium:YAG is used to fragment stones in the ureter. The argon and krypton lasers are used in retinal surgery. Carbon dioxide is used for neurosurgical and reconstructive surgeries.

80. **(D)** Necrotizing fasciitis that is confined to the perineum and scrotum is Fournier's gangrene.

81. **(A)** A stoma pouch is used to provide a leakproof system to collect body fluids while maintaining a healthy wound around the stoma opening.

CHAPTER 24

Thoracic

THORACIC

- The thoracic cavity is enclosed by the ribs, spine, sternum, and diaphragm
- Ribs—12
  - 1–12—ALL connected to the vertebrae
  - 1–7—connected anteriorly to the sternum directly or indirectly by costal cartilage
    - True ribs—they are attached directly to the sternum
  - 8–10–connected to the rib cage by the costal cartilage
    - False ribs—not directly attached to the sternum but attached by the costal cartilage to the sternum
  - 11–12—floating ribs are attached posteriorly only
- Sternum consists of the:
  - Manubrium
  - Body
  - Xiphoid process
- The thoracic cavity contains:
  - The heart
  - Lungs
  - Great vessels
- The great vessels include:
  - Superior and inferior vena cava
  - Pulmonary artery
  - Pulmonary vein
  - Aorta
- The lungs are a pair of air-filled organs located in the chest
  - Right lung—three lobes; left lung—two lobes
  - Air is inhaled through the mouth > to the trachea > into the lungs > into the bronchi > which divide into smaller branches called bronchioles > and then into clusters of air sacs called alveoli

- Alveoli—air and CO_2 exchange takes place here
- Visceral pleura—covering of the lung
- Parietal pleura—covers the thoracic cavity
- Lungs work on negative pressure for proper pulmonary function
- Mediastinum—area between the two lungs; this includes:
  - Thymus
  - Thoracic aorta
  - Heart and great vessels
  - Esophagus and trachea
- Diaphragm—separation between the peritoneal cavity and thoracic cavity
- A double endotracheal tube is commonly used in thoracic surgery
  - This provides expansion for the good lung and collapse of the lung on the surgical side
- Thoracotomy instruments include:
  - Bronchus clamp—Sarot clamp
  - Lebsche rib shears
  - Davidson scapula retractor
  - Allison lung retractor
  - Bailey rib approximator
  - Duval lung clamp
  - Tuffier rib retractor
  - Finochietto rib retractor
- Any time the pleural space is entered, you must use a Pleur-evac/closed water seal drainage system
  - Closed water seal drainage is hooked up to suction at the end of the surgical procedure. When moving the patient, it is removed from the suction and kept below the patient's chest level to prevent drainage from going back into the lung and causing an infection. Once patients are in the postanesthesia care unit

(PACU), they are immediately hooked up to suction again
- ○ Chest tube is placed and hooked up to the drainage system to reestablish negative pressure
- ○ When two chest tubes are used, the superior chest tube is used to evacuate air, and the inferior chest tube is used to drain fluid and/or blood
- Bronchoscopy—a bronchoscope is inserted through the nose or mouth to provide a view of the tracheobronchial tree. It is also used to collect bronchial and lung secretions. Tissue biopsies can also be done
  - ○ There are two types of scopes; they include:
    - Rigid—this scope is commonly used for foreign body retrieval
    - Flexible—this is used on patients who cannot hyperextend their neck
- Mediastinoscopy—this procedure is performed to view areas of the mediastinum. This is the cavity between the lungs; it contains:
  - ○ Thymus
  - ○ Thoracic aorta
  - ○ Heart and great vessels
  - ○ Esophagus and trachea
- The incision is made in the notch of the neck
- Biopsy of the lymph nodes is performed for the staging of lung cancer
- Thymus gland—located in the space between the lungs called the mediastinum
  - ○ Thymomas are slow-growing tumors. The prognosis is excellent when they are discovered in the early stages
  - ○ The most commonly associated condition with thymoma is myasthenia gravis
    - Myasthenia gravis—an autoimmune disease that affects neuromuscular tissue causing weakness of the muscles
  - ○ Thymectomy—removal of the thymus gland. The incision is a median sternotomy
- Mediastinal shift—caused by a loss of negative pressure on one side of the pleural cavity, which causes the other side to shift the mediastinum in order to equalize the pressure
- Thoracoscopy—insertion of a chest tube hooked up to a closed drainage system to provide negative pressure to the thoracic cavity
- Thoracoscopy—performed for direct visualization of the pleural cavity, mediastinum, and

pericardium. This is performed to diagnose buildup of fluid, pus, or blood and to biopsy lung tumors and biopsy specimens
- VATS procedure/video-assisted thoracic surgery—a minimally invasive surgical procedure used to diagnose and treat diseases of the thoracic cavity. Indications include:
  - ○ Biopsy for tissue diagnosis
  - ○ Surgery of the esophagus
  - ○ Surgery on the lung
- Video equipment and endoscopic instruments are needed
- Anesthesia requires a double endotracheal tube
- Endoscopic linear staplers
- Have available thoracic and vascular instruments
- Position is posterolateral, lateral, anterolateral, or supine
- Thoracoabdominal
- Rib resection—performed for reconstructive procedures of the face, ear, etc.
- Pneumothorax—collapsed lung
- Blebs—thin-walled air sacs located on the apex (top) of the lung; if ruptured, they can cause a pneumothorax
- Pectus deformities—congenital deformities of the chest wall. These deformities can cause pressure on the heart, respiratory distress, dyspnea, and/or chest pain
  - ○ Pectus carinatum—chest bows outward
  - ○ Pectus excavatum—funnel chest
- Thoracotomy—incision into the chest wall
- Lung resection—performed for diseased lung. All or part of the lung can be resected
  - ○ Pneumonectomy—removal of the entire lung. This is usually performed for a malignancy
  - ○ Hemoptysis—a condition where the patient is coughing up blood. This can be caused by an irritation of the bronchial tree or something more serious, such as a lung malignancy
  - ○ Lobectomy—removal of one lobe of the lung
    - The nerves that are preserved during a pneumonectomy include:
      - □ Vagus
      - □ Left recurrent laryngeal
      - □ Phrenic
  - ○ Wedge resection—a small wedge portion is removed from one lobe of a lung

- ○ Segmental resection—same as above except the portion removed is a little larger than the wedge
- ○ Scalene nodes/supraclavicular nodes are used to detect metastatic cancer from the lung
- ○ Pulmonary function tests are a group of tests that measure how well the lungs take air in and out and oxygenate the body
  - ▪ Total lung capacity—the total amount of air that you can inhale into your lungs. Forced expiratory volume—this test determines how much air is forced out (exhaled)
  - ▪ Tidal volume—the amount of air that enters the lungs during normal inhalation
  - ▪ Vital capacity—the highest amount of air that can be expelled from the lungs after taking a deep breath
  - ▪ Spirometer—an instrument used to measure the air capacity inhaled and exhaled from the lungs
- • Lung volume reduction surgery (LVRS)—a surgical procedure performed to remove diseased lung tissue caused by emphysema
  - ○ Emphysema—the alveoli at the end of the bronchiole tree become enlarged and cause destruction of the air sacs. This causes the lung to overinflate
- • Decortication of the lung—this procedure is performed to remove the surface layer of the lung. It is the fibrous layer. The layer becomes thick and restricts the lung from expanding
  - ○ Dissection can be performed with a Metzenbaum scissor and blunt dissection with the surgeon's fingers and/or peanuts
- • Thoracic outlet syndrome—the thoracic outlet is between the collarbone and first rib. This is caused by trauma or an extra rib
  - ○ The nerves and blood vessels in the thoracic outlet become compressed and irritated and cause pain in the arms, shoulder, and neck. You also have tingling and/or numbness along your arm and fingers
  - ○ This can also be a result of an extra first rib or a problem with the clavicle that causes the space to become too small for the vessels and nerves
- • Thoracentesis—this procedure is performed to remove blood or air in the pleural cavity by introducing a needle and syringe for aspiration

- ○ Pleural effusion is a buildup of excess fluids, including blood, caused by infection or tumor. A thoracentesis is performed for a diagnosis of the pleural effusion
- ○ Once the fluid is removed, talcum powder or antibiotic solution is inserted to dry out the space and aid in eliminating the space from preventing further fluid buildup
- ○ This helps the patient to breathe easier
- • Hiatal hernia—the stomach protrudes through the diaphragm into the pleural cavity
  - ○ This procedure can be performed with an abdominal approach or through the thoracic cavity
- • Lung transplant—performed for patients with severe lung disease
  - ○ Lungs can be donated by cadaver lung donors and live donors
  - ○ One lung, both lungs, or a lobe of a lung from multiple donors may be taken for the transplant
  - ○ Collin's solution is one solution that can be used to preserve the donor kidney prior to transplantation
  - ○ The heart-lung machine is used
  - ○ Chest tube and closed chest drainage are used
  - ○ Single-lung transplant—unilateral
    - ▪ Incision is made on the side of the chest that is being transplanted
    - ▪ Lung is removed and replaced with the donor lung
    - ▪ Donor—supine position
    - ▪ Recipient—supine or lateral position
  - ○ Double lung transplant—bilateral
    - ▪ The incision is made across the entire chest from below the breast "clamshell incision"
    - ▪ The procedure is performed on one side and then the other side
    - ▪ Donor—supine
    - ▪ Recipient—supine
    - ▪ The side chosen is based on the lung requiring the lesser perfusion
- • There are three anastomoses in order to provide an effective lung transplant; they include:
  - ○ From the most posterior:
    - ▪ Bronchus
    - ▪ Pulmonary artery
    - ▪ Atrial cuff

Questions

1. The thoracic cavity contains all EXCEPT:

   (A) vertebrae
   (B) heart
   (C) lungs
   (D) great vessels

2. What instrument is used to view lymph nodes or masses in the space that medially separates the pleural cavities?

   (A) Bronchoscope
   (B) Mediastinoscope
   (C) Endoscope
   (D) Colonoscope

3. The procedure of choice for removal of a foreign body in a child's tracheobronchial tree is:

   (A) bronchoscopy
   (B) mediastinoscopy
   (C) fluoroscopy
   (D) telemetry

4. A cytological specimen collector used in bronchoscopy is:

   (A) Ellik
   (B) Toomey
   (C) Jackson
   (D) Lukens

5. All of the following are true regarding disposable chest drainage units EXCEPT:

   (A) provides drainage collection from intrapleural space
   (B) maintains a seal to prevent air from entering the pleural cavity
   (C) provides suction control determined by water level
   (D) aids in reestablishing positive pressure in the intrapleural space

6. Compression of the subclavian vessels and the brachial plexus usually caused by the first rib is surgically known as:

   (A) cervical sympathectomy
   (B) thoracic outlet syndrome
   (C) thoracic sympathectomy
   (D) decortication

7. A reduction of negative pressure on one side of the thoracic cavity that causes the negative pressure on the normal side to pull in an effort to equalize pressure is called:

   (A) vital capacity
   (B) mediastinal shift
   (C) subatmospheric pressure
   (D) pneumothorax

8. Surgical removal of fibrinous deposits on the visceral and parietal pleura is called:

   (A) posterolateral thoracoplasty
   (B) talc poudrage
   (C) decortication of the lung
   (D) anterior thoracoplasty

9. What substance is introduced through a thoracoscope to deal with recurrent pleural effusion attributable to advanced cancer?

   (A) Chemotherapeutics
   (B) Talc
   (C) Tetracycline
   (D) Hemostatic agents

10. What instrument is used to reapproximate the ribs following an open thoracotomy?

    (A) Doyen
    (B) Bailey
    (C) Alexander
    (D) Bethune

11. What cold solution is used to preserve a donor lung before transplant into a recipient?

    (A) Ringer's lactate
    (B) Saline
    (C) Collin's
    (D) PhysioSol

12. How many anastomoses must be completed to effect a single-lung transplant?

    (A) One
    (B) Two
    (C) Three
    (D) Four

13. What is the preferred solution used for bronchial washings?

    (A) Sterile water
    (B) Sterile saline
    (C) Heparinized saline
    (D) Ringer's lactate

14. During the mechanical process of breathing, the diaphragm contracts during _____ and relaxes during _____.

    (A) inhalation, exhalation
    (B) exhalation, inhalation
    (C) compression, expansion
    (D) normal respiration, maximum respiration

15. Biopsy of which node is performed before a thoracotomy to stage cancer or to confirm a diagnosis?

    (A) Axillary
    (B) Mediastinal
    (C) Iliac
    (D) Scalene

16. The most important laboratory test done to measure pulmonary function is:

    (A) CBC (complete blood count)
    (B) ABGs (arterial blood gases)
    (C) hemoglobin and hematocrit
    (D) WBC (white blood cell count)

17. Which of the pulmonary function tests measures the amount of air that moves into or out of the lungs with each respiratory cycle?

    (A) Forced vital capacity
    (B) Total lung capacity
    (C) Vital capacity
    (D) Tidal volume

18. All of the following are TRUE regarding the rigid bronchoscope EXCEPT:

    (A) used for procedures that require a large-bore endoscope
    (B) used for removal of a tissue mass and foreign bodies
    (C) used in patients who have difficulty hyperextending the neck and difficult jaw manipulation
    (D) complications include injury to the tracheobronchial structures if patient moves

19. A thymectomy is commonly performed for malignant tumors and:

    (A) myasthenia gravis
    (B) Graves' disease
    (C) muscular dystrophy
    (D) pneumothorax

20. What nerves are carefully preserved during a pneumonectomy?

    (A) Vagus, left recurrent laryngeal, and phrenic
    (B) Vagus, pneumatic, and phrenic
    (C) Vagus, pneumatic, and epigastric
    (D) Phrenic, right recurrent laryngeal, and vagus

21. When performing a thoracotomy, the wound edges are covered to protect them from bruising with what?

    (A) Nothing is used to prevent losing something
    (B) Moist lap pads or towels
    (C) To-and-fros
    (D) 4 × 4's

22. The lung is divided into anatomical regions. The right lung has _____ lobes and the left lung has _____ lobes.

    (A) two, two
    (B) three, two
    (C) three, three
    (D) two, three

23. In which surgery would a closed drainage system be used?

    (A) Thoracoscopic lung biopsy
    (B) Open thoracotomy
    (C) Lung volume reduction surgery
    (D) All of the above

24. Bleeding arising from the respiratory tract is called:

    (A) empyema
    (B) pleural effusion
    (C) hemoptysis
    (D) blebs

25. Regarding positioning for a single-lung transplant, the donor patient is _____ and the recipient patient is _____.

    (A) supine, lateral
    (B) supine, supine
    (C) lateral, lateral
    (D) lateral, supine

26. Place the three anastomoses that provide an effective lung transplant in the order in which they must be done.

    (A) Atrial cuff, pulmonary artery, bronchus
    (B) Pulmonary artery, atrial cuff, bronchus
    (C) Bronchus, pulmonary artery, atrial cuff
    (D) Bronchus, atrial cuff, pulmonary artery

27. When performing a bilateral lung transplant, the first lung to be transplanted is determined:

    (A) by the amount of blebs present
    (B) by whether the donor was a live or cadaver donor
    (C) based on the lung requiring lesser perfusion
    (D) all of the above

28. The incision performed for a bilateral lung transplant is:

    (A) median sternotomy
    (B) clamshell
    (C) right subcostal
    (D) midline

29. When two chest tubes are placed in the chest, the superior chest tube is used to:

    (A) drain air
    (B) drain blood
    (C) prevent a mediastinal shift
    (D) all of the above

30. The approach to repairing a hiatal hernia includes:

    (A) abdominal approach
    (B) thoracic approach
    (C) both A and B
    (D) mediastinal approach

31. The procedure performed for pleural effusion is termed:

    (A) Nissen fundoplication
    (B) decortication of the lung
    (C) thoracentesis
    (D) vagotomy

32. When performing a decortication of the lung, the fibrous lining can be planed with:

    (A) peanuts
    (B) surgeon's fingers
    (C) Metzenbaum scissors
    (D) all of the above

33. Lung volume reduction surgery can be performed for:

    (A) chronic bronchitis
    (B) emphysema
    (C) clots
    (D) thoracic outlet syndrome

34. The disease caused when the alveoli at the end of the bronchiole tree become enlarged and destroy the air sacs and cause the lung to overinflate is termed:

    (A) hemothorax
    (B) pneumothorax
    (C) emphysema
    (D) pleural effusion

35. Pulmonary function tests include all EXCEPT:

    (A) total lung capacity
    (B) tidal volume
    (C) ABGs
    (D) vital capacity

36. A spirometer is an instrument used to:

    (A) measure the amount of fluid in the lung
    (B) measure the amount of fluid in the mediastinum
    (C) measure the air capacity inhaled and exhaled from the lungs
    (D) assist in breathing

37. A _____ is removal of the entire lung. A _____ is removal of a lobe of the lung, and a _____ is removal of a portion of the lobe of the lung.

    (A) segmental resection, wedge resection, pneumonectomy
    (B) lobectomy, segmental resection, pneumonectomy
    (C) lobectomy, pneumonectomy, segmental resection
    (D) pneumonectomy, lobectomy, segmental resection

38. The congenital pectus deformity of the chest also known as funnel chest is:

    (A) excavatum
    (B) carinatum
    (C) mediastinal shift
    (D) scoliosis

39. Blebs are:

    (A) fluid buildup in the lungs
    (B) thin-walled air sacs on the apex of the lung
    (C) enlarged alveoli at the end of the bronchial tree
    (D) fluid-filled sacs within a lobe of the lungs

40. Pressure in the thoracic cavity is:

    (A) positive
    (B) left lung positive
    (C) right lung negative
    (D) negative

41. The thymus gland is located in the:

    (A) mediastinal cavity
    (B) pericardial cavity
    (C) clavicular notch of the neck
    (D) endocardial space

42. The retractor commonly used to retract the lung is:

    (A) Bailey
    (B) Finochietto
    (C) Tuffier
    (D) Allison

43. All are parts of the sternum except:

    (A) manubrium
    (B) xyphoid
    (C) apex
    (D) body

44. There are 12 pairs of ribs. The ribs known as the floating ribs are attached:

    (A) anteriorly to the sternum
    (B) posteriorly to the vertebrae
    (C) anteriorly to the costal cartilage
    (D) both anteriorly and posteriorly to the sternum and vertebrae

45. The great vessels include all EXCEPT:

    (A) aorta
    (B) pulmonary artery and vein
    (C) superior and inferior vena cava
    (D) jugular vein

46. Where in the lung does the exchange of air and CO_2 take place?

    (A) Visceral pleura
    (B) Parietal pleura
    (C) Alveoli
    (D) Mediastinum

47. The membrane covering the wall of the thoracic cavity is the _____, and the membrane covering the lungs is the _____.

    (A) parietal pleura/visceral pleura
    (B) visceral pleura/parietal pleura
    (C) pericardium/hilum
    (D) endocardium/transversus thoraces

48. The procedure performed to remove blood or air in the pleural cavity by introducing a needle and syringe for aspiration is termed:

    (A) hiatal hernia
    (B) thoracentesis
    (C) Lung volume reduction
    (D) Decortication

49. A collapsed lung is termed _____, and when a part of the lung is affected, it is termed _____.

    (A) atelectasis/pneumothorax
    (B) pneumonectomy/pneumothorax
    (C) pneumothorax/atelectasis
    (D) pleural effusion/atelectasis

50. Following a pneumothorax, which of the following drainage systems helps to maintain negative pressure in the thoracic cavity?

    (A) Closed water seal drainage system
    (B) Pleur-evac
    (C) Underwater seal drainage system
    (D) All of the above

51. Air, pus, and blood located in the lung are known as pulmonary infiltrates. They are diagnosed by:

    (A) tidal volume pulmonary function test
    (B) ABG
    (C) chest x-ray
    (D) ultrasound

52. What separates the peritoneal cavity and the thoracic cavity?

   (A) Rib cage
   (B) Sternum
   (C) Diaphragm
   (D) Stomach

53. What is the closed procedure performed for a collapsed lung?

   (A) VATS procedure
   (B) Pneumonectomy
   (C) Thoracotomy
   (D) Thoracoscopy

Answers and Explanations

1. **(A)** The heart, lungs, and great vessels are located in the thoracic cavity.

2. **(B)** The mediastinoscope is used to view the lymph nodes or masses in the superior mediastinum.

3. **(A)** A rigid bronchoscope is the instrument of choice for removal of foreign bodies in infants and children.

4. **(D)** A Lukens or a Clerf is used to hold secretions as they are sucked through the aspirating tube. They collect bronchial washings, which are sent to cytology.

5. **(D)** Disposable chest drainage collects drainage, maintains a water seal, and provides suction control. It is aimed at providing a conduit for air, blood, and other fluids as well as the reestablishment of negative pressure in the intrapleural space.

6. **(B)** Decompression for thoracic outlet syndrome is done to correct either a congenital deformity or traumatic injury resulting in anatomical changes in the skeletal structure of the first rib.

7. **(B)** A reduction of negative pressure on one side causes the negative pressure on the normal side to pull on the mediastinum in an effort to equalize the pressure. This is referred to as mediastinal shift; it tends to compress the lung, causing dyspnea.

8. **(C)** Removal of the fibrinous deposit or restrictive membrane on the visceral and parietal pleurae that interfere with pulmonary function is called decortication of the lung.

9. **(B)** Pleural effusions are a significant cause of morbidity, particularly in patients with advanced cancer. Instillation of talc is done to dry up excessive fluid that accumulates in the pleural cavity. Excessive fluid impairs breathing and causes limited expansion, which leads to a pneumothorax.

10. **(B)** All instruments are used to effect an open thoracotomy. A Doyen is a rib elevator, an Alexander is a rib raspatory, a Bethune is a rib shear, and a Bailey is a rib approximator.

11. **(C)** After harvesting of the lung is complete, the trachea is stapled shut, and the donor lung is placed in cold Collin's solution.

12. **(C)** Three anastomoses are completed for a single-lung transplant: bronchus to bronchus, pulmonary artery to pulmonary artery, and recipient pulmonary veins to donor atrial cuff.

13. **(B)** Sterile saline is the solution used for bronchial washings.

14. **(A)** Breathing is a complex physiological and mechanical process controlled by the autonomic nervous system also under voluntary control. During inhalation, the diaphragm contracts, and it relaxes during exhalation.

15. **(D)** Lung cancer spreads through the intrathoracic and mediastinal lymphatics to the supraclavicular nodes, which are the last nodes in the drainage chain. The scalene fat pad is biopsied in conjunction with a thoracotomy to diagnose and stage malignant and nonmalignant thoracic disease.

16. **(B)** With ABGs, the blood is assessed for oxygen, carbon dioxide, and pH acid-base balance. This is the most important laboratory test done to measure pulmonary function.

17. **(D)** Tidal volume is the amount of air you move in and out during normal quiet breathing when there is no extra effort used.

18. **(C)** The flexible bronchoscope is preferred over the rigid bronchoscope for patients who have difficulty hyperextending their neck or when jaw manipulation is difficult or impossible.

19. **(A)** Myasthenia gravis is a neuromuscular disease that involves the muscles and the nerves that control them. Removal of the thymus gland may result in permanent remission and lessens the need for medication.

20. **(A)** The vagus, left recurrent laryngeal, and phrenic nerves are retracted with vessel loops or moist umbilical tape to protect them.

21. **(B)** When performing a thoracotomy, the edges of the wound are covered with lap pads or towels to prevent bruising.

22. **(B)** The right lung has three lobes and the left lung has two lobes.

23. **(D)** After spontaneous or traumatic air leak or surgery is performed in which the pleural cavities are opened, negative air pressure must be restored in order for the lungs to expand. Chest tubes and a closed chest drainage system are used.

24. **(C)** Hemoptysis is one of many pathological indications for a bronchoscopy. It is bleeding arising from the respiratory tract.

25. **(A)** The donor patient is placed in supine because this allows the best exposure of organs to be excised, and the recipient patient is placed laterally with the operative side up.

26. **(C)** The correct order in which the anastomoses must be done is bronchus, pulmonary artery, and then atrial cuff.

27. **(C)** The lung requiring less perfusion is the first lung to be transplanted.

28. **(B)** The clamshell incision is used for a bilateral lung transplant. This incision is placed under bilateral submammary areas that are connected in the middle.

29. **(A)** When two chest tubes are placed into the chest, the superior chest tube is used to drain air. The inferior tube is used to drain the blood.

30. **(C)** Approaches used to repair a hiatal hernia are an abdominal approach and a thoracic approach.

31. **(C)** Thoracentesis is performed to drain fluid surrounding the lungs. A Nissen is used for a hiatal hernia. Decortication of the lung includes scraping the fibrous connective tissue off of the lung, and a vagotomy is done to reduce gastric secretions.

32. **(D)** When a decortication of the lung is needed, the surgeon can use peanuts, his or her fingers, or a Metzenbaum scissor.

33. **(B)** Lung volume reduction is performed for emphysema.

34. **(C)** Emphysema is the disease caused by alveoli becoming enlarged, which destroy the air sacs and cause the lung to over inflate. Hemothorax is blood in the lungs. Pneumothorax is a collapsed lung, and pleural effusion is a fluid buildup in the lungs.

35. **(C)** Pulmonary function tests include checking total lung capacity, tidal volume, and vital capacity. ABGs check arterial blood to see how well the patient's lungs move O_2 to the blood and remove CO_2.

36. **(C)** A spirometer is used to measure the air capacity inhaled and exhaled from the lungs.

37. **(D)** Removal of the entire lung is termed a pneumonectomy, removal of a lobe of the lung is termed a lobectomy, and removal of a

portion of a lobe of the lung is termed a segmental resection.

38. **(A)** Pectus excavatum is a deformity of the chest also known as funnel chest. Pectus carinatum is a condition where the chest bows outward. Mediastinal shift is a movement of one side to the other, and scoliosis is a condition of a curved spine.

39. **(B)** Blebs are thin-walled air sacs on the apex of the lung.

40. **(D)** The pressure in the thoracic cavity is negative.

41. **(A)** The thymus gland is located in the mediastinal cavity.

42. **(D)** The Allison is the retractor commonly used for exposure of the lung. Baley is a rib approximator, a Finochietto and Tuffier are rib retractors.

43. **(C)** The apex is not a part of the sternum. It is the area in the superior portion of the lungs.

44. **(B)** The floating ribs are attached posteriorly to the vertebrae.

45. **(D)** The great vessels are located in the thoracic cavity. They include the aorta, pulmonary artery and vein, and the superior and inferior vena cava. The jugulars are paired veins located in the neck.

46. **(C)** The blood exchange of oxygen and CO_2 takes place in the alveoli. They are tiny clusters of air sacs located at the end of the bronchioles.

47. **(A)** The parietal pleura is the covering of the thoracic cavity, and the visceral pleura is the covering of the lungs themselves. The pericardium is the membrane covering the heart. The endocardium is the membrane that lines the inner chambers of the heart. The hilum of the lung is the region located on the medial surface of the lung where the bronchi, arteries, veins, and nerves enter and exit the lungs. The transverse thoracis is a thin muscle located in the anterior chest wall.

48. **(B)** Thoracentesis is performed to remove blood or air in the pleural cavity by introducing a needle and syringe for aspiration.

49. **(C)** A collapsed lung is caused by air entering the pleural cavity; if the entire lung is affected, it is a pneumothorax. If only part of the lung is affected, it is termed atelectasis. This more commonly occurs when there is a blockage of air causing a partial collapse.

50. **(D)** Following a pneumothorax, you must reestablish negative pressure in the thoracic cavity in order to allow the lungs to expand. The Pleur-evac, closed water seal drainage system, and underwater seal drainage system help body fluids and air to drain, prevent backflow into the pleural cavity, and return negative pressure to the cavity.

51. **(C)** Pulmonary infiltrates are commonly associated with diseases of the lungs. They can be observed on a chest x-ray.

52. **(C)** The diaphragm separates the peritoneal cavity from the pleural/thoracic cavity.

53. **(D)** An open lung procedure is called a thoracotomy. A pneumonectomy is removal of a lung. You can perform a thoracotomy procedure for a pneumonectomy. A VATS procedure is a minimally invasive procedure using smaller incisions, scopes, endoscopic instruments, and a video camera. A thoracotomy is an incision into the thoracic cavity. A thoracoscopy is a diagnostic procedure where the surgeon uses video imaging technology for visualization of the thoracic cavity.

CHAPTER 25

Cardiac

- The heart is located in the mediastinum
- Pericardium—covering of the heart. It has two layers:
  - Outer layer—fibrous pericardium
  - Inner layer—serous pericardium
- The wall of the heart consists of three layers:
  - External layer—epicardium
  - Middle layer—myocardium
  - Inner layer—endocardium
- Blood flow through the heart:
  - Blood enters the heart through the veins (deoxygenated blood) > into the superior and inferior vena cava > into the right atrium > through the tricuspid valve > into the right ventricle > through the pulmonary valve (semi-lunar valve) > into the pulmonary artery > flows out through the lungs (becomes oxygenated) > oxygenated blood flows back through the pulmonary vein > into the left atrium > through the bicuspid valve > into the left ventricle > through the aortic valve into the aorta > to the body through the arteries
- SA (sinoatrial) node of the heart—"pacemaker of the heart"
- AV (atrioventricular) node—major element in the cardiac conduction system; controls heart rate
- Cardiac conduction system—the main components include:
  - SA node—"pacemaker of the heart"
  - AV node
  - Bundle of His
  - Purkinje fibers
- Tachycardia—rapid heart rate over 100 bpm
- Bradycardia—slow heart rate less than 60 bpm
- Coronary artery disease—narrowing of the arteries caused by plaque formation
- Arrhythmia—an abnormal heart rhythm

- Endocarditis—inflammation of the inner lining of the heart
- Pericarditis—inflammation of the pericardial lining of the heart
- Pericardial effusion—fluid buildup of the pericardial cavity
- Fibrillation—irregular muscle contractions
- Atrial fibrillation—abnormal rhythm of the heart. The electrical impulse does not travel properly through the atrium
- Ventricular arrhythmia—rapid heart rate occurring in the ventricles
- Ventricular fibrillation—erratic rapid impulses. It is caused when the ventricle quivers instead of pumping blood
- Cardiac arrhythmias can be treated with defibrillation
- Electrocardiogram—traces the electrical activity of the heart
- Echocardiogram—shows the heart muscle using ultrasound
- Arteriogram—x-ray of the arteries using contrast media
- Angiogram—x-ray of veins using contrast media
- AED—automated external defibrillator—portable electronic device that evaluates the heart for arrhythmias and delivers a shock to the heart to bring it back to a normal rhythm
- Pacemaker—implanted device to regulate the heart beat when you have irregular heart beats
  - Cardiac catheterization—procedure performed to visualize your arteries and how your heart is functioning to diagnose heart disease
- Catheter is introduced through the femoral or brachial artery to your heart and injected with contrast media

- Angioplasty—this procedure is performed during cardiac catheterization. A balloon catheter is inserted and the vessel is dilated; then, a stent is placed to keep the artery open
- Aneurysm—enlargement of an artery wall caused by weakening of the wall
- Ventricular aneurysm—bulge and weakening in the wall of the ventricle. These occur in patients who have had a heart attack
- Angina—chest pain caused by lack of blood flow to the heart
- Cardiac transplantation—this is performed for end-stage heart disease. A cadaver heart is transplanted into the recipient. The recipient's heart is either removed or left to support the transplanted heart
- Cardiopulmonary bypass (CPB):
  - During cardiac surgery, the CPB takes over the function of the heart and lungs for the patient
  - Also called the heart-lung machine
  - Used in cardiac surgery to stop the heart from beating and create a bloodless surgical field so the surgery can be performed. It is difficult to operate on a moving target. It provides blood to the body organs while also providing a bloodless surgical field
  - It filters and oxygenates the blood
  - This is a form of extracorporeal circulation (circulation outside the body)
  - The machine is operated by a perfusionist
  - It is also used for induction of hypothermia (lowering the body temperature), which requires less oxygen intake
  - Cooling the heart allows the surgeon to stop the heart for long periods of time without damaging it
    - The bypass machine cools the blood flowing back into the body
    - Cool saline solution can be used
    - Cardioplegia—solution (potassium solution) stops the heart and prevents cell death during cross-clamping of the aorta
- Cardiac cannulation—this is needed for cardiopulmonary bypass
  - A cannula is placed to retrieve, filter, oxygenate, and warm or cool the blood and return it to the body through a second cannula
  - Purse-string suture is used to secure the cannulas

- To retrieve the blood, a cannula can be placed in the:
    - Right atrium
    - Vena cava
    - Femoral vein
  - To return the blood, the cannula is placed in the:
    - Ascending aorta
    - Femoral artery
- Important parts to the heart-lung machine:
  - Oxygenator—removes CO_2 and adds oxygen to the blood
  - Heat exchanger—controls blood temperature and can heat or cool the blood
  - Pump—acts as the heart muscles and pushes the blood through the tubes on the machine
- The position used for heart procedures is supine/dorsal recumbent
- The prep extends from the chin to the toes of both feet, abdomen laterally on both sides, and both legs circumferentially
- Incision extends from the sternal notch to the xyphoid process
- Specialty cardiac instrumentation:
  - Vascular instruments
  - Thoracic instruments
  - General surgery
  - Sternal saw
  - Sternal retractor
  - Lebsche knife
  - Herrick kidney clamps
  - Satinsky clamps
- Coronary artery bypass graft (CABG) surgery—this surgery is performed to replace diseased or blocked arteries. The bypass forms a new route for the blood to flow through the heart
  - Autograft vessels are taken from another part of the patient's body and used to replace the diseased vessels
  - The vessels used to bypass the diseased ones include:
    - Internal mammary arteries
    - Greater saphenous veins
- CABG—requires the heart-lung machine
- MIS—minimally invasive surgery/MID-CABG—minimally invasive direct coronary artery bypass graft—this procedure does not require the heart lung machine. Surgery is performed on a beating heart

- OPCAB—off-pump coronary artery bypass graft—this procedure does not require the heart-lung machine, and the procedure is performed on a beating heart
- IABP—intra-aortic balloon pump—this is a polyethylene balloon catheter inserted through the femoral artery to the aorta to increase cardiac output. The balloon inflates during diastole and deflates during systole with the change in the patient's condition; it is controlled by a machine
- VAD—ventricular assist device—the pump is surgically placed inside the chest and connected to your heart. The pump controller is attached and secured to the abdomen. This takes control of the heart's pumping action and is also used for the patient who has difficulty coming off the heart-lung machine
- Cardiac valve replacement—the mitral/bicuspid, tricuspid, and aortic valves can be replaced
- Aortic valve replacement—when the aortic valve does not function properly as a result of a leaky valve or stenosis, the valve is replaced with an artificial valve
- Mitral valve replacement—the mitral valve connects the left atrium to the left ventricle. With this disease, the valve does not open properly. It is commonly caused by rheumatic fever. The valve can be replaced or repaired
- Patent ductus arteriosus—the ductus arteriosus (blood vessel) does not close at birth. Treatment includes medication; if it does not work, surgery is required to close the ductus
- Tetralogy of Fallot—a combination of four cardiac defects. There are variations including ventricular septal defect (VSD), infundibular or pulmonary valve stenosis, an aorta that overrides the VSD, and right ventricular hypertrophy. Of the four above, the first three are congenital, and the right ventricular hypertrophy is acquired as a result of pressure within the right ventricle. This is the most common cyanotic heart defect in children
- Atrial septal defect—a defect in which the septum of the heart's upper chambers that separates the atria remains open after birth
- Ventricular septal defect—the septum separating the left and right ventricles fails to close
- Coarctation of the aorta—narrowing of the aorta where the vessel should be normal

- Cardiac medications:
  - Warfarin/Coumadin—anticoagulants, which lower the risk of blood clots. People who have atrial fibrillation (A-fib or AF) are at risk for blood clots because their heart does not beat normally. These are medications taken by mouth
  - Heparin—an anticoagulant (blood thinner) that prevents the formation of blood clots. These are administered via IV
  - Protamine sulfate—reverses the anticoagulant effects of heparin
  - Papaverine—relaxes the blood vessels and prevents vasospasms
  - Lidocaine hydrochloride/Xylocaine—used to treat ventricular fibrillation
  - Streptokinase—used to dissolve blood clots that have formed in the coronary artery vessels and lungs
  - Tissue plasminogen activator—a protein used in the breakdown of blood clots
  - Cardioplegia—used to cause temporary cessation of the heart during cardiac surgery. The main component is potassium
- Thymus gland—located in the mediastinal cavity. It is part of the immune system and produces T cells
- Cardiac ablation—a procedure performed to correct cardiac arrhythmias by scarring or destroying cardiac tissue that causes the arrhythmias. A long flexible catheter is inserted into the heart. It uses extreme cold or heat to destroy the tissue that is causing the arrhythmia
- Skin prep for cardiac surgery—this prep goes well beyond the perimeters of the incision site depending on the procedure. It includes an anterior full body prep, including the limbs and upper thorax, in order to access the saphenous veins and the axillary veins. For a valve repair, chin to mid-thigh must be prepped. If access to the femoral veins is required, a groin prep is also done
- Medulla oblongata—part of the lower half of the brainstem within the central nervous system. It controls heart rate, blood pressure, and breathing. Damage to the medulla is life threatening
- Aortic punch—a type of vessel cutter used to make a hole in an artery for an anastomosis of another vein or artery. It is commonly used on cardiac procedures such as CABG

Questions

1. The action to be taken if a patient is experiencing a cardiac arrhythmia, specifically a ventricular fibrillation, would be to:

   (A) start an IV
   (B) defibrillate
   (C) order blood to replace blood volume
   (D) administer intravenous lidocaine

2. Dextran is used parenterally to:

   (A) expand blood plasma volume
   (B) renourish vital tissue
   (C) carry oxygen through the system
   (D) decrease blood viscosity

3. Which drug can be added to saline for irrigation during a vascular procedure?

   (A) Protamine
   (B) Epinephrine
   (C) Sublimaze
   (D) Heparin

4. The intraoperative diagnostic test that measures tissue perfusion is:

   (A) blood volume
   (B) respiratory tidal volume
   (C) arterial blood gases
   (D) hematocrit

5. Passage of a sterile catheter into the heart via the brachial or femoral artery for the purpose of image intensification is called:

   (A) angiography
   (B) arteriography
   (C) cardiac catheterization
   (D) cardioscopy

6. Hypothermia is employed in cardiac surgery:

   (A) to reduce oxygen consumption
   (B) to reduce elevated temperature
   (C) to slow metabolism
   (D) to induce ventricular fibrillation

7. Which vessels are harvested for a coronary artery bypass?

   (A) Pulmonary vein and external mammary vein
   (B) Portal vein and hepatic artery
   (C) Saphenous vein and internal mammary artery
   (D) Pulmonary artery and pulmonary vein

8. The term used to denote the function accomplished by the cardiopulmonary bypass machine is:

   (A) diversion
   (B) dialysis
   (C) perfusion
   (D) profusion

9. In balloon angioplasty, the dilating balloon is inflated with:

   (A) diluted heparin
   (B) diluted solution of contrast media
   (C) saline
   (D) Ringer's lactate solution

10. What position is commonly used for cardiac procedures?

   (A) Supine
   (B) Lateral
   (C) Prone
   (D) Sims

11. A drug used intraoperatively for its antispasmodic effect on the smooth muscle of the vessel wall is:

   (A) Ringer's lactate
   (B) papaverine hydrochloride
   (C) PhysioSol
   (D) protamine sulfate

12. The technique applied to the patient who is unable to be weaned from cardiopulmonary bypass is:

   (A) Intra-aortic balloon pump (IABP)
   (B) Ventricular assist devices (VADs)
   (C) Pacemaker
   (D) both A and B

13. What is the most commonly acquired valvular lesion?

   (A) Mitral regurgitation
   (B) Mitral stenosis
   (C) Tricuspid valve regurgitation
   (D) Aortic insufficiency

14. What drug is used to effect coronary thrombolysis in the cardiac catheterization laboratory?

   (A) Tissue plasminogen activator
   (B) Heparin
   (C) Streptokinase
   (D) both A and C

15. Electrical impulses that stimulate the heart muscle are achieved with:

   (A) pacemaker
   (B) arterial defibrillation
   (C) electrosurgical unit (ESU)
   (D) alligator clamp

16. Fibrillation is described as:

   (A) fast heart rate
   (B) involuntary muscle contraction
   (C) slow heart rate
   (D) coronary artery occlusion

17. The cardiac phase when the ventricles contract is:

   (A) systole
   (B) diastole
   (C) fibrillation
   (D) relaxation

18. Bradycardia is defined as _____ bpm.

   (A) 40–60
   (B) 80–100
   (C) higher than 110
   (D) 100–110

19. The most commonly used incision for surgical procedures of the heart is:

   (A) right lateral
   (B) left lateral
   (C) anterior thoracotomy
   (D) median sternotomy

20. The aortic valve maintains one-way blood flow to the aorta from the:

   (A) right atrium
   (B) left atrium
   (C) left ventricle
   (D) right ventricle

21. The only arteries in the body that carry deoxygenated blood to the lungs are:

   (A) carotid
   (B) subclavian
   (C) coronary
   (D) pulmonary

22. During dialysis, the patient's blood is shunted to the outside of the body. The term referring to outside the body is:

    (A) in situ
    (B) angiogram
    (C) extracorporeal
    (D) intracorporeal

23. The relaxation phase of the cardiac cycle is:

    (A) systole
    (B) infarction
    (C) diastole
    (D) intraoperative vasospasm

24. A precipitous drop in the patient's blood or fluid volume is:

    (A) hypovolemia
    (B) hypervolemia
    (C) hypertension
    (D) ischemia

25. If you require surgery on your thymus gland, the surgeon would enter the:

    (A) pleural cavity
    (B) mediastinal cavity
    (C) pericardial cavity
    (D) peritoneal cavity

26. Which surgery requires the use of a heart-lung machine?

    (A) Coronary artery bypass grafting (CABG)
    (B) Abdominal aortic aneurysm (AAA)
    (C) Inferior vena cava (IVC) filter umbrella
    (D) Video-assisted thoracoscopic surgery (VATS)

27. The heart is located in which cavity?

    (A) Mediastinal cavity
    (B) Endocardial cavity
    (C) Myocardial cavity
    (D) Both B and C

28. The inner layer of the heart is the:

    (A) endocardium
    (B) myocardium
    (C) epicardium
    (D) pericardium

29. The semilunar valve is also known as:

    (A) tricuspid
    (B) bicuspid
    (C) pulmonary
    (D) SA

30. All are components of the cardiac conduction system EXCEPT:

    (A) AV node
    (B) SA node
    (C) Purkinje fibers
    (D) pericardium

31. Arrhythmia is defined as:

    (A) rapid heart rate
    (B) slow heart rate
    (C) abnormal heart rhythm
    (D) None of the above

32. What medication is used for ventricular arrhythmias?

    (A) Xylocaine
    (B) Marcaine
    (C) Heparin
    (D) Both A and B

33. Pericardial effusion is defined as:

    (A) inflammation of the inner lining of the heart
    (B) irregular muscle contractions
    (C) fluid buildup surrounding the heart
    (D) inflammation of the pericardial lining of the heart

34. Which of the following shows the heart using ultrasound?

    (A) Echocardiogram
    (B) Arteriogram
    (C) Angiogram
    (D) None of the above

35. What arteries are used during a cardiac catheterization?

    (A) Femoral
    (B) Brachial
    (C) Carotid
    (D) Both A and B

36. What vessel increases cardiac blood flow to the heart following a CABG?

    (A) Carotid
    (B) Brachial
    (C) Internal mammary
    (D) Saphenous vein

37. What diagnostic procedure visualizes the cavity between the lungs, aorta, and vena cava?

    (A) Angiogram
    (B) Mediastinoscopy
    (C) VATS
    (D) Echocardiogram

38. Levophed:

    (A) increases cardiac output
    (B) decreases venous return to the heart
    (C) increases urine secretion
    (D) restores and maintains blood pressure

39. A drug used to treat metabolic acidosis is:

    (A) Inderal
    (B) Pronestyl
    (C) sodium bicarbonate
    (D) Isuprel

40. When performing a mediastinoscopy procedure, the incision is made in the:

    (A) manubrium
    (B) xiphoid
    (C) suprasternal notch
    (D) trachea

41. What congenital cardiac anomaly is commonly known as the cyanotic heart defect?

    (A) Tetralogy of Fallot
    (B) Patent ductus arteriosus
    (C) Atrial septal defect
    (D) Ventricular septal defect

42. What disease is a defect in the septum of the heart's upper chambers that separates the atria causing it to remain open after birth?

    (A) Tetralogy of Fallot
    (B) Atrial septal defect
    (C) Patent ductus arteriosus
    (D) Ventricular septal defect

43. How many pulmonary veins are there?

    (A) Two
    (B) Three
    (C) Four
    (D) Six

44. Which of the following is not a cardiac valve?

    (A) Aortic
    (B) Mitral
    (C) Septal
    (D) Tricuspid

45. The mitral valve is also known as the:

    (A) semilunar valve
    (B) bicuspid valve
    (C) pulmonary valve
    (D) cardiac valve

46. Which heart valve is commonly associated with a heart murmer?

    (A) Bicuspid
    (B) Mitral
    (C) Tricuspid
    (D) Both A and B

47. A disease that affects the mitral valve is:

    (A) neurovirus
    (B) parasite
    (C) rheumatic fever
    (D) all of the above

48. A _____ traces the electrical activity of the heart, and a _____ shows the heart with ultrasound.

    (A) arteriogram, electrocardiogram
    (B) echocardiogram, angiogram
    (C) electrocardiogram, echocardiogram
    (D) angiogram, echocardiogram

49. The procedure that is used to scar small areas in the heart by using extreme cold or heat energy, which corrects cardiac abnormalities by preventing the abnormal electrical signals or rhythms from moving through the heart, is termed:

    (A) cardioplegia
    (B) cardiac conduction
    (C) cardiac ablation
    (D) cardiac catheterization

50. What is the term for a congenital defect where there is a stricture of the aorta in pediatric patients?

    (A) Coarctation
    (B) Stenosis
    (C) Arteriosus
    (D) Prolapse

51. With ventricular fibrillation, the lower chambers of the heart quiver. This is considered the most serious of cardiac arrythmias. This causes the heart to beat erratically and fast. During this time, the heart:

    (A) does not fill the chamber with blood
    (B) does not empty blood from the chamber
    (C) does not pump the blood adequately
    (D) completely stops beating

52. Cardiac skin prep may include:

    (A) full anterior body prep
    (B) peripheral limbs
    (C) chin to mid-thigh
    (D) all of the above

53. What part of the central nervous system controls heart rate, blood pressure, and breathing by providing nerve impulses?

    (A) Phrenic nerves
    (B) Medulla oblongata
    (C) Vagus nerve
    (D) Parasympathetic fibers

54. When performing an anastomosis on the aorta using a vein graft (CABG), a Satinsky or DeBakey occluding clamp is used on the aorta. A #11 blade is used to make a small incision, and the _____ is used to enlarge the opening.

    (A) Potts–Smith scissors
    (B) ESU needle tip
    (C) aortic punch
    (D) tenotomy scissors

55. When a cardiac procedure is performed on a beating heart, a/an _____ is used to secure the vessel being worked on to prevent damage because it is very difficult to work on a moving target.

    (A) aortic punch
    (B) heart stabilizer
    (C) cardiac cannula
    (D) Cooley anastomosis clamp

56. Grafts used in cardiac surgery:

(A) come available in various sizes

(B) can be straight or bifurcated

(C) can consist of Teflon, Dacron, or PTFE

(D) all of the above

57. Parts of the cardiopulmonary machine include all EXCEPT:

(A) venous reservoir

(B) oxygenator

(C) cannulator

(D) arterial pump

58. Complications of a CABG include:

(A) ventricular/atrial arrhythmia

(B) clotting

(C) stroke

(D) all of the above

59. Which autograft is the ideal graft used for arterial bypass in a CABG procedure?

(A) Saphenous

(B) Femoral

(C) Brachial

(D) Jugular

60. When there is excessive buildup of fluid in the pericardial sac causing compression of the heart, it is called:

(A) pericarditis

(B) tamponade

(C) infarction

(D) cardiomyopathy

61. Blood enters the heart through the veins (deoxygenated blood) into the:

(A) superior and inferior vena cava

(B) bicuspid valve

(C) right atrium

(D) right ventricle

62. From the right atrium, blood flows through the tricuspid valve into the:

(A) left ventricle

(B) right ventricle

(C) pulmonary artery

(D) pulmonary vein

63. Blood flows from the right ventricle through the:

(A) pulmonary valve

(B) semilunar valve

(C) pulmonary artery

(D) both A and B

64. From the pulmonary artery, blood flows out through the lungs and becomes _____ blood; this blood flows back through the pulmonary vein into the left atrium.

(A) oxygenated

(B) deoxygenated

65. Blood flows into the left atrium through the bicuspid valve into the _____ through the aortic valve into the aorta to the body through the arteries.

(A) left ventricle

(B) right ventricle

(C) pulmonary artery

(D) right atrium

Answers and Explanations

1. **(B)** Ventricular fibrillation requires prompt defibrillation and cardiopulmonary resuscitation. It is rapidly fatal because respiratory and cardiac arrests follow quickly unless successful defibrillation is effected.

2. **(A)** Dextran is used to expand plasma volume in emergency situations resulting from shock or hemorrhage. It acts by drawing fluid from the tissues. It remains in the circulatory system for several hours.

3. **(D)** Heparin may be used locally or systemically to prevent thrombosis during vascular operative procedures. When a vessel is completely occluded during surgery, heparin is often injected directly. Heparinized saline irrigation may also be used. The dosage and concentration may vary according to the surgeon's preference. The saline used must be injectable saline.

4. **(C)** Serial monitoring of blood gases is indispensable in evaluating pulmonary gas exchange and acid-base balance. Either or both arterial or venous blood gas determination can be monitored. It is a chemical analysis of the blood for concentrations of oxygen and carbon dioxide.

5. **(C)** Cardiac catheterization is used to diagnose coronary artery disease. It involves a sterile setup and fluoroscopy to diagnose ischemic heart disease. The brachial or femoral artery is used to effect this procedure.

6. **(A)** Hypothermia deliberately reduces body temperature to permit reduction of oxygen consumption by about 50%.

7. **(C)** Coronary artery bypass grafting (CABG) involves harvesting of the saphenous vein and internal mammary artery (IMA).

8. **(C)** Perfusion is the technique of oxygenating and perfusing the blood by means of a mechanical pump-oxygenator.

9. **(B)** The goal is to restore internal patency of a vessel by creating a channel through the diseased artery and then introducing a balloon catheter. The dilating balloon is inflated with fluid consisting of a dilute solution of the contrast media.

10. **(A)** Supine is the position most commonly used for cardiac procedures.

11. **(B)** Vasospasm may be of particular concern in working with small vessels during a procedure. Papaverine HCl may be added to saline solution for its direct antispasmodic effect on the smooth muscle of the vessel wall.

12. **(D)** IABP is a technique that employs the principle of counterpulsation. It increases the cardiac output and may permit separation of the patient from cardiopulmonary bypass (CPB). VADs are designed to augment cardiac output if patients cannot be weaned from CPB with IABP.

13. **(B)** Mitral stenosis, the most commonly acquired valvular lesion, is usually caused by rheumatic fever. It causes a rise in pressure and dilatation of the left atrium.

14. **(D)** The cardiac catheterization laboratory has also become the site for more aggressive interventional therapies related to evolving

and acute myocardial infarctions. Coronary thrombolysis with streptokinase and tissue plasminogen activator can dissolve fresh blood clots and reopen the artery.

15. **(A)** An artificial pacemaker is implanted in the body to correct cardiac arrhythmia caused by disease in the conduction system.

16. **(B)** Fibrillation is a small local involuntary muscle contraction due to spontaneous activation of single muscle cells or muscle fibers.

17. **(A)** Contraction of the ventricles during which blood is forced into the aorta and the pulmonary artery is the systolic phase.

18. **(A)** Bradycardia is a heart rate from 40–60 bpm.

19. **(D)** A median sternotomy is the most common incision used in heart surgery.

20. **(C)** The aortic valve maintains one-way blood flow to the aorta from the left ventricle.

21. **(D)** Arteries are vessels that carry oxygenated blood away from the heart to the rest of the body except the pulmonary arteries. They carry deoxygenated blood.

22. **(C)** The term extracorporeal refers to outside the body.

23. **(C)** Diastole is the phase when there is maximum cardiac relaxation.

24. **(A)** With hypotension, there is a drop in blood pressure. There is a fluid shift between spaces in the body also caused by shock and infection.

25. **(B)** Your thymus gland is located in the mediastinal cavity. Your lungs are located in the pleural cavity. Your abdominal organs are in the peritoneal cavity, and the pericardial cavity contains pericardial fluid.

26. **(A)** CABG patients must be put on the heart-lung machine. This machine is not necessary for AAA, IVC, or VATS.

27. **(A)** The heart is located in the mediastinal cavity. The endocardium is the inner layer of the heart. The myocardium is the middle layer.

28. **(A)** The inner layer of the heart is the endocardium. The myocardium is the middle, epicardium is the outermost, and the pericardium encases the heart.

29. **(C)** The pulmonary valve is also known as the semilunar valve.

30. **(D)** The pericardium is the membrane that covers the heart. It has nothing to do with conduction.

31. **(C)** An arrhythmia is an abnormal heart rhythm. A rapid heart rate is tachycardia, and a slow heart rate is bradycardia.

32. **(A)** Xylocaine is used to treat ventricular arrhythmias.

33. **(C)** Pericardial effusion is fluid buildup between the lining of the heart. Endocarditis is the inflammation of the inner lining of the heart. Irregular muscle contractions are called fibrillation, and pericarditis is inflammation of the pericardium of the heart.

34. **(A)** An echocardiogram examines the heart using ultrasound. Arteriogram is an x-ray of the arteries using contrast media, and an angiogram is an x-ray of veins using contrast media.

35. **(D)** The femoral and brachial arteries can both be accessed during a cardiac catheterization.

36. **(C)** The internal mammary increases cardiac blood flow to the heart following a CABG.

37. **(B)** A mediastinoscopy visualizes the cavity between the lungs, aorta, and vena cava. An angiogram is the x-ray of veins using contrast media, and a VATS procedure visualizes the thoracic cavity with a scope. Echocardiogram examines the heart using ultrasound.

38. **(D)** Levophed (norepinephrine) restores and maintains blood pressure following peripheral vascular collapse or as a result of severe hypotensive or cardiogenic shock.

39. **(C)** Sodium bicarbonate treats acidosis. It should not be mixed in an IV line.

40. **(C)** The incision for the mediastinoscopy procedure is made in the suprasternal notch. The manubrium and the xiphoid process are parts of the sternum.

41. **(A)** Tetralogy of Fallot is a congenital heart defect. It involves a combination of four cardiac defects including ventricular septal defect, pulmonary valve stenosis, right ventricular hypertrophy, and an overriding aorta.

42. **(B)** Atrial septal defect is a defect in the septum of the heart's upper chambers that remains open after birth.

43. **(C)** There are four pulmonary veins. They carry oxygenated blood from the lungs to the left atrium of the heart.

44. **(C)** The aortic, mitral, and tricuspid are the three heart valves.

45. **(B)** The mitral valve is also known as the bicuspid valve. The pulmonary and aortic valves are also known as the semilunar valve, and the tricuspid valve is the atrioventricular valve.

46. **(D)** A heart murmur is a sound that is auscultated by using a stethoscope. The bicuspid/mitral valve is commonly associated with a heart murmur.

47. **(C)** Rheumatic fever is a type of inflammatory disorder that causes inflammation around the mitral valve of the heart.

48. **(C)** An electrocardiogram records the electrical signals that cause the heart to beat. These signals present themselves as waves on a monitor. An echocardiogram is an ultrasound of the heart used to diagnose cardiac problems.

49. **(C)** Cardiac ablation is a procedure performed to correct cardiac arrhythmias by scarring or destroying heart tissue that causes the cardiac arrhythmias.

50. **(A)** Coarctation of the aorta is a congenital heart problem where there is decreased blood flow to the lower part of the body caused by a narrowing of the aorta.

51. **(C)** Ventricular fibrillation causes the heart to quiver and beat fast and erratically. When this happens, the lower chamber of the heart does not pump the blood adequately to the lower part of the body. Treatment includes defibrillation.

52. **(D)** The skin prep for cardiac procedures goes well beyond the perimeter of the incision site depending on the procedure. It can include an anterior full-body prep, including the peripheral limbs and upper thorax in order to have access to the saphenous veins and axillary veins. Prep is chin to mid-thigh for a valve repair. If access to the femoral vein is required, a groin prep is also required.

53. **(B)** The medulla oblongata is part of the lower half of the brainstem within the central nervous system. It controls heart rate, blood pressure, and breathing. Damage to the medulla is very serious and can be life threatening.

54. **(C)** An aortic punch is a type of vessel cutter used to make a hole in an artery for an anastomosis using another vein or artery. This is commonly used in cardiac procedures such as CABG.

55. **(B)** A heart stabilizer is an instrument used to reduce the cardiac surface motion during anastomosis of a vessel. It immobilizes the target vessels when suturing during CABG surgery. An aortic punch is used to enlarge an incision in a vessel for anastomosis of another vein or artery. A cardiac cannula is used with the heart-lung machine for filtering the blood out and back into the body. A Cooley anastomosis clamp is a vascular clamp.

56. (D) Grafts are available in various sizes. They can be straight or bifurcated. They are made from Teflon, Dacron, and PTFE (polytetrafluoroethylene). The most common grafts used are the knitted and woven grafts for large arteries. Grafts made of Teflon and PTFE are commonly used for patch grafts.

57. (C) Cannulation is used to remove, filter, heat, or cool blood and then infuse it back into the body. It is used with the heart-lung machine. Parts of the machine include the venous reservoir (blood collected), oxygenator (removes CO_2 and adds oxygen to the blood), heat exchanger (controls blood temperature), and arterial pump (acts as the heart muscles and pushes the blood through the tubes on the machine).

58. (D) Complications of a cardiopulmonary bypass graft include ventricular and/or atrial arrhythmia, clotting, stroke, infection, cardiac ischemia, and myocardial infarction.

59. (A) The saphenous vein is the ideal autograft used for an arterial bypass on a CABG procedure.

60. (B) Cardiac tamponade is excessive fluid buildup in the pericardial sac causing compression on the heart. Some of the causes of cardiac tamponade include kidney failure, infection (pericarditis), and cancer.

61. (A) Blood enters the heart through the superior and inferior vena cava.

62. (B) Blood flows from the right atrium through the tricuspid valve into the right ventricle.

63. (D) Blood flows from the right ventricle through the pulmonary valve/semilunar valve into the pulmonary artery.

64. (A) From the pulmonary artery, blood flows out through the lungs and becomes oxygenated blood. This blood flows back through the pulmonary vein into the left atrium.

65. (A) Blood flows into the left atrium through the bicuspid valve into the left ventricle through the aortic valve into the aorta to the body through the arteries.

CHAPTER 26

Vascular

- Peripheral vascular surgery includes surgeries of the veins and arteries outside of the brain and heart
- Arteriosclerosis—hardening/stenosis of the arterial wall
- Atherosclerosis—the most common form of arteriosclerosis. It is a thick yellowish plaque that causes a blockage in the artery and lack of blood flow to a particular part of the body
- Thromboembolic disease
  - Embolus—a clot of blood, air, or organic material that moves freely in the vascular system
  - Thrombus—stationary clot
- Three layers of blood vessels include:
  - Tunica intima—innermost
  - Tunica media—muscular middle layer
  - Tunica externa/adventitia—composed of fibrous tissue
- Arteries—carry oxygenated blood from the heart to body
  - Pulmonary artery—the only artery that carries deoxygenated blood
  - Blood is moved by the pumping action of the heart
  - Blood loss is rapid and severe
- Veins—carry deoxygenated blood to the lungs
  - Pulmonary vein—the only vein that carries oxygenated blood
  - Blood is moved by contractions of the skeletal muscles
  - Veins have valves
- Venous stasis—pooling of blood
- Varicosity—abnormally dilated veins caused by venous stasis
  - When the valve in the vein malfunctions, it causes venous stasis, which then causes the vein to dilate, and causes a varicosity. This can also cause a thrombus
- Arteries branch into → arterioles → capillaries → venules → veins
- Aorta—the largest artery in the body; begins from the arch of the heart
  - Thoracic descending aorta → abdominal aorta → iliac arteries → femoral arteries → popliteal artery → tibial artery
- Three major arteries that arise from the aorta and supply blood to the upper extremities include:
  - Brachiocephalic
  - Common carotid
  - Left subclavian
- Angiography—contrast medium is used to get a radiographic image of the vessel
- Angioscopy—performed with a fiberoptic angioscope to visualize the inside of a vessel and diagnose what is causing the blockage
- Doppler scanning—can be used intraoperative and postoperatively. Probe is used to hear the blood flowing through the vessel
- Ultrasonography
- Arterial plethysmography—performed for small arterial disease. It is used to find a stricture at a particular point on the leg. Three pressure cuffs are placed at different points on the leg. They are inflated, and the pressure readings should be the same; the one that varies is where the stricture is
- Arterial catheter—used to measure blood pressure on extremely ill patients and also to instill dyes and chemotherapeutic (chemo) agents
- Central venous catheters—used to administer IV fluids, drugs, and nutritional solutions and to withdraw blood

- Angioplasty—this procedure involves opening up a clogged artery by inserting a balloon catheter to help widen the artery. A stent is placed following the procedure to maintain patency of the vessel
  - Groshong catheter—used for more long-term IV therapy and chemo. The catheter is introduced into the subclavian vein to the vena cava
  - Hickman catheter—used for chemo, blood withdrawal, medications, and/or dialysis. The catheter is introduced into the jugular vein to the superior vena cava
  - Broviac catheter—similar to a Hickman catheter, it has a very small lumen; can be used for children. Introduced same as above
- Blood pressure
  - Systolic pressure—occurs during contraction of the ventricles (top number)
  - Diastolic pressure—occurs during relaxation phase of the cardiac cycle (bottom number)
- Hypotension—low blood pressure
- Hypovolemia—low blood volume (loss of blood)
- Shock—occurs when the tissues of the body do not receive enough oxygen and can lead to cellular death—organ failure—death
  - Clinical symptoms of shock are:
    - Hypovolemia
    - Hypotension
    - Tachycardia
- Hypertension—high blood pressure
- Medications:
  - Heparin—prevents blood from coagulating/thins the blood
    - Mixed with saline for irrigation
    - Is given by the anesthesiologist 3–4 minutes before cross-clamping an artery
  - Protamine sulfate—antagonist for heparin
  - Papaverine hydrochloride—prevents vessels from spasm
  - Thrombin—topical hemostatic agent. Never inject topical thrombin directly into a vessel
  - Gelfoam/Gelfilm/Avitene—absorbable hemostatic agent that helps control bleeding
- Vascular grafts
  - Synthetic—knitted Dacron grafts: preclotted. This is performed to cut down on bleeding
    - Polyester
    - Gore-Tex
  - Natural materials include:
    - Autografts (eg, saphenous)
    - Banked human umbilical
    - Bovine
- Sutures
  - Polypropylene—most common
  - Polytetrafluoroethylene—PTFE
  - Ethibond
  - Silk
- Suture gauges for vascular surgery:
  - Aorta 3-0/4-0
  - Iliac 4-0/5-0
  - Femoral 5-0/6-0
  - Popliteal 5-0/6-0
  - Tibia 6-0/7-0
  - Carotid 6-0/7-0
  - Brachial 6-0/7-0
  - Radial ulnar 6-0/7-0
- Suture boots—placed on mosquitos and used to hold one end of a double-armed suture. They prevent kinks in the suture that a normal clamp would cause; when pulling through a vessel, the kink could increase the size of the hole and increase bleeding
- Vessel loops—used to identify structures, retract vessels, and occlude vessels
- Pledgets—small Teflon-coated cottonoids attached with sutures. They are used to reinforce the anastomosis and are commonly used on an abdominal aortic aneurysm
- Rummel tourniquet—used to occlude a vessel. Dacron tape is wrapped around a vessel and threaded through a small silastic bolster and tightened
- Arterial embolectomy—performed to remove clots. A Fogarty embolectomy catheter is used with a tuberculin syringe
- Hemodialysis—this procedure is performed on patients in renal failure because their blood is no longer being properly filtered by the kidney. They need extracorporeal hemodialysis (blood removed from the body and filtered outside the body in a machine and infused back to the patient)
- Arteriovenous fistula—direct anastomosis between an artery and vein
  - When performing this procedure, the vein and artery used are:
    - Forearm—radial artery to cephalic vein
    - Upper arm—brachial artery to basilic vein

- Brachial artery to cephalic vein
  - The large cannulation bore hole needles are injected into the vein three times a week for dialysis
  - The arterial pressure enlarges the vein for dialysis access
  - A Doppler is used intraoperatively (sterile) and postoperatively
  - Bruit/brui—the pulse in the fistula/graft is called signal/thrill/buzzing (swishing sound)
- Arteriovenous shunt—a graft is used to connect the artery and vein instead of a direct (no graft) connection between the artery and vein
  - can be synthetic grafts, patients own vein or bovine carotid artery or human umbilical vein
    - Gore-Tex grafts are commonly used. Gore-Tex—PTFE
- Vascular anastomosis includes:
  - Side to side
  - End to end
  - End of vein to side of the artery
  - End of artery to side of vein
- Tenckhoff catheter insertion—performed for renal dialysis—it filters the patient's blood. This is used for peritoneal dialysis
  - A silicone catheter is inserted into the abdominal cavity
  - A special fluid (dialysate) is infused into the abdominal cavity and remains for 3–6 hours and then drained
  - The intestines and peritoneal membrane act as a filter between the fluid and the bloodstream
  - Waste products and excess water are removed from the body
- Venus catheter—used for quick short-term dialysis—this type of central venous catheter can be inserted into the:
  - Internal jugular vein
  - Subclavian vein
  - Femoral vein
- Vena cava filter placement—performed to prevent clots from traveling to the lungs (pulmonary embolism)
- This is caused by deep vein thrombosis (DVT), which is the formation of clots in the deep veins of the body
  - Fluoroscopy is used
  - The vena cava filter can be inserted through:
    - Femoral vein
    - Jugular vein
  - The filter is placed in the inferior vena cava
- Vein stripping and ligation—varicose veins are large dilated veins caused by venous stasis (pooling of blood)
  - The most common vein affected is the saphenous vein and its branches in the leg
  - A vein stripper is used to remove the saphenous vein
  - Smaller veins are clamped and tied with clamps
- Sclerotherapy—a procedure used to eliminate varicose veins. It is an injection of a salt solution directly into the vein. The solution destroys the lining of the blood vessel and causes the vessel to swell and become stenosed
- Endarterectomy—performed to remove plaque from an artery
  - Freer elevator is used to dissect plaque from the arterial wall
- Carotid endarterectomy—performed to remove plaque from the carotid artery. The three carotid vessels are:
  - Internal/external/common
  - The order in which the carotids must be clamped off:
    - First: internal carotid
    - Second: external carotid
    - Third: common
  - The order in which the clamps must be removed is the opposite:
    - First: common
    - Second: external
    - Third: internal
  - Primary indication for surgery is cerebral ischemia (small pieces of plaque break off from the vessel and travel to the brain, causing stroke)
  - Remove plaque from the carotid artery to increase blood flow to the brain
  - Javid and Argyle shunts are the most common carotid shunts
- Claudication—disabling pain during rest. A condition in which cramping pain in the leg is caused by ischemia
- Cross clamping—two vascular clamps are placed on a vessel to occlude the vessel so they can work in a bloodless field
- Abdominal aortic aneurysm (AAA)

- Aneurysms—weakened areas on an arterial wall; atherosclerotic plaque builds up and can cause the wall to dissect or rupture. There are two types; they include:
  - Saccular—ballooning of one area on the arterial wall
  - Fusiform—involves the entire circumference of the artery wall
- Dissecting aneurysm—blood seeps through the walls of the aneurysm
- Grafts for the AAA include:
  - Bifurcated if the iliacs are involved (low aneurysm)
  - Tubular Dacron knitted—needs to be preclotted
- Cell saver—intraoperative cell salvage machine—a salvage device that suctions, washes, and saves the blood cells so they can be transfused directly back into the patient. It is used on patients with religious objections to receiving blood transfusions and patients who do not want to use banked blood
  - Commonly used on AAA
  - The cell saver should not be used on patients with metastatic cancer, if any hemostatic agent (Avitene) is in use, or when there is the presence of amniotic fluid
- Hemolysis—buildup of fluid in a vessel causing the red blood cells (RBCs; erythrocytes) to rupture. The surgeon must be careful with the heparin when using the cell saver
- Disseminated intravascular coagulation (DIC)—a disorder in the blood. There is an overstimulation of blood clotting in the blood vessels, which causes bleeding within the body. Activation of the clotting cascade occurs, and normal clotting is disrupted, which causes widespread bleeding and organ death
- Endotoxins—bacterial toxins located within the blood that can cause sepsis. Sepsis can stimulate blood clotting and cause DIC
- Endovascular AAA repair—minimally invasive procedure performed in interventional radiology under fluoroscopy
  - The incision is in the femoral artery
  - A metal stent that is covered with fabric and has holes that allow the blood to flow freely is inserted through the femoral artery. The endograft is fitted inside the aneurysm, not sewn
  - Can be bifurcated or tubular
- Femoral-popliteal bypass—performed for blockage in femoral artery. It restores blood flow to the leg
  - Can use a synthetic or the saphenous vein (from the patient's own leg)
  - Incisions are in the femoral area and popliteal area
  - A tunneler is used to pass the graft from one incision to the other (actually looks like a tube/tunnel)
- Saphenous vein in situ—contained in its original position
  - All tributaries are tied off with 4-0 silk free ties
  - Once the vein is out, both ends are occluded, and heparinized saline is injected to check for leaks
  - The saphenous vein is placed in situ (original position)
- Femoral-tibial bypass—performed for blockage in the femoral artery/popliteal artery
  - Incisions in the femoral artery and the tibial artery
- Femoral-femoral bypass—performed for blockage in the iliac artery
  - Incisions in both femoral arteries
- Aortofemoral bypass—performed for blockage in the iliacs
  - Incisions are made in each of the femoral arteries and the aorta
- Axillofemoral bypass—blockage can be in the aorta/iliacs where blood flow to the lower extremities is compromised
  - Incisions in the axilla and the femoral artery
- Collateral circulation/blood flow—the rerouting of blood circulation around a blocked artery or vein. This is often a result of anastomoses of branches between adjacent blood vessels
- Amputation—performed for vascular insufficiency caused by plaque/clots; the limb becomes ischemic and necrotic and must be removed
  - It can be below the knee or above the knee
  - Above the knee is performed when there is not good vascular flow below the knee and the wound will not heal

- o Soft tissue instruments and orthopedic instruments needed:
  - Power saw/Gigli saw/rasps/rongeurs
- o Limbs are wrapped and sent to morgue and refrigerated
- Phantom pain—described as a sharp burning pain in the amputated limb. As time goes by, the pain diminishes

- Stripping and ligation—performed for varicose veins. The saphenous vein is the most common vein involved
  - o Vein stripper with various sizes of acorn tips for stripping the vein
  - o Inner layer—endocardium

Questions

1. In which procedure could a Fogarty catheter be utilized?

   (A) Embolectomy
   (B) Gastrectomy
   (C) Craniotomy
   (D) Thoracotomy

2. Amputated extremities are:

   (A) sent to the pathology laboratory, as with other specimens
   (B) preserved in formaldehyde
   (C) wrapped and refrigerated in the morgue
   (D) placed in a dry container

3. If a knitted graph is preclotted, it:

   (A) minimizes bleeding
   (B) makes a graft more pliable
   (C) facilitates attachment
   (D) prevents rejection

4. The antagonist to heparin sodium is:

   (A) epinephrine
   (B) mannitol
   (C) sodium bicarbonate
   (D) protamine sulfate

5. Pedal pulses are assessed with a:

   (A) Berman locator
   (B) Doppler
   (C) Mobin–Uddin device
   (D) polytetrafluoroethylene (PTFE) prosthetic

6. Heparin is utilized during vascular surgery:

   (A) to coagulate blood
   (B) to correct acidosis
   (C) to constrict arteries
   (D) to prevent thrombosis

7. The prime consideration in a ruptured abdominal aortic aneurysmectomy is:

   (A) shunting blood flow
   (B) hemorrhage control
   (C) bypassing occlusion
   (D) removal of thromboembolic material

8. In which surgery would a tunneler be used?

   (A) Abdominal aortic aneurysm (AAA)
   (B) Angioplasty
   (C) Embolectomy
   (D) Femoral-popliteal bypass

9. Which piece of equipment would be placed on an embolectomy setup for the purpose of removing clots through an arteriotomy?

   (A) Wishard
   (B) Swan–Ganz
   (C) Fogarty
   (D) Garceau

10. The goal of a carotid endarterectomy is to:

    (A) remove a thrombus
    (B) provide a shunt for blood flow
    (C) bypass the affected area
    (D) remove plaque

11. Plaque removal from a vessel is termed:

    (A) embolectomy
    (B) thrombectomy
    (C) shunt
    (D) endarterectomy

12. Placement of a vascular graft proximal to and inclusive of the common iliac vessels will necessitate the use of a/an:

    (A) autogenous graft
    (B) straight Teflon graft
    (C) bifurcated graft
    (D) polytetrafluorethylene graft

13. The most common vessels used for hemodialysis in the forearm are:

    (A) radial artery to cephalic vein
    (B) radial artery to basilica vein
    (C) cephalic vein to basilica vein
    (D) both A and B

14. Migrating clots that have formed in the lower extremities can be intercepted on the way to the heart or lungs by a:

    (A) Greenfield filter
    (B) Pudenz shunt
    (C) Scribner shunt
    (D) LeVeen shunt

15. Retraction of fine structures and blood vessels during vascular surgery is accomplished by use of:

    (A) Senn retractor
    (B) Penrose drain
    (C) malleable ribbon retractor
    (D) vessel loops

16. Fluoroscopy is required for all of the following vascular procedures EXCEPT:

    (A) Greenfield filter
    (B) endocardial pacing electrode
    (C) myocardial pacing electrode
    (D) arteriovenous fistula creation

17. Compression of subclavian vessels and the brachial plexus at the superior aperture of the thorax is known as:

    (A) thymoma
    (B) pectus excavatum
    (C) thoracic outlet syndrome
    (D) pectus carinatum

18. In vascular surgery, the term in situ graft references the use of a/an:

    (A) autogenous graft
    (B) heterogeneous graft
    (C) allograft
    (D) synthetic graft

19. The surgery scheduled as "Greenfield filter insertion" indicates a diagnosis of:

    (A) emboli formation
    (B) venous stasis
    (C) arteriovascular occlusion
    (D) kidney failure

20. During a vascular procedure, monitoring the activated clotting time intraoperatively provides useful data for judging the need for reversal or addition of:

    (A) Angiovist
    (B) papaverine
    (C) heparin
    (D) protamine sulfate

21. A low-molecular-weight protein that, when combined with heparin, causes a loss of anticoagulant activity postoperatively is:

    (A) papaverine
    (B) protamine sulfate
    (C) tromethamine
    (D) Angiovist

22. What is the purpose for the surgical creation of an arteriovenous fistula?

(A) Hemodialysis
(B) Insertion of Greenfield filter
(C) Peritoneal dialysis
(D) Placement of Javid shunt

23. Conservative treatment of occlusive disease involving recanalization to restore the lumen of a vessel is called:

(A) PTFE
(B) percutaneous transluminal angioplasty (PTA)
(C) Greenfield filter
(D) endarterectomy

24. What procedure is used intraoperatively and postoperatively to determine blood flow in a vessel?

(A) Arteriogram
(B) Swan–Ganz
(C) Doppler ultrasound
(D) Angioscopy

25. Which vessels are responsible for exchange of oxygen and metabolic waste?

(A) Arteries
(B) Veins
(C) Capillaries
(D) Venules

26. An abnormal localized dilatation of an artery resulting from mechanical pressure of blood on a weakened wall is called:

(A) atherosclerosis
(B) arteriosclerosis
(C) collateral circulation
(D) aneurysm

27. What are urokinase and streptokinase used for in vascular pathology?

(A) Vasoconstriction
(B) Vasodilation
(C) Hemostasis
(D) Lysis of embolus

28. What intraoperative test determines the need for reversal or addition of heparin?

(A) Arterial blood gases (ABGs)
(B) Activated clotting time (ACT)
(C) Activated partial thromboplastin time (aPPT)
(D) None of the above

29. What drug is used intraoperatively in a topical manner for its direct effect on the muscle of the vessel wall?

(A) Papaverine hydrochloride
(B) Heparin
(C) Topical thrombin
(D) Protamine sulfate

30. Following a vascular case, the patient is washed and dried and dressing is applied. What is the next step the STSR should do?

(A) Push the back table, Mayo stand, and basin away from the patient and break it down
(B) Push the back table, Mayo stand, and basin away from the patient and keep it sterile
(C) Leave the back table, Mayo stand, and basin close to the patient in case they are needed again
(D) There is no specific recommendations as long as the patient is safe

31. The buildup of fat residue on a vessel wall is:

(A) atherosclerosis
(B) lipidosis
(C) vasodilation
(D) vasoconstriction

32. The self-retaining retractor used when performing a femoral-popliteal bypass is:

    (A) DeBakey
    (B) Finochietto
    (C) Weitlaner
    (D) Alm

33. Chronic cerebral ischemia can often lead to a stroke. The procedure performed to correct this and restore blood flow to the brain is:

    (A) femoral endarterectomy
    (B) carotid endarterectomy
    (C) electroencephalogram
    (D) electrocardiogram

34. AAAs commonly occur:

    (A) above the renal arteries
    (B) below the renal arteries
    (C) above the iliac arteries
    (D) below the iliac arteries

35. Occluding peripheral vessels is achieved with the use of:

    (A) Glassman
    (B) Leland–Jones
    (C) Bulldog
    (D) Myergils

36. When performing an arteriotomy, the surgeon will require a #11 blade and:

    (A) Potts–Smith scissor
    (B) Metzenbaum
    (C) Lahey
    (D) Stevens

37. Removal of plaque during a carotid endarterectomy requires:

    (A) Cobb elevator
    (B) Hurd dissector
    (C) Freer elevator
    (D) None of the above

38. Which of the following is the correct order from outermost to innermost layers of blood vessels: (1) tunica adventitia, (2) tunica media, (3) tunica intima.

    (A) 1, 2, 3
    (B) 3, 2, 1
    (C) 3, 1, 2
    (D) 1, 3, 2

39. A Javid shunt is used during a/an:

    (A) arteriovenous fistula
    (B) carotid endarterectomy
    (C) femoral-femoral bypass
    (D) abdominal aortic aneurysm

40. The procedure that is performed for dialysis that produces a direct anastomosis between an artery and a vein is:

    (A) Gore-Tex graft insertion
    (B) arteriovenous shunt
    (C) endarterectomy
    (D) arteriovenous fistula

41. When performing a carotid endarterectomy, the suture commonly used is:

    (A) 3-0/4-0 Vicryl SH
    (B) 4-0 chromic SH
    (C) 6-0/7-0 RB polypropylene
    (D) 4-0 RB polypropylene

42. Thick plaque that causes blockage in the arteries is:

    (A) atherosclerosis
    (B) arteriosclerosis
    (C) thrombus
    (D) embolus

43. All are true regarding venous stasis EXCEPT:

    (A) the valves in the vein malfunction
    (B) the vein becomes dilated
    (C) blood pools
    (D) it requires a vena cava filter

44. The major arteries that arise from the aorta and supply blood to the upper body are:

(A) brachiocephalic

(B) common carotid

(C) left subclavian

(D) all of the above

45. All apply to central venous catheters EXCEPT:

(A) they are introduced into an artery

(B) medications can be instilled directly into the catheter

(C) they can be accessed to infuse chemotherapy

(D) they can be accessed to draw blood

46. Symptoms of shock include:

(A) hypovolemia

(B) hypotension

(C) bradycardia

(D) both A and B

47. A common suture gauge used on a carotid endarterectomy procedure is:

(A) 3-0 and 4-0

(B) 4-0 and 5-0

(C) 6-0 and 7-0

(D) 10-0

48. All of the following pertain to a Rummel tourniquet EXCEPT:

(A) used to occlude a vessel

(B) used with Dacron tie threaded through a silastic bolster

(C) used in cardiac and vascular surgery

(D) used to identify a vascular structure

49. Hemodialysis:

(A) is necessary for patients with end-stage renal failure

(B) is extracorporeal filtration of blood

(C) may require arteriovenous shunt or arteriovenous fistula

(D) all of the above

50. A Tenckhoff catheter is:

(A) used for peritoneal dialysis

(B) inserted into the thoracic cavity

(C) used for filtering blood extracorporeally

(D) inserted through the fistula

51. The minimally invasive procedure performed to destroy varicose veins by introducing a salt solution directly into the vein is:

(A) vein stripping and ligation

(B) ligation of saphenous vein

(C) sclerotherapy

(D) endarterectomy

52. Following a carotid endarterectomy, clamps must be removed in which order?

(A) Internal, external, common

(B) Common, external, internal

(C) External, common, internal

(D) External, internal, common

53. The type of aneurysm that forms circumferentially is called:

(A) saccular

(B) dissecting

(C) leaking

(D) fusiform

54. All are true regarding a cell saver machine EXCEPT:

(A) it is a type autologous transfusion

(B) it collects the patient's own blood, filters it, and infuses it back into the same patient during the surgical procedure

(C) hemostatic agents, such as Avitene, suctioned and mixed with the patient's blood can be infused back into the patient

(D) pleural effusion and amniotic fluid cannot be infused back into the patient

55. The following statements are true regarding disseminated intravascular coagulation EXCEPT:

    (A) it is caused by exotoxins
    (B) it is caused by endotoxins
    (C) it causes widespread bleeding
    (D) it can cause organ death

56. When reinfusing blood back into the patient, the primary blood bag must be disconnected from the machine and air evacuated to prevent:

    (A) hemorrhage
    (B) emboli
    (C) venous stasis
    (D) aneurysm

57. Which aneurysm usually develops between the renal and iliac arteries?

    (A) ascending thoracic
    (B) aortic arch
    (C) descending thoracic
    (D) abdominal aortic

58. All apply to the Rummel tourniquet EXCEPT:

    (A) used to occlude vessels
    (B) Dacron tape and a silastic band are used
    (C) used only to occlude the aorta
    (D) a hemostat is used to clamp the ends of the Dacron tape

59. Arteriovenous fistula:

    (A) is a direct anastomosis between an artery and vein
    (B) is when a graft is used to bypass an obstruction
    (C) is when a balloon catheter is used to dilate an obstruction
    (D) can be performed with a Tenckhoff catheter

60. During vascular surgery, a pledget would be used to:

    (A) mechanically control bleeding
    (B) control bleeding caused by a needle during the anastomosis
    (C) occlude a vessel
    (D) both A and B

61. Transient cerebral ischemic episodes are treated surgically by:

    (A) angioplasty
    (B) carotid endarterectomy
    (C) coronary artery bypass
    (D) AAA

62. A Swan–Ganz catheter is:

    (A) a catheter used to monitor the function of the heart
    (B) used to monitor oxygen saturation
    (C) used to infuse chemotherapy
    (D) used to monitor the heart rhythm

63. All are true pertaining to veins EXCEPT:

    (A) they carry blood back to the heart from the peripheral tissue
    (B) they are thin walled
    (C) blood loss can be rapid and severe
    (D) blood moves through the veins by pumping action of skeletal muscles

64. Which arteries are formed by the bifurcation of the abdominal aorta?

    (A) femoral
    (B) renal
    (C) mesenteric
    (D) iliac

65. The STSR is requesting suture for an anastomosis of a femoral-popliteal bypass. What type of suture material would be requested?

    (A) Absorbable multifilament
    (B) Nonabsorbable monofilament
    (C) Nonabsorbable multifilament
    (D) Absorbable monofilament

66. When the saphenous vein is used for a bypass procedure (in situ saphenous femoropopliteal bypass), all are true EXCEPT:

    (A) it is used as an alternative to a synthetic graft
    (B) it is performed to bypass a diseased femoral artery
    (C) the incision is continuous and made along the entire saphenous vein
    (D) the leg is prepped from the knee to the ankle circumferentially

67. The three basic types of central venous catheters include:

    (A) tunneled catheter
    (B) nontunneled catheter
    (C) port
    (D) all of the above

68. The term used to describe the rerouting of blood circulation around a blocked artery or vein is called:

    (A) collateral circulation
    (B) in situ
    (C) en bloc
    (D) embolization

69. What is another name for the inanimate artery?

    (A) Brachiocephalic trunk
    (B) Left common carotid
    (C) Jugular vein
    (D) Aorta

70. What is done with the aneurysm sac when repairing an AAA?

    (A) The sac is sent to pathology.
    (B) The sac is discarded.
    (C) The wall of the artery is sutured over the graft.
    (D) The wall is inverted and attached to the graft.

71. Prior to making an arterial incision on a carotid endarterectomy, the anesthesiologist administers:

    (A) protamine sulfate
    (B) systemic heparin
    (C) antibiotics
    (D) lidocaine

72. The most common cause of a hemolytic reaction is:

    (A) malignant hyperthermia crisis
    (B) vascular surgery
    (C) blood transfusion
    (D) hemorrhage

73. When performing a vein stripping and ligation, the vein is stripped by:

    (A) pulling the vein stripper through the distal opening in the leg at the level of the knee
    (B) pulling the vein stripper through the proximal opening in the leg in the groin
    (C) grasping the saphenous vein with a clamp and pulling it through a small incision in the calf
    (D) making numerous stab incisions and dividing up the vein

74. Diagnostic procedures performed for vascular disease include:

    (A) arterial plethysmography
    (B) Doppler studies
    (C) angiography
    (D) all of the above

75. What is the largest vein in the body?

    (A) Iliac
    (B) Aorta
    (C) Carotid
    (D) Vena cava

Answers and Explanations

1. **(A)** In an embolectomy, a Fogarty catheter is inserted beyond the point of clot attachment. The balloon is inflated, and the catheter is withdrawn along with the detached clot.

2. **(C)** Amputated extremities are wrapped before sending them to a refrigerator. The morgue is the usual place that receives them, unless hospital policy dictates otherwise. They must be tagged and labeled properly.

3. **(A)** A knitted graft is prepared before inserting to minimize blood loss from seepage through graft interstices. The patient's own blood may be used, immersing the graft in a small quantity.

4. **(D)** Protamine sulfate reverses heparin.

5. **(B)** Pedal pulse can be assessed manually or with an ultrasonic instrument (Doppler). It assesses movement of blood through a vessel.

6. **(D)** Heparin can be used locally or systemically to prevent thrombosis during an operative procedure. It can be directly inserted into the IV or used as heparinized saline irrigation (eg, 5,000 units in 500 mL of saline).

7. **(B)** The prime surgical consideration when a dissection or rupture occurs is control of the hemorrhage by occluding the aorta proximal to the point of rupture.

8. **(D)** A femoral-popliteal bypass is the restoration of blood flow to the leg with a graft bypassing the occluded section of the femoral artery with either a saphenous vein or a graft. The tunneler is passed from the popliteal fossa to the groin, and the graft is pulled through.

9. **(C)** A Fogarty arterial embolectomy catheter is used on an embolectomy to remove the clots.

10. **(D)** A carotid endarterectomy is performed to remove an atheroma/plaque from the carotid artery. A temporary shunt is placed, plaque is removed, and blood flow is restored.

11. **(D)** Endarterectomy is the removal of arteriosclerotic plaque from an obstructed artery. It occurs frequently at the bifurcation of the vessel.

12. **(C)** A graft placed proximal to and inclusive of the common iliac vessels will necessitate the use of a bifurcation into the common iliac branches.

13. **(B)** The most common vessels in the forearm used to create an arteriovenous (AV) fistula for hemodialysis are the radial artery to the cephalic vein or the radial artery to the basilica vein. When performing the AV fistula in the upper arm, the vessels used are the brachial artery to the basilica vein or the brachial artery to the cephalic vein.

14. **(A)** A filter device may be inserted (in its collapsed form) through a cut-down in a large vein, usually the right internal jugular. The Greenfield filter is shaped like an umbrella. It is designed to allow blood to pass through the vena cava while filtering clots.

15. **(D)** To prevent undue trauma, umbilical tapes or vessel loops are used for retraction and vascular control.

16. **(D)** AV fistulas do not require fluoroscopy.

17. **(C)** The cause of this compression of the sub-clavian vessels, known as thoracic outlet syndrome, is usually a congenital deformity or traumatic injury to the first rib.

18. **(A)** The term in situ in vascular surgery refers to the position of placement of the saphenous vein for the bypass. The in situ femoral-popliteal bypass is performed to restore blood flow to the leg by bypassing an occluded portion of the femoral artery with the patient's own vein. The advantages of a saphenous vein bypass procedure include graft availability, improved patency, and less tissue reaction.

19. **(A)** Greenfield vena cava filter insertion entails the partial occlusion of the inferior vena cava (IVC) with an intravascular filter that maintains a patent vena cava but prevents pulmonary embolism by trapping emboli at the apex of the device.

20. **(C)** Heparin is the most common drug used in vascular surgery. It may be given as an intravenous bolus to systemically anticoagulate the patient. It is given just before the placement of the vascular clamp and is monitored regularly during surgery to determine its level in the body.

21. **(B)** A low-molecular-weight protein that, when combined with heparin, causes a loss of anticoagulant activity is called protamine sulfate. It is administered by the anesthesiologist IV after bypass is complete.

22. **(A)** A direct anatomic arteriovenous fistula provides a dilated vein valuable for direct cannulation with large-bore needles for hemodialysis.

23. **(B)** PTA is a conservative treatment for localized or segmental stenosis or occlusive vascular disease. PTA recanalizes the vessel to allow for better flow. PTFE is a microporous graft for bypass. Greenfield filters are placed to catch venous thrombi, and endarterectomy requires the opening and scraping of a vessel to remove plaque.

24. **(C)** After vascular closure is completed, a Doppler pulse detector (ultrasound) is used to check patency of a vessel and ultimate blood flow.

25. **(C)** Capillaries are tiny vessels that branch out from arterioles. They help to connect arteries and veins. They function to help with the exchange of oxygen, nutrients, and waste between the blood and tissues.

26. **(D)** An aneurysm is when the wall of a vessel becomes weakened. This localized abnormal dilatation results from mechanical pressure of blood on a vessel wall.

27. **(D)** Streptokinase and urokinase are drugs used to dissolve clots.

28. **(B)** Monitoring the ACT intraoperatively provides useful data for judging the need for reversal or addition of heparin.

29. **(A)** Papaverine hydrochloride may be added to a heparinized saline for its direct antispasmodic effect on the smooth muscle of the vessel wall and its vasodilating properties.

30. **(B)** According to best practices, the correct step to take is to push the back table, Mayo stand, and basin set away from the patient and keep them sterile until the patient is in the postanesthesia care unit.

31. **(A)** Atherosclerosis is the buildup of fat residue on a vessel wall.

32. **(C)** A Weitlaner is a retractor used to retract during a femoral-popliteal bypass.

33. **(B)** Chronic cerebral ischemia often leads to a stroke; the procedure used to treat this is a carotid endarterectomy. This is removal of the atherosclerotic plaque in the carotid arteries and restoration of blood flow to the brain.

34. **(B)** AAA commonly occurs below the renal arteries.

35. **(C)** Bulldogs are used to occlude peripheral vessels.

36. **(A)** An arteriotomy is performed using a #11 blade and a Potts–Smith scissor.

37. **(C)** A Freer elevator is used to peel plaque off of the carotid artery during endarterectomy.

38. **(A)** Tunica adventitia is outermost, tunica media is the middle, and tunica intima is the innermost.

39. **(B)** During a carotid endarterectomy, a Javid shunt is used to provide continuous blood flow to the brain. The shunt is inserted into the internal and common carotid arteries.

40. **(D)** The two techniques used for hemoaccess are an AV fistula, which is a direct connection between an artery and a vein, and an AV shunt, which is a Gore-Tex graft that is used to connect the cephalic vein and the brachial artery.

41. **(D)** A femoral-femoral bypass is performed for atherosclerotic disease in the iliac arteries. For a femoral-popliteal bypass, the disease is in the femoral artery.

42. **(C)** A 6-0/7-0 polypropylene double-armed renal bypass suture is commonly used for the anastomosis of the carotid artery during a carotid endarterectomy procedure.

43. **(D)** A vena cava filter is inserted to stop blood clots from entering the lungs. With venous stasis, the valves are incompetent, the veins become dilated, and the blood pools.

44. **(D)** All mentioned arteries supply blood to the upper body.

45. **(A)** Central venous catheters are introduced into veins not arteries. Medication can be instilled into the catheter including chemotherapy, and blood can be drawn from the catheter.

46. **(D)** Patients in shock experience both hypovolemia and hypotension.

47. **(C)** 6-0 and 7-0 sutures are used in carotid endarterectomy surgery.

48. **(D)** Rummel tourniquets are not used to identify vascular structures.

49. **(D)** Hemodialysis is necessary for end-stage renal failure. The filtration of blood takes place extracorporeally accessing an AV shunt or AV fistula.

50. **(A)** A Tenckhoff catheter is used for peritoneal dialysis. It is inserted through the abdomen and not a fistula. This does not filter blood extracorporeally.

51. **(C)** Sclerotherapy is a minimally invasive procedure that involves injecting a salt solution into the smaller dilated veins and spider veins in the leg to improve the symptoms and cosmetic appearance of the leg.

52. **(B)** Clamps must be removed in the following order following a carotid endarterectomy: common, external, and then internal carotids.

53. **(D)** A fusiform aneurysm forms circumferentially. A saccular aneurysm balloons in one area. A dissecting aneurysm is one that is slowly tearing through the arterial walls, and a leaking aneurysm is a slow leak of blood from the artery.

54. **(C)** Contraindications for infusing the patient's own blood back into their body when using the cell saver system include use of hemostatic agents, patients with metastatic cancer, amniotic fluid, pleural effusion, and polymethyl methacrylate (PMMA).

55. **(A)** Disseminated intravascular coagulation (DIC) is not caused by exotoxins.

56. **(B)** When using the cell saver machine, you must disconnect the primary infusion blood bag from the machine and also evacuate air to prevent an embolism.

57. **(D)** An abdominal aortic aneurysm develops below the renal arteries and below the iliac arteries.

58. **(C)** A Rummel tourniquet is used to compress/occlude a vessel. Dacron tape is passed around a vessel. Both ends are threaded through a small catheter (commonly a red rubber catheter) and secured with a hemostat clamp.

59. **(A)** An AV fistula is an anastomosis between an artery and a vein for hemodialysis. An AV shunt would be used for the same purpose of hemodialysis, except a graft is used to connect the artery to the vein. A balloon catheter is used for a balloon angioplasty to unblock a blood vessel. A Tenckhoff catheter is inserted into the abdomen for peritoneal dialysis.

60. **(D)** A pledget is the most effective mechanical method used to control bleeding caused by a needle hole during an anastomosis.

61. **(B)** Transient ischemic attacks are strokes that last only a few minutes and can be an indication of a future stroke. They are commonly caused by a blockage in the carotid arteries. The procedure to correct this and restore blood flow to the brain is a carotid endarterectomy.

62. **(A)** A Swan–Ganz catheter is a thin catheter with four ports. It is used to measure the pressure of the blood flow through the right side of the heart as well as pressure in the pulmonary artery. It can also check blood oxygen levels and administer cardiac medications.

63. **(C)** Veins have thin walls and move blood by the pumping action/contraction of skeletal muscles. They function to carry blood back to the heart from peripheral tissue. Loss of function of a vein is not as severe as loss of function of an artery. When a vein is severed, it bleeds slowly. If an artery is severed, blood loss is rapid and severe.

64. **(D)** The iliac arteries are formed by the bifurcation of the abdominal aorta. As they travel down the leg, they become the femoral arteries. The renal artery comes off the kidney, and the superior and inferior mesenteric arteries supply blood to the intestines.

65. **(B)** The suture preferred for use on a vascular anastomosis would be a nonabsorbable monofilament.

66. **(D)** The prep for a femoropopliteal bypass encompasses the entire leg circumferentially from the umbilicus to the feet. The leg is prepped and draped to allow the surgeon to reposition the leg during the procedure.

67. **(D)** The three basic types of central venous catheters are as follows: (1) A tunneled catheter is when part of the catheter is tunneled under the skin in the subcutaneous tissue. These are used for long-term use. Examples include Groshong, Broviac, and Hickman catheters. (2) Nontunneled catheters are central venous catheters inserted into a vein in the arm rather than a vein in the neck or chest. An example is a peripherally inserted central catheter (PICC) line. (3) A port is a small drum made of plastic or metal with a thin tube (line) going from the drum into a large vein. Ports are permanently placed under the skin of the chest or arm surgically. The drum has a silicone covering across the top, and special needles are stuck through the skin into the septum to use the port.

68. **(A)** Collateral circulation is the rerouting of blood circulation around a blocked artery or vein. This is often a result of anastomoses between adjacent blood vessels. In situ is defined as in its original position. For example, cancer in situ is when abnormal cells have not spread beyond where they first formed. En bloc refers to removing tissue in one piece instead of breaking it up and causing seeding. Embolization refers to development of an embolus.

69. **(A)** Another name for the brachiocephalic trunk is the inanimate artery.

70. **(C)** The graft is anastomosed and the arterial wall is sutured over the graft.

71. **(B)** Systemic heparin is administered intravenously. This prevents clotting and reduces the risk of an embolus. Protamine sulfate reverses the effects of heparin, and lidocaine may be used to prevent bradycardia and hypotension.

72. **(C)** A hemolytic transfusion reaction is a serious complication that can occur with a blood transfusion. Red blood cells are destroyed, which is termed hemolysis. The action to be taken is to stop the blood transfusion and test the blood for compatibility.

73. **(A)** When performing a stripping and ligation, the saphenous vein is removed by pulling the vein stripper and stripping the vein through the distal opening in the leg by the knee. The smaller superficial veins are removed by making numerous stab incisions and grasping them with a mosquito clamp and pulling them through the incision.

74. **(D)** Arterial plethysmography is used to assess vascular patency, most commonly in the legs. Blood pressure cuffs are placed and inflated, and blood flow is compared between each of the cuffs to determine where the reduced blood flow is. A Doppler is used to hear sounds of blood flowing through a vessel. The sound is intensified and reflects the pressure, volume, and rate of blood flow. An angiography is used to visualize blood flow. Contrast media is injected into the vessel under fluoroscopy to view the inside of the lumen to see if the vessel is stenosed, blocked, or enlarged, which would mean further studies are needed.

75. **(D)** The largest vein in the body is the vena cava. It is divided into inferior and superior branches.

CHAPTER 27

Neurosurgery

- The nervous system is divided into two systems; they include:
  - CNS—central nervous system—the spinal cord and the brain
  - PNS—peripheral nervous system—includes the nerves from the brain and the spinal nerves that originate from the spinal cord
- The peripheral nervous system is further divided into:
  - Somatic (voluntary system)
  - Autonomic (involuntary system)
- Somatic nervous system—voluntary
  - Skeletal muscles control body movement
  - Contain afferent/efferent nerve impulses
    - Afferent—carry impulses to the brain (eg, a burn from your hand to your brain)
    - Efferent—provide instructions from the brain to the rest of the body in order to react
- Mnemonic—afferent arrives/efferent exits
- Autonomic nervous system—involuntary—this is the subconscious; it includes:
  - Breathing, heartbeat, digestion
  - It is broken down even further into:
    - Sympathetic—"fight or flight"
      - Associated with the adrenal secretion of epinephrine
      - Increased heart rate
      - Increased blood flow to the brain and muscles
      - Raised sugar levels
      - Sweaty palms
      - Dilated pupils

- - - Parasympathetic—calms you down when the emergency is over so you can get back to healing the immune system

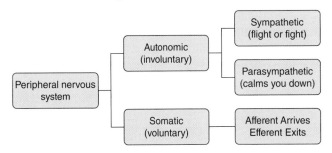

- Skull—provides protection for the brain. The bones of the skull are flat bones
- Cranial bones/bones of the face—these bones are irregular
- Galea—a tough fibrous layer of tissue, that covers the pericranium (outer layer of the skull)
- The bones of the skull are connected by seams called sutures; they include:
  - Sagittal suture—joins the two parietal bones
  - Squamous suture—joins the temporal and parietal bones
  - Coronal suture—joins the frontal and parietal bones
  - Lambdoid suture—joins the occipital bone and the parietal bones
- The bones connected by sutures have nonmoveable joints called synarthrotic joints

- Craniosynostosis—the most common pediatric skull deformity. This results from a premature closure of the cranial suture lines
  - This procedure is performed between 6 weeks and 6 months of age. At this time, the infant's skull bones are still malleable and easier to work with
- Cranioplasty—a surgical procedure used to repair a cranial defect. It is used to treat craniosynostosis
- Meninges—the covering of the brain and spinal cord. It has three layers; they include:
  - Dura mater—in direct contact with the skull
  - Arachnoid mater—web-like membrane
  - Pia mater—the innermost layer; it is closest to the brain
- Subdural space—space between the dura mater and the arachnoid space
- Subarachnoid space—space between the arachnoid space and the pia mater
- Brain—encephalon—is made up of gray and white matter
- The brain is divided into three basic parts:
  - Forebrain
  - Midbrain
  - Hindbrain
- Hindbrain—the part of the brain that controls respiration and heart rate; it includes:
  - The upper part of the spinal cord
  - Brainstem
  - Cerebellum
- Midbrain—the uppermost part of the brainstem that controls some reflex actions and eye movements and other voluntary movements
- Forebrain—the largest part of the brain; it consists of the cerebrum
- Diencephalon—the thalamus and hypothalamus are located here
  - Hypothalamus—controls body temperature
  - Thalamus—controls hunger, thirst, emotions
- Cerebral hemisphere—divided into right and left sides
  - Right cerebral hemisphere—controls the left side of the body
  - Left hemisphere—controls the right side of the body
  - They are connected by the corpus callosum
- Each cerebral hemisphere can be divided into lobes; they include:
  - Frontal lobes—directly behind the forehead
  - Parietal lobes—side of the head
  - Occipital lobes—back of the head
  - Temporal lobes—side of the forehead
- Blood supply to the brain is provided by:
  - Carotids
  - Vertebral arteries
  - Basilar arteries
- Circle of Willis—the circular connection of arteries that supplies blood to the brain
- Brainstem—extends from the cerebral hemisphere to the spinal cord
- Pons—responsible for horizontal eye movement and facial movement
- Cerebrum—largest part of the brain
- Cerebellum—responsible for balance and coordination
  - Suboccipital approach is used for procedures on the cerebellum
- Medulla oblongata—responsible for cardiac and respiratory functions
- Ventricles—cavities within the brain are filled with cerebrospinal fluid
  - The first two ventricles are the lateral ventricles
  - The third ventricle
  - The fourth ventricle
- Aqueduct of Sylvius—connects the third and fourth ventricles
- Cerebrospinal fluid (CSF)—clear fluid that cushions, nourishes, and bathes the brain
  - CSF is produced in the choroid plexus
- Intracranial tumors—brain tumors
  - Astrocytoma—most common of all brain tumors
  - Glioblastoma—cancerous and fast growing
  - Medulloblastoma—common in children
- Vestibular schwannomas/acoustic neuromas—tumors of the eighth cranial nerve. These tumors affect balance and hearing
  - As the tumor grows, it causes pressure on the eighth cranial nerve (acoustic nerve, vestibular nerve), causing one-sided hearing, dizziness, and problems with balance
  - The tumor can also cause pressure on the seventh cranial nerve (facial nerve), causing facial numbness and pain
- Meningiomas—tumors of the meninges begin in the covering of the brain

- Encephalocele—cranial defect causing a sac-like protrusion through the skull that contains CSF, meninges, and brain tissue
  - This defect results from failure of the neural tube to close
- Anencephaly—infants with this condition are born without formed brains or without all parts of their skull
- Spina bifida—an incomplete closure of the vertebral arches in the spine causing damage to the spine and nerves
- CSF—clear colorless fluid that nourishes, bathes, and protects the brain and spinal cord
  - It is formed in the choroid plexus of the third and fourth ventricles
  - It is aspirated by performing a lumbar puncture
- Hydrocephalus—a condition where there is an excessive amount of CSF in the brain
  - Causes pressure in the brain
  - Hydrocephalus can be congenital or acquired. The congenital condition found in infants and children causes an enlargement of the child's head
  - Hydrocephalus can also present itself as a blockage of CSF in one of the ventricles of the brain and can cause stroke
- Ventriculoperitoneal (VP) shunt—a shunt placed in the lateral ventricle of the brain to the peritoneal cavity to shunt the excess CSF away from the lateral ventricles of the brain to another location in the body, which, in this procedure, is the peritoneum
  - These shunt procedures are performed to reduce intracranial pressure
- Ventriculoatrial shunt—performed for the same reason as the VP shunt, except the CSF is shunted into the right atrium
- Manometer—an instrument used to measure CSF fluid pressure in the brain
- Ventriculoscopy—performed for an enlarged ventricle in the brain to drain excess CSF
  - A hole is created within the ventricle for drainage
  - Usually from the third ventricle
- Aneurysms—weakening in the arterial wall of a cerebral vessel
  - May be congenital or acquired as a result of high blood pressure, infection, or trauma
  - The vessels most often involved include the:
    - Vertebral arteries
    - Basilar arteries
  - Most common approach for aneurysm repair in the brain is frontotemporal area
  - Types of aneurysm repair equipment are:
    - Coils
    - Stents
    - Aneurysm clips
- Hematomas—abnormal collections of clotted blood in an area of the brain. They can be caused by:
  - Leakage of vessels
  - Head injury
  - Bleeding disorders
- Epidural hematoma—hematoma between the skull and the dura
  - Commonly caused by a blow to the head
  - The procedure to correct this involves making burr holes to drain excess fluid
- Subdural hematoma—this type of hematoma is bleeding in the space between the dura (covering of the brain) and the brain itself
  - Causes increased intracranial pressure
  - The procedure to treat this hematoma involves making burr holes
- Burr holes—performed to drain blood from the cranial cavity to reduce intracranial pressure
  - They can be enlarged with a double-action rongeur or Kerrison rongeur
  - Bleeding is controlled with bone wax
- Cranial nerves
  - I—olfactory—sense of smell (nose to brain)
  - II—optic—visual information to the brain (retina to brain)
  - III—oculomotor—controls muscles around the eye; constricts the pupil
  - IV—trochlear—supplies only the superior oblique muscle
  - V—trigeminal—sensory nerve that controls the sensation of the face, forehead, mouth, nose, and top of the head and chewing
  - VI—abducens—controls lateral movement of the eye
  - VII—facial—motor nerve that controls the muscles in the face and scalp, as well as tears and salivation
  - VIII—vestibulocochlear—acoustic—controls hearing and equilibrium

o IX—glossopharyngeal—controls the sense of taste and pharyngeal movement, as well as the parotid gland and salivation
o X—vagus—stimulates the pharyngeal and laryngeal muscles, heart, pancreas, lungs, and digestive systems
o XI—accessory—has two parts:
  ▪ The cranial portion helps control the pharyngeal and laryngeal muscles
  ▪ The spinal portion controls the trapezius and the sternocleidomastoid muscle
o XII—hypoglossal—stimulates the muscles of the tongue

- Computed tomography (CT) scan—the standard used for brain and spinal cord injury. Studies can be done with or without contrast media
- Magnetic resonance imaging (MRI)—performed to diagnose tumors, abscesses, ligament damage, and herniated discs
- Angiography—injection of contrast medium into the blood vessels to diagnose vascular abnormalities
- Myelography—contrast medium is injected into the subarachnoid space in the spine, and fluoroscopy is used to view the spinal cord, nerve roots, and spinal column
- Lumbar puncture—a spinal needle is placed in the subarachnoid space to get CSF; the pressure can be measured to determine if there is increased pressure surrounding the brain and spinal cord
- Electroencephalogram (EEG)—electrodes are placed on the scalp or on the brain itself that measure electrical brain activity

OPERATING ROOM BED AND ATTACHMENTS

- Jackson table/Andrews table—used for posterior spine surgery
- Headrests: used to stabilize the head during surgery (separate sterile setup is used to insert the headrest)
  o Mayfield headrest
  o Three-pin suspension skull clamps
  o Gardner–Wells tongs
- Ultrasonic aspirator—Cavitron ultrasonic surgical aspirator (CUSA)— used for precise dissection, irrigation, and aspiration of brain tumors without affecting surrounding tissue
- Craniotome—has a perforator drill for creating burr holes with a dura guard attachment

to protect the dura. Bleeding is controlled with bone wax
- Gigli saw—handheld saw used to remove bone flap on a craniotomy
- Midas Rex—high-speed pneumatic (compressed air–powered drill) power drills contain a variety of instrument attachments

NEUROLOGY INSTRUMENTS

- Titanium plates and wires (used to reattach bone flap)
- Bipolar cautery
- Metal Frazier suction tips
- Leyla–Yasargil—self-retaining retractor for brain tissue
- Penfield dissector—used to separate the dura from the cranium (five with different tips)
- Raney scalp clips—applied to the scalp and galea using a clamp or gun to provide hemostasis
- Dandy clamps—hemostatic clamp with a sideways curve
- Adson–Beckman retractor—self-retaining retractor
- Cerebellar retractor—self-retaining retractor
- Meyerding handheld retractor
- Padded brain spatulas
- When marking the skin for a craniotomy, you should never use methylene blue on a cotton-tipped applicator because it is damaging to neurological tissue. Skin markers are the ink of choice

HEMOSTATIC AGENTS

- Bone wax (formed into a little ball and placed on the tip of a freer elevator or a Penfield dissector)
- Cottonoid strips/patties
- Gelfoam—can be used dry or soaked in topical thrombin. Gelfoam is followed by a patty to add extra compression to the bleeder
- Surgicel/Fibrillar—absorbable hemostatic agent that contains bacterial properties
- Bone instruments

SUTURES

- The dura mater can be closed with silk, polypropylene, and nylon
- Never use a chromic suture because of the alcohol solution it is preserved in; this could damage neurological tissue

- Wires, plates, screws, and methylmethacrylate bone cement are used to suture cranial bones back in place
  - Small holes are drilled into the bone flap, and skull wire is passed through them and twisted together with a wire tightener
- Skin staples are used for skin
- When performing micro neurosurgery, microscopes and/or loops are used; it is important for the STSR to carefully place the instruments in the surgeon's hands as they are to be used because the surgeon's field of vision is restricted
- Craniotomy—surgical opening into the cranium; they are performed for:
  - Tumors
  - Aneurysms
  - Hemorrhage
  - Insert electrodes can also be placed
- Supratentorial craniotomy
  - Includes the temporal, parietal, frontal, and occipital lobes
  - Position—supine/dorsal recumbent
- Infratentorial craniotomy
- Includes the areas of the brainstem (midbrain, pons, medulla, cerebellum)
- Position for the infratentorial craniotomy varies from prone to Fowler's position
- Craniectomy—removal of a section of the cranium. The bone flap is not replaced
  - Burr holes are made, and the flap is extended with a craniotome (it cuts from burr hole to burr hole)
  - When the bone flap is removed, it is safely placed in antibiotic solution
  - The bone flap is sutured back in place with wires or plates and screws
- Cranioplasty—performed to repair a skull defect; the skull bone is replaced with a bone graft and/or synthetic graft
  - Performed to improve the patient's cosmetic appearance
    - Method 1—mesh is used to make a mold, and methylmethacrylate is molded over the mesh and hardens
      - Holes are drilled into the cement and skull bone, and the bone flap is sutured in place with wire
    - Method 2—the defect is measured prior to surgery with a CT scan, and a synthetic flap

is made and attached with micro-plates and screws
- Arteriovenous malformation—an abnormal connection between veins and arteries in the brain causing hemorrhage. This is caused by a congenital defect or trauma
  - Cerebral aneurysms are commonly found by the circle of Willis
  - Embolization—performed to treat arteriovenous malformation; it is repaired with:
    - Coils
    - Glue
    - Microscopic plastic particles
    - Bipolar cautery
    - Laser
- Decompression of the trigeminal nerve—performed to treat trigeminal neuralgia, which is severe pain in the face caused by compression of the trigeminal nerve (fifth cranial nerve)
- Transsphenoidal hypophysectomy—performed to remove all or a part of the pituitary gland and the tumor. These tumors are endocrine-dependent malignant tumors. This procedure helps control the hormones and therefore helps to slow the cancer cells
  - Transsphenoidal approach—approach used for a transsphenoidal hypophysectomy. Incision is made through the nose or through the upper gum line
  - This procedure can also be performed endoscopically
  - Performed for tumors of the pituitary gland, which rests on the sella turcica
  - To perform this procedure, a neurosurgeon and otorhinolaryngologist work together
- Stereotactic procedures/stealth craniotomy—this procedure uses the technique of MRI and a CT scan with geometric coordinates (magnetic markers) to provide a three-dimensional picture of the brain, specifically targeting the tissue of concern
  - This procedure allows a small probe, needle, or laser beam to be guided to the target tissue without damaging other tissue
- Carpel tunnel syndrome—caused by compression of the median nerve by the carpel ligament in the wrist. This causes pain, tingling, and numbness in the hand
  - The incision is on the palmer surface of the hand

- o The ligament is cut and the tendons are released
- Ulnar nerve transposition—performed to move the ulnar nerve from behind the medial epicondyle (inner side of the elbow) to a better position to prevent irritation and impingement on the nerve
- Spinal nerves—the spinal nerves come in pairs and branch off to both sides of the body. They include:
  - o 7 pairs of cervical
  - o 12 thoracic
  - o 5 lumbar
  - o 5 sacral
  - o 4 coccygeal
- Meninges—the vertebrae and the meninges protect the spinal cord
  - o The dura mater, arachnoid mater, and pia mater of the spinal cord are continuous with those of the brain
  - o CSF is in the subarachnoid space
- Brain
  - o Consists of the central nervous system
  - o The rest of the body is the peripheral nervous system
- Vertebral disc
  - o Atlas—first cervical vertebra
  - o Axis—second cervical vertebra
  - o Intervertebral discs—fibrocartilage joints that act as cushions in between the vertebrae. Examples include: C3, T5, L4
  - o Annulus fibrosis—the tough outer part of the disc
  - o Nucleus pulpous—the soft gel-like substance in the center of the disc
  - o Ligamentum flavum—elastic tissue that runs between the lamina
- Spina bifida—a birth defect caused by failure of the neural tube in the spine to close during embryonic development.
- Meningocele—a type of spina bifida. A fluid-filled sac protrudes through an opening in the spine. There is usually little or no nerve damage. This type of spina bifida can cause minor disabilities
- Myelomeningocele—a fluid-filled sac that contains the spinal cord and nerves protrudes through part of the spinal cord; these nerves and cord are damaged, which causes disabilities

ranging from loss of feeling in the legs and feet to being paralyzed
  - o This is the most serious form of spina bifida
- Benign spinal tumors—include:
  - o Meningiomas
  - o Schwannomas
  - o Osteoblastomas
- Malignant tumors—include:
  - o Chondrosarcomas
  - o Ewing's sarcomas
  - o Osteosarcomas
- Diagnostic tests include:
  - o MRI
  - o Myelography/myelogram—x-ray of the spine with contrast media
- Disc disease—the central canal of the spine can become narrow and cause compression on the spinal cord. If the pressure begins to cause symptoms, a decompression is performed by removing segments of bone at the affected site. Prolonged pressure on the cord can cause permanent nerve damage
- Lumbar laminectomy and fusion
  - o Lumbar laminectomy is a surgical procedure to relieve pressure on the spinal nerve. The back part of the vertebra called the lamina is removed to relieve the spinal stenosis and take pressure off the spinal nerves
- Anterior cervical decompression and fusion—performed to treat cervical disc herniation or cervical spondylosis (degeneration of the spine)
  - o The incision is made in the front of the neck and the herniated disc is removed
  - o Following removal of the disc, a fusion is performed. Bone is taken from the iliac crest and placed above and below the diseased disc for support
  - o There are two preps: one for the iliac crest and the other for the anterior cervical incision
- Artificial disc replacement—performed for degenerative disc disease/and spinal stenosis
  - o The mechanical implant replaces the disc and restores movement to the spine
- Rhizotomy—surgical procedure where the spinal nerve roots are cut to relieve intractable pain, providing relief from chronic back pain and muscle spasms
- Cordotomy—this surgical procedure is performed for relief of spinal nerve pain due to

terminal cancer or other debilitating diseases. The nerve fibers on one or both sides of the spinal cord are cut to prevent nerve impulses from traveling to the brain

- Kyphoplasty—performed to repair an injured or collapsed vertebra; this procedure restores the original shape and position of the vertebra, relieves pain, and restores height
  - A balloon instrument is inserted in between the injured vertebra to create a space, and bone cement is put in the vertebra to repair the vertebra and restore height
- Scoliosis—a deformity of the spine in which a person's spine is curved from side to side
- Lordosis—the deformity is in the lower back; the spine curves inward
- Kyphosis—this deformity of the spine is in the upper back; hunchback

- Instrumentation includes:
  - Weitlaner
  - Osteotomes/oscillating saw used to remove the bone graft.
  - Cobb periosteal elevators
  - Penfield dissectors
  - Bipolar cautery
  - Kerrison
  - Pituitary rongeur
  - Curettes
  - Nerve root retractors
- Thoracic outlet syndrome
  - Brachial plexus—composed of nerves and arteries that pass between the clavicle and first rib. When these structures become impinged, it causes muscle tightness, irritation, and poor alignment—this is termed thoracic outlet syndrome

Questions

1. Raney clips are:

   (A) skin clips
   (B) hemostatic clips
   (C) aneurysm clips
   (D) hemostatic scalp clips

2. Which of the following are tongs providing skeletal traction for cervical fracture/dislocation?

   (A) Yasargil
   (B) Cushing
   (C) Gigli
   (D) Crutchfield

3. A surgical procedure used most frequently to control intractable pain of terminal cancer is called a:

   (A) sympathectomy
   (B) neurectomy
   (C) cordotomy
   (D) thermocoagulation

4. Which operative procedure facilitates the draining of a subdural hematoma?

   (A) Cranioplasty
   (B) Hypophysectomy
   (C) Craniosyntosis
   (D) Burr holes

5. Hemostasis in neurosurgery is achieved by using Gelfoam saturated with saline solution or:

   (A) heparin
   (B) topical thrombin
   (C) mannitol
   (D) epinephrine

6. A tumor arising from the covering of the brain is a/an:

   (A) hemangioblastoma
   (B) angioma
   (C) meningioma
   (D) glioma

7. Which of the following is used to control bleeding beneath the skull and around the spinal cord?

   (A) Webril
   (B) Gauze sponges
   (C) Cottonoid
   (D) Kitners

8. A large, encapsulated collection of blood over one or both cerebral hemispheres that produces intracranial pressure is known as a/an:

   (A) epidural hematoma
   (B) intracerebral hematoma
   (C) subdural hematoma
   (D) subarachnoid hematoma

9. A surgical procedure in which a nerve is freed from binding adhesion for relief of pain and restoration of function is termed a:

   (A) neurexeresis
   (B) neurorrhaphy
   (C) neurotomy
   (D) neurolysis

10. Surgical creation of a lesion in the treatment of a disease such as Parkinson's is called:

(A) cryosurgery

(B) diathermy

(C) rhizotomy

(D) pallidotomy

11. During neurosurgical procedures, venous stasis in the lower extremities and maintenance of blood pressure may be aided by all of the following EXCEPT:

(A) Esmarch bandage wrapped groin to toe

(B) elastic bandages wrapped toe to groin

(C) sequential compression devices

(D) special tensor stockings (TED) stockings

12. All pertain to the autonomic nervous system EXCEPT:

(A) it is the subconscious

(B) it is sympathetic

(C) it is parasympathetic

(D) it controls walking

13. All of the following are used for hemostasis in a neurosurgical procedure EXCEPT:

(A) bone wax

(B) compressed cotton strips

(C) bipolar coagulation

(D) monopolar coagulation

14. Upon craniotomy closure, the bone flap is sutured on with:

(A) stainless steel suture

(B) silk

(C) absorbable suture

(D) nonabsorbable suture

15. Removal of an anterior cervical disc with accompanying spinal fusion is termed a:

(A) Schwartz procedure

(B) Cloward procedure

(C) Torkildsen operation

(D) stereotactic procedure

16. In laminectomy, herniated disc fragments are removed with a:

(A) bayonet

(B) Cloward punch

(C) Scoville

(D) pituitary rongeur

17. When using the perforator to create burr holes, heat is counteracted by:

(A) irrigating drill site as hole is drilled

(B) surrounding the area with cool lap pads

(C) dipping perforator in water

(D) working quickly and stopping often

18. A ventriculoperitoneal shunt treats:

(A) Parkinson's disease

(B) hydrocephalus

(C) Meniere's disease

(D) trigeminal neuralgia

19. Cardiac muscles are controlled by which division of the nervous system?

(A) afferent

(B) somatic

(C) autonomic

(D) central

20. Neurosurgical sponges soaked in solution are placed within the reach of the surgeon and displayed on a/an:

(A) inverted emesis basin

(B) dry sterile towel

(C) plastic drape

(D) both A and C

21. All of the following statements are true about knee-chest positioning for laminectomy EXCEPT:

(A) decreased bleeding

(B) better exposure of laminae

(C) increased operating time

(D) increased ease of ventilation

22. What is the most common congenital lesion encountered that requires neurosurgical intervention?

    (A) Meningomyelocele
    (B) Arteriovenous (AV) malformation
    (C) Aneurysm
    (D) Neurofibroma

23. All are true of afferent nerve impulses EXCEPT:

    (A) carry nerve impulses to the brain
    (B) carry nerve impulses away from the brain
    (C) part of the somatic nervous system
    (D) voluntary

24. What instrument is used to excise the laminae overlying the herniated disc during its removal in a laminectomy procedure?

    (A) Cloward
    (B) Leksell
    (C) Kerrison
    (D) Beckman–Adson

25. Malabsorption of cerebrospinal fluid (CSF) and resultant hydrocephalus are corrected by a neurosurgical:

    (A) ventriculoperitoneal (VP) shunt
    (B) AV shunt
    (C) ventriculoatrial (VA) shunt
    (D) both A and C

26. Neurosurgical procedures done for the purpose of locating and destroying target structures in the brain are called:

    (A) stereotactic
    (B) cranioplasties
    (C) craniosynostosis
    (D) trigeminal rhizotomies

27. What is the incisional approach used to effect a transsphenoidal hypophysectomy?

    (A) Middle of the upper gum
    (B) Bifrontal approach
    (C) Frontal approach
    (D) Frontotemporal approach

28. Dorsal sympathectomy entails removal of which of the following chains of the sympathetic division of the autonomic nervous system?

    (A) Thoracolumbar
    (B) Cervicothoracic
    (C) Lumbar
    (D) Cervical

29. The thalamus controls _____, and the hypothalamus controls _____.

    (A) body temperature; hunger, thirst, and emotions
    (B) the processing center for sensory and motor information; body temperature
    (C) balance and coordination; body temperature
    (D) cardiac function; balance

30. Which of the following meninges lies closest to the brain?

    (A) Dura mater
    (B) Pia mater
    (C) Arachnoid
    (D) Subarachnoid

31. What cranial nerve is responsible for the sense of smell?

    (A) I
    (B) II
    (C) III
    (D) IV

32. The diagnostic test used to measure electrical activity of the brain is:

   (A) electrocardiogram
   (B) myelogram
   (C) electromyography
   (D) electroencephalogram

33. Imaging studies used to visualize the spinal cord are an MRI and:

   (A) myelography
   (B) electromyography
   (C) ultrasound
   (D) discography

34. A fatal disease of the nervous system that is caused by a prion (infectious protein) that cannot be destroyed by normal disinfection and sterilization is:

   (A) Parkinson's disease
   (B) Creutzfeldt–Jakob disease
   (C) Meniere's disease
   (D) hydrocephalus

35. Incomplete closure of the spine is:

   (A) scoliosis
   (B) intervertebral disc disease
   (C) subdural hematoma
   (D) spina bifida

36. A slow-growing tumor of the vestibular branch of the eighth cranial nerve is:

   (A) acoustic neuroma
   (B) glioma
   (C) seizure disorder
   (D) meningioma

37. A type of malignant brain tumor is:

   (A) meningioma
   (B) glioma
   (C) sacrococcygeal tumor
   (D) teratoma

38. What medication is used to prevent increased intracranial pressure and reduce cerebral or spinal edema?

   (A) Papaverine
   (B) Lidocaine
   (C) Mannitol
   (D) Topical thrombin

39. The cerebral cortex covering of the brain is _____. It has grooves that are termed _____, and the higher ridges are termed _____.

   (A) convoluted, gyri, sulci
   (B) sulci, gyri, convoluted
   (C) convoluted, sulci, gyri
   (D) gyri, convoluted, sulci

40. The system controlling the "fight or flight" response of the body is:

   (A) sympathetic
   (B) parasympathetic
   (C) autonomic
   (D) both A and B

41. The most common site for a bone graft is:

   (A) iliac crest
   (B) femur
   (C) vertebral spine
   (D) acetabulum

42. For surgery on a pituitary tumor, which sinus would be entered?

   (A) Sphenoid
   (B) Ethmoid
   (C) Frontal
   (D) Maxillary

43. What self-retaining retractor is used to maintain traction of brain tissue?

   (A) Craniotome
   (B) Raney
   (C) Gelpi
   (D) Yasargil

44. A Gigli saw is used during a:

    (A) laminectomy
    (B) Cloward
    (C) cordotomy
    (D) craniotomy

45. The following are types of brain tumors EXCEPT:

    (A) meningioma
    (B) glioma
    (C) ependymoma
    (D) hematoma

46. During a craniotomy, a Penfield dissector or a Woodson dissector is used to release the _____ from cranial bone.

    (A) dura mater
    (B) galea
    (C) rami
    (D) gyri

47. What type of bone is the cranium?

    (A) Irregular
    (B) Round
    (C) Sesamoid
    (D) Flat

48. During cranial surgery, the patient's hair is:

    (A) discarded
    (B) sent to pathology
    (C) saved with the patient's chart
    (D) there is no standard procedure

49. What is the congenital cranial deformity in which the suture lines of the infant's cranium fail to close?

    (A) Myelomeningocele
    (B) Craniosynostosis
    (C) Scoliosis
    (D) Anencephaly

50. What suture is used for dural retraction and closure?

    (A) Chromic
    (B) Nylon
    (C) Silk
    (D) Both A and B

51. A brain tumor causing decreased muscle coordination and balance would be found in the:

    (A) cerebellum
    (B) circle of Willis
    (C) medulla oblongata
    (D) fourth ventricle

52. What surgeon works alongside the neurosurgeon on a pituitary tumor using the transsphenoidal approach?

    (A) Ophthalmologist
    (B) Cardiovascular surgeon
    (C) Otorhinolaryngologist
    (D) Endodontist

53. What is the area of the brain that controls respirations?

    (A) Pituitary
    (B) Cerebrum
    (C) Circle of Willis
    (D) Medulla oblongata

54. Cerebral aneurysms are commonly found in the:

    (A) choroid plexus
    (B) circle of Willis
    (C) hypothalamus
    (D) none of the above

55. Put the layers of the skull in the correct order from the outside layers to the inside meningeal layers of the brain: (1) galea aponeurotica, (2) skull bone, (3) dura mater, (4) arachnoid mater, (5) pia mater.

    (A) 1, 2, 3, 4, 5
    (B) 2, 3, 4, 5, 1
    (C) 3, 4, 5, 1, 2
    (D) 3, 1, 2, 4, 5

56. The autonomic nervous system controls:

    (A) breathing
    (B) heartbeat
    (C) fight or flight
    (D) all of the above

57. The tough fibrous tissue that covers the pericranium is termed:

    (A) dura mater
    (B) pia mater
    (C) galea
    (D) arachnoid mater

58. The corpus callosum:

    (A) divides the right and left half of the brain
    (B) controls the right side of the body (left hemisphere)
    (C) controls the left side of the body (right hemisphere)
    (D) is located in the medulla oblongata

59. Blood supply to the brain is provided by all EXCEPT:

    (A) carotids
    (B) vertebral arteries
    (C) basilar arteries
    (D) ventricles

60. The aqueduct of Sylvius connects:

    (A) the third and fourth ventricles
    (B) lateral ventricles
    (C) choroid plexus
    (D) cerebrum to the pons

61. Equipment for neurological procedures includes all EXCEPT:

    (A) Mayfield headrest
    (B) CUSA
    (C) Midas Rex
    (D) Alvarado

62. The pituitary gland rests on the:

    (A) third ventricle
    (B) aqueduct of Sylvius
    (C) sella turcica
    (D) forebrain

63. The technique that uses geometric coordinates to provide a three-dimensional picture of the brain for surgery is:

    (A) stereotactic
    (B) embolization
    (C) myelography
    (D) fusion

64. What is the term for the extension of the pia mater that is a continuation of the end of the spinal cord attached to the coccygeal sections and whose function is to suspend the end of the spinal cord?

    (A) Cauda equina
    (B) Filum terminale
    (C) Vertebral body
    (D) Nucleus pulposus

65. The surgical procedure where the spinal nerve roots are cut to relieve intractable pain is called:

    (A) kyphoplasty
    (B) cordotomy
    (C) rhizotomy
    (D) anterior cervical fusion

66. The procedure that uses a balloon instrument inserted in between injured vertebra and infuses bone cement to repair the vertebra and restore height is termed:

(A) rhizotomy

(B) laminectomy

(C) kyphoplasty

(D) none of the above

67. The instrument used for precise dissection, irrigation, and aspiration of brain tumors is a:

(A) Midas Rex

(B) craniotome

(C) perforator

(D) CUSA

68. What is the largest part of the brain?

(A) Cerebellum

(B) Cerebrum

(C) Pons

(D) Medulla oblongata

69. When performing a stealth craniotomy, MRI and CT scans are used with magnetic markers called _____. They produce detailed three-dimensional images in the brain using geometric coordinates.

(A) neurosurgical markers

(B) diodes

(C) fiducials

(D) stereotaxis

70. The neural tube defect that occurs during embryonic development and results in the absence of a portion of the brain or meningeal covering is called:

(A) spina bifida

(B) anencephaly

(C) encephalocele

(D) meningioma

71. What is the tough band that surrounds the nucleus pulposus?

(A) Annulus fibrosis

(B) Cauda equina

(C) Intervertebral foramina

(D) Corpus callosum

72. What is the term for the bundle of spinal nerves that is found at the end of the spinal cord?

(A) Corpus callosum

(B) Filum terminale

(C) Cauda equina

(D) Foramen magnum

73. The four major regions of the brain are:

(A) cerebellum, cerebrum, diencephalon, brainstem

(B) pons, cerebellum, hindbrain, meninges

(C) cerebrum, brainstem, medulla oblongata, ventricles

(D) pituitary, cerebrum, cerebellum, pons

74. The _____ make(s) up the central nervous system, and the _____ make up the peripheral nervous system.

(A) brain and spinal cord; cranial nerves and spinal nerves

(B) neuromuscular junctions; brain and spinal nerves

(C) spinal nerves and cranial nerves; nerve roots

(D) brain; spinal nerves

75. What carries nerve impulses toward the cell?

(A) Axon

(B) Soma

(C) Dendrites

(D) Body

Answers and Explanations

1. **(D)** Hemostatic scalp clips include Michel, Raney, Adson, and LeRoy clips.

2. **(D)** Head and neck stabilization in a patient with a cervical fracture and/or dislocation is effected by use of Vinke or Crutchfield tongs for skeletal traction.

3. **(C)** Cordotomy is division of the spinothalamic tract for the treatment of intractable pain.

4. **(D)** Burr holes are placed to remove a localized fluid collection beneath the dura mater in a subdural hematoma.

5. **(B)** Gelfoam is supplied in powder and also a compressed sponge. The sponge form can be applied to an oozing surface, dry or saturated, with saline solution or topical thrombin.

6. **(C)** Meningioma arises from the arachnoid space tissue, the middle covering of the brain. It is slow growing and very vascular. Removal may be difficult.

7. **(C)** Cottonoid pledgets or strips or "patties" are used because they are gentler on the fragile tissue located here. They are counted items.

8. **(C)** A subdural hematoma, one that occurs between the dura and the arachnoid, is usually caused by a laceration of the veins that cross the subdural space.

9. **(D)** Neurolysis is the freeing of an adhered nerve to restore function and relieve pain. Carpal tunnel syndrome is an example in which the median nerve is entrapped in the carpal tunnel of the wrist.

10. **(A)** Cryosurgery utilizes subfreezing temperatures to create a lesion in the treatment of disease, such as Parkinson's disease. This brain lesion destroys diseased cells of the brain and reduces the tremors associated with the disease.

11. **(A)** Preoperatively, elastic bandages (toe to groin), TED, or sequential compression stockings may be applied to help prevent venous stasis in lower extremities and also to help maintain blood pressure.

12. **(D)** Walking is part of the somatic nervous system. It involves the skeletal muscles that control body movement. The sympathetic and parasympathetic nervous systems control involuntary functions, such as breathing. The autonomic nervous system is the subconscious.

13. **(D)** Bipolar units are commonly used in neurosurgery. They provide a completely isolated output with negligible leakage of current between the tips of the forceps, permitting use of coagulation current in proximity to structures where ordinary unipolar coagulation would be hazardous.

14. **(A)** In craniotomy, the bone flap may be anchored with stainless steel suture.

15. **(B)** A Cloward procedure is done to relieve pain in the neck, shoulder, or arm caused by cervical spondylosis or herniated disc. It involves removal of the disc with fusion of the vertebral bodies.

16. **(D)** Herniated disc fragments are removed in laminectomy with a pituitary rongeur.

17. **(A)** A great deal of heat is generated by the friction of the perforator against the bone. For this, irrigation of the drilling site counteracts the heat and removes bone dust.

18. **(B)** In hydrocephalus, there is an increase in CSF in the cranial cavity caused by excessive production, inadequate absorption, or obstruction of flow. The shunt procedures divert CSF from ventricles to other body cavities from which it is absorbed.

19. **(C)** Cardiac muscles are controlled by the autonomic nervous system.

20. **(D)** Neurosurgical sponges, thoroughly soaked with saline or Ringer's lactate solution, may be displayed near the surgeon's hand on an inverted basin, plastic drape, Vi-Drape, or small bowl. A dry towel absorbs the solution before its use.

21. **(C)** All are advantages of the knee-chest position except the increase in operating room time. Knee-chest actually reduces operating time.

22. **(A)** The most common congenital lesion encountered is a lumbar meningocele or meningomyelocele. The fluid-filled, thin-walled sac often contains neural elements. Surgical correction is necessary when the sac wall is so thin that there is a potential or actual CSF leak.

23. **(B)** All of the above pertain to afferent nerve impulses except they do carry impulses to the brain. Efferent nerve impulses carry impulses away from the brain. A mnemonic to help you remember is afferent/arrives and efferent/exits.

24. **(C)** The edges of the laminae overlapping the interspace with a herniated disc are defined with a curette. A partial hemilaminectomy of these laminal edges extending out into the lateral gutter of the spinal canal is performed with a Kerrison rongeur.

25. **(D)** Hydrocephalus is a pathologic condition in which there is an increase in the amount of CSF in the cranial cavity because of inadequate absorption or obstruction through the ventricular system. Ventriculoatrial (VA) shunts and ventriculoperitoneal (VP) shunts are used for absorption of excess CSF.

26. **(A)** The use of complex mechanisms to locate and destroy target structures in the brain is known as stereotactics. Common target areas include obliterating tumors and aneurysms, abolishing movement disorders, and alleviating pain.

27. **(A)** Bifrontal, frontal, and frontotemporal approaches are frequently used for removal of craniopharyngiomas, optic gliomas, and other suprasellar and parasellar tumors. A transsphenoidal hypophysectomy approaches the pituitary gland through the upper gum margin into the floor of the sella turcica.

28. **(B)** Sympathetic denervation of the upper extremities and heart may be accomplished by cervicothoracic sympathectomy (dorsal). The vasospastic phenomenon of Raynaud's disease is relieved by this procedure.

29. **(B)** The thalamus and hypothalamus make up the diencephalon, which is one of the major regions of the brain. The thalamus relays the sensory information in the brain. The hypothalamus controls body temperature, blood pressure, and hormones.

30. **(B)** The meninges have three protective coverings. The outermost is the dura mater, the middle is the arachnoid mater, and the pia mater is closest to the brain.

31. **(A)** Cranial nerve I is the olfactory nerve and is responsible for the sense of smell.

32. **(D)** Electroencephalogram (EEG) is the diagnostic test used to measure the electrical activity of the brain.

33. **(A)** Myelography uses contrast medium injected into the subarachnoid space of the

cervical or lumbar spine, and plain x-rays are taken to produce images.

34. **(B)** Creutzfeldt–Jakob disease is a disease of the nervous system that is caused by a prion that cannot be destroyed by normal disinfection and sterilization. Recommendations include using disposable instruments, which are isolated and incinerated upon disposal.

35. **(D)** An incomplete closure of the spine is spina bifida.

36. **(A)** A slow-growing tumor of the vestibular branch of the eighth cranial nerve is an acoustic neuroma. It is composed of Schwann cells. It is also known as a vestibular schwannoma.

37. **(B)** A glioma is a malignant tumor of the brain composed of glia cells.

38. **(C)** Mannitol acts on the kidneys to remove fluid from the tissues.

39. **(C)** The cerebral cortex is the covering of the brain. It is convoluted. This means it has many folds and creases. The sulci are the groves and depressions that make up the cerebral cortex, and the gyri are the higher ridges of the cerebral cortex.

40. **(A)** The sympathetic system controls thermoregulation, heart rate, peristalsis, and vascular constriction or dilation.

41. **(A)** The iliac crest is the most common bone grafting donor site.

42. **(A)** The approach to remove a pituitary tumor would be the transsphenoidal approach. This is performed with a neurosurgeon and an otorhinolaryngologic surgeon. The incision is accessed from the nose and sphenoid sinus into the brain.

43. **(D)** A self-retaining retractor used to maintain traction of brain tissue is a Yasargil.

44. **(D)** During a craniotomy, burr holes are connected with a craniotome or a Gigli saw.

45. **(D)** A hematoma is a collection of blood in the tissue.

46. **(A)** A Penfield dissector or a Woodson dissector is used to release the dura mater from the cranial bone.

47. **(D)** The ribs, cranial bones, scapula, and sternum are examples of flat bones.

48. **(C)** The patient's hair is personal property and should be shaved and sent with the patient's chart.

49. **(C)** Craniosynostosis is the congenital deformity where the suture lines of the infant's cranium fail to close. A myelomeningocele is a defect in the spine where the spinal cord and meninges protrude through the spine. Scoliosis is a side-to-side curvature of the spine. Anencephaly is when a baby is born without a fully formed brain or the entire skull.

50. **(D)** Both 4-0 silk and 4-0 nylon can be used to retract and close the dural tissue.

51. **(A)** The cerebellum is responsible for balance and coordination. The circle of Willis is the circular connection of arteries that supply blood to the brain. The medulla oblongata is responsible for cardiac and respiratory functions. The fourth ventricle is the cavity within the brain filled with CSF.

52. **(C)** When removing a pituitary tumor, an otorhinolaryngologist works with the neurosurgeon because a transsphenoidal approach is used.

53. **(D)** The medulla oblongata is responsible for cardiac and respiratory function. The pituitary is an endocrine gland that influences growth and development. The cerebrum is the largest part of the brain. The circle of Willis is the circular connection of arteries that supply blood to the brain.

54. **(B)** Cerebral aneurysms are commonly found at the circle of Willis. The choroid plexus is

where CSF is produced. The hypothalamus is responsible for body temperature.

55. **(A)** Beneath the skin is the galea aponeurotica, which is the dense fibrous covering of the skull bone. The first layer of connective tissue that makes up the meninges of the brain is the dura mater. The second is the arachnoid mater, and the direct meningeal covering of the brain is the pia mater.

56. **(D)** The autonomic nervous system controls breathing, heartbeat, and the fight-or-flight response.

57. **(C)** The tough fibrous tissue that covers the pericranium is termed the galea. The dura mater is the layer of the meninges that has direct contact with the skull. The pia mater is the closest layer of the meninges to the brain. The arachnoid mater is the middle layer.

58. **(A)** The corpus callosum divides the right and left halves of the brain. The left hemisphere controls the right side of the body. The right hemisphere controls the left side of the body. The medulla oblongata controls respiration and cardiac functions.

59. **(D)** The carotids and vertebral and basilar arteries all supply blood to the brain.

60. **(A)** The aqueduct of Sylvius connects the third and fourth ventricles. The lateral ventricles are the first two ventricles. The choroid plexus produces CSF. The pons is responsible for horizontal eye movement and face movement, and the cerebrum is the largest part of the brain.

61. **(D)** The Alvarado is a knee holder. The others are equipment used during neurological procedures.

62. **(C)** The pituitary gland rests on the sella turcica. The third ventricle is one of four chambers in the brain containing CSF. The aqueduct of Sylvius connects the third and fourth ventricles. The forebrain is the largest part of the brain and contains the cerebrum.

63. **(A)** The stereotactic technique uses geometric coordinates that provide three-dimensional pictures of the brain prior to treatment.

64. **(B)** The filum terminale is an extension of the pia mater that is a continuation of the end of the spinal cord attached to the coccygeal sections. It functions to suspend the end of the spinal cord. The cauda equina is a bundle of nerve roots at the end of the spinal cord. The vertebral body is the thick bone that makes up the front of the vertebra. The nucleus pulposus is the inner part of the vertebral disc and also the specimen in the spine case.

65. **(C)** A rhizotomy is the surgical procedure where the roots of the spinal nerves are cut to relieve intractable pain. A kyphoplasty is performed for a collapsed vertebra. A cordotomy is the procedure performed for spinal pain from terminal cancer.

66. **(C)** A kyphoplasty is the procedure that uses a balloon instrument in between injured vertebra to infuse bone cement to repair the vertebra and restore height. A rhizotomy is the procedure where the spinal nerve roots are cut to relieve intractable pain. A laminectomy is a procedure to relieve pressure from a nerve in the spine that is affected.

67. **(D)** The Cavitron ultrasonic surgical aspirator (CUSA) is the instrument used for precise dissection, irrigation, and aspiration of brain tumors. The Midas Rex is a high-speed pneumatic drill. A craniotome is a perforating drill used to drill the skull during a craniotomy. The perforator is the drill attachment that is used to create burr holes.

68. **(B)** The cerebrum is the largest part of the human brain. It has right and left hemispheres. It begins at the frontal bone and extends to the back of the skull to the occipital bone. It controls motor and sensory impulses. The cerebellum is located at the back of the skull. It is responsible for balance. The pons is a bridge between the cerebrum and cerebellum. It controls eye movement and respiratory function. The medulla oblongata

is a continuation of the spinal cord and the pons. It is responsible for respirations and cardiac function.

69. **(C)** Fiducials are magnetic markers. Along with MRI and CT scans, these are used to produce detailed, three-dimensional images in the brain using geometric coordinates. They look like Life Savers candies and are placed at different locations on the head such as the forehead, face, and behind the ear.

70. **(B)** Anencephaly is the neural tube defect causing an infant to be born without a portion of the brain. This is a very serious defect, and the infant usually does not live long. Spina bifida is an incomplete closure of the vertebral arches in the spine. This cranial defect is a sac-like protrusion through the skull that allows CSF, meninges, or brain tissue to herniate through the skull. A meningioma is a tumor of the meninges.

71. **(A)** The annulus fibrosis is the outer circular portion of the intervertebral disc that surrounds the nucleus pulposus.

72. **(C)** The cauda equina is the bundle of nerve roots found at the distal end of the spinal cord.

73. **(A)** The four major regions of the brain are the cerebellum, cerebrum, diencephalon, and brainstem.

74. **(B)** The brain and spinal cord make up the central nervous system, and the parts of the nervous system outside of the brain make up the peripheral nervous system. This includes the cranial nerves and spinal nerves.

75. **(C)** The dendrites carry nerve impulses toward the cell/afferent. The soma is the area that sends and receives nerve impulses. The axon carries nerve impulses away from the cell/efferent.

CHAPTER 28

Orthopedics

- The skeleton is divided into:
  - Axial skeleton—skull/ribcage/vertebrae
  - Appendicular skeleton—bones that make up the limbs
- Axial skeleton—the skull or cranium is connected by connective tissue called sutures
  - Skull bones—the bones on the top of the head—flat bones
  - Cranial, facial bones—bones of the face—irregular bones; they include:
    - Facial bones include nasal sinus, orbit of the eye, and jaw (mandible, zygoma)
- Spinal nerves—the spinal nerves come in pairs and branch off to both sides of the body. They include:
  - 7 pairs of cervical—true ribs—connected by costal cartilage anteriorly to the sternum and directly to the vertebra posteriorly
    - Ribs 8, 9, 10—false ribs—these ribs are connected to the sternum by the lowest true ribs and directly to the vertebra posteriorly
  - 12 thoracic—floating ribs—ribs 11 and 12 are not connected anteriorly and to the vertebra posteriorly
  - 5 lumbar
  - 5 sacral
  - 4 coccygeal
- Sternum—forms anterior chest:
  - Manubrium
  - Body
  - Xiphoid
- Long bones
  - Humerus
  - Radius
  - Ulna
  - Femur
- Tibia
- Fibula
- Giant cell tumor—a tumor of the epiphysis of long bones that commonly occurs between the ages of 20 and 40
- Osteogenic sarcoma—a malignant tumor that occurs in long bones; it also metastasizes to the lungs
- Epiphysis—the end of the long bone
- Diaphysis—the shaft of the long bone
- Short bones
  - Bones in the hand—carpels
  - Foot—tarsals
- Flat bones
  - Scapula
  - Patella
  - Pelvic girdle
  - Sternum
- Irregular bones
  - Vertebrae
  - Cranial bones/facial
- Bone marrow—the innermost substance of bone; it is classified as either red or yellow. Bone marrow is responsible for the formation of red blood cells and certain white cells
  - Plasma cell myeloma—a malignant bone tumor found in the plasma cells of bone marrow
- Ewing sarcoma tumor—bone tumor common to children; it can occur in the bone and soft tissue
- Cortical/compact bone—outer layer of bone; it is hard connective tissue
- Cancellous bone—middle layer is soft spongy bone
- Periosteum—a strong fibrous membrane that covers bone

- Bone healing—bone healing takes place in five stages; they are:
  - The inflammatory stage/hematoma formation begins immediately following the injury and can last for 2 days.
  - The cellular proliferation stage/fibrin mesh formation begins the second day to help seal the approximated edges.
  - The callus formation stage lasts about 3–4 weeks. Osteoblasts form collagen and help the fracture site to unite the two ends of the bone.
  - The fourth stage of bone healing is the ossification stage. This begins 3–4 weeks following the fracture and can last for about 3–4 months. The osteoblasts calcify and unite the bone.
  - The final stage of bone healing is the remodeling stage. The bone has healed, and now begins the maintenance of the normal bone.
- Hematoma formation
  - Blood collects at the break site
  - Phagocytosis (white blood cells destroy necrotic tissue)
- Callus formation
  - Fibrin and collagen form
- Calcification process
  - Calcification begins
- Remodeling phase
  - Bone begins to gain its normal structure
- Cartilage—a fibrous connective tissue at the articulating surface of joints and a smooth gliding surface for joint movement
  - It does not have a direct blood supply, lymphatic supply, or vascular supply
  - Chondroma—a benign tumor of cartilage
- Muscles—cover bones and provide movement to the skeletal system. They are classified as:
  - Smooth—involuntary
  - Cardiac
  - Striated—voluntary
- Ligaments—attach bone to bone
  - Tendons—attach muscle to bone
- Joints—joint articulation is where two bones come together
  - Joints have a membranous lining called the synovial membrane; it secretes synovial fluid to lubricate the joint
  - There are many different types of joints, and they are classified according to structure and their ability to move. They include:

- Synarthrotic—immovable—examples include suture lines in the cranium
- Amphiarthrotic—slightly moveable and are connected by cartilage—examples include pubis symphysis, intervertebral joints
- Diarthrotic—have one or more range of motion and are lined with a synovial membrane. They include:
  - Ball-and-socket joint—provides the widest range of motion
    - Examples are the hip and shoulder joints
  - Condyloid joint—movement is in one plane with some lateral movement
    - Example is the temporomandibular joint
  - Gliding joint—provides a side-to-side movement and a twisting movement
    - An example is the carpals of the wrist
  - Hinge joint—this joint has movement in one plane, like the hinge on a door
    - An example is the elbow
  - Pivot joint—the movement is rotational around an axis
    - The proximal end of the radius is an example of a pivot joint
  - Saddle joint—movement is in a variety of planes
- Arthralgia—joint pain
- Arthritis—joint inflammation
- Rheumatoid arthritis
  - Autoimmune disease—the body produces antibodies that fight against the body's own natural antibodies
  - This disease mainly affects the synovium in the joint, causing inflammation and joint stiffness and pain
  - An example is the thumb
- Abduction—moving a body part away from the midline
- Adduction—moving a body part toward the midline of the body
- Circumduction—moving a particular body part without moving the entire body part
- Rotation—moving a body part around a central axis
- Dorsiflexion—bending the foot upward at the ankle joint
- Plantar flexion—bending the foot downward at the ankle joint
- Eversion—turning the foot outward

- Inversion—turning the foot inward at the ankle joint so the sole of the foot is pointing inward
- Flexion—bending a joint
- Extension—straightening a joint
- Pronation—pointing a body part downward (eg, the palm of the hand downward)
- Supination—pointing a body part upward
- Diagnostic testing includes:
  - Arthrogram—an x-ray of a joint after an injection of contrast medium
  - Electromyography—a recording of the electrical activity of muscle by using electrodes attached to the skin or inserted into the muscle
  - Magnetic resonance imaging (MRI)
  - Computed tomography (CT) scan
  - X-rays/fluoroscopy
  - Bone scans—a visual image of bone following an injection of contrast medium
- Fractures—a fracture is the medical term for a broken bone
  - Displaced fracture—the bone breaks into two or more parts and moves so that the two ends are not lined up straight
  - Nondisplaced fracture—the bone breaks either part of the way or all of the way through but maintains its proper alignment
  - Closed fracture/simple fracture—the bone breaks but it does not puncture through the skin
  - Open fracture/compound fracture—bone breaks and protrudes through the skin
  - Greenstick fracture—one side of the bone is broken and the other side is bent. This type of fracture occurs most often in children
  - Transverse fracture—a fracture at a right angle to the bone's axis
  - Oblique fracture—a fracture in which the break has a curve; it breaks diagonally
  - Comminuted fracture—a fracture in which the bone breaks into several pieces
  - Impacted fracture/buckle fracture—at the point of the break, the bones' ends are jammed into each other
  - Colles' fracture—fracture of the distal radius
  - Pathologic fracture—caused by a disease that weakens the bones and causes them to break
  - Avulsion fracture—occurs when a tendon or ligament comes away from the bone and pulls a small piece of bone with it

- Stellate fracture—occurs at a central point on the bone and radiates outward from the fracture site
- Subluxation—partial dislocation
- Dislocation—displacement of one particular surface from another
- Equipment includes:
  - Fracture table—used to stabilize the patient and provide traction
  - Andrews table—used for spine surgery
  - Jackson table—provides skeletal traction
  - Alvarado foot holder for total joints
  - Shoulder attachments used for open procedures or arthroscopic procedures
  - Arthroscopic holder knee attachments
  - Pneumatic tourniquet—provides a bloodless surgical field
- Traction can be used preoperatively, intraoperatively, or postoperatively
  - Various traction techniques include:
    - Skin—strips of tape
    - Straps
    - Elastic bandages—all are attached directly to skin
  - Manual—traction is done by hand to pull on the bone being realigned
  - Skeletal—traction is applied directly to the bone using pins
    - Skeletal traction is often done on the fracture table using pins to reduce long bone fractures
- Casting is the most common bone immobilization technique for a fractured bone. Casting materials include:
  - Plaster
  - Synthetic
  - Fiberglass
  - To apply a cast:
    - The limb is covered with Webril padding
    - Fill a bucket with room temperature water
    - Vertically hold the cast material until all the bubbles rise to the top
  - Examples of various casts include:
    - Walking cast
    - Hip spica
    - Minerva jacket
    - Abduction pillows are used on hip cases to prevent the hip from dislocating and rotating inward

- Complications of bone healing include:
  - Delayed union—delay in healing
  - Malunion—the fracture does not heal in its original position
  - Nonunion—the fracture does not heal and come together
- Osteoma—bone tumor
- Osteoarthritis—disease of the joint; the cartilage wears away, causing bone friction
- Osteomyelitis—bone infection; staphylococci are the bacteria commonly associated with this disease
- Osteonecrosis/avascular necrosis—lack of blood supply to bone caused by infection or trauma
- Osteomalacia—metabolic bone disease that causes softening of bones
- Osteogenesis imperfecta—genetic congenital condition of the connective tissue causing brittle bones that easily fracture
- Osteoporosis—a disease caused by a lack of calcium, which causes a loss of bone density; the bone becomes hard and porous and easily fractures
- Compartment syndrome—after an injury, blood or edema accumulates in the area of the break and causes increased pressure. The fascia cannot expand and pressure builds, preventing blood flow to tissues in the area. Severe tissue damage and tissue death can occur
- Positions
  - Lateral position
  - Prone position
    - Prone position is a challenge for anesthesia; it is very important that positioning is performed properly and the chest has room to expand with respirations, and to protect the endotracheal tube
  - Supine position—when the patient is positioned in supine, it is important not to use the draw sheet and tuck the patient's arms under the mattress but under the patient's body
- Bone cement—PMMA—polymethylmethacrylate
  - Used to secure an implant
  - Used on pathological fractures to fill in bone tumors; the cement is made into beads, and they are placed with bone graft material into the fracture
    - When mixing the cement, it is attached to suction to remove the fumes because they are toxic to mucous membranes and the liver
    - Bone cement is extremely toxic to pregnant women
- Problems with bone cement include:
  - Hypotension
  - Pulmonary embolus
  - Thrombophlebitis
  - Allergic reaction
- Lasers—CO_2/Nd:YAG—used on arthroscopies/total joints/lumbar laminectomies
- Sutures
  - Surgical steel—bone to bone/sternum
  - Ethibond (polyester)—tendon to bone
  - Prolene (polypropylene)—tendon to bone
  - Nylon (Neurolon)—tendon to bone
  - Chromic—periosteum
    - Vicryl (polyglactin)—periosteum
- Antibiotics used for irrigation include:
  - Polymyxin
  - Bacitracin
    - These antibiotics and irrigations can be administered by Asepto syringe or a pulse lavage irrigation system (pulsating irrigation)
- Steroids—dexamethasone (injected into the joint)
- Hemostatic agents include:
  - Bone wax
  - Gelfoam/thrombin
  - Microfibullar
- Bone grafts are used to:
  - Fill cavities after removal of bone that will help to improve the stability of the bone
  - Fill bony defects
  - Promote healing of a bone fracture
- Bone grafts include:
  - Autograft—patient's own bone commonly taken from the iliac crest
  - Allograft—bone from a tissue bank
    - Allograft bone is used when there is insufficient bone from the patient

SURGICAL PROCEDURES

- Closed reduction—the surgeon manipulates the bone manually with his hands
  - Closed reduction may be attempted before an open reduction
  - Reduction may be performed under fluoroscopy

- Skeletal traction—this technique uses a pulling force directly applied to bone via a pin in the bone using weights and pulleys
- Manual—done by the surgeon's hand pulling on the bone being realigned
- External fixation includes:
  - Bone-anchoring devices
    - Threaded Steinmann pins
    - K-wires
    - Smooth rods/stabilizing bars

INTERNAL FIXATION DEVICES

- Treatment of choice for long bones and hip region includes:
  - Compression plate and screw
  - Pins
  - Intramedullary rods, nails
  - Wiring
- Types of screws include:
  - Cortical—the threads run the entire length of the screw and cut a path into the bone; they are also blunt ended
  - Cancellous—threads run further apart and bone collects in threads to form a union; cancellous screws are self-tapping
- Closed reduction—the fracture is reduced by manual manipulation, and traction is applied with percutaneous insertion of pins, nails, and/or rods
- Open reduction and internal fixation (ORIF)—performed by open method at the fracture site and repairing it with fixation devices
  - The fracture is reduced
  - Bone holder and fixation device are placed
  - Screws are inserted; the procedural steps include:
    - Drill
    - Measure
    - Tap
    - Place screw
- Acromioclavicular joint separation—this joint begins at the end of the collar bone (clavicle) and connects to the acromion process of the shoulder blade (scapula)
  - The fracture is repaired with Steinmann pins and/or screws
- Correction of a sternoclavicular dislocation—this joint is between the clavicle and sternum. This dislocation is treated by manipulation and manual traction

- Rotator cuff tear—the rotator cuff is a large tendon that is made up of four muscles that form a cuff over the head of the humerus. The muscles include:
  - Supraspinatus
  - Infraspinatus
  - Subscapularis
  - Teres minor
  - Repair of this procedure includes:
    - Supine position/semi-sitting position
    - Minor tear repair can be performed with heavy nonabsorbable suture
    - Major tears are repaired with bone-anchoring devices and power equipment
- Recurrent anterior shoulder dislocation—the shoulder joint is a ball-and-socket joint that connects humeral head with the shallow socket in the scapula called the glenoid cavity
  - A dislocation occurs when the humeral head comes completely out of the socket and stays out
  - A subluxation occurs when the humeral head comes partly out of the socket and then slips back in
  - The two common procedures performed on the shoulder include:
    - Bankart procedure
    - Putti–Platt
      - The anterior capsule is reattached to the rim of the glenoid fossa with heavy suture
      - Glenoid fossa rim is scraped with curette or rasp to provide raw surface to attach capsule
      - Capsule may be attached by anchors
      - The shoulder is immobilized, and padding is placed between the skin fractures of the humeral shaft
- Fractures of the humeral head can be repaired with an intramedullary rod/compression plate/lag screw or locking nail with distal screws. A bone graft may be needed
- Olecranon fracture—elbow fracture
  - The elbow joint consists of the humerus in the upper arm and the radius and ulna in the forearm; it is a hinge joint
  - The olecranon process is the bony prominence on the upper end of the ulna in the elbow

- Transposition of the ulna nerve—ulnar nerve entrapment occurs when the ulnar nerve in the arm becomes compressed or irritated
  - The most common place where the nerve gets compressed is behind the elbow
- Excision of the head of the radius—a severe comminuted fracture of the radial head. The radial head is important for rotation of the forearm, and elbow loss of motion is a complication of this surgery
- Ganglion cyst—a ganglion cyst is a swollen, closed, fluid-filled sac under the skin. The sac may arise from the sheath of a tendon or joint
  - The ganglion can be on your hand, wrist, foot, or other part of your body
- Fracture of the carpel bones—carpal bones are the small bones that make up the wrist; they connect the hand to the forearm
  - Scaphoid bone is the most commonly fractured bone of the carpels
  - Fixation is performed with K-wires, small compression screws, mini-fragment plates, and screws
  - When performing surgery on the hand, a tourniquet is used and Webril is placed below the tourniquet to protect the skin
  - An Esmarch is used to exsanguinate the limb prior to surgery to create a bloodless field; the Esmarch is wrapped distal to proximal
- Acetabulum—the socket of the hipbone in which the head of the femur fits
- Pelvis—the pelvis is made up of:
  - Ilium
  - Ischium
  - Pubis
  - Acetabulum

HIP FRACTURES

- Intertrochanteric fracture—occurs near the hip joint in the femur
  - Free-Lock compression plate and lag screw are used for the repair
- Hemiarthroplasty is an operation that is used most commonly to treat a fractured femoral head. Also called an Austin Moore prosthesis
  - The operation is similar to a total hip replacement, but it involves only half of the hip
  - The hemiarthroplasty replaces only the ball portion of the hip joint, not the socket portion.

In a total hip replacement, the socket is also replaced
  - The prosthesis is composed of a metal stem that fits into the hollow marrow space of the femur; it also has a metal ball that fits into the acetabular socket
- Two types of prosthesis are used:
  - Unipolar
    - Unipolar—solid metal ball that replaces the femoral head along with the stem is one component
  - Bipolar
    - Bipolar—the bipolar implant has a femoral head that swivels and attaches to the stem
- Instrumentation includes:
  - Rasp/femoral broach—used to ream the femoral canal
  - Acetabula reamer
  - Hibbs retractor
  - Townley caliper—used to measure the femoral head
  - Acetabular trials/femoral trials
  - Acetabular powered reamers
  - Powered reamer driver/saws
    - Sagittal—side to side on the sagittal plane
    - Reciprocating—front/back motion, push/pull
    - Oscillating—the blade runs along the same axis as the handle, and the motion is back and forth
    - When working with power equipment, the STSR should irrigate the tip of the power equipment being used to prevent heat damage of surrounding tissue throughout the procedure
  - Femoral neck elevator—used during femoral broaching
  - Bone hook—used to dislocate the hip
  - Cement mixer
  - Cement restrictor—inserted prior to placing the cement in the femoral canal for the implant
- Coxa valga—outward turning of the hip
- Coxa vara—inward turning of the hip joint
- Tibial plateau fracture—a bone fracture in the proximal part of the tibia or shinbone. A fracture here affects stability and motion of the knee
  - Repair of this fracture includes:
    - Intramedullary nails
    - Plates and screws

- Buttress plate—a curved plate; fits over curved bones
- Commonly used on tibial plateau fractures
- Patella—a broken kneecap occurs when the small round bone (patella) that sits over the front of your knee joint breaks
  - The patella is a sesamoid bone
  - Repair of the patella consists of:
    - Wires and screws
- Ligaments—tough bands of tissue that connect the ends of bones together
  - Stability of knee depends on all four ligaments
  - There are two collateral ligaments—they provide side-to-side motion of the knee
    - Medial collateral ligament (MCL) is found on the side of the knee closest to the other knee
    - Lateral collateral ligament (LCL) is found on the opposite side of the knee
  - The anterior cruciate ligament (ACL) keeps the tibia from sliding too far forward
    - ACL tears are caused by pivoting or side-stepping movements and landing off-kilter
  - The posterior cruciate ligament (PCL) sits in front of the ACL. It prevents the tibia from sliding too far back
    - PCL tears are caused by a direct hit to the front of the knee while the knee is bent
  - Medial cruciate ligament (MCL)—injury to MCL is caused to a hit from the outside of the knee
  - Lateral cruciate ligament (LCL)—tear of LCL is caused by twisting
- Repairs are performed by replacing the torn ligament
  - The common ligament used for the repair is the patient's own patellar tendon (autograft)
  - Continuous passive motion (CPM) machine—provides continuous motion; it straps to the postoperative leg and electronically bends and straightens the leg to prevent joint stiffness
- Baker's cyst—swelling caused by fluid from the knee joint bulging to the back of the knee in the popliteal fossa. These cysts are caused by degenerative changes
  - Treatment includes:
    - Rest
    - Drainage
    - Cortisone injection
    - Ice packs

- Pott's fracture/bimalleolar ankle fracture—occurs in the tibia near the ankle and in the medial malleolus in the tibia
- Trimalleolar fracture—fracture of the ankle that involves the lateral malleolus, medial malleolus, and distal posterior aspect of the tibia. This is a fracture of all three bones
  - This can be repaired with plates and screws
- Triple arthrodesis—arthrodesis is the medical term for fusion, and with this procedure, it refers to fusing of three joints:
  - Talocalcaneal
  - Talonavicular
  - Calcaneocuboid
  - The goal of a triple arthrodesis is to relieve pain from arthritis, congenital deformities, and unstable joints
    - Congenital deformities include:
      - Clubfoot
      - Polio
- Bunionectomy—hallux valgus—the bump at the base of the big toe and the lateral deviation of the big toe
  - Bunions are caused by a combination of uncomfortable shoes and heredity
  - Procedures performed to repair the bunion are called:
    - Keller
    - McBride
  - Exostosis (overgrowth of bone)—the surgeon removes the overgrowth of bone and realigns the big toe
  - K-wires, power wire driver, and microsagittal saw
- Hallux varus—big toe turns toward the midline
- Hammer toe—when a person has hammer toe, the end of their toe bends downward and the middle joint curls up. Eventually, the toe gets stuck in a stiff, claw-like position
  - Hammer toe usually affects the second toe (the toe next to the big toe), but it can affect other toes too
- Talipes valgus—congenital deformity where the foot is turned inward and the person walks on the inside of the foot
- Talipes varus—congenital deformity where the heel is turned inward; it is a type of clubfoot

- Metatarsal fracture—metatarsal bones are the long bones in the foot above the toes
  - Repair with K-wires, screws, or plates
- Metatarsal resection—performed to replace head due to arthritis or injury
- Knee arthroscopy—minimally invasive procedure performed for:
  - Diagnosis
  - Removal of foreign bodies that can cause pain and obstruct movement
  - Meniscal repair
- Meniscus—a fibrous cartilage between the joints of the knee
  - A meniscal tear is one of the most common knee injuries
    - Bucket handle tear—common meniscal tear
    - Joint mice—loose particles of bone and cartilage within the knee joint. These particles become trapped and cause pain and irritation and limit movement
  - Instrumentation includes:
    - Ringer's lactate or sterile normal saline is the medium used to inflate the knee
    - Arthroscope
    - Tubing
    - Trocar and cannula
    - Shaving/cutting instruments
    - Biopsy punch
    - Probes, hooks, scissors, knives
  - Patient position is supine with the knee positioned at a 90-degree angle
- Total knee replacement—performed for a diseased knee joint. There are three components to a total knee replacement; they include:
  - Tricompartmental (most common) total knee replacement
    - Femoral component
    - Tibial component
    - Patellar component
- Partial knee replacement—resurfaces one or two bones of the knee
  - Unicompartmental includes one of the following components:
    - Medial unicondylar component
    - Lateral unicondylar component
    - Femoral-patellar component
  - Bicompartmental knee replacement—replaces both medial and lateral surfaces of femur and tibia
- Genu valgum—the knees are closed in and the space at the ankles is further apart. Knock-kneed
- Genu varum—the space between the knees is further apart and bows closer at the ankles. Bowlegged
- Total shoulder replacement—performed for severe pain and stiffness caused by arthritis or degenerative joint disease
  - Position is beach chair
  - Implants include a ball and stem for the humeral component and a plastic socket
- Shoulder arthroscopy—performed for diagnosis, frozen shoulder, or rotator cuff repair
  - Position—beach chair
  - Glenohumeral joint is distended with saline
- Above the knee amputation/below the knee amputation is performed for:
  - Trauma
  - Diabetic patients
  - Vascular disease
  - Tumors
  - The goal of the procedure is to preserve as much movement to the limb as possible so a prosthesis can be used
  - Amputated limbs are sent to the morgue

Questions

1. Which nutrient is responsible for providing bone strength and is monitored as you get older to preserve strong bones?

   (A) Iron
   (B) Vitamin C
   (C) Calcium
   (D) Zinc

2. What is the proper wrapping procedure utilizing an Esmarch bandage?

   (A) Start at the distal end of the extremity
   (B) Start at the proximal end of the extremity
   (C) Start after the cuff is inflated
   (D) Start at the incision site

3. Baker's cysts are found in the:

   (A) popliteal fossa
   (B) interdigital fossa
   (C) intercarpal joints
   (D) olecranon fossa

4. Benign outpouchings of synovium from intercarpal joints are called:

   (A) ganglia
   (B) exostosis
   (C) polyps
   (D) synovitis

5. Compression of the median nerve at the volar surface of the wrist is known as:

   (A) Dupuytren's contracture
   (B) carpal tunnel syndrome
   (C) ganglia
   (D) Volkmann's contracture

6. A fixation device that provides maximum holding and rigid fixation of a fracture by tightening bone fragments together is called a/an:

   (A) compression plate and screws
   (B) intramedullary nailing
   (C) Ilizarov technique
   (D) interlocking nail fixation

7. In a total hip replacement, which structure is reamed?

   (A) Acetabulum
   (B) Greater trochanter
   (C) Lesser trochanter
   (D) Femoral head

8. The ideal candidate for a noncemented total hip arthroplasty is:

   (A) young and healthy
   (B) young with arthritis
   (C) old and healthy
   (D) old with osteoporotic bone disease

9. A total hip replacement would be indicated when the patient has:

   (A) degenerative hip joint disease
   (B) hip fracture
   (C) congenital hip dislocation
   (D) hip cancer

10. Joint reconstruction is known as:

    (A) arthrodesis
    (B) arthroplasty
    (C) arthrotomy
    (D) arthropexy

11. Osteogenesis or bone growth can be induced by:

    (A) bone grafting, autogenous
    (B) bone grafting, homogeneous
    (C) hormone installation
    (D) electrical stimulation

12. An infection in bone is termed:

    (A) osteomalacia
    (B) osteomyelitis
    (C) osteitis
    (D) osteoporosis

13. A surgical procedure designed to stiffen or fuse a joint is called:

    (A) arthropexy
    (B) arthroplasty
    (C) joint fixation
    (D) arthrodesis

14. A lateral curvature of the spine is:

    (A) kyphosis
    (B) scoliosis
    (C) lordosis
    (D) orthosis

15. Harrington rods are used to treat:

    (A) femoral fracture
    (B) scoliosis
    (C) talipes deformity
    (D) congenital hip dislocation

16. The congenital deformity known as clubfoot is surgically referred to as:

    (A) talipes valgus
    (B) talipes varus
    (C) hallux valgus
    (D) exostosis

17. The most frequent site of cartilage tears in the knee joint is at the:

    (A) collateral ligament
    (B) cruciate ligament
    (C) lateral meniscus
    (D) medial meniscus

18. An abduction pillow would be used to:

    (A) immobilize hip joints after hip surgery
    (B) stabilize a femoral fracture
    (C) immobilize the tibia after surgery
    (D) rotate the hips outward after hip reconstruction

19. A Free-Lock compression screw system is indicated for correction of a/an _____ fracture.

    (A) hip
    (B) wrist
    (C) elbow
    (D) cervical

20. Decreased bone mass results in a condition called:

    (A) osteoporosis
    (B) osteomyelitis
    (C) ossification
    (D) ecchymosis

21. Place the stages of bone healing in the correct order: (1) inflammatory stage, (2) remodeling stage, (3) ossification stage, (4) cellular proliferation stage, (5) callus formation stage.

    (A) 1, 4, 5, 3, 2
    (B) 1, 2, 3, 4, 5
    (C) 5, 3, 4, 2, 1
    (D) 2, 5, 4, 3, 1

22. An olecranon fracture occurs in the:

    (A) wrist
    (B) knee
    (C) elbow
    (D) finger

23. All of the following are considered good methods of maintaining strict asepsis within an orthopedic surgical suite EXCEPT:

    (A) ultraviolet light
    (B) laminar flow rooms
    (C) charcoal masks
    (D) space suits

24. A common method to immobilize a fracture is to apply a cast. When applying a cast:

    (A) a bucket of lukewarm water is required
    (B) the cast material is held vertically in the water until the bubbles stop rising to the surface
    (C) flat sheets of cast material are used for a splint
    (D) all of the above

25. Orthopedic surgery prepping:

    (A) is done under sterile conditions
    (B) is done the day before surgery
    (C) is eliminated
    (D) is increased in time only

26. What type of cast is applied to the trunk of the body to immobilize the spine?

    (A) Cylindrical
    (B) Minerva jacket
    (C) Montgomery
    (D) Spica

27. In orthopedic surgery, the x-ray viewing of the progression of a procedure in real time is known as:

    (A) fluoroscopy
    (B) radiography
    (C) portable filming
    (D) x-ray

28. Surgery on the medial malleolus would be surgery of the:

    (A) fibula
    (B) jaw
    (C) tibia
    (D) radius

29. Plaster is ready for application:

    (A) when air bubbles cease to rise
    (B) when air bubbles begin to rise
    (C) after 2 minutes of submersion
    (D) after 10 minutes of submersion

30. A greenstick fracture:

    (A) is a common fracture found in children under 10 years of age
    (B) is when the bone bends and cracks on one side but is not totally broken in two
    (C) more commonly occurs in the arm than leg
    (D) all of the above

31. Which orthopedic hip procedure is indicated for patients with degenerative joint disease or rheumatoid arthritis?

    (A) AO external fixation
    (B) Total hip arthroplasty
    (C) Femoral endoprosthesis
    (D) Modular endoprosthesis

32. What skeletal traction requires the use of sterile supplies for application of a traction appliance?

    (A) Thomas splint
    (B) Russell
    (C) Crutchfield
    (D) Buck's extension

33. An infectious musculoskeletal condition affecting the bone and marrow is:

    (A) osteomalacia
    (B) osteoporosis
    (C) osteomyelitis
    (D) Paget's disease

34. Polymethylmethacrylate, commonly called bone cement, can have toxic effects and cause complications. They include:

    (A) pulmonary embolus
    (B) implantation syndrome
    (C) hypotension
    (D) all of the above

35. The fundamentals of screw placement involved in ORIF surgical procedures include the following stems. Place them in the correct order of procedural steps: (1) tap, (2) place screw, (3) drill, and (4) measure.

(A) 1, 2, 3, 4
(B) 3, 4, 1, 2
(C) 2, 3, 4, 1
(D) 3, 2, 4, 1

36. All of the following are indications for external fixation EXCEPT:

(A) infected joints
(B) clean long bone fractures
(C) highly comminuted closed fractures
(D) major alignment and length deficits

37. A procedure done to correct recurrent anterior dislocation of the shoulder that involves reattachment of the rim of the glenoid fossa is called a:

(A) Bankart
(B) Putti–Platt
(C) Bristow
(D) Monteggia

38. The most commonly fractured carpal bone is the:

(A) scaphoid
(B) lunate
(C) trapezium
(D) capitate

39. Compression force of the distal femur upon the tibia produces varying types of fractures of the:

(A) patella
(B) tibial plateau
(C) femoral condyle
(D) head of the femur

40. Surgery that requires incision of the long extensor tendon of the interphalangeal joint of the four lateral toes and subsequent fusion is called:

(A) exostectomy
(B) Keller procedure
(C) hammer toe correction
(D) McBride procedure

41. The rare use of laser during orthopedic surgery may be seen in the use of the CO_2 laser during a revision arthroplasty to:

(A) remove a cemented implant
(B) vaporize protein
(C) weld tissue for collagen bonding
(D) create hemostasis

42. After surgery on a shoulder, the arm may be bound against the side of the arm for:

(A) comfort
(B) abduction
(C) immobilization
(D) mobilization

43. The most commonly used implants in hand surgery are made of flexible:

(A) polypropylene
(B) Silastic
(C) tantalum
(D) polyethylene

44. Before the insertion of cement into the femoral medullary canal during a total hip arthroplasty, which of the following is placed with an inserter to occlude the femoral medullary canal?

(A) Polyethylene insert
(B) Cement restrictor
(C) Broach
(D) Distal centralizer

45. Femoral prostheses such as the Austin Moore and Thompson are used to correct all of the following diagnoses EXCEPT:

(A) avascular necrosis

(B) nonunion fractures

(C) displaced femoral neck fractures

(D) rheumatoid arthritis

46. Orthopedic implants are covered by all of the following rules EXCEPT:

(A) different metals should not be mixed because they may react chemically

(B) if the implant is driven by force, a driver with a metal head must be used

(C) a template must be used for sizing purposes

(D) handle as little as possible before insertion

47. Galvanic corrosion is a process that occurs postoperatively because of:

(A) poor handling of device during implant

(B) mixed use of metals for implant

(C) misplacement of implant

(D) damage of an implanted device

48. Bunionectomy is also known as:

(A) metacarpal arthroplasty

(B) hallux valgus

(C) triple arthrodesis

(D) hammer toe

49. A Colles' fracture is a fracture of the:

(A) distal radius

(B) femur

(C) patella

(D) fibula

50. The Keller and McBride procedures are types of:

(A) bunionectomy procedures

(B) shoulder repairs

(C) ankle repairs

(D) patellectomy procedures

51. The three phases of bone healing in order are:

1. Remodeling
2. Inflammatory phase
3. Reparative phase

(A) 1, 2, 3

(B) 2, 1, 3

(C) 2, 3, 1

(D) 3, 1, 2

52. The patella is what type of bone?

(A) Flat

(B) Short

(C) Sesamoid

(D) Round

53. Polymethylmethacrylate (PMMA) is a type of bone cement most commonly used in what procedure?

(A) Arthroplasty procedures

(B) Keller procedures

(C) ACL repair

(D) Triple arthrodesis

54. The proper position for the patient undergoing arthroscopic knee surgery is:

(A) skeletal traction on fracture table

(B) lateral position, foot of table flexed at 45 degrees

(C) the Alvarado knee holder

(D) supine position, foot of table flexed at 90 degrees

55. Orthopedic saws are identified by the movement of the blade. Which saw blade is mounted along the same axis as the handle and moves back and forth?

(A) Sagittal

(B) Reciprocating

(C) Oscillating

(D) Rotating

56. An orthopedic screw is the most commonly used type of orthopedic implant. All are orthopedic screws EXCEPT:

(A) cancellous

(B) lag

(C) self-tapping

(D) depth

57. The three main components of a knee arthroplasty are:

1. Femoral
2. Acetabular
3. ibial base plate
4. Patella component

(A) 1, 3, 4

(B) 1, 2, 3

(C) 2, 3, 4

(D) 4, 2, 1

58. Which graft is used to replace the ACL during an ACL repair?

(A) Patella tendon

(B) Cadaver

(C) Hamstring or quadriceps

(D) All of the above

59. A Putti–Platt is used to correct the:

(A) ankle

(B) wrist

(C) patella

(D) shoulder

60. What connects bone to bone?

(A) Ligament

(B) Tendon

(C) Muscle

(D) Bursa

61. The shaft of the long bone is the _____, and the end of the long bone is the _____.

(A) diaphysis, epiphysis

(B) epiphysis, diaphysis

(C) symphysis, diaphysis

(D) symphysis, epiphysis

62. A fracture that consists of multiple bone fragments is:

(A) comminuted

(B) greenstick

(C) spiral

(D) impacted

63. Bone healing is termed:

(A) osteoporosis

(B) osteoplasty

(C) osteogenesis

(D) osteomalacia

64. A hemostatic agent used on bone is:

(A) heparin

(B) bone wax

(C) lidocaine

(D) Cottonoid

65. A pneumatic tourniquet is placed:

(A) as soon as the patient enters the operating room

(B) directly after the patient is prepped and draped

(C) before the patient is prepped and draped

(D) as soon as anesthesia says it is okay

66. Equipment needed to repair a femoral neck fracture using a compression screw and sliding plate includes all of the following EXCEPT:

(A) fracture table

(B) C-arm (fluoro)

(C) K-wires

(D) pneumatic tourniquet

67. A pressurized solution of antibiotics or saline, commonly used for wound debridement and irrigation, is called:

(A) pulse lavage system

(B) ancillary system

(C) inactive irrigation system

(D) topical irrigation system

68. Traction that requires surgical insertion of metal rods or pins through bone that are attached to a traction device that applies force or is attached to a weighted pulley is known as:

(A) skin traction
(B) applied traction
(C) manual traction
(D) skeletal traction

69. During a procedure involving a power saw in use, the surgical technician in the scrub role should:

(A) clean the blade
(B) lightly apply irrigation to the blade in use
(C) suction bone debris
(D) do nothing

70. The condition where fibrous bands cause contractures in the fingers, commonly the ring finger and the little finger, is called:

(A) compartment syndrome
(B) Dupuytren's
(C) exostosis
(D) ganglion

71. Bone tumors include all EXCEPT:

(A) Ewing's sarcoma
(B) osteogenic sarcoma
(C) chondroma
(D) Wilms' tumor

72. The surgical repair of a torn tendon is:

(A) triple arthrodesis
(B) percutaneous tendonectomy
(C) tendonitis
(D) tenorrhaphy

73. The tendon involved when there is inability to plantar flex the foot is the:

(A) Achilles tendon
(B) lateral metatarsal tendon
(C) capsular tendon
(D) digitorum tendon

74. Mrs. Smedley was scheduled to have a right total hip replacement with an anterior approach. What position would she be placed in?

(A) supine
(B) right lateral
(C) left lateral
(D) Fowler's

75. The responsibility of the STSR when applying the cast is to keep the foot in a plantar flexed position (toes downward) in order to:

(A) keep good blood supply to the foot
(B) keep the muscle hyperextended
(C) keep stress off the new suture line
(D) allow the local to penetrate the surgical site

76. A stellate fracture is:

(A) when the bone breaks in a central point and radiates outward, like a cracked mirror
(B) when the fracture curves around the bone due to twisting motion
(C) a bone fracture where the bone remains attached by a ligament
(D) when the bone is driven inward

77. Dorsal flexion is where the foot is turned _____, and plantar flexion is where the foot is turned _____.

(A) upward, downward
(B) downward, upward
(C) inward, outward
(D) outward, inward

78. When the joint is freely movable and is lined with a synovial membrane, it is termed:

(A) amphiarthrosis
(B) diarthrosis
(C) synarthrosis
(D) none of the above

79. All apply to compartment syndrome EXCEPT:

    (A) the wound is closed following an incision and drainage with a pulse lavage system
    (B) an incision is made and the wound is left open until swelling is reduced
    (C) it commonly occurs in the leg
    (D) the fascia cannot easily expand, causing the pressure to build up in the compartment of the limb; this causes pressure on the vessels and nerves, causing inadequate blood flow to the tissues

80. When the calcaneocuboid, talonavicular, and talocalcaneal bones are fused together, the procedure to correct this is:

    (A) McBride
    (B) arthroscopy
    (C) triple arthrosis
    (D) arthroplasty

81. Subluxation is:

    (A) complete fracture
    (B) incomplete dislocation
    (C) malunion fracture
    (D) nonunion fracture

82. The procedure performed for a rotator cuff tear is:

    (A) Keller
    (B) acromioplasty
    (C) arthroscopy
    (D) ORIF

83. All pertain to intertrochanteric fracture EXCEPT:

    (A) occurs on the femur
    (B) occurs at the lesser trochanter
    (C) repaired with a dynamic hip screw
    (D) occurs at the acetabular head

84. The bones of the palm of the hand are referred to as:

    (A) phalanges
    (B) carpals
    (C) metacarpals
    (D) calcaneus

85. The gastrocnemius is the chief muscle of the:

    (A) calf of the leg
    (B) stomach
    (C) stomach's greater curvature
    (D) thigh

86. In adults, red bone marrow that produces red blood cells is mainly found in which type of bone?

    (A) Flat and irregular
    (B) Femur/long
    (C) Sesamoid
    (D) Irregular

87. The medial bone of the forearm, which is located on the small finger side of the hand, is called the:

    (A) ulna
    (B) radius
    (C) humerus
    (D) fibula

88. The bone located in the neck between the mandible and the larynx, which supports the tongue and provides attachment for some of its muscles, is the:

    (A) palatine bone
    (B) vomer
    (C) pterygoid hamulus
    (D) hyoid bone

89. The adult vertebral column has:

    (A) 33 bones
    (B) 28 bones
    (C) 26 bones
    (D) 32 bones

90. How many cervical vertebrae are there?

    (A) 7
    (B) 12
    (C) 5
    (D) 4

91. The bone in the axial skeleton that does not articulate with any other bone is the:

(A) sternum
(B) trochlea
(C) talus
(D) hyoid

92. A slender, rod-like bone that is located at the base of the neck and runs horizontally is the:

(A) scapula
(B) shoulder blade
(C) clavicle
(D) sternum

93. The upper, flaring portion of hipbone is the:

(A) ischium
(B) pubis
(C) ilium
(D) femoral head

94. The larger, weight-bearing bone of the lower leg is the:

(A) humerus
(B) talus
(C) fibula
(D) tibia

95. The bone that fits into the acetabulum, forming a joint, is the:

(A) tibia
(B) femur
(C) fibula
(D) patella

96. The infraspinatus, teres minor, subscapularis, and supraspinatus muscles make up the:

(A) rotator cuff
(B) pelvic girdle
(C) sternal notch
(D) vertebra

97. The longest bone in the body is the:

(A) femur
(B) fibula
(C) tibia
(D) humerus

98. A rounded protuberance found at a point of articulation with another bone is called a:

(A) trochanter
(B) trochlea
(C) tubercle
(D) condyle

99. In which joint would a bucket handle tear be found?

(A) Shoulder
(B) Knee
(C) Hip
(D) Wrist

100. Which of the following is NOT a muscle classification?

(A) Smooth
(B) Elastic
(C) Cardiac
(D) Skeletal

101. What is the most commonly used donor tendon for a free flexor tendon graft?

(A) Palmaris longus
(B) Plantaris tendon
(C) Abductor pollicis longus
(D) Both A and B

102. Joints are classified by their structure and their ability to move. Which is a ball-and-socket joint?

(A) Elbow
(B) Carpel bones of the wrist
(C) Skull bones
(D) Hip

103. An example of a saddle joint is the:

(A) shoulder

(B) elbow joint

(C) thumb joint

(D) radius

104. A recording of the electrical activity of muscle tissue by using electrodes attached to the skin or inserted into the muscle is termed:

(A) electrocardiogram

(B) positron emission tomography

(C) electromyography

(D) computed tomography

105. What type of operating room tables are commonly used for orthopedic procedures?

(A) Fracture table

(B) Andrews table

(C) Jackson table

(D) All of the above

Answers and Explanations

1. **(C)** Calcium, vitamin D, and phosphorus are needed to maintain strong bones and make up the bone matrix.

2. **(A)** Prior to using a tourniquet, the wrapping of the extremity is implemented using an Esmarch bandage, wrapping the limb distal to proximal.

3. **(A)** Baker's cysts are found in the popliteal fossa. They are frequently painful and can become large. Excision requires prone position.

4. **(A)** Ganglia are benign outpouchings of synovium from the intercarpal joints that become filled with synovial fluid. They often resolve spontaneously but occasionally must be excised.

5. **(B)** In carpal tunnel syndrome, the median nerve becomes compressed at the volar surface of the wrist because of thickened synovium, fractures, or aberrant muscles.

6. **(A)** Rigid fixation by compression plate and screws uses heavy and strong compression plates to give maximum hold and rigid fixation. Tightening the nut on compression instruments brings bone fragments together.

7. **(A)** The femoral head is removed and replaced with a prosthesis. The acetabulum is reamed to the configuration of the acetabulum component, which is then fixed in the socket.

8. **(A)** Young active individuals with strong healthy bones are ideal candidates for non-cemented total hip replacement. Elderly patients with osteoporosis and patients with poor quality bone are usually candidates for cement because their bones may lack the compressive strength to support weight-bearing forces.

9. **(A)** Total hip replacement is indicated for patients with hip pain caused by degenerative joint diseases or rheumatoid arthritis.

10. **(B)** Reconstruction of a joint (arthroplasty) may be necessary to restore or improve range of motion and stability or to relieve pain.

11. **(D)** Electrical stimulation is artificially applied electrical current that induces or influences osteogenesis. This accelerates fracture healing. Bone growth stimulation is also used in treating infected nonunions because the electrical stimulation retards bacterial growth.

12. **(B)** Osteomyelitis, or an infection in bone, occurs after bone is injured in an accident or is involved in surgical repair. It may cause nonunion of fractures. Microorganisms reach the bone via the bloodstream. *Staphylococcus aureus* is commonly the causative agent.

13. **(D)** Arthrodesis is most commonly employed to relieve pain by eliminating motion, to provide stability where normal ligament stability has been destroyed, or to correct deformity by realignment at the level of fusion.

14. **(B)** Scoliosis is a lateral curve and rotation of the spine.

15. **(B)** Harrington rods are used with spinal fusion to treat scoliosis.

16. **(B)** Talipes varus, the condition known as club-foot, refers to the inversion of the forefoot.

17. **(D)** Tears in the menisci (semilunar cartilage) are the most common knee injuries occurring most frequently in the medial meniscus.

18. **(A)** An abduction pillow aids in immobilizing hip joints after surgery.

19. **(A)** Internal fixation of a hip can be accomplished with a Free-Lock compression hip screw fixation system allowing earlier ambulation and thus fewer complications.

20. **(A)** Osteoporosis is an age-related disorder characterized by increased susceptibility to fractures as a result of decreased levels of estrogen.

21. **(A)** The inflammatory stage/hematoma formation begins immediately following the injury and can last for 2 days. The cellular proliferation stage/fibrin mesh formation begins the second day to help seal the approximated edges. The callus formation stage lasts about 3–4 weeks. Osteoblasts form collagen and help the fracture site to unite the two ends of the bone. The fourth stage of bone healing is the ossification stage. This begins 3–4 weeks following the fracture and can last for about 3–4 months. The osteoblasts calcify and unite the bone. The final stage of bone healing is the remodeling stage. The bone has healed, and normal bone is maintained.

22. **(C)** An olecranon fracture occurs in the elbow.

23. **(C)** When used in the operating room, charcoal masks restrict inhalation of vaporized particles of viruses such as venereal warts. All of the others are varying degrees of specialized units that address the principle of "strict surgical asepsis" for orthopedic surgery.

24. **(D)** When applying a cast, first the limb is covered and skin is protected with Webril padding or a stockinette. The width of the cast material is determined by the surgeon. The position of the limb is determined by the surgeon. The position of the limb is determined by the surgeon, and the cast material is submerged in the water. When ready, it is applied distal to proximal and is held until it hardens. When applying a splint, sheets of cast material are used and molded into the proper position, and the limb is then wrapped with an Ace bandage.

25. **(A)** A primary concern in orthopedic surgery is the prevention of infection, thus calling for meticulous technique with the operative scrub, carried out under sterile conditions.

26. **(B)** A Minerva jacket/body jacket cast is used to immobilize the spine and is applied to the trunk of the body. A cylindrical cast is used for immobilization of the knee and is applied from the ground to the ankle. Montgomery straps are a type of abdominal surgical dressing. A spica cast/hip spica is applied to the trunk and the leg of the affected side and is used for hip and femoral fractures.

27. **(A)** In many different types of surgical procedures, especially orthopedics, where moving images need to be viewed in real time, a fluoroscopy machine/image intensification is used. An x-ray beam passes through the target tissue and displays continuous images on a monitor.

28. **(C)** Ankle fractures include fractures of the medial malleolus (tibia), lateral malleolus (fibula), and posterior malleolus (posterior distal tibia).

29. **(A)** When preparing plaster rolls or splints, they are submerged in room temperature water (70–75°F). Water above this temperature will speed up the process and make the cast application ineffective. When bubbles cease to rise to the surface, the rolls are removed, lightly compressed, and used.

30. **(D)** A greenstick fracture is an incomplete fracture. The bone is bent and only partly breaks on one side. It is commonly found in children because their bones have not yet fully calcified.

31. **(B)** The hip procedure indicated for degenerative joint disease or rheumatoid arthritis

is total hip arthroplasty, cemented or noncemented. All of the others are femoral head components used to treat fractures that have not achieved union in a conventional manner.

32. **(C)** Some cervical spine fractures or injuries may require Crutchfield or Gardner–Wells tongs inserted into the skull to stabilize the vertebrae and reduce spinal cord damage. Application of traction requires the use of sterile supplies, including a bow, pins, and drill.

33. **(C)** An infectious musculoskeletal condition affecting the bone and the marrow is osteomyelitis. This infection may develop from bloodborne pathogens deposited at the site. The infection develops as pathogenic organisms become trapped in small arteries in the metaphyseal area.

34. **(D)** PMMA (bone cement) is commonly used to secure implants in the body, fill in pathological bone tumors, and replace skull flaps. There are adverse reactions that may occur when using it. They include hypotension, cardiac arrythmias, stroke, pulmonary embolus, and/or severe allergic action. It is highly toxic to pregnant women.

35. **(B)** The sequence of screw placement is: drill, measure, tap, and place the screw

36. **(B)** This method of fracture management provides rigid fixation and reduction with the ability to manage severe soft tissue wounds.

37. **(A)** A Bankart procedure involves reattachment of the anterior capsule to the rim of the glenoid fossa. A Putti–Platt is similar; in addition, it requires the lateral advancement of the subscapularis and produces a barrier against dislocation of the shoulder.

38. **(A)** The scaphoid is the most commonly fractured carpal bone. Internal fixation is generally accomplished with Kirschner wires, small compression screws, or minifragment compression plates and screws.

39. **(B)** Tibial plateau fractures have historically been attributed to bumper or fender injuries. Compression force of the distal femur upon the tibia produces varying types of plateau fractures.

40. **(C)** A hammer toe flexion deformity develops at the proximal interphalangeal joint of the four lateral toes. It is treated by incising the long extensor tendon and fusing the middle joint.

41. **(A)** Although not used as commonly as in other surgical specialties, lasers are used in some orthopedic procedures. Methylmethacrylate can be vaporized with a carbon dioxide laser to remove a cemented implant. Nd:YAG laser can be used in arthroscopy to vaporize protein as well as to weld tissue by bonding collagen.

42. **(C)** After a shoulder procedure, the arm may be bound against the side for immobilization. An absorbent pad or a large piece of cotton or sheet wadding is placed under the arm to keep skin surfaces from touching because they may macerate.

43. **(B)** The most commonly used implants in hand surgery are flexible implants made of Silastic. They are available for arthroplasty within the scope of hand surgery, such as finger joints, wrist joints, carpal trapezium, lunate, and navicular.

44. **(B)** After reaming of the femoral canal has been accomplished, a trial component is fitted. After removal of the trial, the canal is lavaged and brushed to accommodate the femoral component. A cement restrictor is inserted into the femoral canal. The cement is injected, and the femoral component with proximal and distal centralizers is inserted.

45. **(D)** These implants are a single unit including stem and head, which require limited rasping and canal preparation. Currently, this is the accepted treatment for nonunion fractures, avascular necrosis, rheumatoid arthritis, and osteoarthritis. Total hip replacement

is generally indicated for patients with degenerative joint disease or rheumatoid arthritis.

46. **(B)** Metal implants are extremely expensive. Once an implant has been scratched, it cannot be used. All personnel should follow these rules: store separately, handle as little as possible, use a driver with a Teflon head to drive the implant, do not bend, and use a template for sizing purposes.

47. **(B)** Many different alloys are used in the manufacture of implants. However, the implantation of devices with different metallic composition must be avoided to prevent galvanic corrosion; internal fixation devices used during an orthopedic procedure should be of the same metal.

48. **(B)** A bunionectomy is removal of an enlarged metatarsal head, hallux valgus. The bunion is reduced or removed. The goal of this surgery is to alleviate pain and increase mobility.

49. **(A)** A Colles' fracture is an angulated fracture of the distal radius.

50. **(A)** Keller and McBride are variations of bunionectomy procedures.

51. **(C)** The three phases of bone healing in order are inflammatory, reparative, and remodeling.

52. **(C)** Patella is a type of sesamoid bone. They are irregularly shaped bones.

53. **(A)** Implants used in arthroplasties (joint replacement) may be cemented in place with PMMA.

54. **(D)** The patient is placed in supine position, and the foot of the table may be flexed at 90 degrees.

55. **(C)** The oscillating blade is mounted along the same axis as the handle and moves back and forth.

56. **(D)** Orthopedic screws come in different sizes, shapes, and designs. They are made of titanium, stainless steel, or bioabsorbable material. They include cancellous, cortical, lag, Herbert, locking, cannulated, and self-tapping.

57. **(A)** The three components are the metal femoral component inserted over the distal femur, tibial base plate placed over the proximal tibia, and a polyethylene patellar component.

58. **(D)** A graft can be taken from the central portion of the patellar tendon, hamstring or quad, or a cadaver.

59. **(D)** The Putti–Platt procedure is used to correct a recurrent anterior dislocation of the shoulder.

60. **(A)** A ligament is a band of fibrous connective tissue connecting to the articular ends of bones and serving to bind bones together.

61. **(A)** Each long bone has a geographic landmark. The shaft of the long bone is the diaphysis, and the end of the long bone is the epiphysis.

62. **(A)** This type of fracture consists of multiple bone fragments and fractured bone. It also may require repair of both soft tissue and bone.

63. **(C)** Osteogenesis is bone healing.

64. **(B)** During surgery, a waxy preparation called bone wax is pressed into the bleeding area of bone to control bleeding.

65. **(C)** The tourniquet cuff is placed proximal to the surgical site before the patient is prepped and draped.

66. **(D)** A pneumatic tourniquet is used on extremity surgery. A fracture table is used to reduce the fracture. Fluoroscopy is used to view the fracture, and K-wires are used to stabilize a fracture.

67. **(A)** The pulse lavage system uses antibiotic solution or saline solution to apply a pulsed

stream of pressurized solution to the wound for debridement and irrigation.

68. **(D)** Using metal rods or pins through the bone is skeletal traction.

69. **(B)** Power instruments generate heat due to friction of saw on bone. To prevent surrounding tissue injury, the STSR should irrigate the tip of the blade with an Asepto syringe and sterile saline (with surgeon's approval).

70. **(B)** Dupuytren's contracture is when fibrous bands cause contractions in the fingers, usually the ring finger and little finger. They are seldom painful; however, they cause restriction of extension but not flexion because they do not involve the flexor tendon.

71. **(D)** Ewing's sarcoma and osteogenic sarcoma are malignant bone tumors. A chondroma is a slow-growing benign tumor. A Wilms' tumor is also known as a nephroblastoma. This is a malignant tumor found in the kidney. It is commonly found in children.

72. **(D)** Tenorrhaphy is the surgical repair of a tendon.

73. **(A)** Achilles tendon rupture presents with the inability to plantar flex the foot.

74. **(A)** Supine position is used for a total hip replacement with an anterior approach because the hip is accessed from the front. The incision is made from the iliac crest to the top of the thigh on the affected side.

75. **(C)** The responsibility of the STSR is to keep the foot plantar flexed and keep stress off the new suture line.

76. **(A)** A stellate fracture is a bone that breaks in a central point and radiates outward like a shattered mirror. Fractures caused by a twisting motion are spiral fractures. A bone fracture where the bone remains attached by a ligament is an avulsion. A cranial fracture is when the bone is driven inward.

77. **(A)** Dorsal flexion is an upward motion of the foot, and plantar flexion is when the foot is turned downward.

78. **(B)** Joints that are freely movable, have one or more range of motion positions, and are lined with a synovial membrane are diarthroses. Amphiarthrosis is a slightly movable joint, and synarthrosis is an immovable joint.

79. **(A)** Compartment syndrome incisions are never closed. All others pertain to compartment syndrome.

80. **(C)** A triple arthrodesis is done when the calcaneocuboid, talonavicular, and talocalcaneal bones are fused together. McBride procedure relates to podiatry. Arthroscopy is a scoping of an area. Arthroplasty is a total joint repair. All others pertain to the shoulder.

81. **(B)** Subluxation is an incomplete dislocation.

82. **(B)** Acromioplasty is performed for a rotator cuff repair.

83. **(D)** The acetabular head does not pertain to the intertrochanteric fracture. This involves only the femur and lesser trochanter and can be repaired with a dynamic screw.

84. **(C)** The metacarpal bones form the palm of the hand. There are five on each side. The heads of the metacarpal are commonly called the knuckles.

85. **(A)** The gastrocnemius is the chief muscle of the calf of the leg. It is a large muscle on the posterior part of the leg. It extends the foot and helps to flex the knee upon the thigh.

86. **(A)** Bone marrow is found within all bones but is primarily found in the medullary cavity of flat bones.

87. **(A)** The forearm is the ulna. It is on the same side as the little finger. On the proximal end is the olecranon process, which forms the prominence of the elbow.

88. **(D)** The hyoid bone is located in the neck between the mandible and the larynx. It supports the tongue and provides an attachment for its muscles. It does not articulate with any other bone.

89. **(C)** In an infant, there are 33 separate bones in the vertebral column. Five of these bones eventually fuse to form the sacrum, and four others join to become the coccyx. As a result, an adult vertebral column has 26 parts.

90. **(A)** There are 7 cervical vertebrae in the neck, 12 thoracic vertebrae, and 5 lumbar vertebrae (lower back).

91. **(D)** The single hyoid bone does not articulate with any other bone. It supports the tongue, providing attachment sites for muscles of the tongue, neck, and pharynx.

92. **(C)** The clavicles are slender, rod-like bones with an elongated "S" shape. They are located at the base of the neck and run horizontally between the sternum and the shoulders. Another name is collarbone.

93. **(C)** The upper, flaring portion or prominence of the hipbone is the ilium. Its superior border is the iliac crest. The internal surface is the iliac fossa.

94. **(D)** The tibia is the larger medial bone of the lower leg. It bears the major portion of the weight on the leg. Another name is shinbone.

95. **(B)** The head of the femur fits into a lateral depression in the os coxae (the acetabulum), forming a joint. It is held in place by a ligament and by a tough fibrous capsule surrounding the joint.

96. **(A)** The infraspinatus, teres minor, subscapularis, and supraspinatus make up the rotator cuff.

97. **(A)** Long bones consist of a rod-like shaft with knob-like ends. The longest bone in the body is the femur. Another name is the thighbone.

98. **(D)** A condyle is a rounded protuberance found at the point of articulation with another bone. The distal end of the femur has large condyles. These condyles articulate with the tibia at the knee joint.

99. **(B)** A bucket handle tear is commonly found in the meniscus of the knee, and it actually looks like a bucket with a handle. It commonly occurs in the medial meniscus.

100. **(D)** Muscles are classified as smooth, cardiac, and skeletal.

101. **(D)** The most commonly used donor tendon for a free graft is the palmaris longus tendon of the wrist and forearm. The plantaris tendon in the leg is also frequently used.

102. **(D)** The hip is a ball-and-socket joint. The carpel bones of the wrist are gliding joints. Skull bones are considered synarthrotic joints because they have very little movement, and the elbow is a hinge joint.

103. **(C)** The thumb is a saddle joint. The elbow is a hinge joint, and the shoulder is a ball-and-socket joint. The radius is a pivot joint.

104. **(C)** A recording of the electrical activity of muscle tissue by using electrodes attached to the skin or inserted into muscle tissue is electromyography. An EKG/ECG is an electrocardiogram. It measures the electrical activity of the heart. PET scan is positron emission tomography. PET uses radioactive radiotracers to provide three-dimensional pictures of your body and is used to diagnose many conditions, including cancer, before they show up on another test. A CT scan is a computed tomography scan. It is used in orthopedics to detect bone and joint problems, specifically bone fractures and tumors.

105. **(D)** The fracture, Andrews, and Jackson tables are commonly used for orthopedic and spine surgical procedures.

CHAPTER 29

Pediatrics

- Pediatric patients are between the age of birth and 18 years old
- Neonate—the first 28 days outside the mother
- Infant—1–18 months
- Preschool—30 months–5 years
- School age—6–12 years
- Adolescent—13–18 years
- Fears of the pediatric patient include anesthesia and separation from their parents. In order to reduce their anxiety, we can:
  - Let them bring a toy or stuffed animal to the operating room with them
  - Introduce them to the surgical team
  - Let the parents accompany them to the operating room
  - Allow the parents to come into the postanesthesia care unit (PACU) at the appropriate time
- Radiation—transfer of heat between the body and objects that are not in direct contact with each other. Example: linens, walls of the room, and windows. If infants are placed too close to the cool object, they will loose heat
- Evaporation—when wet surfaces are exposed to air, heat loss occurs. When the solutions used on the infants begin to dry, heat loss also occurs. It is important to warm solutions and bath water and to dry the infant immediately.
- Conduction—when the infant's skin comes in contact with cold surfaces
- Convection—when the air surrounding the infant is cool, heat is lost. Examples include air conditioning as well as people simply walking around the infant
- Airway obstruction is a major complication of extubation
- Hypothermia—when the infant's body temperature drops below 36.5°C/97.7°F

- Infants lack the ability to shiver. To reduce the risk of hypothermia in infants, you can:
  - Increase the operating room temperature prior to the surgical procedure
  - Use heat lamps
  - Warm blankets
  - Wrap the infant's limbs
  - Warm solutions
- The umbilical artery is used for an intra-arterial monitor on a neonate during surgery
- Central venous catheters are placed in the external jugular vein
- Pyloromyotomy—performed for pyloric stenosis
- Laparoscopic Nissen fundoplication—performed on infants and children who experience severe gastroesophageal reflux
- Pectus excavatum—a genetic defect. Funnel chest is a defect of the sternum and the ribs
- Erythroblastosis fetalis—a fatal blood disorder in infants where the mother's blood is incompatible with the infant
- Esophageal atresia—a serious birth defect in which the esophagus is closed off at some point between the mouth and the stomach
- Tracheoesophageal fistula—a birth defect where the trachea is connected to the esophagus
- Intussusception—the intestines telescope into one another
- Volvulus—twisting of the intestines causing obstruction
- Hirschsprung's disease—a congenital defect caused by the absence of ganglion cells in the intestines. This affects the peristaltic contractions of the intestines
- Imperforate anus—a congenital defect where there is no anus but a fistula between the anus and vulva or bladder

- A common hernia in infants and children is an umbilical hernia
- Omphalocele—a congenital defect where the organs of the body are covered in an amniotic sac and protrude through a defect in the umbilical ring
- Spina bifida—congenital defect in the spine where part of the spinal cord and the meninges are exposed through an opening in the backbone
- Myelomeningocele—failure of the neural tube to close. Causes the meninges and spinal cord to protrude through the skin within a sac
- Bariatric surgery can be performed on children who are diagnosed as obese with a body mass index (BMI) of 40 combined with life-threating medical conditions
- The bariatric patient should be placed in reverse Trendelenburg position immediately following the surgical procedure
- A hernia is a complication of gastric bypass surgery
- Complications of bariatric surgery are diagnosed with a laparoscopy
- Cleft lip—the upper lip does not totally form properly and leaves an opening in the skin between the nose and lip
- The cleft lip repair is performed in stages, and a Z-plasty repair is performed
- Cleft palate—the roof of the mouth does not completely close. This deformity causes complications with eating and speech
- Wilms' tumor—also known as a nephroblastoma—intra-abdominal tumor
- Neuroblastoma—cancerous tumor commonly found in the retroperitoneum and adrenal medulla
- Sacrococcygeal teratoma—this tumor is located near the sacrum and coccyx. It is made up of different cells during early development. It can be solid or cystic
- Epispadias repair—the urethral meatus is on the dorsum of the penis
- Hypospadias repair—the urethral meatus is on the ventral surface of the penis
- Circumcision—procedure performed to remove the prepuce/foreskin from the glans penis
- Hydrocele—an abnormal accumulation of fluid in the scrotum. It can cause an infection. A scrotal incision is made and the fluid is suctioned out

- Orchiopexy—procedure performed to bring the testicle to its normal position in the scrotum after the testicle has traveled up into the inguinal canal
- Cryptorchidism—an undescended testicle
- Ventriculoatrial and ventriculoperitoneal shunts—procedures performed for hydrocephalus
  - Ventriculoatrial shunt—fluid is shunted from the lateral ventricle of the brain to the atrium
  - Ventriculoperitoneal shunt—fluid is shunted from the lateral ventricle to the peritoneal space
- Two types of shock common to children are:
  - Septic—commonly caused by a bacterial infection
  - Hypovolemic—dehydration is the cause of hypovolemic shock in children
- Gastrostomy feeding tubes are commonly used on the pediatric patient following gastrointestinal (GI) procedures
- Percutaneous endoscopic gastrostomy (PEG)—the PEG tube is the most common gastrostomy tube used. It is used for gastric decompression and external feedings
- Child abuse includes:
  - Shaken baby syndrome
  - Neglect
  - Sexual abuse
  - Unexplained falls and/or skin, facial, or thermal injuries and fractures
- Head trauma is the leading cause of injury of the pediatric patient. Causes include car accidents, falls, bicycle accidents, drowning, burns, and poisonings
- Atrial septal defect—a congenital defect where there is a hole in the atrial septum causing blood to flow from the left atrium to the right atrium
- Ventricular septal defect—incomplete closure of the septum between the right and left ventricle
- Tetralogy of Fallot—a combination of a few congenital defects. These babies are cyanotic—blue in skin color. The congenital defects include:
  - Pulmonary stenosis
  - Ventricular septal defect
  - Right ventricular hypertrophy
  - Dextroposition of the aorta
- Patent ductus arteriosus—a heart defect that happens when the ductus arteriosus does not close at birth. The ductus arteriosus is the

temporary fetal blood vessel that connects the aorta and the pulmonary artery

- Pediatric medications are prescribed according to the child's weight in kilograms
- Fetal surgery—surgical intervention to repair a birth defect while the fetus is still in the uterus. These surgical procedures can be repaired percutaneously with a fetoscope or as an open procedure
- Craniosynostosis—premature closure of the cranial suture lines. It can occur along one or more suture lines. The procedure performed is a craniectomy
- Crouzon's syndrome—includes premature closure of cranial suture lines causing skull and facial deformities
- Apert's syndrome—congenital disorder that causes craniofacial deformities and can also include syndactyly
- Club foot—congenital deformity of one or both feet. The affected foot rotates inward. Treatment varies from braces and tapes to surgical intervention

- Tendon lengthening—one type of surgical procedure performed for club foot. It is also used for patients with cerebral palsy. It helps to release contractures
- Otoplasty—performed to correct protruding ears from traumatic injury or a congenital deformity
- Microtia—small ears—congenital defect in which all or part of the external ears are missing. The rib is used as a graft for the patient's ear
- Passive immunity (natural)—can occur naturally such as when an infant receives a mother's antibodies through the placenta or breast milk.
- Passive immunity (artificial)—when antibodies are injected into the patient
- Active immunity (natural)—when a person acquires an infection and builds their own antibodies
- Artificial acquired active immunity—vaccines

Questions

1. The telescoping of the proximal intestine into the lumen of the distal intestine is called:

   (A) volvulus
   (B) intussusception
   (C) pyloric stenosis
   (D) ileal atresia

2. An imperforation or closure of a normal opening is called a/an:

   (A) hypertrophy
   (B) atresia
   (C) stenosis
   (D) atrophy

3. Failure of the intestines to encapsulate within the peritoneal cavity of a newborn is called:

   (A) umbilical hernia
   (B) omphalocele
   (C) hydrocele
   (D) intestinal exstrophy

4. A congenital malformation of the chest wall with a pronounced funnel-shaped depression is called:

   (A) truncus arteriosus
   (B) pectus excavatum
   (C) pectus carinatum
   (D) costochondral separation

5. Newborn vomiting, free of bile and projectile in nature, is indicative of:

   (A) atresia of the esophagus
   (B) pyloric stenosis
   (C) volvulus
   (D) intussusception

6. The surgical pediatric patient with an increased metabolic rate requires all of the following EXCEPT:

   (A) oxygen
   (B) caloric intake
   (C) blood transfusions
   (D) fluids

7. Hirschsprung's disease is synonymous with:

   (A) bowel obstruction
   (B) malrotation
   (C) ileal stenosis
   (D) Meckel's diverticulum

8. The condition evidenced by incomplete closure of the vertebral arches in newborns is:

   (A) hydrocephalus
   (B) encephalocele
   (C) spina bifida
   (D) myelomeningocele

9. The condition involving premature closure of infant cranial suture lines is referred to as:

   (A) cranioplasty
   (B) stereotactic surgery
   (C) craniosynostosis
   (D) transsphenoidal hypophysectomy

10. An imperforate anus means:

   (A) anal opening is absent
   (B) anus is closed
   (C) anal sphincter is too tight
   (D) anal sphincter is too loose

11. A Wilms' tumor, the most common intra-abdominal childhood tumor, is known as a/an:

   (A) nephroblastoma
   (B) neuroblastoma
   (C) aganglionic colon
   (D) intussusception

12. Nonclosure at birth of the duct that carries blood from the pulmonary artery directly to the aorta is termed:

   (A) tetralogy of Fallot
   (B) coarctation of the aorta
   (C) patent ductus arteriosus
   (D) anomalous venous return

13. The most common congenital cardiac anomaly in the cyanotic group is:

   (A) tricuspid atresia
   (B) tetralogy of Fallot
   (C) patent ductus arteriosus
   (D) truncus arteriosus

14. The mechanical strength of a weak eye muscle due to strabismus in a pediatric patient can be corrected by all of the following EXCEPT:

   (A) tucking
   (B) advancement
   (C) recession
   (D) resection

15. What surgery is performed to treat otitis media?

   (A) Myringotomy
   (B) Adenoidectomy
   (C) Tympanoplasty
   (D) Tonsillectomy

16. What problem is most commonly seen in the pediatric postoperative patient?

   (A) Hypotension
   (B) Airway impairment
   (C) Hypothermia
   (D) Metabolic depression

17. During surgery on the pediatric patient, which intervention(s) is/are performed to maintain the patient's temperature?

   (A) The OR is prewarmed prior to the patient arriving.
   (B) A warm air blanket is used during the procedure.
   (C) Heating lamps are used preoperatively or at any time they are needed.
   (D) All of the above

18. Pediatric medications are prescribed according to the patient's weight in:

   (A) kilograms
   (B) pounds
   (C) grams
   (D) neograms

19. What procedure is performed to reconstruct the external ear?

   (A) Rotation flap
   (B) Lobuloplasty
   (C) External auditory fixation
   (D) Otoplasty

20. The procedure performed to open a stricture at the gastric outlet on an infant is:

   (A) gastrectomy
   (B) pyloromyotomy
   (C) pyloric stenting
   (D) Ramstedt

21. Intestinal obstruction by twisting of the intestines is:

   (A) pyloric stenosis
   (B) volvulus
   (C) neuroblastoma
   (D) encephalocele

22. Orchiopexy is performed to treat:

   (A) testicular cancer
   (B) torsion of the testicle
   (C) congenital undescended testicle
   (D) both B and C

23. The most common defects that occur when the embryonic development of the central nervous system (spinal cord and brain) is incomplete are spina bifida, anencephaly, and encephalocele. This condition is called:

    (A) tetralogy of Fallot
    (B) ventricular septal defect
    (C) vertebral recession
    (D) neural defect

24. A medical term used for the condition characterized by fusion of the fingers and toes is:

    (A) club hand and foot
    (B) syndactyly
    (C) mermaid syndrome
    (D) trigger finger

25. An untreated condition in infants that causes the skull to enlarge is called:

    (A) hydrocephalus
    (B) cerebral defect
    (C) cerebral aneurysm
    (D) meningioma

26. A ventriculoatrial shunt, a ventriculoperitoneal shunt, and an in vitro shunt are performed for the condition called:

    (A) decompression of the cranial nerves
    (B) hydrocephalus
    (C) cranial neuroma
    (D) intracranial aneurysm

27. The transfer of heat between the body and objects when they are not in direct contact with each other is:

    (A) evaporation
    (B) conduction
    (C) radiation
    (D) convection

28. A major complication in the pediatric patient upon extubation is:

    (A) hyperthermia
    (B) airway obstruction
    (C) hypothermia
    (D) aspiration

29. The artery used for intra-arterial monitoring on a neonate during surgery is the:

    (A) carotid artery
    (B) brachial artery
    (C) umbilical artery
    (D) femoral artery

30. The central venous pressure (CVP) catheter is placed in which vein in the neonate?

    (A) External jugular
    (B) Internal jugular
    (C) Subclavian
    (D) Brachiocephalic

31. Which procedure is performed on infants and children for severe gastroesophageal reflux?

    (A) Pyloromyotomy
    (B) Billroth I
    (C) Gastrojejunostomy
    (D) Nissen fundoplication

32. Erythroblastosis fetalis is a disorder:

    (A) where the mother's blood is incompatible with the infant
    (B) of too many red blood cells
    (C) of too few red blood cells
    (D) of too few platelets

33. The most common hernia in a child is:

    (A) umbilical
    (B) inguinal
    (C) femoral
    (D) hiatal

34. Failure of the neural tube to close, causing the meninges and spinal cord to protrude through the skin in a sac, is called:

    (A) omphalocele
    (B) spina bifida
    (C) imperforate anus
    (D) myelomeningocele

35. Bariatric surgery can be performed on children who are so obese that their BMI is greater than:

    (A) 60
    (B) 40
    (C) 20
    (D) 10

36. What position should the postoperative pediatric/bariatric patient be placed in?

    (A) Trendelenburg
    (B) Dorsal recumbent
    (C) Reverse Trendelenburg
    (D) Left lateral

37. The Z-plasty procedure is used to correct:

    (A) cleft palate
    (B) protruding ears
    (C) cleft lip
    (D) microtia

38. What is the cancerous tumor commonly found in the retroperitoneal adrenal medulla?

    (A) Neuroblastoma
    (B) Nephroblastoma
    (C) Glioma
    (D) Astrocytoma

39. The tumor located near the sacrum and made up of different cells during early development is a:

    (A) leiomyoma
    (B) sacrococcygeal teratoma
    (C) nephroblastoma
    (D) none of the above

40. The condition where the urethral meatus is on the ventral side of the penis is called:

    (A) epispadias
    (B) cryptorchidism
    (C) phimosis
    (D) hypospadias

41. A patient is considered a pediatric patient until what age?

    (A) Birth to 12 years
    (B) Birth to 18 years
    (C) 6 years to 12 years
    (D) 30 months to 5 years

42. Septic shock in children is caused by:

    (A) viral infection
    (B) bacterial infection
    (C) dehydration
    (D) both A and B

43. A PEG tube is used for:

    (A) gastric decompression
    (B) external feeding
    (C) internal feeding
    (D) both A and B

44. Child abuse injuries include:

    (A) shaken baby syndrome
    (B) malnutrition
    (C) thermal injuries
    (D) all of the above

45. When a fetus is born with their blood flowing from the left atrium to the right atrium, this is called:

    (A) atrial septal defect
    (B) ventricular septal defect
    (C) coarctation of the aorta
    (D) patent ductus arteriosus

46. Which disease involves premature closure of the cranial suture lines with skull and facial deformities?

    (A) Craniosynostosis
    (B) Crouzon's syndrome
    (C) Apert's syndrome
    (D) Microcephaly

47. The congenital deformity that causes the affected foot or feet to rotate inward is called:

    (A) ruptured Achilles
    (B) hallux valgus
    (C) drop foot
    (D) club foot

48. The procedure to correct protruding ears is a/an:

    (A) Z-plasty
    (B) cheiloplasty
    (C) mentoplasty
    (D) otoplasty

49. The position of the pediatric patient following a tonsillectomy and adenoidectomy is:

    (A) dorsal recumbent
    (B) lateral
    (C) lateral with head slightly elevated
    (D) Sims

50. A congenital defect where the abdominal contents are outside the body at birth is:

    (A) hiatal hernia
    (B) diverticular disease
    (C) Crohn's disease
    (D) omphalocele

51. If a pregnant woman requires surgery, in which trimester is it best to perform the surgery?

    (A) First trimester
    (B) Second trimester
    (C) Third trimester
    (D) All trimesters are equal

52. The childhood virus that affects the salivary glands/parotid glands is:

    (A) chickenpox
    (B) mumps
    (C) hydrocephalus
    (D) smallpox

53. What type of immunity does a vaccination provide?

    (A) Artificial acquired passive immunity
    (B) Artificial acquired active immunity
    (C) Natural acquired passive immunity
    (D) Natural acquired active immunity

54. What type of instrument is commonly used to retrieve an aspirated foreign object that a child has swallowed?

    (A) Flexible bronchoscope
    (B) Endotracheal tube
    (C) Rigid bronchoscope
    (D) Laryngoscope

55. What fetal disease occurs when the mother's blood type is incompatible with the fetus and causes the mother's immune system to produce antibodies that work against the fetus?

    (A) Erythroblastosis
    (B) Bacterial infection
    (C) Dehydration
    (D) Shaken baby syndrome

56. The most common type of shock found in children is hypovolemic shock. This is caused by:

    (A) viral infection
    (B) bacterial infection
    (C) dehydration
    (D) shaken baby syndrome

57. The roof of the mouth consists of the:

    (A) hard palate
    (B) soft palate
    (C) hyoid
    (D) both A and B

58. Craniofacial deformities that include early fusion of the skull bones, facial deformity, syndactyl, and mental disabilities are seen in:

    (A) Craniosynostosis
    (B) Crouzon's syndrome
    (C) Apert's syndrome
    (D) Hirschsprung's disease

59. Infants lose heat quickly because:

    (A) they lack the ability to shiver
    (B) they have little subcutaneous fat
    (C) they have little body mass
    (D) all of the above

60. If a pregnant woman requires surgery, it is best performed in the second trimester because:

    (A) the uterus is not too large at this time and will not get in the way
    (B) there is less chance of miscarriage after the first trimester
    (C) there is less risk of premature delivery
    (D) all of the above

Answers and Explanations

1. **(B)** Intussusception is the telescopic invagination of a portion of intestine into an adjacent part with mechanical and vascular impairment frequently at the ileocecal junction.

2. **(B)** Atresia is an imperforation or closure of an opening. Atresia and stenosis (a narrowing of an opening) are the most common causes of obstruction in a newborn.

3. **(B)** Failure of the intestines to become encapsulated within the peritoneal cavity during fetal development results in herniation through a midline defect in the abdominal wall at the umbilicus. This is termed omphalocele.

4. **(B)** A congenital malformation of the chest wall, pectus excavatum, is characterized by a pronounced funnel-shaped depression over the lower end of the sternum.

5. **(B)** The first sign of pyloric stenosis is projectile vomiting free of bile. The surgical procedure for repair is a pyloromyotomy. The muscles of the pylorus are incised to relieve the stenosis.

6. **(C)** Oxygen, calories, and fluids must be increased because of the increased demands of surgical stress. Blood is not given unless there is a need.

7. **(A)** The goal for Hirschsprung's is resection and reconstruction of the distal colon to restore functional peristalsis and to prevent a further bowel obstruction. The diagnosis is confirmed with a rectal biopsy.

8. **(C)** A newborn anomaly that is evidenced by incomplete closure of the vertebral arches, with or without herniation of the meninges, is called spina bifida.

9. **(C)** In craniosynostosis, the suture line of an infant has closed prematurely. A synthetic material (such as silicone) is used to keep the edges of the cranial sutures from reuniting and preventing brain growth.

10. **(B)** In imperforate anus, the anus remains closed during fetal development and must be opened soon after birth.

11. **(A)** A Wilms' tumor, also known as nephroblastoma, is the most common intra-abdominal childhood tumor. It presents as a painless mass whose enlargement may laterally distend the abdomen.

12. **(C)** During fetal life, the ductus arteriosus carries blood from the pulmonary artery to the aorta, bypassing the lungs. After birth, this duct closes in the first hours. Nonclosure is termed patent ductus arteriosus and requires surgical closure.

13. **(B)** Tetralogy of Fallot is the most common congenital cardiac anomaly in the cyanotic group. It is the result of shunting unoxygenated blood into the systemic circulation.

14. **(C)** Recession is a procedure done for strabismus where the muscle is overactive. All other procedures listed deal with the underactive (weak) eye muscle.

15. **(A)** Secretory otitis media is the most common chronic condition of childhood. Fluid accumulates in the middle ear from Eustachian tube obstruction. This condition is

corrected by myringotomy, an incision in the tympanic membrane.

16. **(B)** Airway problems are the most common concern on emergence from surgery and immediately postoperative. At the conclusion of the operation, the oropharynx and stomach are suctioned. All monitors are left in place until the patient is fully awake and extubated.

17. **(D)** The methods used to maintain a pediatric temperature include prewarming the operating room and using a warm water-filled blanket, heat lamps, a solution warmer, warm IV solution, and prewarmed surgical sponges.

18. **(A)** The patient's weight is measured in kilograms.

19. **(D)** Otoplasty is performed to reconstruct the external ear after trauma or to correct protruding ears.

20. **(B)** Pyloromyotomy is surgery to correct an infantile hypertrophic pyloric stenosis.

21. **(B)** A volvulus is a rotation of the intestine around itself or the attached mesentery.

22. **(C)** The goal of surgery for the undescended testicle is to restore the testicle to its normal position in the scrotum.

23. **(D)** The neural tube is an embryonic structure that gives rise to the nervous system. Defects in this neural tube occur when this tube fails to close completely.

24. **(B)** Syndactyly is a congenital condition in which the digits of the hand and/or feet are joined from birth.

25. **(A)** Hydrocephalus occurs when the flow of cerebrospinal fluid (CSF) is blocked or obstructed. This results in an increased amount of fluid in the ventricles of the brain.

26. **(B)** All three shunts are performed for hydrocephalus. A ventriculoatrial shunt is from the ventricle to the atrium, a ventriculoperitoneal shunt is from ventricle to the peritoneal cavity, and an in vitro shunt is done while the fetus is in vitro.

27. **(C)** The transfer of heat between the body and objects, which are not in direct contact with each other, is radiation. An example is linens. Evaporation occurs when wet surfaces are exposed to air. Heat loss occurs. Conduction is when the infant's skin comes in direct contact with cold surfaces. Convection is when the air surrounding the infant is cool and heat is lost. An example is air conditioning.

28. **(B)** Airway obstruction is a major complication during extubation of pediatric patients. Hyperthermia is an increase in body temperature. Hypothermia is a decrease in body temperature below 36.5°C/97.7°F, and aspiration is when the infant swallows fluid directly into the trachea.

29. **(C)** The umbilical artery is used for intra-arterial monitoring on a neonate during surgery.

30. **(A)** A CVP is placed in the external jugular vein.

31. **(D)** A laparoscopic Nissen fundoplication is performed on infants and children who have severe gastroesophageal reflux.

32. **(A)** Erythroblastosis fetalis is when the mother's blood is incompatible with the blood of the fetus.

33. **(A)** Umbilical hernias are common hernias in infants and children.

34. **(D)** Myelomeningocele is failure of the neural tube to close, which causes the meninges and spinal cord to protrude through the skin in a sac. An omphalocele is a congenital defect where the organs of the body are covered in an amniotic sac and exposed through a defect in the umbilical ring. Spina bifida is a congenital defect of the spine where part of the spinal cord and the meninges are exposed through an opening in the backbone.

Imperforate anus is the absence of an opening into the anus.

35. **(B)** BMI >40 is an indication for bariatric surgery.

36. **(C)** The pediatric/bariatric patient should be placed in reverse Trendelenburg position immediately following surgery.

37. **(C)** A cleft lip is a condition where the upper lip does not totally form, leaving an opening in the skin between the nose and the lip. Protruding ears are large ears. A cleft palate is when the roof of the mouth does not completely close, and microtia is the term for small ears.

38. **(A)** Neuroblastoma is a cancerous tumor commonly found in the retroperitoneal space in the adrenal medulla. The nephroblastoma, also called a Wilms' tumor, is a kidney tumor. Glioma and astrocytoma are both cancerous brain tumors.

39. **(B)** Sacrococcygeal teratoma is a tumor located near the sacrum and coccyx. It is made up of different cells during early development.

40. **(D)** Hypospadias is when the urethral meatus is on the ventral side of the penis. Epispadias is when the urethral meatus is on the dorsal side of the penis. Phimosis is a congenital narrowing of the opening of the foreskin. Cryptorchidism is a condition when one or both testes fail to descend from the abdomen to the scrotum.

41. **(B)** A patient is considered a pediatric patient from birth to age 18 years.

42. **(D)** Septic shock is commonly caused by a viral or bacterial infection. Dehydration is a common cause of hypovolemic shock in children.

43. **(D)** PEG tubes are used for gastric decompression and external feedings.

44. **(D)** Shaken baby syndrome, malnutrition, and thermal injuries are all examples of child abuse and neglect.

45. **(A)** Atrial septal defect is a congenital disorder where there is a hole in the atrial septum causing the blood to flow from the left atrium to the right atrium. Normal blood flows from the left atrium to the left ventricle. Ventricular septal defect is an incomplete closure of the septum between the right and left ventricle. Coarctation of the aorta is a congenital condition where the aorta is narrow. Patent ductus arteriosus is a heart defect that occurs when the ductus arteriosus does not close at birth.

46. **(B)** Crouzon's syndrome is a premature closure of cranial sutures with skull and facial deformities. Craniosynostosis is premature closing of cranial sutures. Apert's syndrome is a congenital disorder that causes cranial and facial deformities and also includes syndactyly. Microcephaly is an abnormally small head and incomplete brain formation.

47. **(D)** A club foot is a congenital deformity of one or both feet causing the foot to rotate inward.

48. **(D)** Otoplasty is a surgical correction of protruding ears. A Z-plasty is a type of plastic surgery closure. Cheiloplasty is surgery of the lip, and mentoplasty is plastic surgery on the chin.

49. **(C)** The position for the postoperative tonsillectomy patient is lateral with the head of the bed slightly elevated.

50. **(D)** Omphalocele is a congenital defect where the abdominal contents are outside of the body at birth.

51. **(B)** Surgery for a pregnant woman should always be avoided if possible, but when it is required, it is safest to perform in the second trimester. In the second trimester, there is less risk of miscarriage and preterm delivery. In addition, the uterus is not too large in the second trimester, and this is the best time to receive general anesthesia.

52. **(B)** Mumps is a viral infection that causes swelling of the parotid glands. It is spread

through saliva. Chickenpox is a virus caused by the varicella-zoster virus, which causes an itchy, blistery rash on the body. Hydrocephalus is a buildup of cerebrospinal fluid in the brain characterized by an enlarged head. The excess fluid causes pressure on the brain tissue. Smallpox was a severe viral infection characterized by flulike symptoms that was eradicated worldwide in the early 1980s.

53. **(B)** A vaccine provides artificially acquired active immunity. Artificial acquired passive immunity is when antibodies are injected. Natural acquired passive immunity occurs naturally, such as when an infant receives a mother's antibodies through placenta or breast milk. Natural acquired active immunity is when you get the disease and build up antibodies by fighting the infection.

54. **(C)** A foreign body obstruction is more common in the right bronchus than the left because it is shorter and wider. The rigid bronchoscope is commonly used to retrieve the object. A flexible bronchoscope is commonly used for patients who have a short neck or difficulty hyperextending the neck or jaw. The laryngoscope is used to facilitate intubation, and an endotracheal tube is used to maintain a patient's airway.

55. **(A)** Erythroblastosis is a condition that occurs when the mother and fetus have different blood types and the mother's antibodies work against the fetus. Hirschsprung's disease affects the large intestine and is caused by problems with the peristaltic contractions. Sickle cell disease is caused by abnormally shaped red blood cells (RBCs) that break down. Anemia is a lack of RBCs that carry oxygen to the body tissue.

56. **(C)** The most common type of shock found in children is hypovolemic shock. This is caused by dehydration. Septic shock is caused by a bacterial or viral infection. Shaken baby syndrome is a type of child abuse where the infant is shaken and the brain bounces around in the skull, causing brain damage and death.

57. **(D)** The roof of the mouth is made up of the hard palate, which includes the palatine process of the maxilla and the horizontal plate and paired palatine bones, and soft palate. The hyoid bone supports the tongue and larynx.

58. **(C)** Apert's syndrome is characterized by fused skull bones (craniosynostosis), syndactyl (fused fingers), and facial deformities with mental disabilities. Crouzon's syndrome is also characterized by craniosynostosis. This premature closure of the skull bones affects the shape of the face and causes facial deformities. Hirschsprung's is a disease that affects the intestines.

59. **(D)** Infants lack the ability to shiver until about 6 months. They also have little subcutaneous fat, which results in poor thermal insulation, and less body mass. This makes it difficult for infants to retain and generate heat.

60. **(D)** Surgery on a pregnant woman should always be avoided if possible. When it is required, it is safest to perform surgery in the second trimester when there is less risk of miscarriage and preterm delivery. The uterus is not very large during this trimester, and it is the safest time to administer anesthesia.

CHAPTER 30

Biomedical Science (Electricity, Hemostasis, Lasers, and Computers)

- ELECTRONS—negatively charged particles
- NEUTRONS—neutral particles
- PROTONS—positively charged particles
- NUCLEUS—center of an atom. Protons and neutrons are found in the nucleus of an atom, and electrons travel in an orbit around the nucleus
- FREE ELECTRON—an electron that is not attached to an atom and is free to move to another atom
- MASS—any matter that occupies space
- POWER—rate at which work is done (energy is used). Power is measured in watts
- SPEED—how fast an object moves
- VELOCITY—how fast something is moving without concentration or direction
- FREQUENCY—the rate at which something occurs or is repeated over a particular period of time. The number of cycles or completed alternations per unit time of a wave. Frequency is measured in Hertz
- CURRENT—the movement/flow of electricity. Current is measured in amps
- ACCELERATION—change in velocity over a period of time
- WORK—the force that causes an object to change direction
- VOLTAGE—the pressure that pushes electricity. Voltage is controlled by a power source
- MATTER—anything that has mass and occupies space
- CONDUCTORS—allow electrical current to flow freely; examples include metals such as copper and aluminum
- NONCONDUCTIVE—means that it will not accept electrical current
- INSULATORS—materials that do not conduct electricity. An example of this is the covering on some laparoscopic instruments. When the current reaches the insulator, it does not completely stop but finds an alternative route to take; when there is no alternative route, the current will stop and cause heat
- NEWTON'S LAWS OF MOTION
  - Newton's first law states that a body at rest will remain at rest, and a body in motion will remain in motion with a constant velocity, unless acted upon by a force. This law is also called the law of inertia
  - Newton's second law—acceleration is produced when a force acts on a mass. The greater the mass (of the object being accelerated), the greater the amount of force needed to accelerate the object
  - Newton's third law states that for every action, there is an equal and opposite reaction. Thus, if one body exerts a force on a second body, the first body also undergoes a force of the same strength but in the opposite direction
- There are two types of electrical currents, direct current and alternating current
  - DIRECT CURRENT—the current flows in one direction. An example is a battery
  - ALTERNATING CURRENT—the current moves in one direction and can reverse its direction
  - The voltage used in hospitals is 110 or 120 V

METHODS OF HEMOSTASIS

- BIPOLAR ELECTROCAUTERY/BIPOLAR CAUTERY—the current is delivered to the surgical site and returned to the generator by forceps. The current passes between the tips of the forceps. One tip is active, and the other is inactive
- MONOPOLAR ELECTROSURGERY—current flows from the generator to the active electrode (Bovie handpiece) to the patient to the inactive dispersive electrode and back to the generator
- COAGULATING CURRENT—a current that passes through the active electrode (Bovie handpiece) with intense heat to burn and control bleeding vessels
- CUTTING CURRENT—the current used to cut tissue
- BLENDED CURRENT—a current that can be used to provide hemostasis to tissue and cut tissue
- GENERATOR—the power source; the machine that produces the current by using high-frequency radio waves
- INACTIVE DISPERSIVE ELECTRODE—the pad used to return the current back to the generator. Also referred to as the grounding pad, inactive electrode, or return electrode
- ACTIVE ELECTRODE—the handpiece or active electrode directs the current to the target tissue
- CRYOSURGERY—liquid nitrogen and CO_2 are used to provide extreme cold/freezing to remove tissue and control bleeding
- ULTRASONIC SCALPEL—the scalpel blade uses ultrasonic motion to cut and coagulate diseased or abnormal tissue without damage to other tissue
- LIGASURE—bipolar device that seals vessels and tissue
- HARMONIC SCALPEL—uses ultrasonic wave energy to seal and cut tissues and vessels
- MORCELLATOR—a device that cuts and fragments tissue into strips, which are then suctioned through the instrument. This instrument is contraindicated in the presence of cancer

LASERS

- LASER—LIGHT AMPLIFICATION BY STIMULATED EMISSION OF RADIATION
- The laser light beam is monochromatic (one color or one wave length)
- All the wavelengths are coherent (they wave together and are lined up)
- Laser light waves travel in the same direction and are parallel to each other
- Lasers can emit their light beam in brief spurts (pulsate), or they can produce continuous light beams
- An active medium is needed to produce a laser beam; they can be gases, solids, crystals, liquid, dyes, and free electrons
- You need an energy source; it may be electrical or radiofrequency
- It contains an amplification system so the beam can change direction
- It contains a wave guide to aim and control the beam (pulsing or continuous)
  - It has backstops to prevent the beam from going beyond its target. They include wet towels, sponges, titanium, or quartz rods
  - It emits a beam from invisible to infrared

TYPES OF LASERS

- ARGON LASER
  - The medium used is argon gas
  - Blue-green beam
  - Argon lasers are used to treat retinal tears and also in urology for bladder tumors
- CO_2 LASER
  - The medium used is carbon dioxide gas
  - The laser beam is invisible, so a helium–neon laser beam is lined up with the CO_2 beam so the surgeon can aim the beam
  - The beam is delivered through an articulated arm whereby a handpiece can be attached
  - The CO_2 laser cannot be used on tissue with high water content because it absorbs the beam
  - It can be used like a scalpel, or the beam can be defocused to ablate soft tissue
  - It is commonly used in plastic, gynecological, neurological, orthopedic, cardiovascular, and general surgery
- EXCIMER LASER
  - The laser beam is an ultraviolet color
  - The medium used is a mixture of gases
  - This beam ablates or disintegrates tissue instead of cutting or burning
  - Used for LASIK surgery to reshape the cornea; also used for angioplasty

- YAG—HOLMIUM:YTTRIUM–ALUMINUM–GARNET LASER
  - Uses water as the medium and is commonly used in orthopedics for arthroscopic surgery except for the spine
  - This laser uses a pulse type of a beam
- KRYPTON LASER
  - Uses electrical current as the medium
  - Emits a red-yellow beam
  - Works from electrical power
  - Commonly used in eyes
- KTP/GREENLIGHT LASER
  - Commonly used for benign prostatic hyperplasia (BPH)
- ND:YAG LASER—(YAG—YTTRIUM–ALUMINUM–GARNET)
  - Used in an iridectomy for patients with glaucoma and for liver tumors, skin cancers, and thyroid nodules

LASER SAFETY

- The patient's eyes should be covered and protected from the laser beam
- The skin prep used must be a nonflammable solution
- The immediate area around the target area should be covered with moistened cloth towels (water not saline)
- All sponges and laps should be moistened with water when used around the laser
- Drapes should be nonflammable
- Endotracheal tubes should be insulated (wrapped with a special metallic foil) when the target tissue is on the face and neck
- Eye protection laser glasses must be worn
- Fire-resistant gowns should be worn
- Do not wear metal jewelry—it could absorb heat from the laser and cause a burn

COMPUTERS

- All the components of the computer are termed HARDWARE
- BOOTING—the term used for turning on a computer
- Your name and password are required to log onto the computer for security purposes
- MODEM—part of the computer that helps to send e-mails and access the internet and other programs
- BYTE—this is equal to a letter, a number, or a sign that computers use
- MOUSE—allows you to scroll across the computer; it moves the cursor on the computer screen
- COMPUTER SOFTWARE—the term used for computer programs
- HARD DRIVE—used to store files and computer programs
- 1,000 bytes = 1 kilobyte
- MONITOR—screen of the computer
- KEYBOARD—a separate part of the computer where you type to enter characters and commands into the computer
- SCROLLING—the term used to move up and down on the computer screen using the mouse
- RAM—an acronym for random access memory
- ROM—an acronym for read-only memory
- MEMORY—the location in a computer that can store information
- BULLETS—symbols that help define a list

Questions

1. Anything that has mass and occupies space is termed:

   (A) element
   (B) matter
   (C) conductor
   (D) insulator

2. The center of an atom is called the:

   (A) matter
   (B) mass
   (C) nucleus
   (D) charge

3. The movement of electrical charge through a conductor is called:

   (A) migration
   (B) electrical current
   (C) conduct
   (D) insulation

4. The sterile component of the electrosurgical unit (ESU) is:

   (A) inactive
   (B) active
   (C) ground
   (D) the patient plate

5. Current is measured in:

   (A) volts
   (B) amps
   (C) circuits
   (D) loads

6. The path that electricity travels from its energy source and back again is called:

   (A) resistor
   (B) circuit
   (C) conductor
   (D) ampere

7. Restriction of the flow of current to a source is called:

   (A) magnetism
   (B) resistance
   (C) force field
   (D) power

8. In a simple electrical circuit, the wire that connects to the switch is:

   (A) neutral
   (B) ground
   (C) hot
   (D) none of the above

9. A separate wire that is an essential protection against an electric shock is:

   (A) hot
   (B) neutral
   (C) ground
   (D) active

10. Most outlets in the operating room run on:

    (A) 220 V
    (B) 110 V
    (C) 120 V
    (D) 60 V

11. When current moves in one direction and then reverses to return to the source, it is known as:

    (A) alternating current
    (B) electrical current
    (C) direct current
    (D) optional current

12. One example of a direct current (DC) is:

    (A) an ESU
    (B) a flashlight
    (C) a surgical room light
    (D) an x-ray machine

13. Alternating current has the ability to:

    (A) step down voltage
    (B) step up voltage
    (C) alternate voltage
    (D) all of the above

14. A device that transmits an impulse to a wave-transmitting system is:

    (A) an optical fiber
    (B) a radio transmitter
    (C) an isolated circuit
    (D) a resistor

15. An ESU used for delicate surgery is a:

    (A) monopolar unit
    (B) disposable unit
    (C) bipolar unit
    (D) dispersive electrode unit

16. A plume of vaporized tissue may contain residual ____, and therefore, it is important to protect the staff.

    (A) carcinogens
    (B) blood-borne pathogens
    (C) mutagens
    (D) All of the above

17. An alternating current (AC) cycle is termed a/an:

    (A) wave
    (B) volt
    (C) amp
    (D) hertz

18. Radio waves are considered ____ waves.

    (A) isolated
    (B) direct
    (C) simple
    (D) magnetic

19. When the electrical current passes from the ESU generator through the active electrode, the energy is converted from electrical to:

    (A) mechanical
    (B) chemical
    (C) thermal
    (D) magnetic

20. What material is the best conductor of electricity?

    (A) Rubber
    (B) Salt water
    (C) Copper
    (D) Lead

21. What device is used to control the flow of electricity at the will of the operator?

    (A) Load
    (B) Resistor
    (C) Switch
    (D) Conductor

22. When operating a piece of electrical operating room (OR) equipment, the most vital prong for safety purposes is the:

    (A) ground
    (B) negative
    (C) positive
    (D) safety

23. Which theory explains the flow of electricity?

    (A) Ohm's
    (B) Electron
    (C) Kirchhoff's
    (D) Atomic

24. The standard metric unit of power is:

    (A) amp
    (B) volt
    (C) watt
    (D) hertz

25. A medical imaging technique that reveals the body's dynamic activities is:

    (A) computed tomography (CT)
    (B) positron emission tomography (PET)
    (C) tomogram
    (D) ultrasound

26. Electrosurgery can be used to:

    (A) incise tissue
    (B) coagulate blood vessels
    (C) destroy or remove diseased tissue
    (D) all of the above

27. The proper placement of the patient return electrode or grounding pad should be:

    (A) on the surgical side
    (B) farthest from the surgical site
    (C) near a bony surface
    (D) always on the opposite side

28. Forceps or an instrument that contains two contact points that are used to coagulate tissue is called:

    (A) monopolar
    (B) Ferris–Smith
    (C) bipolar
    (D) Potts forceps

29. Which of the following can be used as a cutting electrode?

    (A) Needle tip
    (B) Spatula
    (C) Wire loop
    (D) All of the above

30. When using the ESU for coagulation, the energy delivered is:

    (A) intermittent waves at a low frequency and high voltage
    (B) intermittent waves at a low frequency and low voltage
    (C) intermediate frequency and intermediate high voltage
    (D) intermediate waves and low voltage

31. Who is ultimately responsible for abiding by all safety protocols during the use of electrosurgery?

    (A) Surgeon
    (B) Circulator
    (C) STSR
    (D) All perioperative personnel

32. All are safety measures when using the grounding pad (also known as the dispersive electrode, return electrode, inactive electrode, or neutral electrode) EXCEPT:

    (A) must always be used for monopolar surgery to prevent patient burns
    (B) apply the pad prior to final positioning
    (C) gel on pad must always be checked to make sure the moisture content and quality are good
    (D) always check the integrity of the patient's skin before applying the pad

33. The tips of the active electrodes used in minimally invasive surgery (MIS) are coated with insulation to:

    (A) prevent glare from coming off the metal instrument
    (B) keep the metal portion of the instrument clean
    (C) prevent the patient from being burned
    (D) none of the above

34. Sealing vessels with electrosurgery requires:

    (A) high frequency
    (B) a bipolar ESU instrument
    (C) physical pressure to create a weld in tissue
    (D) all of the above

35. What type of energy is used with the harmonic system (harmonic scalpel, forceps, scissors)?

    (A) Ultrasonic
    (B) Radiofrequency
    (C) Fulguration
    (D) Monopolar

36. Motion is known as ___ energy.

    (A) mechanical
    (B) total
    (C) potential
    (D) kinetic

37. The rate at which work is done is known as:

    (A) velocity
    (B) energy
    (C) power
    (D) watt

38. ___ border the outer perimeter of an atom and are ___ charged.

    (A) Neutrons, positively
    (B) Electrons, negatively
    (C) Electrons, positively
    (D) Protons, negatively

39. The gain or loss of electrons in an atom is termed:

    (A) hydraulic pressure
    (B) Boyle's law
    (C) ionization
    (D) consolidation

40. The transfer of thermal energy by contact is called:

    (A) greenhouse effect
    (B) radiation
    (C) convention
    (D) conduction

41. A repeated periodic disturbance or variation of energy carried through a medium from point to point is called:

    (A) transfer energy
    (B) wave
    (C) oscillations
    (D) molecular change

42. The frequency of sound is stated in a measurement of:

    (A) amps
    (B) hertz
    (C) waves
    (D) compressions

43. The study of objects in motion is:

    (A) mechanics
    (B) velocity
    (C) speed
    (D) acceleration

44. The three laws of motion that are the basics of classical mechanics are the work of:

    (A) Hooke
    (B) Newton
    (C) Bohr
    (D) Ohm

45. Any time that an object's velocity is changing, we say it is:

(A) accelerating
(B) projecting
(C) orbiting
(D) static

46. The property of matter that causes matter to resist change in motion is called:

(A) speed
(B) inertia
(C) momentum
(D) range

47. Which law states that for every action, there is an equal and opposite reaction?

(A) Newton's first law
(B) Newton's second law
(C) Newton's third law
(D) Hooke's law

48. If an object returns to its original position after force has been applied and then removed, it is said to be:

(A) dynamic
(B) static
(C) elastic
(D) periodic

49. The maximum distance that an object moves from its central position (equilibrium) is called:

(A) frequency
(B) amplitude
(C) cycle
(D) momentum

50. The bending of a light ray as it passes from one substance to another is called:

(A) reflection
(B) refraction
(C) vibration
(D) incidence

51. What scientist, expanding Hooke's wave theory, theorized that light can bend because it is a wave?

(A) Ohm
(B) Einstein
(C) Newton
(D) Young

52. The longer wavelengths of the color spectrum are seen in what color?

(A) Violet
(B) Green
(C) Blue
(D) Red

53. Who first identified a collection of particles of light as "photons"?

(A) Einstein
(B) Newton
(C) Bohr
(D) Young

54. On the surface of the Earth, what causes objects to accelerate downward?

(A) Energy
(B) Excitation
(C) Gravity
(D) Electrical charges

55. What laser has the most power output?

(A) Liquid
(B) Semiconductor
(C) Gas
(D) Solid state

56. The fourth force found only in nature, and not in the nucleus, is known as:

(A) electromagnetic force
(B) gravitational force
(C) binding energy
(D) kinetic energy

57. Nucleons are composed of subatomic particles known as:

    (A) isotopes
    (B) quarks
    (C) protons
    (D) neutrons

58. All of the following are true of lasers EXCEPT:

    (A) LASER is an acronym for light amplification by stimulated emission of radiation
    (B) electricity does pass through the patient during laser surgery
    (C) laser surgery uses intensely hot, precisely focused beams of light to cut and coagulate tissue
    (D) electricity does not pass through the patient during laser surgery

59. When entering a room while the laser is in use, you must:

    (A) wear a lead apron
    (B) wear protective eyewear
    (C) no special precautions are necessary
    (D) wear a special mask

60. Which laser produces a visible blue-green beam?

    (A) Excimer (gas laser)
    (B) YAG
    (C) Argon laser
    (D) CO_2 laser

61. Surgery using an extremely cold instrument to destroy tissue is called:

    (A) laser surgery
    (B) phacoemulsification surgery
    (C) cryosurgery
    (D) ultrasonic surgery

62. Cryoablation uses a high-pressure gas called:

    (A) argon
    (B) CO_2
    (C) excimer
    (D) KTP

63. All waves in a laser are monochromatic. This means that:

    (A) all waves in the laser have the same length and are one color
    (B) all waves move in columns
    (C) the diameter of the beam is the same
    (D) they use the same power settings

64. What is the medium or element activated to transmit photons in a laser beam?

    (A) Gas
    (B) Solid
    (C) Liquid dye
    (D) All of the above

65. All of the following are true of lasers EXCEPT:

    (A) lasers do not need to be locked up when not in use
    (B) laser warning signs should be visible in areas where laser surgery is being performed
    (C) a laser safety officer is required to manage laser risks and define safety protocols
    (D) only flame-retardant drapes are used in laser surgery

66. Endotracheal tubes and other anesthetic equipment can easily ignite in the presence of laser energy and:

    (A) silastic endotracheal tubing
    (B) oxygen-rich anesthetic agents
    (C) pacemakers
    (D) defibrillators

67. Which equipment must be available during a laser laryngoscopy?

    (A) Water and wet cottonoids
    (B) Tracheotomy tray and wet towels
    (C) Bronchoscope and tracheotomy tray
    (D) None of the above

68. Located on the back of the central processing unit (CPU) are special openings called _____ for plugging in cables for adding additional computer components.

(A) drives

(B) cords

(C) ports

(D) networks

69. The device that enables a computer to send and receive information by phone line is called a:

(A) modem

(B) scanner

(C) USB port

(D) lateral port

70. Visual displays on the desktop of shortcuts to available programs are called:

(A) topics

(B) windows

(C) displays

(D) icons

71. When open to the internet, what function can be used to return to a recently opened site that you have not saved on your computer?

(A) Search

(B) History

(C) Favorites

(D) Address book

72. Web research is generally conducted with the help of:

(A) cursors

(B) search engines

(C) a browser

(D) instant access

73. A product used to buffer the computer hardware against high electrical voltages is called a:

(A) zip drive

(B) surge protector

(C) modem

(D) lateral port

74. A hardware component that converts printed text or a picture to digital information for use in documents is called the:

(A) scanner

(B) printer

(C) modem

(D) ethernet card

75. The arrow or small hand that appears on the screen to identify the location of currently addressed information is known as a:

(A) scanner

(B) cursor

(C) icon

(D) taskbar

76. The component of the computer that controls the cursor is called the:

(A) scroller

(B) mouse

(C) index

(D) scanner

77. The paper form of data in computer technology is the:

(A) file

(B) hard copy

(C) disk

(D) database

78. Precautions and guidelines for lasers include all EXCEPT:

    (A) lasers should be locked when not in use
    (B) laser warning signs should be posted on the front door of the OR where the laser will be used
    (C) instructions for laser use should be posted on every machine so that new and unexperienced staff have guidelines to follow and prevent injury and mishaps
    (D) lasers can be used to destroy/vaporize tissue, for dissection, and to seal vessels

79. To prevent damage to adjacent tissue when using a laser, a backstop is needed. Which of the following can be used?

    (A) Titanium or quartz rods
    (B) Wet sponges
    (C) Reflective metal wrap
    (D) Both A and B

80. All apply to an argon laser EXCEPT:

    (A) argon lasers produce a blue-green beam visible to the human eye
    (B) they are commonly used in eye surgery for diabetic retinopathy and dermatology for removal of pigmented lesions
    (C) the argon laser beam can travel through clear tissue without burning the surrounding tissue
    (D) the medium used for an argon laser is a solid crystal

81. All pertain to the CO_2 laser EXCEPT:

    (A) it has a blue-green beam visible to the human eye
    (B) it is used for dermatological procedures, such as skin resurfacing
    (C) a helium-neon beam that produces a red color is added to the CO_2 laser because otherwise it is not visible to the naked eye, and this helps the surgeon hit the target tissue
    (D) precise cutting and coagulation can be accomplished with the CO_2 laser

82. Which of the following is true of the neodymium:YAG (Nd:YAG) laser?

    (A) It is commonly used in urology to destroy bladder tumors and in ophthalmology.
    (B) The medium is a solid crystal (yttrium, aluminum, and garnet).
    (C) A helium-neon beam that produces a red color is added to the Nd:YAG laser because otherwise it is not visible to the naked eye, and this helps the surgeon hit the target tissue
    (D) All of the above

83. Which of the following is used to alert the surgeon if there is an improperly connected return electrode or active electrode?

    (A) The ESU will automatically stop working and shut down.
    (B) The active electrode will vibrate.
    (C) A red light flashes on the machine.
    (D) The ESU will sound an alarm or make a beeping noise.

84. Which of the following represents a complete cycle of monopolar cautery?

    (A) Generator, cautery pencil, target tissue, return electrode, generator
    (B) Generator, active electrode, target tissue, grounding pad, generator
    (C) Active electrode, sterile handpiece, target tissue, return electrode, generator
    (D) Both A and B

85. A laser can be incorporated into:

    (A) hysteroscopes
    (B) colonoscopes
    (C) arthroscopes
    (D) none of the above

86. Direct coupling occurs when:

    (A) bipolar high frequency, low voltage, and physical pressure seal a bleeding vessel

    (B) the dispersive electrode is not placed properly, resulting in a burn

    (C) the tip of the active electrode comes in contact with another instrument or conductor, causing a burn

    (D) the ESU causes interference with an implanted electronic device and the device malfunctions

87. Which type of endoscopy camera produces the truest color?

    (A) One-chip

    (B) Two-chip

    (C) Three-chip

    (D) Four-chip

88. White balancing prior to endoscopic surgeries requires the STS to focus the telescope lens on:

    (A) a utility drape

    (B) the surgeon's gloves

    (C) suture package

    (D) a solid white object

89. Defogging the video camera is usually the responsibility of the:

    (A) circulator

    (B) surgeon

    (C) scrub person

    (D) camera operator

Answers and Explanations

1. **(B)** Matter is anything that has mass and occupies space. All matter consists of atoms, and all atoms contain protons, neutrons, and electrons.

2. **(C)** The center of an atom contains the nucleus, which contains protons and neutrons.

3. **(B)** The electrical current moves through conductors by movement of free electrons.

4. **(B)** The active electrode carries the energy to the patient, goes through the ground pad on the patient into the inactive cord, and then returns back to the machine.

5. **(B)** Current is measured in amperes (amps).

6. **(B)** The path of electricity from energy source to the piece of equipment and back again is called a circuit.

7. **(B)** Restriction of the flow of current to a source is called resistance.

8. **(C)** In a simple electric circuit, the wire that connects to the switch is hot.

9. **(C)** A separate wire that is essential for protection against electric shock is the ground wire.

10. **(B)** Most outlets in the operating room run on 110 V current. X-ray units require the use of 220 V lines.

11. **(A)** Alternating current (AC) describes the flow of current that reverses direction periodically. Direct current (DC) indicates current that flows in only one direction (eg, a flashlight).

12. **(B)** A flashlight is an example of a one-way current or direct current because its power source is a battery. The electrical current of a battery flows in one direction (direct current) from a negative pole to a positive pole.

13. **(D)** Alternating current has the ability to step down, step up, or alternate voltage continuously. Hospitals use a reduced current.

14. **(B)** A device called a radio transmitter carries an impulse or signal to a wave-transmitting antenna system.

15. **(C)** The unit used to perform electrosurgery in delicate areas, such as in ophthalmology, plastic surgery, and neurosurgery, is the bipolar unit. It has reduced power. The circuit is completed within the handpiece.

16. **(D)** Certain surgical procedures that employ the use of electrocautery, laser, and drills can produce a plume of vaporized tissue that may include carcinogens, blood-borne pathogens, and mutagens. Smoke evacuators are frequently used to remove the potentially hazardous smoke.

17. **(D)** An alternating current cycle is a hertz. The number of cycles per second is a frequency.

18. **(D)** Radio waves are magnetic waves. The number of wave cycles is also called a frequency.

19. **(C)** When electrical current passes through the active electrode, it converts electrical energy to thermal energy.

20. **(C)** The best conductor of electricity is copper. Examples that use copper wire as a conductor

in the OR are surgical lamps, ESUs, and power drills.

21. **(C)** A simple electrical circuit is composed of a source of power, conductor, load, and switch. The switch allows the operator to turn the piece of equipment on and off.

22. **(A)** When operating a piece of equipment in the OR, the most important prong is the ground. It safely transfers any leaking electrons to the ground and prevents injury.

23. **(A)** The scientific theory that explains electricity is Ohm's law. It is a mathematical equation that shows the relationship between voltage, current, and resistance.

24. **(C)** Power is defined as the rate at which work is done. Power is measured in watts.

25. **(B)** Positron emission tomography (PET) is the medical imaging of dynamic activities in the body such as blood flow and glucose uptake in tissues.

26. **(D)** All of the options listed are common uses of electrosurgery, including welding tissue together.

27. **(A)** The patient return electrode should always be placed close to the surgical site over a large muscle mass, never over a bony surface, scar, tattoo, hair, or implants. These increase impedance, which can cause burns.

28. **(C)** In bipolar electrosurgery, the surgeon uses a forceps or an instrument that has two contact points or a return point built into a single tip. The current leaves the power unit and travels from one pole to the other, passing only through the tissue between the contact points. Current goes back to the ESU, and no grounding pad is required.

29. **(D)** The needle tip, spatula, and wire loops are all cutting electrodes.

30. **(A)** When using the coagulation mode of an ESU, the energy delivered is intermittent waves at a low frequency and a high voltage. High-frequency waves at a low voltage are used for the cutting mode.

31. **(D)** All perioperative personnel are responsible for preventing accidents involved with electrosurgery.

32. **(B)** You should always check the expiration date and ensure that the gel on the pad has a good moisture content and the quality of the pad is good. The pad is not guaranteed to work properly if it has been overly exposed to air. You must always check the integrity of the patient's skin before securing the pad. Wait to apply it until after the final positioning of the patient. A grounding pad must always be used with the monopolar ESU; it is not used for bipolar surgery.

33. **(C)** Insulators such as Teflon, silicone, polyethylene, and polyvinyl are used to protect the patient from being burned by stray electricity.

34. **(D)** Examples of electrosurgical vessel sealing are LigaSure and Enseal. This system is used during resection procedures that traditionally require sequential clamping, suturing, and a cutting process.

35. **(A)** The harmonic energy system uses ultrasonic energy. This energy is generated by high-frequency vibration and friction. It simultaneously cuts and coagulates tissue by transmitting ultrasonic wave energy through specially designed forceps and scissors.

36. **(D)** Motion is known as kinetic energy. The mechanical energy of an object can be a result of its motion.

37. **(C)** The rate at which work is done is called power. It is expressed as the amount of work per unit of time.

38. **(B)** Electrons border the outer perimeter of an atom and are negatively charged. These outer electrons are known as free electrons, and it is

the movement of free electrons that produces electric current.

39. **(C)** The gain or loss of electrons in an atom is termed ionization. A loss converts an atom into a positively charged ion, whereas a gain converts an atom into a negatively charged ion.

40. **(D)** The transfer of thermal energy by contact is called conduction. Some energy is transferred to molecules of a second object when they collide. Certain substances are better used for this transfer, such as metals, rather than wood or paper.

41. **(B)** A wave may be described as a disturbance in a medium such as air, water, or a solid substance.

42. **(B)** The frequency of sound can be measured in hertz. Multiples of sound are measured in megahertz.

43. **(A)** Mechanics is the study of objects in motion and is normally restricted to a small number of very large objects.

44. **(B)** Isaac Newton's three laws of motion are the basis of classical mechanics, or Newtonian mechanics.

45. **(A)** Acceleration is defined as a change in velocity over time.

46. **(B)** Newton's first of three laws states that "inertia is a property of matter that causes matter to resist change in motion."

47. **(C)** Newton's third law, also known as the "law of conservation of momentum," states that whenever a force is exerted, an equal or opposite force arises in reaction.

48. **(C)** If an object returns to its original position after a force is applied or removed, then it is said to be elastic. An example is a coiled spring.

49. **(B)** Amplitude is the maximum distance that an object moves from its central position (called equilibrium).

50. **(B)** Refraction is the bending of a light ray as it passes from one substance to another. Light travels at differing speeds as it travels through one medium or another (such as water or glass).

51. **(C)** Hooke proposed that light was a wave, but it was Sir Isaac Newton who posited that if light were a wave, it would bend around corners.

52. **(D)** The red wavelengths of light are the longest, whereas the violet wavelengths are the shortest. The view along the color spectrum changes with each color. White is not a color but is perceived when all colors hit the eye at the same time.

53. **(A)** In 1905, Einstein explained details of the photoelectric effect, which requires that light be a collection of particles called "photons." Young continued his work, and Niels Bohr of the University of Copenhagen further refined the research to establish the "complementarity principle of light."

54. **(C)** On the surface of the Earth, gravity causes objects to accelerate downward.

55. **(D)** A solid-state laser creates the most powerful output.

56. **(B)** The gravitational force, which is found only in nature and is one of the four forces affecting matter, does not affect the nucleus of an atom.

57. **(B)** Protons and neutrons act as if they are identical articles and differ only in their electrical charge. The nucleons themselves are made of subatomic particles called "quarks."

58. **(B)** During laser surgery, electricity does not pass through the patient. Therefore, a grounding pad is not necessary.

59. **(B)** The laser beam can cause permanent eye damage if viewed directly or indirectly by reflection.

60. **(C)** Argon gas lasers produce a visible blue-green beam that is absorbed by red and brown pigmented tissue such as hemoglobin. The argon laser is mostly used in dermatological and ophthalmological procedures.

61. **(C)** Cryosurgery uses liquid nitrogen, which freezes almost immediately and eventually will cause tissue to slough; it is mainly used to treat small skin lesions.

62. **(A)** A high-pressure argon gas is injected into the cryoablation probe causing the surrounding tissue to freeze.

63. **(A)** All waves in the laser have exactly the same length. Their peaks and troughs are in exactly the same location. This is called coherency.

64. **(D)** Laser energy is created when light is pumped into a sealed chamber and filled with a medium. Examples are gases, solids, and liquids.

65. **(A)** Lasers are required to be locked up when not in use under the laser precautions and guidelines (Surgical Technology for the Surgical Technologist).

66. **(B)** In the presence of laser energy and oxygen-rich anesthetic agents, anesthesia equipment could easily ignite. To minimize the risk of endotracheal fires, a special metallic foil is wrapped around the endotracheal tube before surgery.

67. **(A)** Sterile water must be available to keep sponges and linens wet in case of fire.

68. **(C)** Located at the back of the computer are ports that allow us to access a connection to the hard drive to attach scanners, printers, and other components to the system.

69. **(A)** A modem is the communication device that sends and receives information over a telephone line, thereby connecting us to the internet.

70. **(D)** Icons that appear on the desktop screen are shortcuts to programs that also can be accessed through the start menu.

71. **(B)** The computer holds the most recently visited sites in a history menu. Clicking on history will return the site to the screen for viewing.

72. **(B)** There are several search engines available to reach the Web—for example, Google and Yahoo.

73. **(B)** A surge protector is a buffer against damaging high-voltage surges of energy.

74. **(A)** A scanner resembles a printer but reproduces the image electronically rather than duplicating the print.

75. **(B)** A cursor is a small arrow that appears on the screen to identify the information to be addressed.

76. **(B)** The mouse moves the cursor to different areas on the screen and selects commands.

77. **(B)** The hard copy of data is a paper printout of the data. Printing out a hard copy is another method of protecting work.

78. **(C)** Anyone who works with lasers should be trained to use the laser properly and safely. Every institution that uses lasers should appoint a laser safety officer to provide information, instruction, and safety precautions to staff.

79. **(D)** To prevent damage to adjacent tissue and limit the absorption of the hot laser, a backstop is used. Backstops can be wet sponges or titanium or quarts rods. Anything reflective should be covered to prevent the beam from reflecting.

80. **(D)** The active medium for an argon laser is a noble gas. A solid crystal is used for an Nd:YAG laser.

81. **(A)** All apply to the CO_2 laser except that there is no color to the beam so a helium–neon beam that produces a red color is added to the CO_2 laser to help guide the surgeon to hit the target tissue.

82. **(D)** All of the listed options pertain to the Nd:YAG laser.

83. **(D)** It is extremely important to have the volume on the cautery machine always on because if the cords are not properly connected, the generator will make a beeping noise. When the ESU is being activated by the surgeon, the generator will make a buzzing noise, which indicates that the machine is in use.

84. **(D)** Terms used to describe the equipment of the ESU include generator, ESU machine, active electrode, cautery handpiece (pencil, sterile handpiece), target tissue, grounding pad, dispersive electrode, return electrode, generator, and ESU machine.

85. **(D)** The Nd:YAG laser can be used with a hysteroscope to treat uterine polyps and small fibroids. An argon or Nd:YAG laser can be used with the colonoscope to treat polyps, to treat bleeding disorders and arteriovenous malformations, and for ablation. Nd:YAG lasers are used in arthroscopic surgery to cut and smooth cartilage and tissue within the joints.

86. **(C)** Direct coupling occurs when the tip of the active electrode comes in contact with another instrument or conductor or if there is a defect in the insulation on the instrument, causing a stray current and resulting in a serious burn to the patient.

87. **(C)** With a three-chip camera, each chip picks up only one of the primary colors. Since each chip sees the entire image, there is no need to infer the color that should appear on the screen. Three-chip cameras provide truer color.

88. **(D)** To balance a video camera, the scrub person must focus the camera on a white wrapper, wall, or sponge to create a fixed point of reference for all other colors.

89. **(C)** Fogging occurs when the light going through the scope warms the air between the eyepiece and the coupler and causes trapped air to evaporate. To avoid fogging, the scrub person must make sure that the entire area is dry before assembling and must use an antifogging agent on the lens.

CHAPTER 31

Occupational Hazards/Fire Safety

HAZARDS IN THE OPERATING ROOM

- These are classified as:
  - Physical injury to the body
  - Chemical injuries from gases, toxic fumes, and/or cleaning agents
  - Biological injuries from infectious waste, cross-microbial contamination from patient to health care worker, needle sticks, smoke plume, and/or latex allergies

ENVIRONMENTAL HAZARDS

- **Operating room (OR) lights**—should be non-glaring and prevent eye fatigue
- **Noise—caused by:**
  - Loud music
  - Talking
  - Banging instruments
  - Monitors
- **Ergonomics**—proper body mechanics for the surgical technologist
  - Stand with legs shoulder length apart, the wider the better. This helps to distribute your weight evenly
  - Avoid leaning on one foot. Shift your weight back and forth
  - Stand next to the OR bed straight with arms loose
  - When sitting, sit up straight and do not lean over the surgical field
  - Push, do not pull, heavy equipment
  - Instruments should not exceed 25 lb
  - Squat to lift; don't bend at the waist
  - Lift with your legs and abdomen, not your lower back
  - Lift with a smooth even motion; ease your head up first

- When turning, turn with your whole body
- Keep your back bowed when lowering supplies and equipment
- **Radiation**
  - OR staff should wear lead aprons and thyroid collars
  - When possible, protect the patient with a lead apron
  - Stand at least 6 ft from the fluoroscopy beam when possible
  - Exposure should be monitored with an x-ray monitoring device
  - Pregnant staff should avoid participating on cases with x-ray if possible. If you must participate, leave the room when the radiation is being used
  - This is discussed in more depth in Chapter 12
- **Electricity**
  - Electrosurgical unit (ESU)
    - The active electrode should always be placed in its holder when not in use to prevent burning drapes or the patient
    - To prevent burns to the patient, the return electrode must be properly placed
  - Defibrillators
  - X-ray machines
  - This is discussed in more depth in Chapter 30
- **Static electricity**
  - Humidity in the OR should be between 20% and 60% to prevent sparks
- **Fiberoptic beam** on laparoscopic and endoscopic cases
  - Prevent the light from resting on the drape sheets to prevent a fire
- Laser plume

STANDARD PRECAUTIONS/UNIVERSAL PRECAUTIONS

- Gloves should be worn at all times when handling blood and bodily fluids. Every patient should be treated as if they are potentially infectious
- Use personal protective equipment (PPE)
- **Neutral zone/hands-free** sharps are passed in a basin to the surgeon instead of hand to hand
- Never recap hypodermic needles
- If stuck with a needle or sharp
  - All personnel at the sterile field should be double gloved to protect against a needle stick
  - Immediately remove the instrument/needle from the sterile field
  - Immediately remove the glove and assess the injury
  - The injury should be washed with soap and water
  - The injury should be assessed, reported, and treated within 2 hours
  - If the injury is in the eye or nasal or oral mucosa, it should be flushed with water or saline
  - Fill out an incident report

LASER AND ELECTROSURGICAL PLUME

- The concerns with laser plume are the cells in the smoke. A special suction should be used that contains a HEPA filter with combined charcoal filter to absorb the plume
- The ESU is not as dangerous as laser smoke; however, it has a strong odor and can be irritating to your eyes and respiratory tract
- It is the job of the STSR to control the suction. The wand should be as close to the area being worked on as possible without blocking the surgeon's view

LATEX ALLERGY

- Latex is made from rubber (trees)
- Halstead was the first surgeon to wear latex gloves during surgery
- Many other items in the operating room contain latex in addition to surgical gloves
- Symptoms of latex allergies include a skin rash and more severe problems like respiratory arrest

- It is very important to know if your patient has a latex allergy. It should be stated on the patient's chart, and all staff must be alerted prior to setting up for the surgical procedure to ensure there is no latex in the room
- A patient with a latex allergy should be the first scheduled case of the day. This allows the room to be free of latex dust from previous cases

CHEMICAL HAZARDS IN THE OR

- The STSR should be aware of the chemicals they work with in the OR. Many of these chemicals are toxic, causing irritation to the mucous membranes, cancer, and genetic changes. Examples include:
  - Formaldehyde/formalin (used to preserve specimens)
  - Glutaraldehyde/Cidex (used for sterilization)
  - ETO (ethylene oxide; used for sterilization)
- **Anesthetic gases**—these gases can escape from the anesthesia machine and can cause cancer and renal, brain, and nerve damage if overexposed
  - Every anesthesia machine should have a gas scavenging system attached to the machine to filter and remove anesthesia gases. The ventilation systems in the OR help with eliminating the gas
- **PMMA—polymethyl methacrylate**—bone cement—a mixture of liquid and powder used to secure prostheses in bone
  - It is very toxic to the mucous membranes, eyes (can damage soft contact lenses), and the respiratory tract
  - Bone cement implantation syndrome—the cement in the bone causes a reaction where emboli can travel through the vessels to the lungs
  - PMMA can also cause hypotension (abnormally low blood pressure)

FIRE SAFETY

Fire safety guidelines:

- **Class A fire**—water—used for wood, paper, and textiles
- **Class B fire**—CO_2—used for flammable liquids, gas, and oils
- **Class C fire**—halon extinguisher—used for lasers and electrical fires

- **PASS**—acronym used for working the fire extinguisher:
  - **P**—pull
  - **A**—aim
  - **S**—squeeze
  - **S**—sweep
- Most ORs use the acronym **RACE** to prepare employees for a potential fire:
  - **R**—rescue/remove anyone from the fire
  - **A**—alert/sound the alarm
  - **C**—contain the fire
  - **E**—extinguish/evacuate

NATURAL DISASTERS

- Avalanche
- Rockslide, landslide
- Winter storm, tropical storms, and hurricanes
- Heat wave—a prolonged period of abnormally hot weather that can cause many conditions including death
  - Heat cramps—painful muscle cramps caused by exercise or working in a hot environment
  - Heat exhaustion—a condition caused by exposure to extreme heat. Symptoms include physical weakness, collapse, nausea, muscle cramps, and dizziness
  - Heat stroke—caused by the body's failure to regulate its temperature when exposed to excessive heat along with dehydration. Symptoms include fever and confusion and can be as serious as unconsciousness and death. This is a life-threatening condition. The body immediately needs to be hydrated and cooled
- Wildfires
- Earthquakes
  - Richter scale is used to determine how powerful an earthquake is
  - Earthquakes can cause tsunamis/tidal waves

MAN-MADE DISASTERS

- These are caused by people; they include:
  - Explosions where chemicals are released into the environment, including chemical weapons and bombs
    - Nerve agents—cause difficulty breathing and death
    - Vesicants/mustard gas—cause damage to the skin, mucous membranes, and respiratory tract
    - Choking agents—cause damage to the respiratory tract and can cause pulmonary edema
- Car, plane, train accidents
- Nuclear devices/nuclear power plants
- Radiological devices
  - **Dirty bomb**—this type of bomb causing damage to the land, radiation sickness, and physical injury, including:
    - Sickness/cancer
    - Lacerations
    - Retinal burns/flash blindness

TERRORISM/BIOTERRORISM

Terrorism—the use of threats and violence to intimidate a population in order to coerce them to take certain actions or beliefs commonly relating to religion or politics

Bioterrorism/germ warfare—a form of terrorism where biological agents are released to cause harm to humans and the environment. They include:

- Anthrax
- Botulism
- Cholera
- Ebola
- Plague
- Smallpox
- Many more
  - These agents enter the body through the skin, mucous membranes, eyes, open wounds, and the respiratory tract

EAP—EMERGENCY ACTION PLAN

HEALTH CARE FACILITY EAP

- All health care workers should know their responsibility in the event of a bioterrorism attack
- **EAP**—should be in place, including a proper chain of command
  - Safe transfer and evacuation of patients to a safe place "safe zone"
  - All health care workers should know their responsibility in the event of a bioterrorism attack
  - PPE
  - Preserving blood, medications
  - Backup generators
  - Laptops/medical records
  - A way to track the patients
  - Status of the patients

A HAZARDOUS EVENT THAT INCLUDES MASS CASUALTY

- PATIENT DECONTAMINATION AREA
  - This area is important for chemical and radio-logical decontamination
  - **Radiological decontamination**
    - Clothing is removed and placed in a sealed bag
    - Wounds are cleaned with saline
    - Body and hair are cleaned with soap and water
  - **Chemical decontamination**
    - Clothing is removed
    - The skin and wounds are treated with sodium hypochlorite (one part bleach/nine parts H_2O)—rinse with normal saline
    - Do not use this solution in the eyes
- **HOT ZONE**—area where the disaster occurred
- **WARM ZONE**—300 ft or more from the hot zone
- **COLD ZONE**—near the warm zone where less severe injuries are evaluated
- **TRIAGE CATEGORIES**—this is a way of sorting patients according to the severity of their injuries

START—SIMPLE TRIAGE AND RAPID TREATMENT

- **DIME—DELAYED/IMMEDIATE/MINIMAL/ EXPECTANT**—these are the four categories in which to place patients during triage. A tag is placed on each patient; they include:
  - **MINOR**—green tag—minor injuries/"walking wounded"
  - **DELAYED**—yellow tag—bleeding controlled, airway open, patient is stable
  - **INTERMEDIATE**—red tag—patient is in serious condition and needs to be treated immediately within the hour, which is the **"GOLDEN HOUR"** in order for the patient to survive
  - **EXPECTANT**—black tag—patient is beyond healing. They are given pain medication for comfort, but supplies are saved for the victims in the other three categories

SURGICAL TECHNOLOGIST'S ROLE IN TRIAGE

- Train for triage
- Perform cardiopulmonary resuscitation (CPR)
- Perform basic first aid
- Transport

Questions

1. Excessive exposure to radiation can cause:

   (A) many types of cancer

   (B) cataracts

   (C) spontaneous abortion

   (D) all of the above

2. Radiation exposure of the staff is monitored with:

   (A) a homing device

   (B) a Holter monitor

   (C) film badges/dosimeter

   (D) a notation on each operative record

3. Ionizing radiation protection is afforded by the use of:

   (A) iron

   (B) ebonized coating

   (C) zinc

   (D) lead

4. Direct coupling occurs when:

   (A) bipolar high frequency, low voltage, and physical pressure seal a bleeding vessel

   (B) the dispersive electrode is not placed properly and the result is a burn

   (C) the tip of the active electrode comes in contact with another instrument or conductor causing a burn

   (D) the ESU causes interference with an implanted electronic device and causes the device to malfunction

5. An OR hazard that has been linked to increased risk of spontaneous abortion in female OR employees is exposure to:

   (A) x-ray control

   (B) radium

   (C) sterilization agents

   (D) waste anesthetic gas

6. While using this mixture, a scavenging system is used to collect and exhaust or absorb its vapors. It is called:

   (A) glutaraldehyde

   (B) polypropylene

   (C) methyl methacrylate

   (D) halon

7. The best measure for staff protection against HIV is:

   (A) handling all needles and sharps carefully

   (B) using barriers to avoid direct contact with blood and body fluids

   (C) immunization of all staff with vaccine

   (D) both A and B

8. Precautions and guidelines for lasers include all EXCEPT:

   (A) lasers should be locked when not in use

   (B) laser warning signs should be posted on the front door of the OR suite where the laser is being used

   (C) instructions for laser use should be posted on every machine so that new unexperienced staff has guidelines to follow and prevent injuries

   (D) lasers can be used to destroy/vaporize tissue for dissection and to seal vessels

9. How is inhalation of the laser plume best prevented?

   (A) Double mask worn by scrub team
   (B) Filter on suction
   (C) Laser on standby whenever possible
   (D) Mechanical smoke evacuator on field

10. What components are required for a fire and are found in an OR setting?

    (A) O_2
    (B) Fuel
    (C) Source of ignition
    (D) All of the above

11. Fuel sources found at the surgical site include:

    (A) dry sponges and drapes
    (B) endotracheal tube
    (C) prep solvents
    (D) all of the above

12. STSR should _____ to prevent buildup of heat created by friction.

    (A) have suction available to remove smoke plume
    (B) check all equipment before cases begin
    (C) irrigate the active tip (high-speed drills)
    (D) not lay the fiberoptic cord directly on the drape

13. A hospital fire plan is based on four immediate actions remembered by the acronym:

    (A) PASS
    (B) CODE
    (C) OFSI
    (D) RACE

14. To activate a fire extinguisher, what is the correct order of the following: (1) sweep, (2) aim, (3) squeeze, (4) pull?

    (A) 1, 2, 3, 4
    (B) 3, 2, 1, 4
    (C) 4, 2, 3, 1
    (D) 4, 3, 2, 1

15. The preferred type of fire extinguisher used for OR fires is:

    (A) water based
    (B) CO_2
    (C) dry powder
    (D) oil based

16. When a magnetic resonance imaging (MRI) scanner is used, the primary risk to the patient is the presence of:

    (A) CO_2
    (B) O_2
    (C) metal
    (D) none of the above

17. When using the laser, in order to prevent damage to adjacent tissue, a backstop is needed. You can use:

    (A) titanium or quartz rods
    (B) wet sponges
    (C) reflective metal wrap
    (D) both A and B

18. Another name for a "no hands" technique is:

    (A) retractable scalpel
    (B) blunt trocars
    (C) Hassan
    (D) neutral zone

19. Sources of latex include:

    (A) wound drain
    (B) catheters
    (C) pneumatic tourniquet
    (D) all of the above

20. Chemical hazards include:

    (A) formaldehyde
    (B) Cidex
    (C) ETO
    (D) all of the above

21. Which of the following is used to extinguish a class A fire?

(A) Water
(B) CO_2
(C) Halon
(D) None of the above

22. Natural disasters include:

(A) avalanche
(B) rockslide
(C) winter storm
(D) all of the above

23. A condition caused by exposure to extreme heat that causes physical weakness, collapse, nausea, and muscle cramps is termed:

(A) heat stroke
(B) heat exhaustion
(C) heat cramps
(D) sunburn

24. A Richter scale measures:

(A) how powerful an earthquake is
(B) category of hurricane
(C) height of a tidal wave
(D) both A and B

25. All apply to a dirty bomb EXCEPT:

(A) causes sickness and cancer
(B) damages land
(C) is radioactive
(D) has nuclear fallout

26. Bioterrorism uses biological agents to cause harm to humans and the environment. These agents include:

(A) anthrax
(B) botulism
(C) Ebola
(D) all of the above

27. Which decontamination process requires the use of sodium hypochlorite?

(A) Chemical decontamination
(B) Radiological decontamination
(C) Atomic decontamination
(D) Thermal decontamination

28. How many feet away from the disaster is the "warm zone"?

(A) 100 ft
(B) 300 ft
(C) 700 ft
(D) 1 mile

29. A triage patient wearing a black tag designates that they are in which category?

(A) Delayed
(B) Minor
(C) Expectant
(D) Intermediate

30. The so-called "golden hour" refers to:

(A) time of death
(B) 1 hour following the disaster
(C) mandatory treatment within 1 hour
(D) 1 hour preceding the disaster

31. Laser media includes:

(A) gas
(B) solids
(C) liquids
(D) all of the above

32. An argon laser:

(A) produces a blue-green beam visible to the human eye
(B) is commonly used in eye surgery and dermatology for removal of pigmented lesions
(C) has a beam that can travel through clear tissue without burning the surrounding tissue
(D) all of the above pertain to the argon laser

33. All pertain to the CO_2 laser EXCEPT:

    (A) it has a blue-green beam visible to the human eye

    (B) it is used for dermatological procedures like skin resurfacing

    (C) a helium-neon beam that produces a red color is added to the CO_2 laser because it is not visible to the naked eye and the colored beam helps the surgeon hit the target tissue

    (D) there is precise cutting and coagulation with the CO_2 laser

34. The neodymium (Nd):YAG laser:

    (A) is commonly used in urology to destroy bladder tumors and in ophthalmology

    (B) uses a medium of solid crystal (yttrium, aluminum, and garnet)

    (C) has a helium-neon beam that produces a red color because it is not visible to the naked eye and the colored beam helps the surgeon hit the target tissue

    (D) all of the above

35. All are safety measures when using the grounding pad/dispersive electrode/return electrode/inactive electrode/neutral electrode EXCEPT:

    (A) it must always be used for monopolar surgery to prevent patient burns

    (B) apply the pad prior to final positioning

    (C) you should always check the gel on the pad to make sure the moisture content and quality are good

    (D) always check the integrity of the patient's skin before applying the pad

36. Potential risks when performing CPR include:

    (A) broken ribs, collapsed lung, tissue damage

    (B) brain death, if you do not deliver the chest compressions as soon as possible to get the heart and respirations going

    (C) damage to the head, neck, and spine

    (D) all of the above

37. During a code in the operating room, the STSR's main responsibility is to:

    (A) call for assistance

    (B) begin chest compressions until additional personnel arrive to assist

    (C) maintain a sterile field

    (D) assist the anesthesiologist

38. Malignant hyperthermia (MH) is a life-threatening acute disorder that can develop during or after anesthesia has been given. A common medication(s) known to induce an MH crisis is/are:

    (A) succinylcholine

    (B) muscle relaxants

    (C) isoflurane

    (D) all of the above

39. Disseminated intravascular coagulation (DIC) may be stimulated by which of the following?

    (A) Severe tissue trauma (eg, head injury, shock, or burns)

    (B) Severe liver disease

    (C) Obstetric complications

    (D) All of the above

40. The term "all hazards preparation" refers to:

    (A) generalized training and emergency preparation for all disaster situations

    (B) man-made disasters such as chemical release accidents

    (C) natural disasters that affect large populations such as a severe heat wave

    (D) an allied health institution

41. All are effects of an earthquake EXCEPT:

    (A) tsunamis

    (B) hurricanes

    (C) avalanches

    (D) floods

42. Natural disasters can contribute to infectious diseases and produce epidemic and pandemic events as a result of:

(A) displaced groups of people

(B) poor sanitation

(C) compromised health care

(D) all of the above

43. A pandemic includes all EXCEPT:

(A) it is a localized infectious disease affecting a specific population

(B) HIV, AIDS, and COVID are examples of pandemics

(C) it is a worldwide disease outbreak

(D) these types of diseases require isolation, strict hand washing, and disinfection

44. Which of the following tags indicates the least critical of patients in a triage situation?

(A) Yellow

(B) Green

(C) Black

(D) Red

45. Which persons are NOT designated first responders to an immediate response to an all hazards event?

(A) Firefighters

(B) Electricians

(C) Health care responders

(D) Public safety personnel

Answers and Explanations

1. **(D)** Ionizing radiation causes changes in genetic material, cells, and protein. Overexposure is known to cause cancer in bone, thyroid, and reproductive organs. It can also cause cataracts and spontaneous abortion in pregnant women, among other birth defects. The best protection for pregnant staff is to avoid being in cases with ionizing radiation. If you are in a room, step out when x-ray is used and always wear a lead apron, thyroid collar, and an extra film badge under the lead apron at waist level to track fetal exposure.

2. **(C)** Film badges/dosimeters are the most widely used monitors measuring total REMS of accumulated exposure. Data are reviewed.

3. **(D)** Shielding with lead is the most effective protection against gamma rays and x-rays in the form of lead-lined walls, portable lead screens, lead aprons, lead-impregnated rubber gloves, lead thyroid-sternal collars, and lead glasses. The best prevention of overexposure of ionizing radiation is to rotate staff through these cases.

4. **(C)** Direct coupling occurs when the tip of the active electrode comes in contact with another instrument or conductor or if there is a defect in the insulation on the instrument causing a stray current and resulting in a serious burn to the patient.

5. **(D)** Waste anesthetic gas is gas and vapor that escape from the anesthesia machine and equipment, as well as gas released through the patient's expiration. The hazards to personnel include an increased risk of spontaneous abortion in females working in the OR, congenital abnormalities in their children as well as in the offspring of unexposed partners of exposed male personnel, cancer in females administering anesthesia, and hepatic and renal disease in both males and females. This problem can be reduced by a scavenging system that removes waste gases.

6. **(C)** Methyl methacrylate, or bone cement, is mixed at the sterile field. Vapors are irritating to eyes and respiratory tract. It may be a mutagen, a carcinogen, or toxic to the liver. It can cause allergic dermatitis. A scavenging system is used to collect vapor during mixing and exhaust it to the outside or absorb it through activated charcoal.

7. **(D)** A patient may come to the OR infected but may not yet test positive. Careful handling of needles and sharps and using barriers to avoid direct contact with blood and body fluids are the best measures to prevent transmission. A vaccine has not been developed for immunization.

8. **(C)** Anyone who works with lasers should be trained to use the laser properly and safely. Every institution that uses lasers should appoint a laser safety officer to provide information, instruction, and safety precautions to staff.

9. **(D)** A mechanical smoke evacuator or suction with a high-efficiency filter removes toxic substances including carcinogens and viruses from the air. Personnel should not inhale the fumes.

10. **(D)** Fire requires three components: oxygen available in the air or in a pure gas, fuel or combustible material, and a source of ignition, usually in the form of heat.

11. **(D)** Any material capable of burning is a potential fuel for fire.

12. **(C)** When high-speed instruments are used such as drills and saws, the active tip should be irrigated to prevent buildup of heat created by friction.

13. **(D)** RACE means rescue, alert, contain, and evacuate (Fuller).

14. **(C)** These steps can easily be remembered by the acronym PASS.

15. **(B)** The preferred type of fire extinguisher used in ORs is CO_2.

16. **(C)** Whenever an MRI is used, the primary risk to the patient is the presence of metal. It can be drawn from its source into the path of the powerful magnetic field.

17. **(D)** To prevent damage to adjacent tissue and limit the absorption of the laser heat, a backstop is used. It can be wet sponges and/or titanium or quartz rods. Anything reflective should be covered to prevent the beam from reflecting.

18. **(D)** This technique uses a hands-free space (designated receptacle) on the sterile field where sharps can be placed and retrieved so that the surgical technologist and the surgeon do not hand instruments directly to each other.

19. **(D)** All of the above are sources of latex.

20. **(D)** Formalin, Cidex, and ETO are all potential hazardous chemicals handled in the OR.

21. **(A)** Water is used to extinguish a class A fire. This includes fires consisting of wood, paper, and textiles. Class B fires require CO_2 to extinguish and include fires from liquids, gas, and oils. Class C fires require a halon extinguisher and include lasers and/or electrical fires.

22. **(D)** An avalanche, a rockslide, and a winter storm are all examples of natural disasters.

23. **(B)** Heat exhaustion is caused by exposure to extreme heat. Symptoms include physical weakness, collapse, nausea, and muscle cramps. Heat cramps are painful muscle cramps caused by exercise or working in an extremely hot environment. Heat stroke is caused by the body's failure to regulate its temperature when exposed to excessive heat and dehydration. Symptoms include fever and confusion and can be as serious as unconsciousness and death.

24. **(A)** A Richter scale is used to determine how powerful an earthquake is.

25. **(D)** A dirty bomb causes sickness and cancer. It also damages the land and is a radioactive type of bomb, not nuclear.

26. **(D)** Anthrax, botulism, Ebola, plague, and cholera are all types of biological agents used in bioterrorism.

27. **(A)** Sodium hypochlorite is used for chemical decontamination (one part household bleach/ nine parts water and must be rinsed with NaCl). Radiological decontamination requires cleaning wounds with saline.

28. **(B)** The "hot zone" is the area where the disaster occurred. The "warm zone" is 300 ft or more from the hot zone. The "cold zone" is near the warm zone where there are less severely injured people.

29. **(C)** Expectant category is the triage category where the patient is tagged with a black tag, meaning beyond healing. These patients are given pain medication for comfort, but no supplies will be used because they will be used on other patients. The minor category is the triage category marked by green tags. These patients have minor injuries. The delayed category patients wear yellow tags, meaning the patient is stable. Intermediate category patients wear red tags and are in serious condition. These patients should be treated within the hour.

30. **(C)** The "golden hour" refers to the patient being treated within the hour following their injury.

31. **(D)** Active laser media include gases, solids, liquids, and semiconductor crystals.

32. **(D)** All of the above pertain to the argon laser.

33. **(A)** All apply to the CO_2 laser except that there is no color to the beam, so a helium-neon beam that produces a red color is added to the CO_2 laser to help guide the surgeon to hit the target tissue.

34. **(D)** All of the above pertain to the Nd:YAG laser.

35. **(B)** You should always check the expiration date and that the gel on the pad has a good moisture content and the quality of the pad is good. It is not guaranteed to work properly if it has been overly exposed to air. You must always check the integrity of the patient's skin before securing the pad and wait to apply the pad until after the final positioning of the patient. A grounding pad must always be used with the monopolar ESU but not for bipolar surgery.

36. **(D)** Although there are potential risks to performing CPR, it is better than not doing anything. You can make a difference and save someone's life. Chest compressions and ventilations will help to deliver oxygenated blood to the brain, tissues, and organs and prevent the patient from dying. All of the above are potential risks of CPR.

37. **(C)** The main role for the STSR during a code in the OR is to maintain a sterile field, immediately secure the back table and mayo stand, and remain sterile until you are asked for assistance.

38. **(D)** The muscle relaxant succinylcholine and anesthetic gases such as halothane, isoflurane, and enflurane are known to cause MH crisis.

39. **(D)** DIC may be stimulated by severe tissue trauma such as head injury, shock, or burns; severe liver disease; obstetric complications; leukemia or cancer; or recent blood transfusion reactions.

40. **(A)** "All hazards preparation" refers to all types of disasters. There are systems in place to respond to the emergency and provide communication, information, and preparedness training.

41. **(B)** Hurricanes are caused by interactions between the atmosphere and the ocean. Earthquakes are caused by the motions of solid earth and can cause tsunamis (tidal waves), floods, and avalanches.

42. **(D)** Infectious diseases can be associated with a natural disaster by spreading through large gatherings of displaced people due to the disaster, lack of medical help and medication, poor sanitary conditions, poor infrastructures, and a lack of food and water.

43. **(A)** A pandemic is not a localized infectious disease affecting specific populations. A pandemic is nondiscriminant.

44. **(B)** The green triage tag would be designated to be the least critical patient. These patients are also known as "the walking wounded" and have minor injuries, sprains, cuts, and bruises.

45. **(C)** Health care responders should NOT be the first to enter a disaster scene; they should wait until it is safe to enter to safely treat the injured and prevent any further casualties to themselves. There could be downed wires, fires, and/or buildings that have major structural damage and are deemed unsafe.

CHAPTER 32

Endoscopy, Minimally Invasive Surgery, and Robotics

MIS—minimally invasive surgery—is performed using a rigid scope and long instruments. The instruments are introduced through small incisions surrounding the operative site.

Trocar/cannula system—telescopic instruments are introduced through small incisions around the operative site by a trocar (sharp trocar fits inside the cannula and is advanced beyond the tip of the cannula and punctures the abdominal wall). The trocar is removed and the cannula is left in place to receive the laparoscopic instruments.

- Port—the incision where the cannula is left in place
- Cannulas—protect the abdominal wall and maintain a seal between the inside of the body and the outside
- Blunt trocar/Hasson—an infraumbilical incision is made and the open method (cut down) is performed. The Hasson blunt trocar is inserted through this incision
- Fiberoptic light source—used to provide a cool illumination in the body cavity
  - The fiberoptic light is designed to remain cool inside the body; however, it should never be placed on the drapes because it can cause a fire
  - The light cord is made up of thousands of glass fibers. It should not be tightly coiled as the cord fibers can break. The cord should be handled carefully and loosely coiled
- Insufflation—this is the method of expanding the body cavity for visualization during MIS/endoscopic surgeries. The term is called

creating a pneumoperitoneum. Expansion medias include:
  - Laparoscopy—CO_2
  - Arthroscopy—irrigation
  - Bladder—irrigation fluid (saline, glycine, sorbitol, etc.)
  - Inguinal hernia repair—balloon dissector

Multiple-Incision MIS

- One port for the camera
- Up to four other ports are placed for surgical instruments

Single-Incision Laparoscopic Surgery

- Also known as SILS
  - The incision is at the umbilicus
  - A large flexible port with three subports is placed into the umbilical puncture
  - Instruments and camera are placed through these ports
  - The disadvantage is that it is a tight space to work

Advantages to MIS

- Reduced trauma
- Reduced blood loss
- Reduced pain
- Quick recovery

Disadvantages/Hazards

- High risk of adhesions if the patient has had previous surgery
- Risk of perforation with the trocar
- Bleeding

- Limited vision and range of motion with the instruments
- All staff must be trained in MIS
- Gas embolism
- Preperitoneal insufflation—improper placement of the Veress needle

Maintaining Patient Normothermia
- The use of CO_2 lowers the body temperature because it cools as it fills the abdominal space
- Distension fluids used elsewhere (uterus, knee, etc.) have the same effect

Conversion to an Open Case
- Any MIS has the potential to become an emergency open case
- The STSR and circulator must have all sterile supplies ready to go in case of a conversion to an open case

Equipment Used in MIS
- Monitor
- Fiberoptic light source and light cord
- Rigid telescope. Care of the telescope includes:
  - Always hold the scope by its head
  - Be careful not to ding or hit the scope
  - Only use lint-free soft material to wipe the scope
  - Always check for damage before use
  - Prevent lens fogging with defogger
  - White balance:
    - Helps to focus the scope
    - When white balancing, you should not use a 4 × 4. It must be a solid white background
    - Evens out the brightness
    - Prevents dark spots
    - Provides better picture quality
- Video camera
  - Pixel—this is the silicone chip located in a camera head or at the tip of the telescope. Pixels determine the clarity of an image. The more pixels there are, the clearer the image
  - Focus ring—turns to clarify the image
  - Endocoupler—connects the camera to the telescope
- Video cables
- Digital output recorder
- Equipment cart
- Specialty scopes

Tissue Expansion Techniques
- Insufflation—CO_2 for the abdominal cavity
- Continuous irrigation/fluid distension—uterus, bladder, joints
- Balloon expansion—expansion of tissue planes used in extraperitoneal hernia repair

Specimen Retrieval
- Morcellator—reduces large tissue specimens to small tissue pulp so it is small enough to be suctioned from the wound. Not used in the presence of cancer
- Tissue shaver—commonly used in endoscopic cases. The shaver sucks tissue into the channel where a burr shaves it down into small pieces before it is suctioned out
- Retractable tissue bag—large tissue specimens are put in a bag and pulled from a laparoscopic port or through a small abdominal incision

Instruments
- The handles are at a distance from the working end
- Instruments are reusable and disposable
  - Retractors—probe, rods, hooks
  - Scissors—come in straight, hooked, curved, electrosurgery and ultrasonic sheers
  - Forceps—grasping instruments; examples include Maryland, Mixter, Allis, and claw grasper
  - Suction and irrigation
  - Hemostatic clips and staples
  - Knot pusher

Sutures
- Various instruments are designed to tie knots and suture tissue
- There are three types:
  - Extracorporeal—the knot is tied outside of the body and pushed into place with a knot pusher
  - Intracorporeal—a surgical loop is used inside the body and tied with two grasping instruments
  - Ligation loop—Surgiwip—ligation ties instead of using a suture

Stapling Guns
- GIA is commonly used and inserted through a 12-mm port
- Laparoscopic hemoclip appliers

Endoscopic Surgery

- Endoscopes are used for diagnosis, biopsy, repair, and removal of foreign bodies
- Endoscopic surgery is performed by inserting instruments into the body through small, narrow incisions or a natural body orifice
- Diagnostic endoscopy—performed with a flexible, semirigid or rigid endoscope that is inserted into a natural body orifice

Flexible Endoscopy

- Endoscope control head (connects to the camera)
- Insertion tube—the part of the scope that enters the patient and also contains the fiberoptic light channel
- Instrument channel—provides access for other instruments to retrieve tissue specimens. Examples include biopsy forceps and brushes

Care for Endoscopes

- Endoscopes must be disassembled before cleaning
- Wash as soon as possible with an enzymatic cleaner
- Make sure all ports and channels are opened and flushed with an enzymatic cleaner
- Use a brush to clean all lumens
- Do not submerge the camera or allow electrical connections to become wet
- Rinse with deionized water or sterile water. All ports must be flushed
- Drain instruments and dry them
- Preclean
- Leak test—determines if there are any leaks in the flexible scope
- Instrument is cleaned and rinsed, and all water is removed from the channels
- The scope is sterilized according to manufacturer's instructions

Sterilization of Endoscopes

- Steam sterilization—includes some parts of the endoscope. Examples are hollow sheaths and obturators
- Ethylene oxide (ETO)—used for scopes and instruments that cannot be exposed to steam sterilization because high temperatures and moisture will breakdown the cement holding the lens
- Cidex—instruments must be able to be submerged and all ports left open. Following the

sterilization process, the instruments must be thoroughly rinsed with sterile distilled water

Direct coupling—occurs when the active electrode comes in contact with another instrument causing the tissue touching the instrument to be burned. Examples include:

- When the surgeon asks you to hold a clamp while he touches the cautery to it to coagulate the tissue
- This can also be unintentional and cause a burn

Capacitive coupling—occurs when there is a stray current that causes an unintentional burn
Lasers used in endoscopic procedures include:

- CO_2 laser—laser of choice for bronchoscopies and arthroscopies
- Nd:YAG—gastrointestinal procedures, bronchoscopies, laparoscopic cholecystectomy, arthroscopies, genitourinary (GU) and gynecological (GYN) procedures, colonoscopies, and neurological procedures
- Stereotactic laser—brain tissue—neurology
- Argon—laparoscopic cholecystectomy, diabetic retinopathy/ophthalmology, and neurosurgery
- KTP—laparoscopic cholecystectomy and ophthalmology
- Excimer—arteries/vascular

Endoscopic and laparoscopic procedures include:

- Fetoscopy—performed for direct visualization of the fetus inside the uterus. It is performed under sonographic visualization
  - A fiberoptic type of needle scope is inserted into the amniotic fluid to:
    - Obtain a biopsy of fetal blood
    - Directly view the fetus for congenital abnormalities
  - This procedure can be performed at 16 weeks of gestation
- Angioscopy—performed to visualize the inside of vessels
  - The angioscope is a fiberoptic scope connected to a camera that is visualized on a monitor screen
- ERCP—endoscopic retrograde cholangiopancreatogram—performed to take a biopsy, remove stones in the common bile duct (CBD), or dilate a stenosis of the bile duct by placing a stent
  - The scope is put through the mouth and gently moved down the esophagus. It extends

into the stomach and duodenum until it reaches the point where the ducts from the pancreas and gallbladder drain into the duodenum. X-rays can then be taken

- Hysteroscopy—performed to diagnose and treat conditions of the uterus. They include:
  - Menorrhagia
  - Fibroids
  - Polyps
  - Endometrial ablation
  - Remove intrauterine devices (IUDs)
    - The uterus is distended with fluid, and a rigid scope is inserted into the uterus
- Sigmoidoscopy/proctoscopy—a rigid or flexible endoscope for visual examination of the rectum and sigmoid colon
  - Can be a flexible or rigid scope
  - Routinely performed before rectal surgeries
  - Has helped in the early detection of tumors and polyps
- Anoscopy—performed to examine the anus
  - A small rigid instrument is inserted a few inches into the anus to evaluate problems of the anal canal
- Gastroscopy—a flexible fiberoptic scope is inserted through the mouth into the stomach
  - This is performed for:
    - Visual diagnosis
    - Bleeding
    - Biopsy
- Bronchoscopy—performed on the tracheobronchial tree
- Esophagoscopy—performed to view the inside of the esophagus and the esophageal orifice of the stomach for:
  - Biopsies and cytological brush biopsies
  - Removing foreign bodies
  - Diagnosis of diseases
  - Diverticula
  - Varices
  - Tumors, lesions
- It can be performed with a rigid or flexible scope
- The STSR's job is to introduce suction, instruments, and bougies
- Endoscopic brow lift—a cosmetic procedure performed to lift the eyebrow. It elevates the drooping eyebrow and removes deep wrinkle lines in the forehead. Three to five small incisions are inserted at the hairline

- Endoscopic sinus surgery—surgical treatment of sinusitis and nasal polyps performed to restore ventilation and drainage
- Cystoscopy—viewing of the GU tract, specifically the bladder
- Ureteroscopy—viewing of the ureters
- TURP—transurethral resection of the prostate
- TURB—transurethral resection of bladder tumors
- Choledochoscopy—provides images of the biliary system
  - It is introduced into the CBD, and normal saline is used as the medium to provide distention for visualization
  - This is commonly performed for removal of stones
  - The Nd:YAG laser can be introduced onto the scope to crush stones in the distal common hepatic duct
- Laparoscopic cholecystectomy—performed with a rigid scope inserted into the abdomen
  - The pneumoperitoneum is created with CO_2
  - This can be performed with a:
    - Trocar and cannula system
    - Hasson blunt trocar
    - SILS
- Laparoscopic hernia repair—there are two basic types; they include:
  - TAPP—transabdominal preperitoneal repair—this is the more conventional approach into the peritoneal cavity with a trocar and cannula. The mesh is inserted through a peritoneal incision to cover the hernia
  - TEP—totally extraperitoneal repair—TEP is different in that the peritoneal cavity is not entered and mesh is used to seal the hernia from outside the peritoneum
    - A dissection balloon is inserted into the preperitoneal space to create a cavity
    - The trocar and cannula are inserted, and the laparoscopic procedure begins
- Laparoscopic Nissen fundoplication—performed to restore the function of the lower esophageal sphincter (the valve between the esophagus and the stomach) by wrapping the stomach around the esophagus
- Laparoscopic liver biopsy—utilizes laparoscopic instrumentation along with a needle biopsy
- Laparoscopic bariatric surgery—the most common procedures performed include:

- Gastric bypass—a portion of the stomach is removed with laparoscopic instrumentation and guns and reconnected to the duodenum
- Sleeve gastrectomy—removal of a portion of the stomach along the greater curvature of the stomach forming a sleeve or tubular stomach
- Adjustable gastric band—an inflatable silicone band surgically implanted around the top of the stomach creating a small pouch that holds a small amount of food

- Laparoscopic appendectomy—performed laparoscopically
- Laparoscopic colon resection—a technique known as minimally invasive laparoscopic colon surgery is performed through small incisions with the laparoscope and instrumentation to resect a segment of the colon
- Laparoscopic GYN procedures use a 10-/12-mm scope with a 0-degree or 30-degree lens inserted into the peritoneal cavity. The pneumoperitoneum is created with CO_2
  - Chromopertubation—performed to determine tubal patency
    - Methylene blue dye mixed with saline is injected into the vagina and observed with the laparoscope going through the fallopian tubes
  - LAVH—laparoscopic-assisted vaginal hysterectomy—performed using a laparoscope and laparoscopic instruments into the abdomen to guide the removal of the uterus and/or fallopian tubes and ovaries through the vagina
  - Laparoscopic ectopic pregnancy—performed laparoscopically to remove the products of conception from the fallopian tube or anywhere outside the uterus
  - Laparoscopic myomectomy—performed laparoscopically to remove uterine leiomyomas, also known as fibroids
  - Laparoscopic oophorectomy—removal of one or both ovaries laparoscopically
  - Laparoscopic salpingectomy—removal of one or both fallopian tubes laparoscopically
- Laparoscopic nephrectomy—removal of a kidney by percutaneous endoscopic technique through the abdomen
- Endoscopic spinal discectomy—this endoscopic procedure is performed to remove herniated disc material that is causing pain in the lower back, legs, arms, and neck

  - Although a scope is not inserted, a trocar system is used under fluoroscopy
  - A cutting type of instrument, called a nucleotome, is inserted through the trocar, and the herniated nucleus pulposus disc material is removed
- Ventriculoscopy—performed through a burr hole in the skull for the treatment of:
  - Hydrocephalus
  - Lesions in the sella turcica (this is a depression in the sphenoid bone where the pituitary gland rests)
  - Cerebral aneurysms
  - The argon laser can be inserted to remove intravascular lesions
  - Nd:YAG laser can be used to remove cysts
- Endovascular abdominal aortic aneurysm (AAA) repair—performed to repair AAAs that begin below the renal arteries through an incision into the femoral artery. The procedure involves the placement of a stent graft into the aorta without opening the abdomen to reach the aorta. The procedure is performed by an interventional radiologist or vascular/cardiac surgeon
- Radiofrequency ablation of varicose veins—uses radiofrequency energy to heat, collapse, and seal blood vessels
- MIDCAB—minimally invasive coronary artery bypass surgery—also known as "beating heart" surgery, which means that stopping the heart (cardioplegia) and the heart-lung machine is not required
- Video-assisted thoracoscopic surgery—also known as VATS
  - It includes pathology of the thoracic cavity and lumbar spine
  - This is performed for the same reason as an open thoracotomy except that:
    - Recovery is quicker
    - Allows entry into the chest cavity without removing a rib or spreading ribs, both of which are painful

Robotics
- The most commonly used robot is the da Vinci robot by Intuitive Surgical
- Provides three-dimensional viewing
- Telechir—the name given to remote-controlled robots

- Instrumentation with better rotation than a surgeon's hand (endowrist instruments) and more precise surgical movements
- They require surgeon control and input by remote control and voice activation
- They can perform procedures from a distance
- Shorter stay in the hospital
- The robot is commonly used in:
  - Cardiac surgery
  - Colorectal surgery
  - General surgery
  - Gynecological surgery
  - Head and neck surgery
  - Thoracic surgery
  - Urological surgery
- Manipulators—the technical term for robotic arms
  - Can move in three dimensions
- Articulated—sections of the robot arms (manipulators)
- Motions of the robot are described in geometric terms
- Degrees of freedom—number of ways the manipulators move in three dimensions (yaw, roll, pitch)
  - Yaw—right and left movement
  - Roll—rotating movement
  - Pitch—up and down movement
  - Grip—open and close
  - Insertion—back and forth
- Degrees of rotation—relates to the manipulators' clockwise and counterclockwise movement around an axis
- Resolute geometry—refers to the robotic arm that can move in three dimensions; it resembles the movements of a human arm
- Resolution—the robot's ability to differentiate between two objects
- Sensitivity—the ability of the robot to see in dim light or detect weak impulses
- Telesurgery—the term used to perform surgery at a distance
- Binaural hearing—gives the robot the ability to hear what direction sound is coming from. The robot has two sound transducers as we have two ears
- Cartesian coordinate geometry—allows the robot to locate a point in three dimensions. This refers to a plane that is perpendicular to another plane and used to graph mathematical functions. Also called rectangular coordinate geometry
- Micromanipulators—the computer translates messages from micromanipulators on the remote console controlled by the surgeon's hand. This translates the surgeon's hand movements to the robotic arm and instrumentation
- Telepresence—refers to the operation of a robot at a distance. The operator is in one location, and the patient and robot are in another

Components of the Robot

- Console—where the surgeon sits to control the manipulators and perform the surgical procedures
- Patient-side cart—this cart system contains the robotic arms that directly contact the patient
- Manipulators—four robotic arms
- High-definition three-dimensional vision system
- Endowrist instruments—instruments placed in the manipulators
  - Cautery
  - Grasping instruments
  - Needle holders
  - Retractors
  - Hemoclip appliers
  - Each insertion into the robot with an instrument represents one use of the instrument. The average amount of uses is 10

Advantages

- Eliminates hand tremors
- Allows the surgeon to perform complex procedures within a small space
- Better visualization through three-dimensional imaging
- 360-degree wrist movement
- Instruments bend and rotate better than the human wrist
- Telepresence—the procedure can be performed from a distance; the patient can be at one hospital and the surgeon at another. This represents virtual reality

Disadvantages

- Very expensive
- Instruments cost thousands of dollars each
- Requires special training

Questions

1. All of the following applications can be performed through an endoscope EXCEPT:

   (A) cavity washings for diagnosis
   (B) video monitoring
   (C) biopsy
   (D) resection of malignant tumors

2. During minimally invasive surgery (MIS), what is used to achieve a pneumoperitoneum?

   (A) Warm saline
   (B) Oxygen
   (C) Carbon monoxide
   (D) Carbon dioxide

3. Not all patients are suitable for MIS. The term used for fibrous bands and scar tissue of the internal organs due to previous surgeries is:

   (A) adhesions
   (B) wound dehiscence
   (C) intestinal polyps
   (D) evisceration

4. Which endoscope is used to perform surgical assessment and operative procedures such as TURP?

   (A) Flexible endoscope
   (B) Rigid endoscope
   (C) Laparoscope
   (D) Sigmoidoscope

5. The system used to accommodate insertion of a laparoscope and endoscopic instruments is called:

   (A) diagnostic endoscope
   (B) trocar and cannula
   (C) Veress needle
   (D) endocoupler

6. When performing MIS in the upper abdomen or the lower esophagus, the patient is positioned in:

   (A) Trendelenburg
   (B) lateral
   (C) reverse Trendelenburg
   (D) prone

7. For a laparoscopic tubal ligation, the patient is placed in:

   (A) lithotomy
   (B) semi-Fowler
   (C) lateral
   (D) reverse Trendelenburg

8. All of the following statements are true of the fiberoptic light cord EXCEPT:

   (A) the cable is composed of thousands of glass or plastic fibers
   (B) the fibers are aligned in parallel longitudinal bundles
   (C) the cord can be overflexed and coiled
   (D) fibers are easily broken

9. The clarity of the image depends on the number of signals or silicone units the chip contains. The name for these silicone units is:

(A) adapter

(B) pixel

(C) endocoupler

(D) Storz

10. All are guidelines for proper handling of a telescope EXCEPT:

(A) take care to prevent scratches or dents in the shaft of the scope

(B) always hold the scope by its shaft

(C) use warm water or a defogger to prevent the lens from fogging during surgery

(D) everyone who handles the scope from processing to end stage is responsible to ensure integrity of the instrument

11. What part of the endoscopic equipment transmits digital data from the camera head to the camera control unit and from the monitor to the output recorder?

(A) Endoscopic lock ring

(B) Focus ring

(C) Video cables

(D) Video printer

12. All of following are true of white balancing EXCEPT:

(A) the light cable must be connected to the telescope

(B) the lens must be directed to a solid white object

(C) you can use the back of sterile drape or a surgical sponge

(D) the white balance registers automatically by the light source

13. Technique used in arthroscopic MIS, hysteroscopy, and cystoscopy to expand the body cavity is:

(A) balloon dissection

(B) continuous irrigation

(C) insufflations

(D) infiltration

14. Injury from continuous irrigation where the fluid enters the vascular system is:

(A) embolization

(B) endoscopic distension

(C) extravasation

(D) ablation

15. In MIS, large specimens and dense tissue are reduced to small pieces by a process called:

(A) morcellation

(B) harmonic ultrasonic energy

(C) ablation

(D) fulguration

16. Guidelines for cleaning endoscopic instruments include all of the following EXCEPT:

(A) soak instruments for 2 hours

(B) before cleaning, open all stop cocks, ports, and channels

(C) look for defects in the surface of the instrument before cleaning

(D) drain and dry all instruments

17. What term identifies the arms of a robot in surgery?

(A) Articulations

(B) Ratchets

(C) Graspers

(D) Manipulators

18. An "up and down" movement of a robot's arm is known as:

(A) roll

(B) yaw

(C) pitch

(D) rotation

19. The "right to left" movement of a robotic arm is called:

    (A) yaw
    (B) roll
    (C) pitch
    (D) x–y–z-axis rotation

20. What term is used when likening "robotic vision" to "human vision"?

    (A) Sensitivity
    (B) Binocular vision
    (C) Depth perception
    (D) Resolution

21. What allows the robotic computer to create and record three-dimensional data of the surgical site?

    (A) Magnetic resonance sites
    (B) Image planning
    (C) Laser scanning
    (D) Computed tomography (CT) scan

22. Which of the following parts for robotic surgery should NOT be sterilized?

    (A) Manipulators
    (B) The collar that connects the endoscope
    (C) The endoscope
    (D) Surgical instrumentation

23. Sterilization of component parts for endoscopic robotic surgery is best accomplished by:

    (A) STERIS system
    (B) steam sterilization
    (C) hydrogen peroxide sterilizer
    (D) ETO gas sterilization

24. The most popular robotic system used today is:

    (A) AESOP
    (B) da Vinci system
    (C) surgical navigation system
    (D) both A and B

25. All are advantages of robotic surgery EXCEPT:

    (A) reduction of hand tremors
    (B) plays a role in distant surgical interventions
    (C) expensive and uses valuable resources
    (D) robotic images are three dimensional

26. What term is used when the surgeon performs the surgical procedure miles away from the patient?

    (A) Expert systems
    (B) Telesurgery
    (C) Coordinate geometry
    (D) Degrees of freedom

27. What term refers to the ability of humans and robots to determine which direction sound is coming from?

    (A) Binaural hearing
    (B) Unidirectional hearing
    (C) Voice activated
    (D) Automated hearing

28. The technical term for the extent that a robotic joint or joints can move clockwise or counterclockwise around an axis is:

    (A) manipulation
    (B) degree of freedom
    (C) roll
    (D) degrees of rotation

29. The ability of a machine, microscope, human, and robot to differentiate between two objects is called:

    (A) resolution
    (B) binaural vision
    (C) cylindrical geometry
    (D) degrees of freedom

30. The goal of deformable modeling is to:

(A) replace magnetic resonance imaging (MRI)
(B) translate a surgeon's hand movements
(C) achieve a three-dimensional model
(D) position the manipulators

31. The ability of the robot to see in dim light is known as:

(A) stereovision
(B) binaural vision
(C) sensitivity
(D) depth perception

32. Which term refers to a rotating movement?

(A) Pitch
(B) Rotation
(C) Roll
(D) A 360-degree turn

33. The position used for a robotic-assisted prostatectomy is a:

(A) lateral kidney
(B) low lithotomy
(C) Pfannenstiel
(D) prone

34. The STSR's responsibility when setting up for a robot case includes:

(A) checking all instruments prior to using
(B) performing white balance and calibrate camera
(C) determining where the third arm will be placed
(D) all of the above

35. Where is the robot positioned during a prostatectomy?

(A) Right side
(B) Left side
(C) Between legs
(D) At the head

36. The #3 arm of the robot moves:

(A) up and down
(B) in and out
(C) right and left
(D) left only

37. The #1 arm of the robot holds:

(A) scope and camera
(B) instruments
(C) insufflation tubing
(D) none of the above

38. STSR's responsibility when changing instruments on the robotic arm is to:

(A) advance the instrument
(B) guide the instrument
(C) choose the next instrument
(D) wash the instrument

39. The robotic system does not engage until:

(A) the surgeon positions the foot switch
(B) the robotic arms are engaged
(C) the surgeon places head in the viewer
(D) the surgeon speaks into microphone in console

40. When performing a cholecystectomy using the robot, the robotic arm is placed on:

(A) right side, midabdomen
(B) patient's left side midabdomen
(C) patient's right thigh level
(D) patient's left thigh level

41. Which anatomical landmark is used to line up the endoscope for a laparoscopic cholecystectomy using a robotic arm?

(A) Umbilicus
(B) Chest line
(C) Iliac crest
(D) Xiphoid process

42. A flexible fiberoptic device used to view a fetus in utero is termed:

    (A) hysteroscope
    (B) laparoscope
    (C) fetoscope
    (D) both A and B

43. A Hasson is:

    (A) a type of instrument used to grasp the gallbladder
    (B) a blunt trocar inserted into the abdomen through an infraumbilical incision
    (C) used on a SILS procedure to hold the instrumentation
    (D) a type of three-point trocar

44. Disadvantages to MIS include all EXCEPT:

    (A) high risk of adhesions if the patient has had previous surgery
    (B) bleeding
    (C) risk of perforation with the trocar
    (D) All of the above

45. The part of the camera that connects the camera to the scope is termed:

    (A) pixel
    (B) coupler
    (C) endocoupler
    (D) focus ring

46. Instruments used in MIS include:

    (A) suction irrigation
    (B) Maryland
    (C) probes
    (D) all of the above

47. Direct coupling refers to:

    (A) the surgeon touching the electrosurgical unit (ESU) to an instrument being held by the STSR
    (B) when the ESU is accidently activated while in contact with another instrument, causing the current to travel to the other instrument and cause a burn
    (C) stray current caused by improper placement of the grounding pad
    (D) none of the above

48. The procedure performed to take a biopsy, remove stones from the CBD, and dilate a bile duct stenosis with a stent is termed:

    (A) ERCP
    (B) laparoscopic Nissen fundoplication
    (C) TAPP repair
    (D) choledochoscopy

49. The laparoscopic bariatric surgery that removes a portion of the stomach and reconnects it to the duodenum is:

    (A) gastric bypass
    (B) sleeve gastrectomy
    (C) gastrectomy
    (D) adjustable gastric band

50. What procedure uses methylene blue dye mixed with saline that is injected into the vagina and observed with the laparoscope going through the fallopian tubes to check for tubal patency?

    (A) LAVH
    (B) Chromopertubation
    (C) Laparoscopic tuboplasty
    (D) Laparoscopic salpingectomy

51. Ventriculoscopy is performed through a burr hole in the skull for the treatment of:

    (A) hydrocephalus
    (B) lesions in the sella turcica
    (C) cerebral aneurysms
    (D) all of the above

52. The procedure that uses radiofrequency energy to heat, collapse, and seal blood vessels is:

    (A) ablation
    (B) cautery
    (C) cryothermy
    (D) none of the above

53. MIDCAB—minimally invasive heart bypass surgery—is also known as:

    (A) beating heart surgery
    (B) bloodless surgery
    (C) ½ CB....surgery
    (D) all of the above

54. MIS procedures are performed through all of the following natural orifices or stomas EXCEPT:

    (A) mouth
    (B) small incision or puncture into the body cavity
    (C) vagina
    (D) anus

55. When performing natural orifice transluminal endoscopic surgery, entry is through the mouth, vagina, or anus. What makes this surgical approach different from just entering through a natural orifice?

    (A) The scope cannot fit into the nose or urethra due to its size.
    (B) Once the scope is inserted through the natural body orifice, an incision can be made into the target tissue and the procedure performed.
    (C) The incision is then made into the stomach, vagina, and other internal organs, avoiding any external incisions.
    (D) Both B and C

56. What is the procedure where a flexible port is placed slightly above the umbilicus and includes three to four lumen ports and no additional abdominal punctures?

    (A) SILS
    (B) Single-incision laparoscopic surgery
    (C) Closed method
    (D) Both A and B

57. The test performed to determine proper placement of the Veress needle in a laparoscopic procedure by filling a syringe with saline that is then injected into the port of the Veress needle to see if the saline flows easily is termed:

    (A) handing drop test
    (B) manometer test
    (C) aspiration test
    (D) all of the above

58. Which device is used for instrument placement for a laparoscopic procedure?

    (A) Trocar and sheath
    (B) Thoracic trocar
    (C) Hasson
    (D) All of the above

59. Media used for expansion on laparoscopic and endoscopic procedures includes:

    (A) Balloon
    (B) Fluid
    (C) Air
    (D) All of the above

60. What is the medium used for a sigmoidoscopy procedure?

    (A) CO_2
    (B) Lactated Ringer's solution
    (C) Air
    (D) Balloon

61. The term that refers to increasing the light intensity on an MIS procedure is:

    (A) gain
    (B) optical angle
    (C) control unit
    (D) video cables

62. Match the names of the parts of the camera to the correct definition:

    The _____ is the hand control that opens the _____ and locks the telescope in place. The _____ clears the image, and the _____ adjusts the color.

    1. Endocoupler
    2. Coupler
    3. White balance
    4. Focus ring

    (A) 1, 2, 3,4
    (B) 2, 3, 4, 1
    (C) 2, 1, 4, 3
    (D) 1, 2, 4, 3

63. Operating rooms that have state-of-the-art ceiling and wall booms instead of having to transport endoscopic and robotic equipment and supplies from room to room are called:

    (A) intuitive surgical rooms
    (B) integrated operating rooms
    (C) ancillary operating rooms
    (D) robot rooms

64. The procedure performed to determine tubal patency is termed:

    (A) LAVH
    (B) chromopertubation
    (C) laparoscopic tubal ligation
    (D) laparoscopic salpingectomy

Answers and Explanations

1. **(D)** Resection of malignant tumors is performed through an open procedure in order to remove the cancerous tissue in one piece (en bloc). The morcellator is contraindicated in resection of malignant tumors because the tumor is broken up into smaller pieces, which can cause seeding and spreading of the cancerous tumor.

2. **(D)** Carbon dioxide is used to achieve a pneumoperitoneum because it is nontoxic, readily absorbed by the body, and nonflammable.

3. **(A)** Patients who have had previous abdominal surgery and have developed scarring of their organs or adhesions are at risk for a perforation of their intestines during insertion of the trocar.

4. **(B)** A rigid endoscope would be used in a TURP. A laparoscope, although rigid, is only used on the abdomen. A flexible endoscope is used to assess regional anatomy and perform tissue biopsies and minor surgeries. It is also used on patients who have limited movement and when patient positioning is compromised.

5. **(B)** A trocar is a solid rod with a tapered or solid end that fits into the hollow tube cannula.

6. **(C)** Reverse Trendelenburg position is used to displace the abdominal viscera for better visualization.

7. **(A)** Laparoscopic GYN cases are commonly performed with the patient in lithotomy position. This allows the surgeon the ability to manipulate the uterus during the procedure.

8. **(C)** You must handle the fiberoptic cables gently. When storing or transporting the cable, you must coil it loosely. Do not hang the cable. It must be stored in a flat position.

9. **(B)** Pixels are located in the head of the camera or the tip of the telescope. The more pixels there are, the clearer the image.

10. **(B)** A scope should always be held by the head, which is the heavier end, and never by the end or the shaft. When holding the scope by the lighter end, the weight of the handpiece can bend the shaft and damage it.

11. **(C)** The video cables are high-quality fiberoptic systems. They transmit data from the camera head to the camera control unit and from the monitor to the output recorder.

12. **(C)** You should not use porous or woven materials such as a surgical sponge because this can produce shadows on the image.

13. **(B)** Continuous irrigation is used to expand the space for visualization and should be nonconductive and salt free.

14. **(C)** When an increase in fluid instillation exceeds a safe level, it can cause extravasation when the fluid enters the vascular system and increases blood pressure.

15. **(A)** The morcellator reduces the tissue to pulp, which can be suctioned from the wound.

16. **(A)** Do not soak instruments for longer than 1 hour or as directed by manufacturer. Do not

submerge or allow fluid to enter electrical connections or units.

17. **(D)** The term used to identify the robotic arms that control the surgical efforts is manipulators.

18. **(C)** Pitch identifies the up and down movement of the robotic arm. The yaw identifies the right and left movements of the robotic arm. The rotating movement of the shaft is called a roll.

19. **(A)** A right to left movement of a robotic arm (manipulators) is called a yaw.

20. **(B)** Binocular machine vision is analogous to human vision, which is also known as stereovision. This vision is similar to the robot's binaural hearing.

21. **(C)** Once an MRI or CT scan is performed to retrieve a layout of the person's anatomy, a laser scan is then done to achieve a set of three-dimensional coordinates on the patient's skin.

22. **(A)** The manipulators that hold the endoscope and the instrumentation are not sterilized; they are covered with a sterile sleeve.

23. **(A)** The STERIS system (peracetic acid) sterilizer is ideal for sterilization of camera, light cord, and other delicate components used for the procedure.

24. **(B)** The primary robotic system used in the operating room today is the da Vinci system.

25. **(C)** Robotics requires a substantial investment in both time and money spent learning coordinating and the imaging system. Instruments cost thousands of dollars and must be discarded after limited use. They cannot be recycled.

26. **(B)** Telesurgery refers to the operation of the robot at a distance; the operator is at one location, and the robot is on site with the patient at another location.

27. **(A)** Binaural hearing is the ability to determine the direction from which the sound is coming. Humans have two ears, and robots are given two sound transducers that provide the same ability.

28. **(D)** Degrees of rotation relate to a manipulator's clockwise and counterclockwise movements around an axis.

29. **(A)** Resolution is the extent to which a machine, microscope, human, or robot can differentiate between two objects.

30. **(C)** The goal of a deformable model is to achieve a realistic three-dimensional simulation of soft tissue behavior under the effect of an external simulator.

31. **(C)** In some instances, a high level of sensitivity is necessary. An example of this is that during an endoscopic case, operating room lights are dimmed or turned off. The robot requires a level of sensitivity to see in such dim lighting.

32. **(C)** The rotating movement of a robot is called a roll.

33. **(B)** The patient is placed in lower lithotomy, and the robotic arms are placed between the patients' knees.

34. **(D)** The STSR's duties include checking instruments, while balancing and calibrating camera and making sure the third arm is properly placed.

35. **(C)** During prostatectomies, the robot is placed between the legs, so the robotic arms come up from the bottom.

36. **(C)** The #3 arm on the robotic system swings right and left.

37. **(A)** The #1 arm on all robots accommodates the scope and camera.

38. **(B)** The STSR's responsibility is to only guide the instrument for the surgeon as his/her eyes

are on the screen. The STSR should NEVER advance the instrument for fear of perforating the colon.

39. **(C)** Before surgery, the surgeon makes adjustments to the seating, optical viewer, and intercom while his/her head is outside the viewer. The system is engaged when the surgeon places his or her head in the viewer.

40. **(C)** The robotic arm is placed on the patients' right thigh level.

41. **(D)** The xiphoid process is used as a landmark prior to starting a laparoscopic cholecystectomy.

42. **(C)** A fetoscope is a flexible fiberoptic device used to view a fetus in utero. A hysteroscope is a thin, lighted instrument that is inserted into the vagina to examine the cervix and inside of the uterus to diagnosis or treat bleeding. A laparoscope is used to perform MIS procedures in the abdomen.

43. **(B)** The Hasson is a blunt trocar inserted into the abdomen through an infraumbilical incision. It is an open method using a cut-down procedure for laparoscopic surgery instead of using the three-point trocar and cannula system.

44. **(D)** Disadvantages of MIS include:
    - High risk of adhesions if the patient has had previous surgery
    - Risk of perforation with the trocar
    - Bleeding
    - Limited vision and range of motion with the instruments
    - All staff must be trained for MIS
    - Gas embolism
    - Preperitoneal insufflation—improper placement of the Veress needle

45. **(C)** The endocoupler connects the camera to the telescope. A pixel is the silicone chip located in a camera head or at the tip of the telescope. These pixels determine the clarity of an image. The higher the pixels, the clearer the image. The focus ring turns to clarify the image.

46. **(D)** All of the above are instruments used in MIS.

47. **(B)** This occurs when the ESU is accidently activated while in contact with another instrument, causing the current to travel to the other instrument and cause a burn.

48. **(A)** ERCP—endoscopic retrograde cholangiopancreatogram—is a procedure performed to take a biopsy, remove stones in the CBD, and dilate a stenosis of the bile duct by placing a stent. A laparoscopic Nissen fundoplication is performed to restore the function of the lower esophageal sphincter by wrapping the stomach around the esophagus. The TAPP (transabdominal preperitoneal) repair is the more conventional approach into the peritoneal cavity with a trocar and cannula. The mesh is inserted through a peritoneal incision over the hernia. Choledochoscopy provides images of the biliary system.

49. **(A)** In a gastric bypass, a portion of the stomach is removed with laparoscopic instrumentation and guns and reconnected to the duodenum. A sleeve gastrectomy is removal of a portion of the stomach along the greater curvature of the stomach forming a sleeve or tubular stomach. A gastrectomy procedure is removal of the stomach for cancer. The adjustable gastric band is an inflatable silicone band surgically implanted around the top of the stomach, creating a small pouch that holds a small amount of food.

50. **(B)** Chromopertubation is performed to determine tubal patency; methylene blue dye is mixed with saline and injected into the vagina and observed with the laparoscope going through the fallopian tubes. LAVH (laparoscopic-assisted vaginal hysterectomy) is a procedure is performed using a laparoscope and laparoscopic instruments to guide the removal of the uterus and/or fallopian tubes and ovaries through the vagina. Laparoscopic tuboplasty is performed to repair patency to the fallopian tube. Laparoscopic salpingectomy is removal of one or both fallopian tubes laparoscopically.

51. **(D)** All of the above procedures can be performed with a ventriculoscope.

52. **(A)** Radiofrequency ablation uses radiofrequency energy to heat, collapse, and seal blood vessels. Cryotherapy uses a method of localized freezing temperatures.

53. **(A)** MIDCAB is a minimally invasive heart bypass surgery. It is also known as "beating heart" surgery. No heart-lung machine is necessary.

54. **(B)** When performing an MIS procedure through a natural orifice or stoma, entry is made into oral, nasal, urethral, ear, or anal canal, including a stoma.

55. **(D)** The body is entered through a natural body orifice, and the endoscopy equipment is put in place. An incision can be made into the target tissue, and an external incision is avoided.

56. **(D)** A SILS (single-incision laparoscopic surgery) is performed through a flexible single port that contains three to four lumen entries. The scope and all instruments enter through here. The instruments are different from other endoscopic instruments. They have a bend at the joint near the tip of the instrument. This prevents the instruments from intersecting with each other and causing damage to the organs and tissue inside the body.

57. **(A)** Although all of the above are tests used to determine proper placement of the Veress needle, the hanging drop test is the one described. The manometer test is performed by placing the CO_2 tubing and filling the cavity with the gas. If the needle is misplaced, the gas reading will be high. In this case, the gas is turned off, and the Veress needle is repositioned. With the aspiration test, the Veress needle is placed and a syringe is attached and aspirated. If the syringe cannot be pulled back, the needle has not been properly placed. It is removed and repositioned.

58. **(D)** The sharp trocar and sheath, thoracic trocar, Hasson, the shielded trocar, and the dilating trocar and sheath can all be used for instrument placement during a laparoscopic procedure.

59. **(D)** A balloon dilator, various types of irrigation fluids, air, and gas are used to create a space for visualization, instrumentation, and equipment used to perform laparoscopic and endoscopic procedures.

60. **(C)** The medium used to expand the sigmoid colon for a sigmoidoscopy procedure is air. CO_2 is used in the peritoneal cavity to create a pneumoperitoneum. Lactated Ringer's solution is used on a hysterectomy procedure. A balloon is used in a TEP laparoscopic hernia repair.

61. **(A)** Gain is the term used to increase light intensity. The optical angle refers to the angle at the tip of the telescope and is measured in degrees. The camera control unit is where the camera is plugged in. The video cable is the camera cable that is plugged into the camera control unit.

62. **(C)** The coupler is the hand switch that you either squeeze open or turn to attach the scope to the endocoupler (camera attachment). The focus ring clears/focuses the image, and the white balance button adjusts the light color.

63. **(B)** The term used for the state-of-the-art operating rooms that have ceiling- and wall-mounted TVs, endoscopic equipment, and robotic equipment including the robot is integrated operating rooms. The intuitive system is responsible for the da Vinci robotic system.

64. **(B)** Chromopertubation is the procedure performed to determine whether the fallopian tubes are patent (open) for an infertility diagnosis. An LAVH (laparoscopically assisted vaginal hysterectomy) is performed using a laparoscope and laparoscopic instruments to guide the removal of the uterus and/or fallopian tubes and ovaries through the vagina. A laparoscopic tubal ligation is performed to ligate the fallopian tubes using various methods to prevent pregnancy. Laparoscopic salpingectomy is performed to remove one or both fallopian tubes. All of the above procedures are performed laparoscopically.

Bibliography

American Heart Association. *BLS for the Healthcare Provider*. Dallas, TX: American Heart Association; 2010.

Association of Surgical Technologists. *Surgical Technology for the Surgical Technologist: A Positive Care Approach*. Littleton, CO: Association of Surgical Technologists; 2008.

Ball KA. *Lasers: The Perioperative Challenge*. 2nd ed. St. Louis, MO: Mosby-Year Book; 1995.

Bergquist LM, Pogosian B. *Microbiology Principles and Health Science Applications*. Philadelphia, PA: W.B. Saunders; 2000.

Burke WM, Gossner G, Goldman NA. Robotic surgery in the obese gynecologic patient. *Clin Obstet Gynecol*. 2011;54(3):420–430.

Frey K, Price P. *Technological Sciences for the Operating Room*. 1st ed. Centennial, CO: Association of Surgical Technologists; 2002.

Fulcher EM, Soto CD, Fulcher RM. *Pharmacology: Principles and Applications. A Worktext for Allied Health Professionals*. 1st ed. Philadelphia, PA: W.B. Saunders; 2003.

Fuller JK. *Surgical Technology: Principles and Practice*. 4th, 5th ed. Philadelphia, PA: W.B. Saunders; 2005, 2010.

Lehne RA. *Pharmacology for Nursing Care*. 4th ed. Philadelphia, PA: W.B. Saunders; 2001.

Meeker M, Rothrock J. *Alexander's Care of the Patient in Surgery*. 14th ed. St. Louis, MO: Elsevier; 2011.

Miller BF, Keane CB. *Encyclopedia and Dictionary of Medicine, Nursing and Allied Health*. 2nd ed. Philadelphia, PA: W.B. Saunders; 1978.

Mosby's Medical, Nursing, and Allied Health Dictionary. 8th ed. St. Louis, MO: Mosby-Year Book; 2009.

Nemitz R. *Surgical Instrumentation: An Interactive Approach*. St. Louis, MO: W.B. Saunders; 2010.

Phillips N. *Berry and Kohn's Operating Room Technique*. 10th, 11th ed. St. Louis, MO: Mosby; 2004, 2007.

Price P, Frey K. *Microbiology for the Surgical Technologist*. Clifton Park, NY: Delmar Learning; 2003.

Rutherford C. *Differentiating Surgical Equipment and Supplies*. Philadelphia, PA: F.A. Davis; 2010.

Rutherford C. *Surgical Equipment and Supplies*. 2nd ed. Philadelphia, PA: F.A. Davis; 2016.

Stryker Endoscopy: Video Endoscopy for Perioperative Nurses—A Study Guide. Denver, CO: Stryker.

Tighe SM. *Instrumentation for the Operating Room: A Photographic Manual*. 8th ed. St. Louis, MO: Elsevier; 2012.

Tortora GJ, Derrickson BH. *Principles of Anatomy and Physiology*. 12th ed. New York, NY: Wiley; 2009.

Tortora G, Funke B, Case C. *Microbiology: An Introduction*. 7th ed. Menlo Park, CA: Benjamin Cummings; 2001.

Venes D. *Taber's Cyclopedic Medical Dictionary*. 21st ed. Philadelphia, PA: F.A. Davis; 2009:329.

Index